Nonallergic Rhinitis

CLINICAL ALLERGY AND IMMUNOLOGY

Series Editors

MICHAEL A. KALINER, M.D.

Medical Director
Institute for Asthma and Allergy
Washington, D.C.

RICHARD F. LOCKEY, M.D.

Professor of Medicine, Pediatrics, and Public Health
Joy McCann Culverhouse Professor of Allergy and Immunology
Director, Division of Allergy and Immunology
University of South Florida College of Medicine
and James A. Haley Veterans Hospital
Tampa, Florida

Clinical Allergy and Immunology

Executive Director : Michael A. Kaliner

Nonallergic Rhinitis

edited by

James N. Baraniuk

Georgetown University Medical Center
Washington, D.C., U.S.A.

Dennis Shusterman

University of Washington
Seattle, Washington, U.S.A.

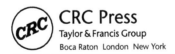

CRC Press

Taylor & Francis Group
Boca Raton London New York

CRC Press is an imprint of the
Taylor & Francis Group, an **informa** business

CRC Press
Taylor & Francis Group
6000 Broken Sound Parkway NW, Suite 300
Boca Raton, FL 33487-2742

© 2007 by Taylor & Francis Group, LLC
CRC Press is an imprint of Taylor & Francis Group, an Informa business

No claim to original U.S. Government works

ISBN-13: 978-0-8493-3991-2 (hbk)
ISBN-13: 978-0-367-38992-5 (pbk)

Visit the Taylor & Francis Web site at
http://www.taylorandfrancis.com

and the CRC Press Web site at
http://www.crcpress.com

Dedicated to the memory of Joe P.M. Braat, a rhinologist lost before his time. The nose was clearly of great importance to this early Aegean civilization (3500 B.C.). The nose was the only organ displayed on the broad faces of their statues.

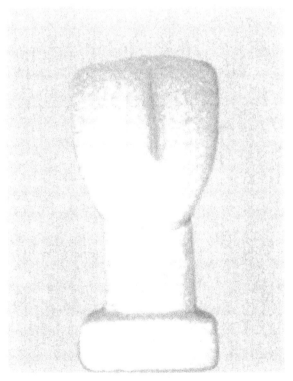

Remembering the past will inspire the future.

Series Introduction

Rhinitis is an incredibly common disease: Everyone suffers from infectious rhinitis, often on an at least yearly basis. Allergic rhinitis affects at least 60 million Americans, and the estimate for nonallergic rhinitis is another 10–20 million. Probably because allergic rhinitis has been recognized for a century or more, and because the symptoms of allergic and nonallergic rhinitis overlap, most clinicians do not distinguish allergic from nonallergic rhinitis. In fact, even among specialists, patients are not carefully classified into allergic, nonallergic or mixed rhinitis (elements of both diseases). Most patients are treated as if they have allergic disease; although both the pathophysiology and effective treatments of these two diseases are quite distinct. In fact, there are multiple causes of nonallergic rhinitis, each of which is distinct. Nonallergic "vasomotor" rhinitis is the most common form, and even rhinologists have difficulty clearly distinguishing which forms of nonallergic rhinitis are present.

To our knowledge, no books have focused on nonallergic rhinitis, elaborating what is known about pathophysiology, epidemiology or treatment. Thus, Baraniuk's and Shusterman's book, "Nonallergic Rhinitis" fills an extremely important clinical gap.

At least one half the patients seen with rhinitis have either nonallergic rhinitis as an exclusive cause of their symptoms or have an important element of nonallergic disease complicating allergic rhinitis. White we believe that the primary group of clinicians interested in this topic will be Allergists and Otolaryngologists, most clinicians would benefit from an increased understanding of the signs, symptoms and pathophysiologic events that separate nonallergic from allergic disease, and many millions of patients would appreciate more effective treatment of their nasal disease if clinicians did understand these important differences.

Thus, it is a pleasure to welcome this book to the "Clinical Allergy and Immunology" series. It accomplishes what we set out to do in this series: bridge basic science with clinical practice, enhancing the treatment of patients.

Michael A. Kaliner, MD
Richard Lockey, MD

Preface

This book is the first iteration stemming from a conversation about the broad differential diagnosis of nonallergic rhinitis (NAR) that began on the long road from Yalta. This conversation has been transformed into an evaluation of rhinopathy that dares not speak its name. This is a topic of significant importance since rhinitis complaints are virtually universal. There is great confusion and misunderstanding about the range of normal nasal sensations and those that indicate inflammatory and noninflammatory nasal disorders. The severity and prevalence of sensations of pruritis, irritation, "fullness," "congestion," limited nasal airflow, anterior and posterior discharge, and facial pain in the general population is poorly understood. Without this information, many patients and physicians may erroneously conclude that an inflammatory rhinitis or rhinosinusitis disease is present when in fact the symptom complex is due to a nonallergic, noninflammatory syndrome. Misdiagnosis, inappropriate medication, and the fact that our pharmacopea for NAR is very limited often leads to "failure" of treatment and frustration on the part of the patient and physician.

One factor contributing to this situation is the tendency to have a "short list" for rhinitis syndromes. Many current rhinitis paradigms are organized by the split between mechanisms of atopic, allergic rhinitis (AR) and all other mechanisms of nasal discomfort and disease, or NAR. This division is based on the presence or absence of symptoms when exposed to seasonal, perennial or occupational allergens, confirmation of IgE – mediated immediate and/or late phase responses to the appropriate offending allergens, and beneficial responses to antihistamines, nasal steroids and allergen injection therapy. The mechanisms of atopy have been extensively studied, with our level of understanding reaching genomic and molecular complexities. This knowledge can be applied to the approximately 20% of the United States population estimated to have allergic rhinitis syndromes.

This intimate knowledge of atopic syndromes is contrasted by lumping all other syndromes and subjects who are nonresponders to current therapies into the derisive garbage can of NAR. The prevalence of NAR is estimated to be 5% to 7%. However, this may be an underestimate based on the broad set of inflammatory and noninflammatory syndromes in the differential diagnosis, and epidemiological survey tools that group subjects with self-reported rhinitis into either AR or NAR without physician confirmation or evaluation of atopic and other inflammatory mechanisms. Surprisingly little is understood about nonatopic rhinitis in childhood, pregnancy, the aging population, and other influence of irritant exposures on AR complaints. We have included several chapters that offer different strategies for distinguishing allergic from nonallergic syndromes, and that expand on the inflammatory and noninflammatory scope of NAR. However, it is clear that NAR mechanisms and complaints also occur in conjunction with AR. The result is the generalized categorization of "pure" AR, "pure" NAR, and "mixed" AR + NAR. This is a necessary step forward in our task of distinguishing between individual syndromes, identifying their mechanisms, and developing new treatment options for patients who do not respond to current drugs and avoidance.

Standing back and reviewing our progress while groping our way into the nature of NAR leads to the realization that the job is only beginning, and that our knowledge base is a glass half-filled. This base is the information we "know". Our more advanced understanding of AR mechanisms contrasts with the less well-developed and at times contradictory descriptions and mechanistic underpinnings of inflammatory and noninflammatory NAR syndromes. However, the glass half empty should not be viewed with sanguine neglect. This void represents an opportunity to carefully observe and define the subsets of NAR based on coherent pathophysiological mechanisms. Newer studies are already moving to this more rigorous approach. We have included discussion of investigations from other organ systems to provide additional insights. Our hope is that this information will generate new hypotheses that can be tested to confirm the discrete nature of selected NAR syndromes. These studies may investigate the nature of other inflammatory and noninflammatory mechanisms that may be recruited in NAR subtypes and also in AR. We anticipate this multidisciplinary approach will lead to a more logical classification of NAR.

From this perspective, our book represents a stepping stone to cross from established dogmas to future insights. One clinical foot is grounded on established evaluations of syndromes such as nonallergic rhinitis with eosinophila (NARES), drug and hormonal rhinitis, and the ultimate statement of futility and frustration in this field – "vasomotor rhinitis" (VMR). Chapters devoted to these topics evaluate the epidemiology, distinguishing clinical features, potential mechanisms and current treatment approaches. They reveal what is known, or often how little is understood about these "classic" NAR syndromes. Controversies will be apparent from the parallel discussions of these disorders provided by leading opinion leaders. The discrepancies should spur efforts at more precise synchronization of NAR syndrome definitions. This section of the book was designed to describe the edge of the envelope of our understanding in order to provoke new thoughts, insights, standardized systematic surveys, and analysis of treatment strategies for each niche of NAR.

Recognizing "what we know" places us in a position to learn "what we need to know." This phase represents the other foot stepping forward into relatively uncharted waters of occupational, inflammatory, and neurological dysfunction. Advances in understanding disorders of the glottis, esophagus and lung have provided new insights into irritant sensitivity, mucosal hyperresponsiveness, increased neural reflex, and mucosal secretory activities. Newer concepts of nonallergic eosinophilic, arachidonic acid, nociceptive, autonomic and central neural, and other mechanisms may seem misplaced in a book on NAR. However, information learned from studies of cough, vocal cord dysfunction, sleep apnea, virus illness, olfactory, and trigeminal chemosensory systems have important implications that can be applied to understanding nasal, sinus and middle ear disease. We hope these interdisciplinary data will cross-pollinate with the standard, largely static dogmas of NAR to generate fertile hybrid concepts that will invigorate investigations into nasal and related disorders. For example, one long term objective is to stimulate a reassessment of long-held beliefs about "vasomotor rhinitis" and the supposed dichotomy of "runners" versus "blockers", and replace these concepts with evidence- and mechanism-based clinical diagnoses.

Some readers may object to our approach, and our authors' analyses and alternative explanations. We feel the degree of debate and analytical reassessment of current dogmatic concepts will be a measure of our success in this effort. Your comments, good and bad, are highly valued and welcomed. Please feel free to contact either of us to further these debates. We hope this intercourse will lead to a blossoming in the emerging field of rhinopathic illnesses, and allow us on to the next stepping stone in understanding airway physiology and pathophysiology.

James N. Baraniuk
Dennis Shusterman

Contents

PART III: NON-EOSINOPHILIC INFLAMMATORY RHINITIS

PART IV: NON-INFLAMMATORY RHINOPATHY

PART V: CLINICAL IMPLICATIONS

PART VI: ASSOCIATED CLINICAL ISSUES

Contributors

Isam Alobid Department of Otolaryngology, Rhinology Unit, University of Barcelona, and Institut d'Investigacions Biomèdiques August Pi i Sunyer (IDIBAPS), Barcelona, Catalonia, Spain

Ron Balkissoon Department of Medicine, National Jewish Medical and Research Center, University of Colorado School of Medicine, Denver, Colorado, U.S.A.

James N. Baraniuk Department of Medicine, Division of Rheumatology, Immunology and Allergy, and Georgetown University Proteomics Laboratory, Georgetown University Medical Center, Washington, D.C., U.S.A.

Fuad M. Baroody Department of Surgery, Section of Otolaryngology—Head and Neck Surgery and Department of Pediatrics, Pritzker School of Medicine, University of Chicago, Chicago, Illinois, U.S.A.

William E. Berger Department of Pediatrics, Division of Allergy and Immunology, University of California, Irvine, California, U.S.A.

Jonathan A. Bernstein Department of Internal Medicine, Division of Immunology/Allergy Section, University of Cincinnati College of Medicine, Cincinnati, Ohio, U.S.A.

Dominique Brandt Department of Internal Medicine, Division of Immunology/Allergy Section, University of Cincinnati College of Medicine, Cincinnati, Ohio, U.S.A.

Begona Casado Georgetown University Proteomics Laboratory, Georgetown University Medical Center, Washington, D.C., U.S.A.

David R. Charnock Department of Surgery, Section of Otolaryngology, University of Vermont College of Medicine, Burlington, Vermont, U.S.A.

Maria Cinta Cid Department of Internal Medicine, Vasculitis Research Unit, Hospital Clínic, University of Barcelona, and Institut d'Investigacions Biomèdiques August Pi i Sunyer (IDIBAPS), Barcelona, Catalonia, Spain

Jacquelynne P. Corey Department of Surgery, Section of Otolaryngology—Head and Neck Surgery, University of Chicago, Chicago, Illinois, U.S.A.

Jonathan Corren Department of Medicine, University of California, Los Angeles, California, U.S.A.

Martin Desrosiers Department of Otolaryngology, McGill University, Montreal, Quebec, Canada

William J. Doyle Department of Otolaryngology, University of Pittsburgh School of Medicine, and Department of Pediatric Otolaryngology, Children's Hospital of Pittsburgh, Pittsburgh, Pennsylvania, U.S.A.

Mark S. Dykewicz Department of Internal Medicine, Division of Allergy and Immunology, St. Louis University School of Medicine, St. Louis, Missouri, U.S.A.

Eva K. Ellegård Department of Otolaryngology, Kungsbacka Hospital, Kungsbacka, Sweden

Lars H. Ellegård Department of Clinical Nutrition, Sahlgrenska University Hospital, Göteborg, Sweden

Anne K. Ellis Department of Medicine, Division of Clinical Immunology and Allergy, McMaster University, Hamilton, Ontario, Canada

Berrylin J. Ferguson Department of Otolaryngology, University of Pittsburgh School of Medicine, Pittsburgh, Pennsylvania, U.S.A.

Wytske Fokkens Academic Medical Centre, Amsterdam, The Netherlands

Deborah A. Gentile Department of Pediatric, Division of Allergy, Asthma, and Immunology, Allegheny General Hospital, Pittsburgh, Pennsylvania, U.S.A.

Peter M. Graf Karolinska University Hospital, Stockholm, Sweden

Johan Hellgren Department of Otolaryngology, Head and Neck Surgery, Capio Lundby Hospital, University of Gothenburg, Göteborg, Sweden

Thomas Hummel Department of Otolaryngology, Smell and Taste Clinic, University of Dresden Medical School ("Technische Universität Dresden"), Dresden, Germany

Nick S. Jones Department of Otolaryngology, Head and Neck Surgery, Queen's Medical Center, University Hospital, Nottingham, U.K.

Rita Kachru Department of Medicine, University of California, Los Angeles, California, U.S.A.

Michael A. Kaliner Institute for Asthma and Allergy, Chevy Chase, Maryland, and George Washington University School of Medicine, Washington, D.C., U.S.A.

N. Göran Karlsson Department of Otolaryngology, Sahlgrenska University Hospital, Göteborg, Sweden

Paul K. Keith Department of Medicine, Division of Clinical Immunology and Allergy, McMaster University, Hamilton, Ontario, Canada

Marek L. Kowalski Department of Immunology, Rheumatology and Allergy, Faculty of Medicine, Medical University of Łódź, Łódź, Poland

Basile N. Landis Department of Otolaryngology, University of Geneva, Geneva, Switzerland

Uyenphuong Ho Le Department of Medicine, Drexel University, Philadelphia, Pennsylvania, U.S.A.

Sonya Malekzadeh Department of Otolaryngology, Head and Neck Surgery, Georgetown University Medical Center, Washington, D.C., U.S.A.

Eva Millqvist Department of Respiratory, Asthma and Allergy Research Group, Medicine and Allergy, The Sahlgrenska Academy at Göteborg University, Göteborg, Sweden

Joaquim Mullol Department of Otolaryngology, Rhinology Unit, University of Barcelona, and Institut d'Investigacions Biomèdiques August Pi i Sunyer (IDIBAPS), Barcelona, Catalonia, Spain

Robert M. Naclerio Department of Surgery, Section of Otolaryngology, Head and Neck Surgery, University of Chicago School of Medicine, Chicago, Illinois, U.S.A.

Mohamed M. Nagi Department of Otolaryngology, McGill University, Montreal, Quebec, Canada

A. Asli Sahin-Yilmaz Department of Surgery, Section of Otolaryngology—Head and Neck Surgery, University of Chicago, Chicago, Illinois, U.S.A.

Mandy Scheibe Department of Otolaryngology, Smell and Taste Clinic, University of Dresden Medical School ("Technische Universität Dresden"), Dresden, Germany

J. Ellen Schonfeld Allergy and Asthma Associates of Southern California, Mission Viejo, California, U.S.A.

Russell A. Settipane Department of Medicine, Brown Medical School, Providence, Rhode Island, U.S.A.

Dennis Shusterman Occupational and Environmental Medicine Program, University of Washington, Seattle, Washington, U.S.A.

David P. Skoner Department of Pediatrics, Drexel University College of Medicine, Philadelphia, Pennsylvania, and Division of Allergy, Asthma, and Immunology, Allegheny General Hospital, Pittsburgh, Pennsylvania, U.S.A.

John C. Sok Department of Otolaryngology, University of Pittsburgh School of Medicine, Pittsburgh, Pennsylvania, U.S.A.

Maria T. Staevska Allergology and Clinical Immunology, Clinic of Asthma, Medical University of Sofia, University Hospital "Alexandrovska," Sofia, Bulgaria

Alkis Togias Department of Medicine, Divisions of Allergy and Clinical Immunology and Respiratory and Critical Care Medicine, Johns Hopkins University School of Medicine, Baltimore, Maryland, U.S.A.

Kjell Torén Department of Occupational and Environmental Medicine, Sahlgrenska University Hospital, Göteborg, Sweden

Roy Gerth van Wijk Department of Internal Medicine, Section of Allergology, Erasmus Medical Center, Rotterdam, The Netherlands

Thomas Zahnert Department of Otolaryngology, Smell and Taste Clinic, University of Dresden Medical School ("Technische Universität Dresden"), Dresden, Germany

1   Nasal and Paranasal Sinus Anatomy and Physiology

Fuad M. Baroody

Department of Surgery, Section of Otolaryngology—Head and Neck Surgery and Department of Pediatrics, Pritzker School of Medicine, University of Chicago, Chicago, Illinois, U.S.A.

INTRODUCTION

When discussing nonallergic rhinitis and the different influences that our environment has on the nose and its function, it is essential to have a clear understanding of the anatomy and physiology of the nasal cavity. This chapter is designed to provide such an understanding of the structure and function of both the nasal cavity and the paranasal sinuses, with the aim of facilitating the appreciation of the impact of the different diseases and treatments discussed in subsequent chapters.

NASAL ANATOMY

External Nasal Framework

The external bony framework of the nose consists of two oblong, paired nasal bones located on either side of the midline, which merge to form a pyramid (Fig. 1). Lateral to each nasal bone is the frontal process of the maxilla, which contributes to the base of the nasal pyramid. The piriform aperture is the bony opening that leads to the external nose.

The cartilaginous framework of the nose consists of the paired upper lateral, lower lateral, and sesamoid cartilages (Fig. 1). The upper lateral cartilages are attached to the undersurface of the nasal bones and frontal processes superiorly and their inferior ends lie under the upper margin of the lower lateral cartilages. Medially, they blend with the cartilaginous septum. Each lower lateral cartilage consists of a medial crus, which extends along the free caudal edge of the cartilaginous septum, and a lateral crus, which provides the framework of the nasal ala, the entrance to the nose (Fig. 1). Laterally, between the upper and lower lateral cartilages are one or more sesamoid cartilages and fibroadipose tissue.

Nasal Septum

The nasal septum divides the nasal cavity into two sides and is composed of cartilage and bone. The bone receives contributions from the vomer, perpendicular plate of the ethmoid, maxillary crest, palatine bone, and the anterior spine of the maxillary bone. The main supporting framework of the septum is the septal cartilage, which forms the most anterior part of the septum and articulates posteriorly with the vomer and the perpendicular plate of the ethmoid bone. Inferiorly, the cartilage rests in the crest of the maxilla, whereas anteriorly, it has a free border

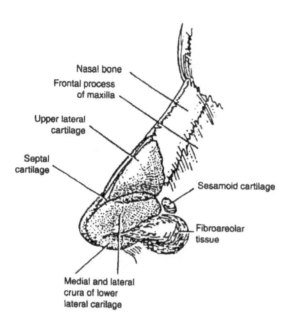

Nasal bone
Frontal process of maxilla
Upper lateral cartilage
Septal cartilage
Sesamoid cartilage
Fibroareolar tissue
Medial and lateral crura of lower lateral carilage

FIGURE 1 External nasal framework. *Source:* From Ref. 1.

when it approaches the membranous septum. The latter separates the medial crura of the lower lateral cartilages from the septal cartilage. The perpendicular plate of the ethmoid bone forms the posterosuperior portion of the septum, and the vomer contributes to its posteroinferior portion. In a study of cadaveric specimens, Van Loosen et al. showed that the cartilaginous septum increases rapidly in size during the first years of life, with the total area remaining constant after the age of two years (2). In contrast, endochondral ossification of the cartilaginous septum resulting in the formation of the perpendicular plate of the ethmoid bone starts after the first six months of life and continues until the age of 36 years. The continuous, albeit slow, growth of the nasal septum until the third decade might explain frequently encountered septal deviations in adults. Other causes for septal deviations may also occur spontaneously or result from previous trauma. Deviations can involve any of the individual components of the nasal septum and can lead to nasal obstruction because of impairment to airflow within the nasal cavities. In addition to reducing nasal airflow, some septal deviations obstruct the middle meatal areas and can lead to impairment of drainage from the sinuses, with resultant sinusitis. Severe anterior deviations can also prevent the introduction of intranasal medications to the rest of the nasal cavity and therefore interfere with the medical treatment of rhinitis (3). It is important to examine the nose in a patient with complaints of nasal congestion to rule out such deviations. It is also important to realize that not all deviations lead to symptoms and that surgery should be reserved for those deviations that are thought to contribute to the patient's symptomatology.

Nasal Vestibule/Nasal Valve

The nasal vestibule, located immediately posterior to the external nasal opening, is lined with stratified squamous epithelium and numerous hairs (or vibrissae) that filter out large particulate matter. The vestibule funnels air toward the nasal valve, which is a slit-shaped passage formed by the junction of the upper lateral cartilages, the nasal septum, and the inferior turbinate. The nasal valve accounts for approximately 50% of the total resistance to respiratory airflow from the anterior nostril to the alveoli. The surface area of this valve, and consequently resistance to airflow, is modified by the action of the alar muscles. An increase in the tone of the dilator naris muscle, innervated by the facial nerve, dilates the nares, increases the cross-sectional area of the nasal valve, and thus decreases resistance to airflow. This occurs in labored breathing, such as during exercise, and is a physiologic mechanism to increase nasal airflow. On the other hand, the nasal valve and the vestibule collapse depending on the pressure gradient between ambient and respired air. As negative pressure in the nose increases to increase airflow, the cartilages collapse in spite of the opposing action of the dilator muscles. An example of these paradoxical actions occurs during sniffing, where resistance to airflow increases across the vestibule/nasal valve complex. Aging results in loss of strength of the nasal cartilages and secondary weakening of nasal tip support and the nasal valve, with resultant airflow compromise (3).

Lateral Nasal Wall

The lateral nasal wall commonly has three turbinates, or conchae: inferior, middle, and superior (Fig. 2). The turbinates are elongated laminae of bone attached along their superior borders to the lateral nasal wall. Their unattached inferior portions curve inwards toward the lateral nasal wall, resulting in a convex surface that faces the nasal septum medially. They not only increase the mucosal surface of the nasal

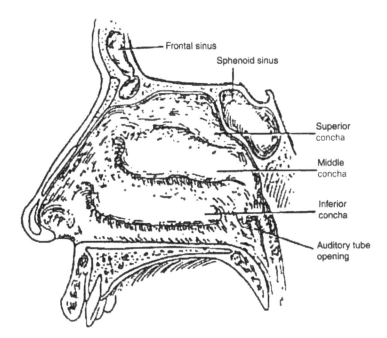

FIGURE 2 A sagittal section of the lateral nasal wall. This shows the three turbinates (conchae), frontal and sphenoid sinuses, and the opening of the Eustachian tube in the nasopharynx. *Source:* From Ref. 4.

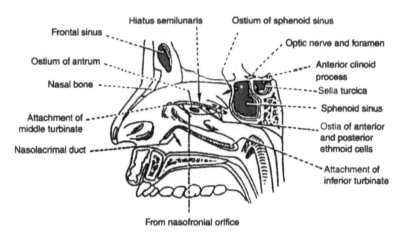

Hiatus semilunaris   Ostium of sphenoid sinus

Frontal sinus

Optic nerve and foramen

Ostium of antrum

Anterior clinoid process

Nasal bone

Sella turcica

Attachment of middle turbinate

Sphenoid sinus

Ostia of anterior and posterior ethmoid cells

Nasolacrimal duct

Attachment of inferior turbinate

From nasofronial orifice

FIGURE 3   A detailed view of the lateral nasal wall. Parts of the inferior and middle turbinates have been removed. The various openings into the inferior, middle, and superior meati are shown. *Source:* From Ref. 6.

cavity to about 100–200 cm^2 but also regulate airflow by alteration of their vascular content and, hence, thickness through the state of their capacitance vessels (5). The large surface areas of the turbinates and the nasal septum allows intimate contact between respired air and the mucosal surfaces, thus facilitating humidification, filtration, and temperature regulation of inspired air. Under and lateral to each of the turbinates are horizontal passages or meati. The inferior meatus receives the opening of the nasolacrimal duct, whereas the middle meatus receives drainage originating from the frontal, anterior ethmoid, and maxillary sinuses (Fig. 3). The sphenoid and posterior ethmoid sinuses drain into the sphenoethmoid recess, located below and posterior to the superior turbinate.

PARANASAL SINUS ANATOMY

The paranasal sinuses are four pairs of cavities that are named after the skull bones in which they are located: frontal, ethmoid (anterior and posterior), maxillary, and sphenoid. All sinuses contain air and are lined by a thin layer of respiratory mucosa composed of ciliated, pseudostratified columnar, epithelial cells with goblet mucous cells interspersed among the columnar cells.

Frontal Sinuses

At birth, the frontal sinuses are indistinguishable from the anterior ethmoid cells and they grow slowly after birth so that they are barely seen anatomically at one year of age. After the fourth year, the frontal sinuses begin to enlarge, and they can usually be demonstrated radiographically in children over six years of age. Their size continues to increase into the late teens. The frontal sinuses are usually pyramidal structures in the vertical part of the frontal bone. They open via the frontal recess into the anterior part of the middle meatus, or directly into the anterior part of the infundibulum. The natural ostium is located directly posterior to the anterior attachment of the middle turbinate to the lateral nasal wall. They are supplied by the supraorbital and supratrochlear arteries, branches of the ophthalmic artery, which in turn is a branch of the internal carotid artery. Venous drainage is via the superior ophthalmic vein into the cavernous sinus. The sensory innervation of the mucosa is via the supraorbital and supratrochlear branches of the frontal nerve, derived from the ophthalmic division of the trigeminal nerve.

Ethmoid Sinuses
At birth, the ethmoid and the maxillary sinuses are the only sinuses that are large enough to be clinically significant as a cause of rhinosinusitis. By the age of 12 years, the ethmoid air cells have almost reached their adult size and formed a pyramid, with the base located posteriorly. The lateral wall of the sinus is the lamina papyracea, which also serves as the paper-thin medial wall of the orbit. The medial wall of the sinus functions as the lateral nasal wall. The superior boundary of the ethmoid sinus is formed by the horizontal plate of the ethmoid bone, which separates the sinus from the anterior cranial fossa. This horizontal plate is composed of a thin medial portion named the cribriform plate and a thicker, more lateral portion named the fovea ethmoidalis, which forms the ethmoid roof. The posterior boundary of the ethmoid sinus is the anterior wall of the sphenoid sinus. The ethmoidal air cells are divided into an anterior group that drains into the ethmoidal infundibulum of the middle meatus and a posterior group that drains into the superior meatus, which is located inferior to the superior turbinate. The ethmoidal infundibulum is a three-dimensional cleft running anterosuperiorly to posteroinferiorly, and the two-dimensional opening to this cleft is the hiatus semilunaris. The bulla ethmoidalis (an anterior group of ethmoidal air cells) borders the ethmoid infundibulum posteriorly and superiorly, the lateral wall of the nose resides laterally, and the uncinate process borders anteromedially. The uncinate process is a thin semilunar piece of bone, the superior edge of which is usually free but can insert into the lamina papyracea or the fovea ethmoidalis and the posteroinferior edge of which usually lies just lateral to the maxillary sinus ostium. The ethmoid sinuses receive their blood supply from both the internal and the external carotid circulations. The branches of the external carotid circulation that supply the ethmoids are the nasal branches of the sphenopalatine artery, and the branches of the internal carotid circulation are the anterior and posterior ethmoidal arteries, derived from the ophthalmic artery. Venous drainage can also be directed via the nasal veins, branches of the maxillary vein, or via the ophthalmic veins, tributaries of the cavernous sinus. The latter pathway is responsible for cavernous sinus thrombosis after ethmoid sinusitis. The sensory innervation of these sinuses is by the ophthalmic and maxillary divisions of the trigeminal nerve.

Maxillary Sinuses
The size of the maxillary sinus is estimated to be 6–8 cm^3 at birth. The sinus then grows rapidly until the third year and then more slowly until the seventh year. Another growth acceleration occurs then until about 12 years of age. By then, pneumatization has extended laterally as far as the lateral wall of the orbit and inferiorly so that the floor of the sinus is even with the floor of the nasal cavity. Much of the growth that occurs after the 12th year is in the inferior direction, with pneumatization of the alveolar process after eruption of the secondary dentition. By adulthood, the floor of the maxillary sinus is usually 4–5 mm inferior to that

of the nasal cavity. The maxillary sinus occupies the body of the maxilla and has a capacity of around 15 mL. Its anterior wall is the facial surface of the maxilla and the posterior wall corresponds to the infratemporal surface of the maxilla. Its roof is the inferior orbital floor and is about twice as wide as its floor, formed by the alveolar process of the maxilla. The medial wall of the sinus forms a part of the lateral nasal wall and has the ostium of the sinus, which is located within the infundibulum of the middle meatus, with accessory ostia occurring in 25% to 30% of individuals. Mucociliary clearance within the maxillary sinus moves secretions in the direction of the natural ostium. The major blood supply of the maxillary sinuses is via branches of the maxillary artery with a small contribution from the facial artery. Venous drainage occurs anteriorly via the anterior facial vein into the jugular vein, or posteriorly via the tributaries of the maxillary vein, which also eventually drains into the jugular system. Innervation of the mucosa of the maxillary sinuses is via several branches of the maxillary nerve (MN), which primarily carry sensory fibers. Another contribution to the innervation via the MN are postganglionic parasympathetic secretomotor fibers originating in the facial nerve and carried to the sphenopalatine ganglion (SG) in the pterygopalatine fossa via the greater petrosal nerve and the nerve of the pterygoid canal.

Sphenoid Sinuses

At birth, the size of the sphenoid sinus is small and is little more than an evagination of the sphenoethmoid recess. By the age of seven years, the sphenoid sinuses have extended posteriorly to the level of the sella turcica. By the late teens, most of the sinuses have aerated to the dorsum sellae and some further enlargement may occur in adults. The sphenoid sinuses are frequently asymmetric because the intersinus septum is bowed or twisted. The optic nerve, internal carotid artery, nerve of the pterygoid canal, MN, and SG may all appear as impressions indenting the walls of the sphenoid sinuses, depending on the extent of pneumatization. The sphenoid sinus drains into the sphenoethmoid recess above the superior turbinate and the ostium typically lies 10 mm above the floor of the sinus. The blood supply is via branches of the internal and external carotid arteries and the venous drainage follows that of the nasopharynx and the nasal cavity into the maxillary vein and the pterygoid venous plexus. The first and second divisions of the trigeminal nerve supply the mucosa of the sphenoid sinus.

Function of the Paranasal Sinuses

Many theories exist related to the function of the paranasal sinuses. Some of these theories include imparting additional voice resonance, humidifying and warming inspired air, secreting mucus to keep the nose moist, and providing thermal insulation for the brain. While none of these theories has been supported by objective evidence, it is commonly believed that the paranasal sinuses form a collapsible framework to help protect the brain from frontal blunt trauma. While the function of the paranasal sinuses might not be completely understood, they are the frequent target of infections, both acute and chronic.

The middle meatus is an important anatomical area in the pathophysiology of sinus disease. It has a complex anatomy of bones and mucosal folds, often referred to as the osteomeatal unit, between which drain the frontal, anterior ethmoid, and maxillary sinuses. Anatomic abnormalities or inflammatory mucosal changes in the area of the osteomeatal complex can lead to impaired drainage from these sinuses which can, at least in part, be responsible for acute and chronic sinus disease. Endoscopic sinus surgery is targeted at restoring the functionality of this drainage system in patients with chronic sinus disease that is refractory to medical management.

NASAL MUCOSA

A thin, moderately keratinized, stratified squamous epithelium lines the vestibular region. The anterior tips of the turbinates provide a transition from squamous to transitional and finally to a pseudostratified columnar ciliated epithelium, which lines the remainder of the nasal cavity except for the roof, which is lined with olfactory epithelium (Fig. 4) (5). All cells of the pseudostratified columnar ciliated epithelium contact the basement membrane, but not all reach the epithelial surface. The basement membrane separates the epithelium from the lamina propria, or submucosa.

Nasal Epithelium
Within the epithelium, three types of cells are identified: basal, goblet, and columnar, which are either ciliated or nonciliated.

Basal Cells
Basal cells lie on the basement membrane and do not reach the airway lumen. They have an electron-dense cytoplasm and bundles of tonofilaments. Among their morphologic specializations are desmosomes, which mediate adhesion between adjacent cells, and hemidesmosomes, which help anchor the cells to the basement

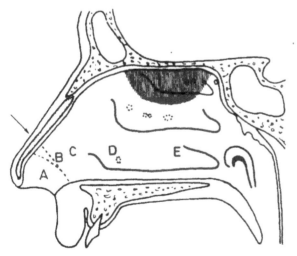

FIGURE 4 Distribution of types of epithelium along the lateral nasal wall. (*Hatched region*) The olfactory epithelium. (*Arrow*) The area of the nasal valve: A, skin; B, squamous epithelium without microvilli; C, transitional epithelium; D, pseudostratified columnar epithelium with a few ciliated cells; and E, pseudostratified columnar epithelium with many ciliated cells. *Source*: From Ref. 7.

membrane (8). These cells have long been thought to be progenitors of the columnar and goblet cells of the airway epithelium, but experiments in rat bron chial epithelium suggest that the primary progenitor cell of airway epithelium might be the nonciliated columnar cell population (9). Currently, basal cells are believed to help in the adhesion of columnar cells to the basement membrane. This is supported by the fact that columnar cells do not have hemidesmosomes and attach to the basement membrane only by cell-adhesion molecules, i.e., laminin.

Goblet Cells

The goblet cells arrange themselves perpendicular to the epithelial surface (10). The mucous granules give the mature cell its characteristic goblet shape, in which only a narrow part of the tapering basal cytoplasm touches the basement membrane. The nucleus is situated basally, with the organelles and secretory granules that contain mucin toward the lumen. The luminal surface, covered by microvilli, has a small opening, or stoma, through which the granules secrete their content. The genesis of goblet cells is controversial, with some experimental studies supporting a cell of origin unrelated to epithelial cells and others supporting either the cylindrical nonciliated columnar cell population or undifferentiated basal cells as the cells of origin (10). There are no goblet cells in the squamous, transitional, or olfactory epithelia of adults and they are irregularly distributed but present in all areas of pseudostratified columnar epithelium (10).

Columnar Cells

These cells are related to neighboring cells by tight junctions apically and, in the uppermost part, by interdigitations of the cell membrane. The cytoplasm contains numerous mitochondria in the apical part. All columnar cells, ciliated and nonciliated, are covered by 300 to 400 microvilli, uniformly distributed over the entire apical surface. These are not precursors of cilia but are short and slender fingerlike cytoplasmic expansions that increase the surface area of the epithelial cells, thus promoting exchange processes across the epithelium. The microvilli also prevent drying of the surface by retaining moisture essential for ciliary function (5). In humans, the ciliated epithelium lines the majority of the airway from the nose to the respiratory bronchioles, as well as the paranasal sinuses, the eustachian tube, and parts of the middle ear.

Inflammatory Cells

Different types of inflammatory cells have been described in the nasal epithelium obtained from normal, nonallergic subjects. Using immunohistochemical staining, Winther et al. identified consistent anti-Human Leukocyte Antigen (HLA-DR) staining in the upper portion of the nasal epithelium as well as occasional lymphocytes interspersed between the epithelial cells (11). There appeared to be more T than B lymphocytes and more T helper than T suppressor cells. The detection of HLA-DR antigens on the epithelium suggested that the airway epithelium may be participating in antigen recognition and processing. Bradding et al. observed rare mast cells within the epithelial layer and no activated eosinophils (12).

Nasal Submucosa

The nasal submucosa lies beneath the basement membrane and contains a host of cellular components in addition to nasal glands, nerves, and blood vessels. In a light microscopy study of nasal biopsies of normal individuals, the predominant cell in the submucosa was the mononuclear cell, which includes lymphocytes and monocytes (13). Much less numerous were neutrophils and eosinophils (13). Mast cells were also found in appreciable numbers in the nasal submucosa as identified by immunohistochemical staining with a monoclonal antibody against mast cell tryptase (12). Winther et al. evaluated lymphocyte subsets in the nasal mucosa of normal subjects using immunohistochemistry (11). They found T lymphocytes to be the predominant cell type with fewer scattered B-cells. The ratio of T helper cells to T suppressor cells in the lamina propria averaged 3:1 in the subepithelial area and 2:1 in the deeper vascular stroma, with the overall ratio being 2.5:1, similar to the average ratio in peripheral blood. Natural killer cells were very rare, constituting less than 2% of the lymphocytes. Recent interest in inflammatory cytokines prompted Bradding et al. to investigate cells containing IL-4, IL-5, IL-6, and IL-8 in the nasal mucosa of patients with perennial rhinitis and normal subjects (12). The normal nasal mucosa was found to contain cells with positive IL-4 immunoreactivity, with 90% of these cells also staining positive for mast cell tryptase suggesting that they were mast cells. Immunoreactivity for IL-5 and IL-6 was present in 75% of the normal nasal biopsies and IL-8 positive cells were found in all the normal nasal tissue samples. A median 50% of IL-5$^+$ cells and 100% of the IL-6$^+$ cells were mast cells. In contrast to the other cytokines, IL-8 was largely confined to the cytoplasm of the epithelial cells.

From the above studies, it is clear that the normal nasal mucosa contains a host of inflammatory cells the role of which is unclear. In allergic rhinitis, most of these inflammatory cells increase in number (14) and eosinophils are also recruited into the nasal mucosa (12). Furthermore, cells positive for IL-4 increase significantly in patients with allergic rhinitis compared to normal subjects (12).

Nasal Glands

There are three types of nasal glands: anterior nasal, seromucous, and intraepithelial. They are located in the submucosa and epithelium.

Anterior Nasal Glands

These serous glands have ducts (2–20 mm in length) that open into small crypts located in the nasal vestibule. The ducts are lined by one layer of cuboidal epithelium. Bojsen-Moller found 50 to 80 crypts anteriorly on the septum and another 50 to 80 anteriorly on the lateral nasal wall (15). He suggested that these glands play an important role in keeping the nose moist by spreading their serous secretions backwards, thus moistening the entire mucosa. Tos, however, was able to find only 20 to 30 anterior nasal glands on the septum and an equal number on the lateral wall (10). The author deduced that the contribution of these glands to the total production of secretions is minimal and that they represent a phylogenetic rudiment.

Seromucous Glands

The main duct of these glands is lined with simple cuboidal epithelium. It divides into two side ducts that collect secretions from several tubules lined with either serous or mucous cells. At the ends of the tubules are acini, which may similarly be serous or mucous. Submucosal serous glands predominate over mucinous glands by a ratio of about 8:1. The glands first laid down during development grow deep into the lamina propria before dividing and thus develop their mass in the deepest layers of the mucosa with relatively long ducts. The glands that develop later divide before growing down into the mucosa and thus form a more superficial mass with short ducts. Vessels, nerves, and fibers develop in between, giving rise to two glandular layers: superficial and deep. The mass of the deep glands is larger than that of the superficial ones and the total number of these glands is approximately 90,000.

Intraepithelial Glands

These glands are located in the epithelium and consist of 20 to 50 mucous cells arranged radially around a small lumen. Many intraepithelial glands exist in nasal polyps. Compared to seromucous glands, intraepithelial glands produce only a small amount of mucus and thus play a minor role in the physiology of nasal secretions.

VASCULAR AND LYMPHATIC SUPPLIES

The nose receives its blood supply from both the internal and the external carotid circulations via the ophthalmic and internal maxillary arteries, respectively (Fig. 5). The ophthalmic artery gives rise to the anterior and posterior ethmoid arteries, which supply the anterosuperior portion of the septum, the lateral nasal walls, the olfactory region, and a small part of the posterosuperior region. The external carotid artery gives rise to the internal maxillary artery, which ends as the spheno-palatine artery, which enters the nasal cavity through the sphenopalatine foramen behind the posterior end of the middle turbinate. The sphenopalatine artery gives origin to a number of posterior lateral and septal nasal branches. The posterolateral branches proceed to the region of the middle and inferior turbinates and to the floor of the nasal cavity. The posterior septal branches supply the corresponding area of the septum, including the nasal floor. Because it supplies the majority of blood to the nose and is often involved in severe epistaxis, the sphenopalatine artery has been called the "rhinologist's" artery. The region of the vestibule is supplied by the facial artery through lateral and septal nasal branches. The septal branches of the sphenopalatine artery form multiple anastomoses, with the terminal branches of the anterior ethmoidal and facial arteries giving rise to Kiesselbach's area, located at the caudal aspect of the septum and also known as Little's area. Most cases of epistaxis occur in this region (17).

The veins accompanying the branches of the sphenopalatine artery drain into the pterygoid plexus. The ethmoidal veins join the ophthalmic plexus in the orbit. Part of the drainage to the ophthalmic plexus proceeds to the cavernous sinus via the superior ophthalmic veins and the other part to the pterygoid plexus via the inferior ophthalmic veins. Furthermore, the nasal veins form numerous anastomoses with the veins of the face, palate, and pharynx. The nasal venous system is valveless, predisposing to the spread of infections and constituting a dynamic system reflecting body position.

The subepithelial and glandular zones of the nasal mucosa are supplied by arteries derived from the periosteal or perichondrial vessels. Branches from these vessels ascend perpendicularly toward the surface, anastomosing with the cavernous plexi (venous system) before forming fenestrated capillary networks next to the respiratory epithelium and around the glandular tissue. The fenestrae always face the respiratory epithelium and are believed to be one of the sources of fluid for

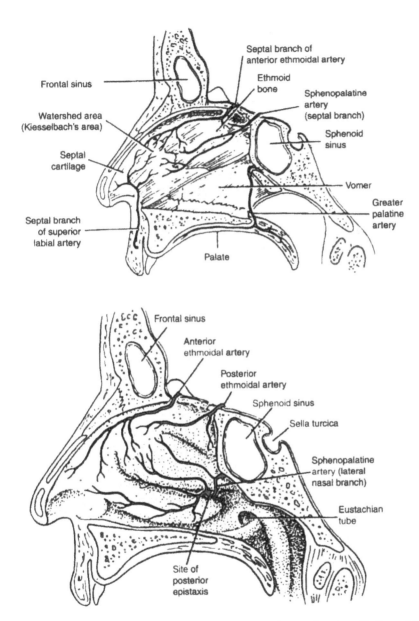

FIGURE 5 Nasal blood supply. (*Top panel*) Supply to the nasal septum. (*Bottom panel*) Supply to the lateral nasal wall. *Source*: From Ref. 16.

humidification. The capillaries of the subepithelial and periglandular network join to form venules that drain into larger superficial veins. They, in turn, join the sinuses of the cavernous plexus. The cavernous plexi, or sinusoids, consist of networks of large, tortuous, valveless, anastomosing veins mostly found over the inferior and middle turbinates but also in the midlevel of the septum. They consist of a superficial layer formed by the union of veins that drain the subepithelial and glandular capillaries and a deeper layer where the sinuses acquire thicker walls and assume a course parallel to the periosteum or perichondrium. They receive venous blood from the subepithelial and glandular capillaries and arterial blood from arteriovenous anastomoses. The arterial segments of the anastomoses are surrounded by a longitudinal smooth muscle layer that controls their blood flow. When the muscular layer contracts, the artery occludes; when it relaxes, the anastomosis opens, allowing the sinuses to fill rapidly with blood. Because of this function, the sinusoids are physiologically referred to as capacitance vessels. Only the endothelium interposes between the longitudinal muscles and the blood stream, making them sensitive to circulating agents. The cavernous plexi change their blood volume in response to neural, mechanical, thermal, psychologic, or chemical stimulation. They expand and shrink, altering the caliber of the air passages and, consequently, the speed and volume of airflow.

Lymphatic vessels from the nasal vestibule drain toward the external nose, whereas the nasal fossa drains posteriorly. The first-order lymph nodes for posterior drainage are the lateral retropharyngeal nodes, whereas the subdigastric nodes serve that function for anterior drainage.

NEURAL SUPPLY

The nasal neural supply is overwhelmingly sensory and autonomic (sympathetic, parasympathetic, nonadrenergic, and noncholinergic) (Fig. 6). The sensory nasal

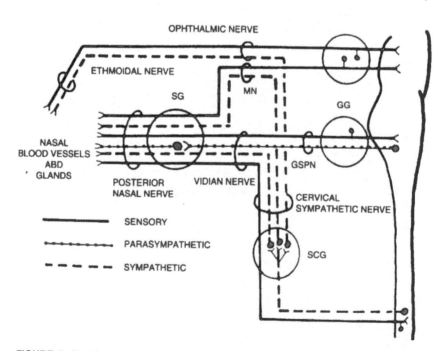

FIGURE 6 Nasal neural supply: sensory, sympathetic, and parasympathetic. *Abbreviations:* SG, sphenopalatine ganglion; MN, maxillary nerve; GG, geniculate ganglion; GSPN, greater superficial petrosal nerve; SCG, superior cervical ganglion. *Source:* From Ref. 7.

innervation comes via both the ophthalmic and the maxillary divisions of the trigeminal nerve and supplies the septum, the lateral walls, the anterior part of the nasal floor, and the inferior meatus. The parasympathetic nasal fibers travel from their origin in the superior salivary nucleus of the midbrain via the nervus intermedius of the facial nerve to the geniculate ganglion where they join the greater superficial petrosal nerve, which in turn joins the deep petrosal nerve to form the vidian nerve. This nerve travels to the SG where the preganglionic parasympathetic fibers synapse and postganglionic fibers supply the nasal mucosa. The sympathetic input originates as preganglionic fibers in the thoracolumbar region of the spinal cord, which pass into the vagosympathetic trunk and relay in the superior cervical ganglion. The postganglionic fibers end as the deep petrosal nerve, which joins the greater superficial nerve to form the vidian nerve. They traverse the SG without synapsing and are distributed to the nasal mucosa.

Nasal glands receive direct parasympathetic nerve supply, and electrical stimulation of parasympathetic nerves in animals induces glandular secretions that are blocked by atropine. Furthermore, stimulation of the human nasal mucosa with methacholine, a cholinomimetic, produces an atropine-sensitive increase in nasal secretions (18). Parasympathetic nerves also innervate the nasal vasculature, and stimulation of these fibers causes vasodilatation. Sympathetic fibers supply the nasal vasculature but do not establish a close relationship with nasal glands, and their exact role in the control of nasal secretions is not clear. Stimulation of these fibers in cats causes vasoconstriction and a decrease in nasal airway resistance. Adrenergic agonists are commonly used in humans, both topically and orally, to decrease nasal congestion.

The presence of sympathetic and parasympathetic nerves and their transmitters in the nasal mucosa has been known for decades but recent immunohistochemical studies have established the presence of additional neuropeptides. These are secreted by unmyelinated nociceptive C fibers [tachykinins, calcitonin gene-related peptide (CGRP), neurokinin A (NKA), gastrin-releasing peptide], parasympathetic nerve endings [vasoactive intestinal peptide (VIP), peptide histidine methionine], and sympathetic nerve endings (neuropeptide Y). Substance P (SP), a member of the tachykinin family, is often found as a cotransmitter with NKA and CGRP and has been found in high density in arterial vessels, and to some extent in veins, gland acini, and the epithelium of the nasal mucosa (19). SP receptors (NK1 receptors) are located in the epithelium, glands, and vessels (19). CGRP receptors are found in high concentration on small muscular arteries and arterioles in the nasal mucosa (20). The distribution of VIP fibers in human airways corresponds closely to that of cholinergic nerves (21). In the human nasal mucosa, VIP is abundant and its receptors are located on arterial vessels, submucosal glands, and epithelial cells (22).

NASAL MUCUS AND MUCOCILIARY TRANSPORT

A 10–15 µm deep layer of mucus covers the entire nasal cavity (23). It is slightly acidic, with a pH between 5.5 and 6.5. The mucous blanket consists of two layers: a thin, low-viscosity, periciliary layer (sol phase) that envelops the shafts of the cilia, and a thick, more viscous, layer (gel phase) riding on the periciliary layer. The gel phase can also be envisioned as discontinuous plaques of mucus. The distal tips of the ciliary shafts contact these plaques when they are fully extended. Insoluble particles caught on the mucous plaques move with them as a consequence of ciliary beating. Soluble materials like droplets, formaldehyde, and CO_2 dissolve in the periciliary layer. Thus, nasal mucus effectively filters and removes near 100% of particles greater than $4\,\mu m$ in diameter (24–26). An estimated 1–2 L of nasal mucus, composed of 2.5% to 3% glycoproteins, 1% to 2% salts, and 95% water, is produced per day. Mucin, one of the glycoproteins, gives mucus its unique attributes of protection and lubrication of mucosal surfaces.

The sources of nasal secretions are multiple and include anterior nasal glands, seromucous submucosal glands, epithelial secretory cells (of both mucous and serous types), tears, and transudation from blood vessels. Transudation increases in pathologic conditions as a result of the effects of inflammatory mediators that increase vascular permeability. A good example is the increased vascular permeability seen in response to allergen challenge of subjects with allergic rhinitis as measured by increasing levels of albumin in nasal lavages after provocation (27). In contrast to serum, immunoglobulins make up the bulk of the protein in mucus; other substances in nasal secretions include lactoferrin, lysozyme, antitrypsin, transferrin, lipids, histamine, and other mediators, cytokines, antioxidants, ions (Cl, Na, Ca, and K), cells, and bacteria. Mucus functions in mucociliary transport, and substances will not be cleared from the nose without it, despite adequate ciliary function. Furthermore, mucus provides immune and mechanical mucosal protection, and its high water content plays a significant role in humidifying inspired air.

Mucociliary transport is unidirectional based on the unique characteristics of cilia. Cilia in mammals beat in a biphasic, or to-and-fro, manner. The beat consists of a rapid effective stroke during which the cilium straightens, bringing it into contact with the gel phase of the mucus, and a slow recovery phase during which the bent cilium returns in the periciliary or sol layer of the mucus, thus propelling it in one direction (Fig. 7).

Metachrony is the coordination of the beat of individual cilia, which prevents collision between cilia in different phases of motion and results in the unidirectional flow of mucus. Ciliary beating produces a current in the superficial layer of the

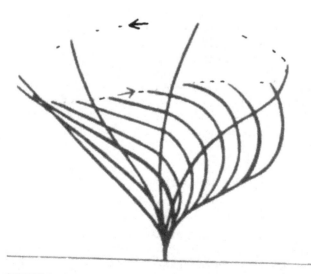

FIGURE 7 A schematic diagram of motion of a single cilium during the rapid forward beat and the slower recovery phase. *Source:* From Ref. 7.

periciliary fluid in the direction of the effective stroke. The mucous plaques move as a result of motion of the periciliary fluid layer and the movement of the extended tips of the cilia into the plaques. Thus, the depth of the periciliary fluid is the key factor in mucociliary transport. If excessive, the extended ciliary tips fail to contact mucous plaques, and the current of the periciliary fluid provides the only means of movement.

Mucociliary transport moves mucus and its contents toward the nasopharynx, with the exception of the anterior portion of the inferior turbinates, where transport is anterior. This anterior current prevents many of the particles deposited in this area from progressing further into the nasal cavity. The particles transported posteriorly toward the nasopharynx are periodically swallowed. Mucociliary transport, however, is not the only mechanism by which particles and secretions are cleared from the nose. Sniffing and nose blowing help in moving airway secretions backward and forward, respectively. Sneezing results in a burst of air, accompanied by an increase in watery nasal secretions that are then cleared by nose blowing and sniffing.

Respiratory cilia beat about 1000 times/min, which translates to surface materials being moved at a rate of 3–25 mm/min. Both the beat rate and propelling speed vary. Several substances have been used to measure nasal mucociliary clearance, and the most utilized are sodium saccharin, dyes, and tagged particles. The dye and saccharin methods are similar, consisting of placing a strong dye or saccharin sodium on the nasal mucosa just behind the internal ostium and recording the time it takes to reach the pharyngeal cavity; this interval is termed "nasal mucociliary transport time." With saccharin, the time is recorded when the subject reports a sweet taste; with a dye, when it appears in the pharyngeal cavity. Combining the two methods reduces the disadvantages of both—namely, variable taste thresholds in different subjects when using saccharin and repeated pharyngeal inspection when using the dye—and makes them more reliable. The use of tagged particles involves placement of an anion exchange resin particle about 0.5 mm in diameter tagged with a 99Tc ion on the anterior nasal mucosa, behind the area of anterior mucociliary movement, and following its subsequent clearance with a gamma camera or multicollimated detectors. This last method permits continuous monitoring of movement.

Studies of several hundred healthy adult subjects by the tagged particle or saccharin methods have consistently shown that 80% exhibit clearance rates of 3–25 mm/min (average = 6 mm/min), with slower rates in the remaining 20% (28). The latter subjects have been termed "slow clearers." The findings of a greater proportion of slow clearers in one group of subjects living in an extremely cold climate raises the possibility that the differences in clearance may be related to an effect of inspired air (28). In diseased subjects, slow clearance may be due to a variety of factors, including the immotility of cilia, transient or permanent injury to the mucociliary system by physical trauma, viral infection, dehydration, or excessively viscid secretions secondary to decreased ions and water in the mucus paired with increased amounts of DNA from dying cells, as in cystic fibrosis.

NASAL AIRFLOW

The nose provides the main pathway for inhaled air to the lower airways, and offers two areas of resistance to airflow (provided there are no gross deviations of the nasal septum): the nasal valve and the state of mucosal swelling of the nasal airway. The cross-sectional area of the nasal airway decreases dramatically at the nasal valve to reach 30–40 mm^2. This narrowed area separates the vestibules from the main airway and account for approximately half of the total resistance to respiratory airflow from ambient air to the alveoli. After bypassing this narrow area, inspired air flows in the main nasal airway, which is a broader tube bounded by the septal surface medially, and the irregular inferior and middle turbinates laterally. The variable caliber of the lumen of this portion of the airway is governed by changes in the blood content of the capillaries, capacitance vessels, and arteriovenous shunts of the lining mucosa, and constitutes the second resistive segment that inspired air encounters on its way to the lungs. Changes in the blood content of these structures occur spontaneously and rhythmically resulting in alternating volume reductions in the lumen of the two nasal cavities, a phenomenon referred to as the nasal cycle. This occurs in approximately 80% of the normal individuals, and the reciprocity of changes between the two sides of the nasal cavity maintains total nasal airway resistance unchanged (29). The duration of one cycle varies between 50 minutes and four hours and is interrupted by vasoconstrictive medications or exercise, which lead to a marked reduction of total nasal airway resistance. Kennedy et al. observed the nasal passages using T2-weighted magnetic resonance imaging and demonstrated an alternating increase and decrease in signal intensity and turbinate size over time in a fashion consistent with the nasal cycle (30). The nasal cycle can be exacerbated by the increase in nasal airway resistance caused by exposure to allergic stimuli, which explains why some allergic individuals complain of alternating exacerbations of their nasal obstructive symptoms.

Swift and Proctor presented a detailed description of nasal airflow and its characteristics (Fig. 8) (31). Upon inspiration, air first passes upwards into the vestibules in a vertical direction at a velocity of 2–3 m/sec, then converges and changes its direction from vertical to horizontal just prior to the nasal valve, where, due to the narrowing of the airway, velocities reach their highest levels (up to 12–18 m/sec). After passing the nasal valve, the cross-sectional area increases and the velocity decreases concomitantly to about 2–3 m/sec. The nature of flow changes from laminar, before and at the nasal valve, to more turbulent posteriorly.

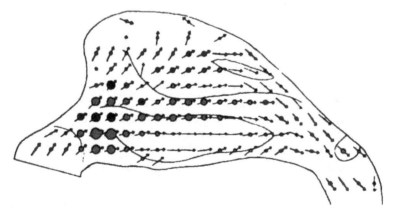

FIGURE 8 Schematic diagram of the direction and velocity of inspired air. The size of the dots is directly proportional to velocity, and the arrows depict direction of airflow. *Source*: From Ref. 7.

As inspiratory flow increases beyond resting levels, turbulent characteristics commence at an increasingly anterior position and, with mild exercise, are found as early as the anterior ends of the turbinates. The airstream increases in velocity to 3–4 m/sec in the nasopharynx, where the direction again changes from horizontal to vertical as air moves down through the pharynx and larynx to reach the trachea. Turbulence of nasal airflow minimizes the presence of a boundary layer of air that would exist with laminar flow and maximizes interaction between the airstream and the nasal mucosa. This, in turn, allows the nose to perform its functions of heat and moisture exchange and of cleaning inspired air of suspended or soluble particles.

NASAL CONDITIONING OF TEMPERATURE AND HUMIDITY OF INSPIRED AIR

Inspiratory air is rapidly warmed and moistened mainly in the nasal cavities and, to a lesser extent, in the remainder of the upper airway down to the lungs (32). Inspired air is warmed from a temperature of around 20°C at the portal of entry to 31°C in the pharynx and 35°C in the trachea. This is facilitated by the turbulent characteristics of nasal airflow, which maximize the contact between inspired and expired air and the nasal mucosal surface (33). After inspiration ceases, warming of the nasal mucosa by the blood is such a relatively slow process that, at expiration, the temperature of the nasal mucosa remains lower than that of expired air. As expiratory air passes through the nose, it gives up heat to the cooler nasal mucosa. This cooling causes condensation of water vapor and, thus, a 33% return of both heat and moisture to the mucosal surface. Because recovery of heat from expiratory air occurs mainly in the region of the respiratory portal, blood flow changes that take place in the nasal mucosa affect respiratory air conditioning more markedly in this region (34).

Ingelstedt showed that the humidifying capacity of the nose is greatly impaired in healthy volunteers after a subcutaneous injection of atropine (32,35). He thus concluded that atropine-inhibitable glandular secretion is a major source of water for humidification of inspired air. In contrast, Kumlien and Drettner failed to show any effect of intranasal ipratropium bromide, another anticholinergic agent, on the degree of warming and humidification of air during passage in the nasal cavity in a small clinical trial using normal subjects and a group of patients with vasomotor rhinitis (36). In addition to glandular secretions, other sources provide water for humidification of inspired air and these include water content of ambient air, lacrimation via the nasolacrimal duct, secretion from the paranasal sinuses, salivation (during oronasal breathing) and secretions from goblet cells and seromucinous glands of the respiratory mucosa, and passive transport against an ionic gradient in the paracellular spaces (35,37). Not inhibited by atropine, but also probably important as a source of water for humidification of inspired air, is transudation of fluid from the blood vessels of the nose. Impairment of the humidifying capacity of the nose is further accentuated when the nasal mucosa is chilled, leading, along with condensation, to the nasal drip so often seen in cold weather.

The ability to warm and humidify air has been investigated using a model system that involves measuring the amount of water delivered by the nose after inhaling cold dry air (38). This is calculated after measuring the temperature and humidity of air as it penetrates the nasal cavity and then again in the nasopharynx by using a specially designed probe. Using this model, the investigators were able to show that the ability to warm and humidify inhaled air is lower in subjects with allergic rhinitis out of season compared to normal controls. The effect of allergic inflammation on the nasal conditioning capacity of individuals with seasonal allergic rhinitis was then investigated by evaluating the ability of the nose to warm and humidify cold dry air in allergies before and after the season as well as 24 hours after allergen challenge (39). These studies showed that allergic inflammation, induced by either the allergy season or an allergen challenge, increased the ability of the nose to warm and humidify inhaled air and the authors speculated that this was related to a change in the nasal perimeter induced by allergic inflammation. In an interesting follow-up study, the same investigators compared the ability of the following groups of subjects to warm and humidify inhaled air: patients with perennial allergic rhinitis, seasonal allergic rhinitis out of season, normal subjects, and subjects with bronchial asthma (40). They showed that subjects with perennial allergic rhinitis were comparable to normals in their ability to condition air and that subjects with asthma had a reduced ability to perform this function compared to normals. Furthermore, the total water gradient, a measure of the ability of the nose to condition air, correlated negatively with severity of asthma assessed by using the Aas score, suggesting that the ability to condition inspired air was worse in subjects with more severe asthma and that this reduced ability might contribute, at least in part, to the pathophysiology of asthma.

OLFACTION

One of the important sensory functions of the nose is olfaction. The olfactory airway is 1–2 mm wide and lies above the middle turbinate just inferior to the cribriform plate between the septum and the lateral wall of the nose. The olfactory mucosa has a surface area of 200–400 mm² and contains numerous odor-receptor cells with thin cilia that project into the covering mucus layer and increase the surface area of the epithelium (41). The olfactory mucosa also contains small, tubular, serous Bowman's glands situated immediately below the epithelium. Each receptor cell is connected to the olfactory bulb by a thin nonmyelinated nerve fiber that is slow conducting but short, making the conduction time as low as 50 m/sec. The impulses from the olfactory bulb are conveyed to the olfactory cortex, which in humans is part of the thalamus, which also receives taste signals.

The area where the olfactory epithelium is located is poorly ventilated as most of the inhaled air passes through the lower aspect of the nasal cavity. Therefore, nasal obstruction, as documented by elevations in nasal airway resistance, leads to an elevation in olfactory thresholds (42). This may be secondary to several conditions such as septal deviations, nasal polyposis, nasal deformities, or increased nasal congestion, one of the characteristic symptoms of allergic rhinitis. Sniffing helps the process of smell by increasing the flow rate of inhaled air and, consequently, raising the proportion of air reaching the olfactory epithelium by 5% to 20%. This results in increasing the number of odorant molecules available to the olfactory receptors and proportionally enhancing odor sensation. In addition to crossing the anatomic barriers of the nose, the odorant molecules must have a dual solubility in lipids and water to be able to reach the olfactory receptors. To penetrate the mucus covering the olfactory mucosa, they solubilize to a certain extent in water. Lipid solubility, on the other hand, enhances their interaction with the receptor membrane of the olfactory epithelial cilia. Lastly, it is to be mentioned that olfactory sensitivity normally decreases with age as evidenced by a recent longitudinal study of men and women between the ages of 19 and 95 followed over a three-year period (43).

VOMERONASAL ORGAN

Many vertebrate species including many mammals have a small chemosensory structure in the nose called the vomeronasal organ (VNO), which is dedicated to detecting chemical signals that mediate sexual and territorial behaviors. A similar structure appears to exist in the human nose and is described as two small sacs about 2 mm deep that open into shallow pits on either side of the nasal septum. Jacob et al. performed a study to characterize the nasal opening of the nasopalatine duct (NPD), which, with the VNO, forms the vomeronasal system (44). Otolaryngologists examined the nose of normal volunteers endoscopically looking for distinct morphologic features of the NPD including the structure's larger fossa or craterlike indentation and its smaller aperture within the fossa. The area examined for presence or absence of the duct was approximately 2 cm dorsal to the nostril opening and less than 0.5 cm above the junction of the nasal floor and septum. The NPD was detected in 94% of 221 nostrils and its nasal opening was consistently located 1.9 cm dorsal to the collumella, 0.2 cm above the junction of the nasal floor and septum. The authors also examined cadaver specimens and found bilateral nasopalatine fossae with apertures in every specimen and VNOs in less than half of the septal regions examined. Thus, while the authors did not establish function, their study confirms the existence of a vomeronasal system, or its anatomical remnants in humans.

In vertebrates, the pair of small sacs is lined by sensory neurons, tucked inside the vomer bone where the hard palate and nasal septum meet. In mice and rats, the VNO is connected to the brain through a neural pathway that is independent from the olfactory pathway, but it is not clear whether the human VNO is connected to the brain. There is renewed interest in researching the anatomy and function of this organ in humans, and this effort is primarily funded by the perfume industry (45).

CONCLUSION

As detailed in this chapter, the nose is an intricate organ with important functions which include filtration, humidification, and temperature control of inspired air in preparation for transit to the lower airways. It is also important in providing the sense of olfaction. It has an intricate network of nerves, vessels, glands, and inflammatory cells, which all help to modulate its function. Chronic inflammation affects multiple end organs within the nasal cavity and will lead to diseases such as rhinitis (allergic and nonallergic) as well as sinusitis. The overview of the anatomy and function of the nose provided in this chapter will hopefully serve as a useful prelude to the coming chapters where different aspects of nonallergic rhinitis are discussed.

REFERENCES

1. Drumheller GW. Topology of the lateral nasal cartilages: the anatomical relationship of the lateral nasal to the greater alar cartilage, lateral crus. Anat Rec 1973; 176:321.
2. Van Loosen J, Van Zanten GA, Howard CV, et al. Growth characteristics of the human nasal septum. Rhinology 1996; 34:78.

3. Gray L. Deviated nasal septum. III. Its influence on the physiology and disease of the nose and ears. J Laryngol 1967; 81:953.
4. Cummings CW, Fredrickson JM, Harker LA, et al. Otolaryngology—Head and Neck Surgery. 2nd ed. St. Louis: Mosby, 1993.
5. Mygind N, Pedersen M, Nielsen M. Morphology of the upper airway epithelium. In: Proctor DF, Andersen IB, eds. The Nose. Amsterdam: Elsevier Biomedical Press BV, 1982.
6. Montgomery WW. Surgery of the Upper Respiratory System. Philadelphia: Lea and Febiger, 1979.
7. Proctor DF, Andersen IB. The Nose-Upper Airway Physiology and the Atmospheric Environment. Amsterdam: Elsevier Biomedical Press, 1982.
8. Evans MJ, Plopper GG. The role of basal cells in adhesion of columnar epithelium to airway basement membrane. Am Rev Respir Dis 1988; 138:481.
9. Evans MJ, Shami S, Cabral-Anderson LJ, et al. Role of nonciliated cells in renewal of the bronchial epithelium of rats exposed to NO_2. Am J Path 1986; 123:126.
10. Tos M. Goblet cells and glands in the nose and paranasal sinuses. In: Proctor DF, Andersen IB, eds. The Nose. Amsterdam: Elsevier Biomedical Press BV, 1982.
11. Winther B, Innes DJ, Mills SE, et al. Lymphocyte subsets in normal airway mucosa of the human nose. Arch Otolaryngol Head Neck Surg 1987; 113:59.
12. Bradding P, Feather IH, Wilson S, et al. Immunolocalization of cytokines in the nasal mucosa of normal and perennial rhinitic subjects. J Immunol 1993; 151:3853.
13. Lim MC, Taylor RM, Naclerio RM. The histology of allergic rhinitis and its comparison to cellular changes in nasal lavage. Am J Respir Crit Care Med 1995; 151:136.
14. Varney VA, Jacobson MR, Sudderick RM, et al. Immunohistology of the nasal mucosa following allergen-induced rhinitis. Am Rev Respir Dis 1992; 146:170.
15. Bojsen-Moller F. Glandulae nasales anteriores in the human nose. Ann Otol Rhinol Laryngol 1965; 74:363.
16. Cummings CW, Fredrickson JM, Harker LA, et al. Otolaryngology—Head and Neck Surgery. Vol. 1. St. Louis: CV Mosby Co., 1986.
17. Cauna N. Blood and nerve supply of the nasal lining. In: Proctor DF, Andersen IB, eds. The Nose. Amsterdam: Elsevier Biomedical Press BV, 1982.
18. Baroody FM, Wagenmann M, Naclerio RM. A comparison of the secretory response of the nasal mucosa to histamine and methacholine. J Appl Physiol 1993; 74(6):2661.
19. Baraniuk JN, Lundgren JD, Mullol J, et al. Substance P and neurokinin A in human nasal mucosa. Am J Respir Cell Mol Biol 1991; 4:228.
20. Baraniuk JN, Castellino S, Merida M, et al. Calcitonin gene related peptide in human nasal mucosa. Am J Physiol 1990; 258:L81.
21. Laitinen A, Partanen M, Hervonen A, et al. VIP-like immunoreactive nerves in human respiratory tract. Light and electron microscopic study. Histochemistry 1985; 82:313.
22. Baraniuk JN, Okayama M, Lundgren JD, et al. Vasoactive intestinal peptide (VIP) in human nasal mucosa. J Clin Invest 1990; 86:825.
23. Wilson WR, Allansmith MR. Rapid, atraumatic method for obtaining nasal mucus samples. Ann Otol Rhinol Laryngol 1976; 85:391.
24. Andersen I, Lundqvist G, Proctor DF. Human nasal mucosal function under four controlled humidities. Am Rev Respir Dis 1979; 119:619.
25. Fry FA, Black A. Regional deposition and clearance of particles in the human nose. Aerosol Sci 1973; 4:113.
26. Lippmann M. Deposition and clearance of inhaled particles in the human nose. Ann Otol Rhinol Laryngol 1970; 79:519.
27. Baumgarten C, Togias AG, Naclerio RM, et al. Influx of kininogens into nasal secretions after antigen challenge of allergic individuals. J Clin Invest 1985; 76:191.
28. Proctor DF. The mucociliary system. In: Proctor DF, Andersen IB, eds. The Nose: Upper Airway Physiology and the Atmospheric Environment. Amsterdam: Elsevier Biomedical Press BV, 1982.
29. Hasegawa M, Kern EB. The human cycle. Mayo Clin Proc 1977; 52:28.
30. Kennedy DW, Zinreich SJ, Kumar AJ, et al. Physiologic mucosal changes within the nose and the ethmoid sinus: Imaging of the nasal cycle by MRI. Laryngoscope 1988; 98:928.

31. Swift DL, Proctor DF. Access of air to the respiratory tract. In: Brain JD, Proctor DF, Reid LM, eds. Respiratory Defense Mechanisms. New York, NY: Marcel Dekker, 1977.
32. Ingelstedt S, Ivstam B. Study in the humidifying capacity of the nose. Acta Otolaryngol 1951; 39:286.
33. Aharonson EF, Menkes H, Gurtner G, et al. The effect of respiratory airflow rate on the removal of soluble vapors by the nose. J Appl Physiol 1974; 37:654.
34. Scherer PW, Hahn II, Mozell MM. The biophysics of nasal airflow. Otolaryngol Clin North Am 1989; 22:265.
35. Ingelstedt S, Ivstam B. The source of nasal secretion in normal condition. Acta Otolaryngol 1949; 37:446.
36. Kumlien J, Drettner B. The effect of ipratropium bromide (Atrovent) on the air conditioning capacity of the nose. Clin Otolaryngol 1985; 10:165.
37. Togias AG, Proud D, Lichtenstein LM, et al. The osmolality of nasal secretions increases when inflammatory mediators are released in response to inhalation of cold, dry air. Am Rev Respir Dis 1988; 137:625.
38. Rouadi P, Baroody FM, Abbott D, Naureckas E, Solway J, NAclerio RM. A technique to measure the ability of the human nose to warm and humidify air. J Appl Physiol 1999; 87:400–406.
39. Assanasen P, Baroody FM, Abbott DJ, Naureckas E, Solway J, Naclerio RM. Natural and induced allergic responses increase the ability of the nose to warm and humidify air. J Allergy Clin Immunol 2000; 106:1045–1052.
40. Assanasen P, Baroody FM, Naureckas E, Solway J, Naclerio RM. The nasal passage of subjects with asthma has a decreased ability to warm and humidify inspired air. Am J Respir Crit Care Med 2001; 164:1640–1646.
41. Berglund B, Lindvall T. Olfaction. In: Proctor DF, Andersen IB, eds. The Nose. Amsterdam: Elsevier Biomedical Press BV, 1982.
42. Rous J, Kober F. Influence of one-sided nasal respiratory occlusion of the olfactory threshold values. Arch Klin Ohren Nasen Kehlkopfheiklk 1970; 196(2):374.
43. Ship JA, Pearson JD, Cruise LJ, et al. Longitudinal changes in smell identification. J Gerontol 1996; 51(2):M86.
44. Jacob S, Zelano B, Gungor A, Abbott D, Naclerio RM, McClintock MK. Location and gross morphology of the nasopalatine duct in human adults. Arch Otolaryngol Head Neck Surg 2000; 126:741–748.
45. Taylor R. Brave new nose: sniffing out human sexual chemistry. J NIH Res 1994; 6:47.

2

Epidemiology of Rhinitis: Allergic and Nonallergic

Russell A. Settipane

Department of Medicine, Brown Medical School, Providence, Rhode Island, U.S.A.

David R. Charnock

Department of Surgery, Section of Otolaryngology, University of Vermont College of Medicine, Burlington, Vermont, U.S.A.

INTRODUCTION

Chronic rhinitis symptoms result from diverse underlying disease mechanisms and are among the most common problems presenting to physicians (1). According to the Joint Task Force Parameters on Allergy, Asthma, and Immunology, rhinitis is defined as inflammation of the mucous membrane lining of the nose, and it is characterized by nasal congestion, rhinorrhea, sneezing, itching of the nose, and postnasal drainage (2). These guidelines further classify rhinitis as allergic or nonallergic, each of which is further subclassified. Allergic rhinitis is divided into seasonal, perennial, episodic, and occupational. Nonallergic rhinitis is a diverse syndrome that encompasses a complex and broad variety of disorders, the subclassification of which shall be reviewed in this chapter.

As simple and straightforward as the above definition and classification scheme of rhinitis may appear, it is not without controversy. Contrary to the above definition, which incorporates inflammation as an essential component, there are thought to exist types of nonallergic rhinitis in which inflammation does not appear to be present (3). Additionally, in response to shortfalls in this classification scheme, a modified classification of rhinitis has been recently proposed that suggests the new term "mixed rhinitis" to describe patients in whom allergic and nonallergic rhinitis disease mechanisms coexist (4).

Before examining the epidemiology of allergic and nonallergic rhinitis, it is important to first review current definitions of rhinitis types.

DEFINITIONS

Allergic rhinitis is defined as an immunologic response modulated by immunoglobulin E (Ig E) and characterized by sneezing, rhinorrhea, nasal congestion, and pruritus of the nose (2). Allergic rhinitis can be classified as seasonal (commonly called hay fever), which most frequently results from IgE-mediated sensitivity to pollen allergens (tree, grass, or weed). Alternatively, allergic rhinitis can be classified as perennial, most commonly caused by allergy to animal dander or dust mites. Other classifications of allergic rhinitis include rhinitis resulting from episodic allergen exposure and rhinitis due to occupational causation. Recently, the allergic rhinitis and its impact on asthma (ARIA) guidelines have proposed a new classification scheme, which proposes that "seasonal/perennial" classification be replaced by "intermittent/persistent." Also a severity classification has been proposed, ranging from "mild" to "moderate/severe" (5).

Nonallergic rhinitis represents a broad classification of nasal diseases that are due to multiple etiologies, none of which involve an immunologic response modulated by IgE. Because symptoms characteristic of nonallergic rhinitis are indistinguishable from those that occur in allergic rhinitis, negative or clinically irrelevant allergy tests for specific IgE sensitivity are necessary to make the diagnosis. There is a lack of consensus in regard to the latter point: some clinicians allow for clinically irrelevant positive allergy tests, whereas other clinicians, particularly researchers, strictly require allergy test results to be completely negative.

The proposed term, "mixed rhinitis," most often describes patients with allergic rhinitis who also experience chronic rhinitis symptoms not entirely explained by the presence of IgE sensitivity (4). An example of mixed rhinitis would be a patient with perennial rhinitis symptoms, aggravated by "classic" vasomotor rhinitis (VMR) provocateurs, who also experiences worsening of rhinitis in the late summer and in whom testing for specific IgE sensitivity is positive only to ragweed and negative to all relevant perennial allergens. Although this scenario may seem fairly straightforward, what remains unresolved is how to classify patients with perennial allergic rhinitis who, in addition to experiencing symptoms triggered by perennial allergens, are also triggered by nonallergic triggers such as weather changes, strong odors, and irritants. Should this be classified as "mixed rhinitis"? Or should this be simply regarded as a manifestation of nasal hyperreactivity resulting from underlying allergic inflammation?

EPIDEMIOLOGY

Allergic Rhinitis

The prevalence of allergic rhinitis has been estimated to range from as low as 9% to more than 40% (6–17). Numerous reports summarizing published prevalence rates are presented in Table 1. Multiple factors contribute to the wide range of reported prevalence rates of allergic rhinitis. These include type of prevalence rate reported (current or cumulative), study selection criteria, age of participants, differences in survey methods, varied geographic locations, and socioeconomic status, any of which are significant enough to confound direct comparison between studies. Some investigators report "current" prevalence rate, which refers to the percentage of the population with the condition during the previous 12 months. Other authors report "cumulative" or "lifetime" prevalence, which is the percentage of a population who have ever had the condition at any time during their life. The cumulative prevalence of hay fever has been reported to be as high as 46% at age 40 years (13).

Problematic is that there is no standard set of diagnostic criteria for allergic rhinitis. In most studies, the criteria for diagnosis are based on the subject's reporting, solely by questionnaire and rarely confirmed by skin testing. Additionally, most studies focus on hay fever, leaving perennial allergic rhinitis underestimated. Sinus imaging is generally not performed and, therefore, rhinosinusitis not differentiated. Finally, it is possible that differences in geographic location and varied populations may be a factor. Local variation in pollens and climate are not the only geographic variables of potential significance. Persistent exposure to air pollution and especially traffic-related particulate matter from motor vehicles has often been

TABLE 1 Prevalence of Allergic Rhinitis

Investigator	Country	Year	Subjects	Rate (%)	Rate type
Freeman and Johnson (6)	United States	1964	12th grade	22	Past year
Broder et al. (7)	United States	1974	16–24 yrs	15	Lifetime
McMenamin (8)	United States	1994	National HIS	9	Past year
Nathan et al. (9)	United States	1997	National Survey	18	Past year
Wright et al. (10)	United States	1994	6 yrs old	42	Lifetime
Gergen and Turkeltaub (NHANES II) (11)	United States	1992	18–24 yrs	9	Past year
Hagy and Settipane (12)	United States	1969	Freshman	21	Lifetime
Settipane and co-workers (13)	United States	1998	Age 41	46	Lifetime
Penard-Morand et al. (14)	France	2005	Ages 9–11	20	Lifetime
				12	Past year
Banac et al. (15)	Croatia	2004	Ages 6–7	16.9	Past year
			Ages 13–14	17.5	Past year
Hannaford et al. (16)	Scotland	2005	≥14	13–15	Past year
Bornehag et al. (17)	Sweden	2005	Ages 1–6	11.1	Past year

Abbreviation: NHANES, National Health and Nutrition Survey.

discussed among the man-made factors likely to be contributing to the development of allergic disease; however a recent review of epidemiologic studies on the long-term effects of exposure to traffic-related air pollution on allergic disease in Europe has found only weak evidence for an increased risk for asthma and hay fever (18). This supports a recent U.S. report by Nathan et al. (9), which found no correlation between the prevalence of allergic rhinitis and geographic location. Nathan et al. also found no correlation with socioeconomic status, which contradicts a recent Swedish report by Almvist et al. (19), who studied 2614 Swedish children from birth to age four, and found that there was a decreasing risk of rhinitis with increasing socioeconomic status.

Another factor likely to be contributing to the wide range in reported prevalence rates of allergic rhinitis is the temporal difference in study performance. Reports spanning the last few decades indicate that the prevalence of allergic rhinitis appears to be increasing. A comparison of British cohorts born in 1958 and 1970 revealed an increase from 12% to 23% (20). Study of an Italian population by Verlato et al. demonstrated an increase in allergic rhinitis from 15% to 18% in only a nine-year period, from 1991 to 2000 (21). Selnes et al. (22) reported that the prevalence of allergic rhinoconjunctivitis in Norway increased steadily from 1995 to 2000. The rise in prevalence of allergic rhinitis in Finland has been particularly striking since 1991, and the trend is still upwards (23). However, there is also evidence that the prevalence of asthma and allergic rhinitis has leveled off in some European countries after several decades of increase (24). In the United States, it is not clear whether the prevalence of allergic rhinitis has changed significantly (25).

If this increasing prevalence of allergic rhinitis is indeed due to the increased development of atopy, then tests for specific IgE sensitivity should reflect this. This is, in fact, what was reported by the Copenhagen Allergy Study where a 50% increase in reported allergic rhinitis symptom prevalence was corroborated by an increased prevalence in sensitization (26). More recent supportive evidence includes comparison of data from the National Health and Nutrition Survey (NHANES) II and NHANES III, which provides evidence that the prevalence of specific IgE sensitivity in the general population seems to be increasing (Table 2) (27). NHANES III (1988–1994) has estimated the prevalence of positive skin tests to be as high as 54.3% of the population. Although methodological differences between the two surveys confound direct comparisons, the prevalence rates of positive testing to each allergen were 2.1 to 5.5 times higher compared to what was found in

TABLE 2 Prevalence of Positive Skin Tests: National Health and Nutrition Survey II vs. National Health and Nutrition Survey III

Allergen	NHANES II 1976–1980 (%)	NHANES III[a] 1988–1994 (%)
Alternaria	4.5	12.9
Cat	3.1	17
Oak	5.8	13.2
Rye grass	11.9	26.9
Bermuda grass	5.2	18.1
Ragweed	12.5	26.2

[a]NHANES III also tested mite, roach, thistle, and peanut.
Abbreviation: NHANES, National Health and Nutrition Survey.
Source: From Ref. 27.

NHANES II (1976–1980). Correlating with this increasing prevalence of specific IgE sensitivity in the general population, there is published evidence for an increasing prevalence of allergic rhinitis in an aging cohort. This is suggested by a 23-year follow-up of college students, which reported the prevalence of allergic rhinitis to increase from 21% at age 18 to 31% at age 40. Also at age 40, the lifetime prevalence of allergic rhinitis was reported to be 42% (13).

Nonallergic Rhinitis

Unfortunately, data regarding the prevalence of nonallergic rhinitis are of substantially lesser quantity and quality than what has been published with regard to allergic rhinitis. Furthermore, the prevalence rates of the various subtypes of rhinitis that comprise this disorder have not been adequately defined. Despite these limitations, enough data exist to allow for an estimation of the prevalence of nonallergic rhinitis.

Five epidemiologic studies have helped to establish the frequency of occurrence of nonallergic rhinitis in comparison to allergic rhinitis (Table 3) (28–32). It is important to note that the majority of these studies have been performed in allergy outpatient settings and that this methodology would be anticipated to skew the reported prevalence rates toward the diagnosis of allergic rhinitis. Mullarkey et al. (28) found that 52% of 142 allergy clinic patients with rhinitis could be classified as having nonallergic rhinitis. Enberg (29) evaluated 152 consecutive adults with nasal symptoms and found a 30% frequency of perennial nonallergic rhinitis. However, in analyzing Enberg's data, it is apparent that this frequency would increase from 30% to 46% if the diagnostic criteria for nonallergic rhinitis had been modified to include subjects with clinically irrelevant positive skin tests. Even though the European Community Respiratory Health Survey (ECRHS) (30) selected 1412 subjects for participation on the basis of their having a history that suggested allergic rhinitis, a 25% frequency of nonallergic rhinitis was reported. Togias (31) classified 17% of 362 allergy clinic patients with rhinitis as having nonallergic rhinitis.

Although these epidemiological data are interesting, consideration also must be given to the fact that most of these studies have limited their classification to only allergic or nonallergic disease while failing to make any attempt to capture the frequency of coexisting allergic and nonallergic rhinitis (mixed rhinitis). A recent assessment, conducted by the National Rhinitis Classification Task Force (NRCTF), is to date the best designed survey that attempted to determine the prevalence of mixed rhinitis in relation to allergic and nonallergic rhinitis (32).

TABLE 3 Rhinitis Prevalence Studies: Allergic vs. Nonallergic Rhinitis

Investigator	N	Allergic (%)	Mixed[a]	Nonallergic (%)
Mullarkey et al. (28)	142	48	Not studied	52
Enberg (29)	128[b]	64	Not studied	36
Togias (31)	362	83	Not studied	17
ECRHS (30)	1142	75	Not studied	25
NRCTF (32)	975	43	34%	23

[a]Mixed counted as "allergic" for total analysis except NCRTF.
[b]Diagnosis determined in only 128 patients.
Abbreviations: ECRHS, European Community Respiratory Health Survey; NRCTF, National Rhinitis Classification Task Force.

This was a retrospective multicenter analysis of 975 patients, selected from 15 different outpatient allergy practice centers, with the goal of determining the prevalence of pure allergic, pure nonallergic, and mixed rhinitis. The determination of rhinitis classification was the following: 43% of patients were classified as pure allergic rhinitis, 23% as pure nonallergic rhinitis, and 34% as mixed rhinitis. Analysis of the data confirmed a surprisingly high prevalence of nonallergic rhinitis, which subsequently raised the awareness of the significant occurrence of this diagnosis. When the mixed rhinitis population was combined with the pure nonallergic population, it was evident that 57% of the population had been classified as having some form of nonallergic rhinitis. Furthermore, as many as 44% of patients with allergic rhinitis were suggested to have a nonallergic rhinitis component to their disease.

Of the five epidemiological studies of nonallergic rhinitis, the NRCTF and the ECRHS are the largest and most significant. The data from both studies suggest that the ratio of allergic rhinitis prevalence (pure and mixed combined) to nonallergic rhinitis prevalence is 3:1. Although subject recruitment in both these studies is likely to have been biased toward allergy, this 3:1 ratio probably is, at the very least, relevant to the allergy specialist's practice. This ratio can be extrapolated to determine a conservative estimate of the prevalence of nonallergic rhinitis in the United States. If the assumption is made that 20% of the U.S. population has allergic rhinitis and on the basis of the most recent U.S. census data indicating a population of 289 million, approximately 58 million people in the United States suffer from allergic rhinitis. Applying the 3:1 (allergic to nonallergic) ratio, approximately 19 million people in the United States suffer from nonallergic rhinitis. Furthermore, applying the 44% rate of concomitant nonallergic rhinitis, an additional 26 million (44% of 58 million with allergic rhinitis) have a nonallergic component (mixed rhinitis). Therefore, 45 million people in the United States may have either pure nonallergic rhinitis or at least a nonallergic component to their rhinitis.

Three interesting demographic observations that have been made with regard to nonallergic rhinitis include those related to age, gender, and perennial occurrence. Togias (31) has observed that 70% of patients diagnosed with nonallergic nasal disease developed their condition in adult life (age > 20 years), whereas 70% of patients diagnosed with allergic rhinitis developed their condition in childhood (age < 20 years).

Gender may be a risk factor for the development of nonallergic rhinitis. In a series of 78 patients studied by Settipane and Klein (33), 58% of the patients with nonallergic rhinitis were female. Enberg (29) found 74% of patients with nonallergic rhinitis to be female. The NRCTF (32) found that 71% of patients with nonallergic rhinitis were female compared with 55% of patients in the allergic rhinitis group. However, a conclusion regarding aging cannot be determined because all three of these studies lacked a control group for comparison.

Sibbald and Rink (34) suggested that patients with nonallergic rhinitis were more likely to experience perennial rather than seasonal symptoms. They reported the following frequencies of negative skin testing: 50% in patients with perennial rhinitis, 32% in patients with combined perennial/seasonal rhinitis, and 22% in patients with purely seasonal allergic rhinitis.

Nonallergic rhinitis may be subclassified based on various characteristics, that include immunologic/cytological features (Table 4) (35), etiology/systemic disease association (Table 5), and frequency of occurrence (Table 6) (36). Clearly,

TABLE 4 Classification of Nonallergic Rhinitis Based on Immunologic and Nasal Cytologic Features

---

Perennial nonallergic rhinitis (inflammatory)
  Eosinophilic nasal disease (NARES and BENARES)
  Basophilic/metachromatic nasal disease
  Infectious
  Nasal polyps
  Atopic rhinitis
  Immunologic nasal disease (non-IgE-mediated or secondary to system
    immunologic disorders)
Noninflammatory, nonallergic rhinitis
  Metabolic
  Rhinitis medicamentosa
  Reflex-induced rhinitis (bright light and other physical modalities)
  Vasomotor rhinitis
  Rhinitis sicca
  Irritant rhinitis
  Cold air rhinitis
Structurally related rhinitis
  Septal deviation
  Neoplastic and non-neoplastic tumors
  Miscellaneous (choanal atresia/stenosis, trauma, foreign body, malformation,
    cleft palate, and adenoid hypertrophy)

Abbreviation: NARES, nonallergic rhinitis with eosinophils syndrome.
Source: From Ref. 35.

VMR is the most common form of nonallergic rhinitis. Settipane and Klein (33) characterized the frequency of occurrence of various nonallergic rhinitis subtypes in 28 patients: VMR was found in 61%, nonallergic rhinitis with eosinophils syndrome (NARES) in 33%, blood eosinophilia nonallergic rhinitis syndrome (BENARES) in 4%, sinusitis in 16%, elevated IgE in 12%, and hypothyroidism in 2% of patients (Table 7). In another series of nonallergic rhinitis patients, Enberg (29) reported that 10% had NARES.

The term "VMR," also referred to as perennial nonallergic rhinitis or chronic noninfectious nonallergic rhinitis, is a designation for a subset of patients with non-allergic rhinitis in whom all other etiologies have been ruled out and there is no cytological evidence of nasal mucosal inflammation (4). It is therefore a diagnosis of exclusion, which is thought to represent a collection of heterogeneous disorders. VMR is the most common subtype of perennial nonallergic rhinitis, representing almost two-third of all cases of nonallergic rhinitis (33). Symptoms of VMR are variable, but are generally indistinguishable from the nasal symptoms of other forms of rhinitis. In a survey of 678 rhinitis patients, nasal blockage was the predominant symptom in the VMR group, whereas the allergic rhinitis patients were more likely to suffer from eye irritation, sneezing, and rhinorrhea (37). Concomitant asthma was more common in the allergic rhinitis group. Subjects with VMR can be divided into two general groups by symptom predominance: "runners" who have rhinorrhea, and "dry" subjects who manifest with predominant blockage to airflow.

The symptoms of VMR are characteristically triggered by "classic" nonaller-gic provocateurs, which include weather and temperature changes as well as respiratory irritants (Table 8). However, there is a considerable amount of controversy regarding which of these triggers or constellation of triggers best

TABLE 5 Classification of Chronic Nonallergic Rhinitis Based on Etiology or Systemic Disease Association

---

Syndromes of unknown etiology
  Basophilic/metachromatic nasal disease
  Nonallergic rhinitis with eosinophils (NARES or BENARES)
  Vasomotor rhinitis
Syndromes of suggested etiology
  Atrophic rhinitis
    Ozena
    Surgical complication
  Chronic sinusitis
    Immunodeficiencies
    Ostiomeatal obstruction
  Drug induced
    Systemic medications
    Topical decongestants
  Metabolic conditions
    Acromegaly
    Estrogen related (oral contraceptive/hormone replacement therapy)
    Hypothyroidism
  Nasal polyps
    Allergic fungal sinusitis
    Aspirin exacerbated respiratory disease
    Chronic sinusitis
    Churg–Strauss syndrome
    Cystic fibrosis
    Kartagener's syndrome (bronchiectasis, chronic sinusitis, and nasal polyps)
    Young's syndrome (sinopulmonary disease, azoospermia, and nasal polyps)
  Neurogenic (3)
    Absent sympathomimetic function
    Bright light–induced hyperactive cholinergic parasympathetic function
    Chronic fatigue syndrome associated
    Food/nocifer-activated cholinergic reflex
    Nociceptive/irritant
    Vidian-neurectomy–induced
  Occupational rhinitis
    Annoyance
    Corrosive
    Immunologic
    Irritant
  Structurally related rhinitis
    Nasal valve dysfunction
    Neoplastic
    Obstructive adenoid hyperplasia
    Septal deviation
    Turbinate deformation
    Trauma (e.g., cerebrospinal fluid rhinorrhea) congenital
  Vasculitides/autoimmune and granulomatous diseases
    Churg–Strauss syndrome
    Relapsing polychondritis
    Sarcoidosis
    Sjogren's syndrome
    Systemic lupus erythematosus
    Wegener's granulomatosis

Abbreviations: NARES, nonallergic rhinitis with eosinophils syndrome; BENARES, blood eosinophilia nonallergic rhinitis syndrome.

TABLE 6 Classification of Nonallergic Rhinitis Based on Frequency of Occurrence

Common	Infrequent
Vasomotor	Aspirin sensitivity
Chronic sinusitis	Hypothyroidism
Structural (septum, turbinates, and valve)	Atrophic
NARES/BENARES	Systemic immunologic disorders
Drug induced	Cerebrospinal-fluid rhinorrhea
Estrogen related	Other structural disorders
Nasal polyps	Foreign body
Physical/chemical/irritant	Ciliary dyskinesia
Nasal mastocytosis	

Abbreviations: NARES, nonallergic rhinitis with eosinophils syndrome; BENARES, blood eosinophilia nonallergic rhinitis syndrome.

define VMR. Historically, certain provocateurs have been recognized as "classic triggers" of VMR. These include respiratory irritants (perfume, soaps, detergent odors, paint fumes, hair spray, cigarette smoke, motor vehicle exhaust, and other strong odors or fumes), temperature and humidity changes (changes in weather conditions, cold drafts, etc.), and consumption of alcoholic beverages. However, could strong odors simply represent an irritant rhinitis or nasal hyperactivity? Does alcohol-induced rhinitis simply represent a vascular response? Although the Food and Drug Administration (FDA) has recently asserted that weather (temperature/relative humidity) triggers best define VMR, this proposal remains without the support of an established consensus of expert opinions. Contributing to this area of controversy is the fact that little is known about the mechanism(s) of response to these various triggers except that nonspecific nasal hyperreactivity occurs on exposure to nonimmunologic stimuli, such as changes in temperature or relative humidity (cold, dry air), strong odors, tobacco smoke, and other airborne irritants. The hyperreactivity of the nasal mucosa to hypertonic saline, methacholine, and histamine has been demonstrated in the laboratory (38–42). If VMR is truly a heterogeneous disorder, perhaps consideration should be given to subclassifying this diagnosis depending on predominant trigger type.

TABLE 7 Diagnosis of 78 Patients with Nonallergic Rhinitis

Diagnosis	Patients (*N*)	Patients considered (*N*)	Percentage of patients
Vasomotor rhinitis	44	72	61
NARES	25	75	33
Sinusitis (radiographs)[a]	11	68	16
Possible allergy[b]	9	76	12
BENARES	3	76	4
Hypothyroidism	1	68	2

[a]Overlapping of diagnosis present.
[b]Elevated serum IgE levels.
Abbreviations: BENARES, blood eosinophilia nonallergic rhinitis syndrome; NARES, nonallergic rhinitis with eosinophils syndrome; IgE, immunoglobin E.
Source: From Ref. 33.

TABLE 8   "Classic Provocateurs" of Vasomotor Rhinitis

Respiratory irritants
  Perfume
  Soaps
  Detergent odors
  Cigarette smoke
  Paint fumes
  Hair spray
  Motor vehicle exhaust
  Other strong odors or fumes
Temperature and humidity (weather) conditions
  Drafts
  Cold air
  Temperature change
  Damp weather
  Changes in weather
Alcoholic beverages

SUMMARY

In summary, the epidemiological data and characterization of allergic and nonallergic rhinitis has been reviewed. Chronic rhinitis symptoms are among the most common problems presenting to physicians. When approaching this problem the diagnostic challenge is to determine the etiology, specifically whether it is allergic, nonallergic, or perhaps an overlap of both conditions. Estimates of the prevalence of allergic rhinitis range from as low as 9% to as high as 42%. Although the prevalence of nonallergic rhinitis has not been studied definitively, it appears to be very common with an estimated prevalence in the United States of approximately 19 million. In comparison, the prevalence of mixed rhinitis is approximately 26 million, and allergic rhinitis ("pure" and "mixed" combined) 58 million. Challenges in the differential diagnosis of rhinitis result from two major factors. Not only are presenting symptoms of allergic, nonallergic, and mixed rhinitis often indistinguishable from one another, but also the differential diagnosis of nonallergic rhinitis is extensive. Nonallergic rhinitis is often characterized by onset after age 20, female predominance, nasal hyperactivity, perennial symptoms, and nasal eosinophilia in approximately one-third of the population. Positive tests for relevant specific IgE sensitivity in the setting of rhinitis do not rule out "mixed rhinitis" and may not rule out nonallergic rhinitis. The significance of symptom exacerbation by nonallergic triggers in the setting of allergic rhinitis remains to be determined.

Goals for the future include reaching a consensus on the definitions of rhinitis and rhinitis subtypes including the establishment of mixed rhinitis, updating guidelines for the interpretation of nonrelevant positive tests for specific IgE sensitivity, and reaching agreement on the nonallergic triggers that best define VMR or VMR subtypes. Only then can the most applicable research results be obtained. The desired result is the delivery of the most appropriate treatment, specifically tailored to the accurate diagnosis of patients with rhinitis.

REFERENCES

1. Turkeltaub PC, Gergen PJ. The prevalence of allergic and nonallergic respiratory symptoms in the U.S. population: data from the second national health and nutrition

examination survey 1976–1980 (NHANES II) [abstr]. J Allergy Clin Immunol 1988; 81:305.

2. Dykewicz MS, Fineman S, eds. Diagnosis and management of rhinitis: complete guidelines of the joint task force on practice parameters in allergy, asthma, and immunology. Ann Allergy Asthma Immunol 1998; 81:478–518.

3. Staevska M, Baraniuk JN. Persistent nonallergic rhinosinusitis. Curr Allergy Asthma Rep 2005; 5:233–242.

4. Settipane RA, Lieberman P. Update on nonallergic rhinitis. Ann Allergy Asthma Immunol 2001; 86:494–508.

5. Bousquet J, Van Cauwenberge P, Khaltaev N, Aria Workshop Group, World Health Organization. Allergic rhinitis and its impact on asthma. J Allergy Clin Immunol 2001; 108:S147–S334.

6. Freeman GL, Johnson S. Allergic diseases in adolescents. Am J Dis Child 1964; 107:549–559.

7. Broder I, Higgins MW, Mathews KP, Keller JB. Epidemiology of asthma and allergic rhinitis in a total community, Tecumseh, Michigan. J Allergy Clin Immunol 1974; 53:127–138.

8. McMenamin P. Costs of hay fever in the United States in 1990. Ann Allergy 1994; 73:35–39.

9. Nathan RA, Meltzer EO, Selner JC, Storms W. Prevalence of allergic rhinitis in the United States. J Allergy Clin Immunol 1997; 99:S808–S814.

10. Wright AL, Holberg CJ, Martinez FD, et al. Epidemiology of physician-diagnosed allergic rhinitis in childhood. Pediatrics 1994; 94:895–901.

11. Gergen PJ, Turkeltaub PC. The association of individual allergen reactivity with respiratory disease in a national sample: data from the second National Health and Nutrition Examination Survey, 1976–1980 (NHANES II). J Allergy Clin Immunol 1992; 90:579–588.

12. Hagy GW, Settipane GA. Bronchia asthma, allergic rhinitis, and allergy skin tests among college students. J Allergy 1969; 44:323–332.

13. Greisner WA, Settipane RJ, Settipane G. Natural history of hay fever: a 23-year follow-up of college students. Asthma Allergy Proc 1998; 19:271–275.

14. Penard-Morand C, Raherison C, Kopferschmitt C, et al. Prevalence of food allergy and its relationship to asthma and allergic rhinitis in schoolchildren. Allergy 2005; 60:1165–1171.

15. Banac S, Tomulic KL, Ahel V, et al. Prevalence of asthma and allergic diseases in Croatian children is increasing: survey study. Croat Med J 2004; 45:721–726.

16. Hannaford PC, Simpson JA, Bisset AF, Davis A, McKerrow W, Mills R. The prevalence of ear, nose and throat problems in the community: results from a national cross-sectional postal survey in Scotland. Fam Pract 2005; 22:227–233.

17. Bornehag CG, Sundell J, Hagerhed-Engman L, et al. 'Dampness' at home and its association with airway, nose, and skin symptoms among 10,851 preschool children in Sweden: a cross-sectional study. Indoor Air 2005; 15(suppl 10):48–55.

18. Heinrich J, Wichmann HE. Traffic-related pollutants in Europe and their effect on allergic disease. Curr Opin Allergy Clin Immunol 2004; 4(5):341–348.

19. Almvist C, Pershagen G, Wickman M. Low Socioeconomic status as a risk factor for asthma, rhinitis and sensitization at 4 years in a birth cohort. Clin Exp Allergy 2005; 35:612–618.

20. Butland BK, Strachan DP, Lewis S, Bynner J, Butler N, Britton J. Investigation into the increase in hay fever and eczema at age 16 observed between the 1958 and 1970 British birth cohorts. Br Med J 1997; 315:717–721.

21. Verlato G, Corsico A, Villani S, et al. Is the prevalence of adult asthma and allergic rhinitis still increasing? Results of an Italian study. J Allergy Clin Immunol 2003; 111:1232–1238.

22. Selnes A, Nystad W, Bolle R, Lund E. Diverging prevalence trends of atopic disorders in Norwegian children. Results from three cross-sectional studies. Allergy 2005; 60:894–899.

23. Latvala J, von Hertzen L, Lindholm H, Haahtela T. Trends in prevalence of asthma and allergy in Finnish young men: nationwide study, 1966–2003. BMJ 2005; 330(7501): 1186–1187.
24. Braun-Fahrländer C, Gassner M, Grize L, et al. No further increase in asthma, hay fever and atopic sensitisation in adolescence living in Switzerland. Eur Respir J 2004; 23:407–413.
25. Sly RM. Changing prevalence of allergic rhinitis and asthma. Ann Allergy Asthma Immunol 1999; 82:233–248.
26. Linneberg A, Nielsen NH, Madsen F, Frolund L, Dirksen A, Jorgensen T. Increasing prevalence of specific IgE to aeroallergens in an adult population: two cross-sectional surveys 8 years apart: the Copenhagen Allergy Study. J Allergy Clin Immunol 2000; 106:247–252.
27. Arbes SJ, Gergen PJ, Elliott L, Zeldin DC. Prevalences of positive skin test responses to 10 common allergens in the US population: results from the third National Health and Nutrition Examination Survey. J Allergy Clin Immunol 2005; 116:377–383.
28. Mullarkey MF, Hill JS, Webb DR. Allergic and nonallergic rhinitis: their characterization with attention to the meaning of nasal eosinophilia. J Allergy Clin Immunol 1980; 65:122–126.
29. Enberg RN. Perennial nonallergic rhinitis: a retrospective review. Ann Allergy Asthma Immunol 1989; 63:513–516.
30. Leynaert B, Bousquet J, Neukirch C, et al. Perennial rhinitis: an independent risk factor for asthma in nonatopic subjects. Results from the European Community Respiratory Health Survey. J Allergy Clin Immunol 1999; 104:301–304.
31. Togias A. Age relationships and clinical features of nonallergic rhinitis. J Allergy Clin Immunol 1990; 85:182.
32. Dykewicz MS, Ledford DK, Settipane RA, Lieberman P. The broad spectrum of rhinitis: etiology, diagnosis, and advances in treatment. Data Presented at the National Allergy Advisory Council Meeting (NAAC), St. Thomas, U.S. Virgin Islands, October 16, 1999.
33. Settipane GA, Klein DE. Nonallergic rhinitis: demography of eosinophils in nasal smear, blood total eosinophil counts and IgE levels. N Engl Reg Allergy Proc 1985; 6:363–366.
34. Sibbald B, Rink E. Epidemiology of seasonal and perennial rhinitis: clinical presentation and medical history. Thorax 1991; 46:895–901.
35. Zeiger RS. Differential diagnosis and classification of rhinosinusitis. In: Schatz M, Zeiger RS, Settipane GA, eds. Nasal Manifestations of Systemic Diseases. Providence, RI: OceanSide Publications, Inc., 1991:3–20.
36. Settipane RA, Settipane GA. Nonallergic rhinitis. In: Kaliner MA, ed. Current Review of Allergic Diseases. Philadelphia, PA: Current Medicine, Inc., 2000:111–123.
37. Lindberg S, Malm L. Comparison of allergic rhinitis and vasomotor rhinitis patients on the basis of a computer questionnaire. Allergy 1993; 48:602–607.
38. Borum P. Nasal methacholine challenge. J Allergy Clin Immunol 1979; 63:253–257.
39. Stjärne P, Lundblad L, Änggard A, et al. Local capsaicin treatment of the nasal mucosa reduces symptoms in patients with nonallergic nasal hyperreactivity. Am J Rhinol 1991; 5:145–151.
40. Togias A, Proud D, Kagey-Sobotka A, et al. Cold dry air (CDA) and histamine (HIST) induce more potent responses in perennial rhinitis compared to normal individuals. J Allergy Clin Immunol 1991; 87:148.
41. Baraniuk JN, Petrie KN, Le U, et al. Neuropathology in rhinosinusitis. Am J Respir Crit Care Med 2005; 171:5–11.
42. Gerth van Wijk R. Nasal hyperreactivity: its pathogenis and clinical significance. Clin Exp Allergy 1991; 21:661.

3

Differential Diagnosis of Persistent Nonallergic Rhinitis and Rhinosinusitis Syndromes

Maria T. Staevska

Allergology and Clinical Immunology, Clinic of Asthma, Medical University of Sofia, University Hospital "Alexandrovska," Sofia, Bulgaria

James N. Baraniuk

Department of Medicine, Division of Rheumatology, Immunology and Allergy, and Georgetown University Proteomics Laboratory, Georgetown University Medical Center, Washington, D.C., U.S.A.

INTRODUCTION

Nonallergic rhinitis (NAR) occurs in 17 million Americans, according to The National Rhinitis Classification Task Force (1). NAR is a diverse syndrome that encompasses a complex and broad variety of disorders (2,3). Approximately half of rhinitis patients in otolaryngology clinics may have allergic rhinitis (AR), and the other half NAR. This discrimination is based on the presence of nasal symptoms with or without positive allergy skin tests (AST), radioimmunallergosorbant test variants of this test, or allergen nasal provocations (4,5). About half of AR patients also complain of nonallergic symptoms that are induced by irritants ("irritant rhinitis") (6). This overlap demonstrates the difficulties of describing syndromes based solely on their clinical or symptomatic characteristics without regard to underlying pathophysiological mechanisms. Our purpose is to outline the many conditions that fall under the rubric of "persistent rhinitis without atopy." We will use the all-encompassing term of NAR, even though some of the conditions may extend into the sinuses ["rhinosinusitis" (7,8)], or be systemic diseases with nasal manifestations. A critical reason for the attention to mechanisms is that targeted treatments can be designed to act against specific mechanisms, but can be very difficult to develop when dealing with a symptom complex.

The general approach used here has been to classify NAR conditions according to the most probable mechanisms. Rhinitis syndromes will be split into inflammatory and noninflammatory groups. The inflammatory group will be further divided according to the predominant or characteristic leukocytic infiltrate: eosinophilic, neutrophilic, or mixed inflammatory cell types. The noninflammatory rhinitides can be divided into anatomical abnormalities, hormonal and medication induced, neural dysfunction, and idiopathic. Our goal has been to identify common mechanisms of disease, and to group clinical syndromes based on these similarities.

EOSINOPHILIC INFLAMMATORY RHINITIS

The eosinophilic group of diseases is united by the release of eosinophil chemoattractants that promote the influx and potential mucosal maturations of these cells (Table 1). The amount of eosinophilia can change with disease activity. This and the differences in eosinophil involvement leads to a fourfold difference in eosinophil

TABLE 1 Differential Diagnosis of Inflammatory Rhinosinusitis Based upon Potential Pathogenic Mechanisms and the Predominant Infiltrating Cellular Components (Eosinophil-Dominant Rhinitis Syndromes)

Eosinophil-predominant syndromes with IgE involvement	Nonatopic eosinophilic rhinitis syndrome
Allergic rhinitis	NARES
Intermittent	BENARS
Perennial	CESS
Food allergy with rhinitis	Nasal polyps with eosinophilia
Allergic fungal sinusitis	Aspirin/NSAID sensitivity
Occupational rhinitis with eosinophilia	Triad asthma
IgE mediated	Asthma
Cigarette smoke–induced atopy-like rhinitis	Chronic rhinosinusitis with nasal polyps
Superantigen rhinitis with eosinophilia	NSAID sensitivity
Localized nasal mucosal allergic responses	Fungal sinusitis syndromes
	Mycetoma
Asymptomatic atopy	Chronic allergic fungal sinusitis
	Chronic allergic fungal sinusitis–like disorder
	Invasive fungal sinusitis
	Occupational rhinitis with eosinophilia Non-IgE–mediated
	Churg–Strauss syndrome with eosinophilic granuloma
	Eosinophilic granuloma

Abbreviations: NARES, nonallergic rhinitis with eosinophilia syndrome; BENARS, blood eosinophilia with nonallergic rhinitis with eosinophilia syndrome; CESS, chronic eosinophilic sinusitis syndromes; NSAID, nonsteroidal anti-inflammatory drug.

cationic protein levels between AR and control subjects (32.6 ± 8.1 ng/mL; mean $\pm$ SEM), and an elevated level with very wide range in NAR subjects (67.0 ± 22.4 ng/mL) (9). These NAR subjects likely represented several distinct syndromes. The inflammatory patterns of T and other cells and their cytokines, and so the mechanisms of disease, differ between AR and NAR (10). These patterns also differ between non allergic rhinitis with eosinophilia syndrome (NARES), nasal polyposis, and aspirin sensitivity. Each topic has a dedicated chapter in this book.

NEUTROPHILIC INFLAMMATORY RHINITIS

In general, neutrophilia is an acute response to injury such as a toxic exposure or bacterial infection (Table 2). Chronic neutrophilia implies chronic infection as in cystic fibrosis. The most potential neutrophil chemoattractants are interleukin (IL)-8 from epithelium, neutrophils, and other cells; lipopolysaccharide (LPS) and related complex lipid–peptide–carbohydrate chemicals; and C3b released when immune complexes form and complement is activated. LPS indicates the importance of tolloid-receptors (toll-receptor 4 for LPS) in mucosal defense against infection. Neutrophilic rhinitis will be discussed in several of our chapters.

Occupational exposures can lead to nasal irritation, including inflammation leading to a "nasal reactive airway disease (NRADS)." Fuel oil ash and vanadium exposures lead to neutrophilic inflammation in nonsmokers (11). This was not apparent in smokers because they demonstrated cigarette smoke-related mucosal

TABLE 2 Inflammatory Rhinitis Syndromes with Neutrophilic and Complex Cellular Infiltration

Neutrophil-predominant	Complex infiltrates
Infectious rhinitis	Common cold syndromes
Acute bacterial sinusitis	Granulomatous and vasculitic diseases
Acute infectious exacerbations of	Wegener's granulomatosis
chronic sinusitis	Malignant midline granuloma
Nasal polyps in cystic fibrosis	Sarcoidosis
HIV/AIDS-related infectious rhinosinusitis	Granulomatous infections
	Tuberculosis
Humoral immunodeficiency	Leprosy
IgA, IgE, IgG subclass, and other	Syphilis
deficiencies	Autoimmune disorders
Common variable hypogammaglo bulinemia	Relapsing polychondritis
	Systemic lupus erythematosis
Young's syndrome of sinopulmonary disease,	Sjogren's syndrome
azoospermia, and nasal polyps	Atrophic rhinitis
Kartagener's syndrome of bronchiectasis, chronic	Postoperative
sinusitis, nasal polyps, and immotile cilia	Senile rhinitis
	Ozena
Foreign body with infection	Basophilic/metachromatic rhinitis
Corrosive occupational rhinitis	Chronic rhinosinusitis without nasal polyps
Superantigen rhinitis with neutrophilia	(glandular hypertrophy)
	Occupational toxic exposure leading to
	transient neutrophilia with persistent
	epithelial metaplasia

Abbreviation: Ig, Immunoglobin.

inflammatory changes. Nonallergic nasal symptoms were found in 33% and 75% of COPD subjects (12,13). About half had significant nasal discharge and sneezing. These symptoms plus the sensations of a blocked nose and itching were more common in city dwellers living close to heavy traffic. Gaseous ammonia and organic dust can lead to atrophic rhinitis (14). In pigs, these exposures are exacerbated by infection with *Pseudomonas multocida* type D. The combination of airborne toxin exposures plus nasal colonization with "exotic" microbes has received little attention in humans, with the exception of *Staphylococcus aureus* (see below).

INFLAMMATORY RHINITIS SYNDROMES WITH OTHER LEUKOCYTIC PATTERNS

T helper (CD4) cells, mast cells, professional antigen presenting cells, epithelium, and other cells may play distinct roles in each of these inflammatory types, and in conditions with mixed or progressively evolving inflammatory cell patterns (Table 2). These involve the granulomatous diseases, vasculitis, and other autoimmune conditions. As more is learned about the underlying sets of triggering mechanisms, T-cell subsets, combinations of cytokines and effector cells present in these disorders, more clearly defined criteria will be developed for diagnosing these syndromes. Allergen-specific CD4+ TH2-lymphocytes in atopy are the sole example of this relationship at this time. The task of determining the role of T-cells may become more complicated as new mechanisms of their immune reactivity become more fully defined and are applied to nasal pathology. The vasculitic and autoimmune syndromes are examples where identification of the precise activities of T-cells may lead to advances in therapy for their nasal manifestations or identification of analogous mucosal conditions.

NONALLERGIC NONINFECTIOUS PERENNIAL RHINITIS

Rhinitis symptoms in the absence of inflammatory cells and with negative allergy tests have been the traditional basis for the diagnosis of NAR. The collection of disorders that meets these criteria has been named on several occasions. Nonallergic noninfectious perennial rhinitis (NANIPER) is one designation that is based on the exclusion of allergic and infectious causes (15).

INFLAMMATORY CONDITIONS INCLUDED IN NANIPER

NANIPER is a syndrome that includes the inflammatory conditions of NARES, occupational irritant, and smoking-induced rhinitis (15).

Passive inhalation of second hand cigarette smoke can lead to an eosinophilic inflammation with TH2 cytokines, elevated IL-4, and increased mucosal immunoglobulin E (IgE)-positive cells in the mucosa (16–18). Nasal symptoms have also been associated with chronic bronchitis and emphysema (12). We recommend these conditions be considered for exclusion from the designation of NANIPER in future classifications.

ATOPY LIMITED TO THE NASAL MUCOSA

Nasal mucosal antigen deposition may stimulate a TH2–IgE–mast cell–eosinophilic reaction that is limited to this organ (19–22). The IgE cannot be detected in blood or by skin testing. This is consistent with local differentiation of B lymphocytes with heavy chain switching from IgM to IgE secretion and the presence of excised IgE circles of DNA that contain the genomic sequences for between the rearranged variable region and the ε heavy chain region (23). The IgE is allergen specific (24). This syndrome can be identified by the presence of allergic symptoms with exposure to allergen; mast cell histaminergic effects of itch and watery, plasmarich rhinorrhea; improvement with antihistamines; intranasal allergen provocation testing; and histological evidence of increased mast cells and eosinophils in the mucosa (25). Intranasal glucocorticoids are likely to be highly effective in controlling this syndrome, and may account for the success of these drugs in studies of undifferentiated "NAR" (i.e., rhinitis with negative skin tests as the only entry criteria).

SUPERANTIGENS

Colonization of the nasal and potentially the sinus mucosa by *Staphylococcus aureus* leads to the local release of staphylococcal enterotoxin superantigens (26,27). Other microbes may secrete similar co-stimulatory virulence macromolecules that co-opt normal host immune responses for the benefit of the microbe. About 25% of the population carry *Staphylococcus aureus* in their nasal vestibule normal flora. These enterotoxins are a family of structurally related, heat-stable, ~27 kD proteins. Five major serological types (A–E) have been complemented by three newly characterized types (G–I) (28). They act as superantigens to stimulate T-cells by cross-linking a region of the variable sequence of T-cell receptor beta chain to Major Histocompatibition Antigen (MHC) class II molecules on accessory or antigen presenting cells (29,30). This cross-linking occurs outside the peptide-binding groove area and does not require an immunogenic peptide to be present. Up to 20% to 25% of naive T-cells (CD45Ra) are activated by this nonspecific mechanism. This contrasts with the activations of only ~0.1% of T-cells by conventional allergen-specific MHC-restricted antigen presentation (31). Closely related toxic shock syndrome toxin-1 upregulated CD40 expression and modulated IgE isotype switching (32–34). Bacterial superantigens may promote antigen presentation by eosinophils (35) and mast cell activation by an interaction with cell bound IgE (36). These actions suggest the microbe has manipulated the host immune response to generate accentuated TH2-atopic responses. This mechanism is inappropriate for elimination of *S. aureus*.

The microbe-induced shift toward a TH2-like immune response also leads to the formation of IgE to Staph superantigens. IgE to fungal antigens has also been identified in nasal lavage and sinus aspirates from chronic rhinosinusitis. Chronic secretion of these proinflammatory bacterial antigens will have the twofold benefit of continuously driving the host immune response to one that is unable to eliminate the microbe, and also providing a steady stream of allergen for processing, binding, and presentation to T-cells with continued stimulation of B-cell production of IgE against the microbe.

This TH2 mechanism is complicated by the concomitant activation of other components of the immune response. Superantigens also activate macrophages to release the neutrophil chemoattractant IL-8 (37), and IL-12 to stimulate antigen-specific TH1 delayed-type hypersensitivity reactions (38). In this fashion, the microbial invader can simultaneously activate multiple limbs of the immune system. TH1 and TH2 mechanisms are generally mutually exclusive because of the cross-inhibition by IL-10 and IL-14/IL-13. However, combined activation of these and other immune mechanisms may lead to the confusing agglomeration of cells and cytokines found in various confusing chronic rhinitis and rhinosinusitis syndromes. It will be necessary to more tediously identify these mechanisms within subsets of these syndromes to classify each more critically and develop optimized treatments aimed at the mechanism(s) active in individual patients. A shotgun approach, such as the use of intranasal steroids (39) or surgery (40) for all forms of inflammatory rhinitis and rhinosinusitis, is doomed to fail under this scenario.

These studies should breed caution into overinterpretation of in vitro superantigen studies. General activation of many conflicting immune mechanisms is a general avoidance and virulence strategy of *S. aureus* and other organisms. Systemic activation of multiple limbs of the immune system would lead to the diverse symptoms of toxic shock and scalded skin syndromes. This would leave the host with fewer immune resources to focus on the development of *S. aureus*-specific antibody formation for complement activation and opsonization, neutrophil chemoattraction localized to the site of infection, and localized bacterial killing. Appropriation of nasal and sinus mucosal immune responses with IgE production to the superantigens and other allergens in these infections would prevent local IgG and IgA subclass production that may eradicate the organism from its mucosal ecological niche. The genes for heavy chains for these subclasses would be eliminated by B-cell heavy chain switching to IgE production. Predisposing conditions such as Ig deficiencies would be anticipated to weaken initial host responses and lead to an increased incidence of chronic infection. This is consistent with the high rate of immune defects found in analyses of chronic rhinosinusitis patients (41–43). We speculate that similar effects occur in excessive allergic responses to fungal antigens in allergic bronchopulmonary aspergillosis and allergic fungal sinusitis. Therapies aimed at interrupting superantigen activation of T, B, eosinophil, macrophage, and other cell populations may prevent and potentially reverse these syndromes by permitting the host to develop the optimal immune response for microbial eradication.

ASYMPTOMATIC ATOPY

Regulatory inhibition of active allergic processes may occur as a result of increased indoleamine 2,3-dioxygenase activity and IL-10 production (44,45). This may account for the group of subjects who have positive skin tests indicating allergen sensitization and circulation of IgE to systemic mast cells, but who have minimal complaints during exposure seasons (46). This syndrome of immune regulation may help explain the protected immune status of the gravid uterus and fetus.

ANATOMICAL ABNORMALITIES

For rhinitis patients with mechanical anomalies, "anatomy is destiny" (Table 3). Deviated nasal septums are common. The deviations may force the narrowing of the middle or inferior turbinate on the side of the deviation, and expansion or hypertrophy of the turbinates into the space vacated by the deviation on the contralateral side. In general, rhinitis symptoms are proportional to the degree of list of the septum (47). However, not all anatomical changes cause symptoms. Magnetic resonance imaging and computed tomography scans taken to evaluate neurological or orbital disease ($n \sim 3000$) revealed high rates of mucosal thickening greater than 4 mm (10–15%), asymptomatic air-fluid levels (2.8–4.6%), and even opacification of one sinus (2.9–3.8%) (48–51).

Collapse of the nasal tip and fleshy swelling of the alae nasi can obstruct the anterior nasal valve and increase nasal airflow resistance. This may be especially important in the elderly (52). Choanal atresia will certainly obstruct nasal airflow. Tumors can range from inverted papillomas to nasopharyngeal carcinoma and cigarette smoke-related squamous cell carcinomas. A role for adenoidal hypertrophy appears established in children, but this finding in adults, and its contribution to sensations of postnasal drip and obstructions, remain largely unexplored. Fracture of the cribriform plate can lead to the leak of clear, glucose-rich cerebrospinal fluid that may mimic NAR.

TURBINATE HYPERTROPHY

Turbinate hypertrophy is a frequent cause of nasal obstruction leading to turbinectomy or other surgical procedures. However, very little is known about the pathophysiology of this condition (53). Hypertrophic turbinate tissue is often used as a "normal" control for studies of nasal polyps. This is inappropriate because turbinate histology depends on the patient pathology (54). Septal deviation with compensatory hypertrophy of the inferior turbinate showed normal glands with some fibrotic areas around vessels when compared to normal tissues. Perennial AR tissue had glandular hypertrophy and interstitial edema. The most striking changes were found in "vasomotor rhinitis" (VMR) where there was a decrease in the size of glands and fibrosis of the lamina propria. This study requires prospective confirmation using patients who have been carefully evaluated preoperatively.

TABLE 3 Differential Diagnosis of Noninflammatory Rhinosinusitis with Structural Abnormalities or Hormonal Pathogenic Mechanisms

Structural anomalies	Hormonal and drug related
Deviated septum	Pregnancy (estrogen and progesterone)
Turbinate hypertrophy (mechanism undefined)	Hypothyroidism
	Acromegaly
OMC anatomical variants	Adrenergic dysfunction
Concha bullosa	Antihypertensive agents
Haller's cells	β-Adrenergic antagonists
Paradoxical curvature of the middle	α-Adrenergic antagonists (reserpine,
turbinate	α-methyldopa, guanethidine, phentolamine,
Glandular hypertrophy	and prazozin)
Early nasal polyposis	*Rhinitis medicamentosa*
Choanal atresia	Chronic topical α-adrenergic agonist
Tumors	abuse
Benign	Cocaine abuse
Neoplastic	Chlorpromazine (neuroleptic)
Adenoidal hypertrophy with potential recurrent	Side effects of eye drops delivered via
infections	nasolacrimal ducts
Complications of excessive surgical excision of	Ketorolac in NSAID sensitivity
mucosa	Glaucoma medications (β-antagonists)
Fracture of cribriform plate	
Cerebrospinal fluid rhinorrhea	
(high glucose)	
Hypertrophy of fleshy components of the anterior	
nasal valve	
Rhinophyma	
Loss of nasal cartilage with sagging	
of the nasal tip with soft tissue obstruction of	
the anterior nasal valve	
Foreign body	

Abbreviations: NSAID, nonsteroidal anti-inflammatory drug; OMC, Otiomeatal complex.

Without similar evaluations, studies using "hypertrophic turbinates" to represent the "normal" state must be viewed with caution.

CEREBROSPINAL FLUID RHINORRHEA

The presence of clear rhinorrhea in patients with recent sinus surgery or head trauma should lead to suspicion of cerebrospinal fluid leak. This occurs in up to 30% of patients after difficult skull-base tumor operations. Cerebrospinal fluid leak can be identified by glucose testing or dipstick, which will indicate a high glucose level nearing that of plasma. Glucose is not normally present in nasal secretion in the levels that are detectable by dipstick. The carbohydrates in normal nasal mucus are present in the oligosaccharide sidechains of mucins and cannot be detected with this test. Another syndrome of nasal stuffiness, rhinorrhea, and sometimes facial flushing may occur following skull-base neurosurgery (55). The symptoms are characteristically exacerbated by exertion or by elevated ambient room temperatures. Lacrimation is typically absent ipsilateral to the nostril with the discharge. This syndrome is pseudo–cerebrospinal fluid rhinorrhea, and is thought to be due to a surgically induced imbalance of the regulatory autonomic supply to the nasal mucosa.

OTHER INFLAMMATORY RHINITIS SYNDROMES

The exclusion of these inflammatory rhinitides leads to the new acronym of non-inflammatory, nonallergic, noninfectious perennial rhinitis (NINANIPER). However, additional mechanisms are still included in this terminology. Hormonal, endocrine, and drug-related rhinitis is also included in this term (Table 3). These are types of rhinitis that should be identified by history with a confirmatory physical examination. Pregnancy is a case in point (56) that is discussed elsewhere.

DRUG-INDUCED RHINITIS

Rhinitis medicamentosa is the state of long-term addiction to intranasal α2-adrenergic vasoconstrictors such as oxymetazoline, xylometazoline, and ephedrine. The nasal mucosa is congested and hyperemic. Vasoconstrictor use leads to rebound vasodilation with obstruction to nasal airflow, and the need for more drug to relieve these symptoms of congestion. The initial reasons given for starting these sprays were: acute upper respiratory infections (29.3%), VMR (21.7%), AR (16.3%), deviated nasal septum (13.0%), nasal polyposis (12%), rhinitis induced by mechanical trauma (4.4%), and hormonal rhinitis (3.3%) (57). It has been proposed that benzalkonium chloride in commercial preparations of these drugs may be responsible for the mucosal injury (58).

Angiotensinogen-converting enzyme inhibitors are associated with chronic cough, urticaria, and can also cause rhinitis. Other antihypertensives that block autonomic preganglionic nicotinic receptors (reserpine and guanethedine), peripheral or central adrenergic receptors (hydralazine, methyldopa, prazosin, and phenotolamine), and β-adrenergic receptor antagonists have all been associated with nasal obstruction. Presumably, this is due to blockade of the sympathetic innervation to the nasal mucosa. Psychotropic drugs such as chlorpromazine, thioridazine, chlordiazepoxide, amitryptiline, and alprazolam, and the immunosuppressive cyclosporine and mycophenoic acid have also been implicated. These effects may occur with oral, intravenous, or ocular preparations of these drugs (59). Epinephrine may be a special case, because topical administration leads to watery rhinorrhea and frequent sneezing (60). These side effects are different from rhinitis medicamentosa and AR. Surprisingly, tranexamic acid, an inhibitor of plasmin, effectively blocked the side effects. The mechanism of norephinephrine's effects, function of plasminogen activator, and potentially effects of traexamic acid that were unrelated to inhibition of plasmin remain open for investigation. Exclusion of these "endocrine" and toxic-irritative rhinopathies, and structural abnormalities (61) narrows our remaining differential down to nonendocrine "normal anatomy" NINANIPER (NENANINANIPER).

NEURAL MECHANISMS

Even still, we have not exhausted our mechanisms of rhinitis. One of the first proposed mechanisms, neurological dysfunction, remains (62). Several lines of evidence suggest that neural mechanisms may explain a large proportion of the remaining NAR subjects (Table 4) (63). These subjects demonstrate systemic dysfunction of their sympathetic and parasympathetic autonomic nervous systems (64,65). Nasal trauma occurred before the onset of symptoms in 11% of a retrospective investigation of 802 NAR subjects (66). We propose that neurological

TABLE 4 Differential Diagnosis of Noninflammatory Rhinosinusitis Based upon Potential Neural Pathogenic Mechanisms

Neural dysfunction	Other
Absent sympathetic function (absent vasoconstriction) Horner's syndrome Hyperactive cholinergic parasympathetic function (excessive mucus exocytosis) Cholinergic rhinitis Food/nocifer-activated cholinergic reflex–mediated rhinitis Gustatory rhinitis, "salsa sniffles" Cold dry air-induced rhinorrhea, "ski bunny rhinitis" Nociceptive rhinitis/irritant rhinitis with increased nociceptive nerve sensitivity to weather changes, perfume, tobacco smoke, and other inhalants Hyperactivity of normal nasal reflexes Bright-light–induced nasal congestion Vidian neurectomy side effects Loss of parasympathetic and sympathetic innervation NAR of chronic fatigue syndrome, fibromyalgia and allied syndromes displaying hyperalgesia	Perennial nonallergic noninfectious rhinitis (includes NARES, cigarette smoke, elderly, and other forms of rhinitis) Nonendocrine, normal anatomy, noninflammatory, nonallergic, noninfectious perennial rhinitis with neurological dysfunction Nasal hyperresponsiveness to mediators Histamine Methacholine Endothelin Bradykinin Hypertonic saline Capsaicin Other pungent botanical products ("spices") Cold dry air Idiopathic rhinitis (vasomotor rhinitis) (exclusion of all other potential causes of NAR)

Abbreviations: NAR, nonallergic rhinitis; NARES, nonallergic rhinitis with eosinophilia syndromes.

dysfunction is responsible for this difficult to treat subset of NAR subjects. This positive criterion of neurological dysfunction adds a suffix to the acronym NENANINANIPERNED.

This group has traditionally been designated as having VMR (3). This term is unsatisfactory because there is no evidence of either a vascular or motor component (67). Use of "VMR" also gives the false impression of a well-defined pathogenesis, when in fact this term is often used as a "garbage can" catch-all designation (68). Its use and misuse may lead to a suboptimal investigation of underlying mechanisms, random prescription of different treatments at each physician visit, and increasing tension and frustration on the part of the "demanding" patient with multiple complaints, and the "failing doctor" who has scraped the bottom of the therapeutic barrel. This all-too-common situation can lead to inappropriate diagnosis and treatment that may have a decidedly negative impact on the care and prognosis of NAR subjects (69). Referral to a specialist in all Allergy and Rhinology has been shown to increase patient satisfaction, Quality of Life scores, and treatment outcomes (70). This may be especially important in pediatric subjects who may be mistaken for chronic rhinosinusitis or immunodeficiency patients (71).

The difficulties with the "VMR" designation were made apparent by a study from the U.S. Agency for Healthcare Research and Quality (AHRQ) (72). They found no prospective studies in the literature that defined precise criteria to explicitly differentiate allergic from "VMR" and other syndromes of NAR (73). Again, this belies the problem of using the presence or absence of atopy as your sole discriminating criteria between AR and NAR, and the lack of understanding about the differential diagnosis of NAR.

"VMR" has traditionally been divided into "runners" who have "wet" rhinorrhea, and "blockers" who have sensations of nasal obstruction with minimal rhinorrhea. The nasal discharge can be blocked with anticholinergic agents, indicating cholinergic rhinitis (74–77). "Blockers" provide a greater challenge because some complain of obstructed nasal airflow because they do not show reductions in nasal airflow resistance. This suggests a disconnection between the subject's perceptions obtained from their mucosal sensory apparatus, and our perceptions of the mythical "vasomotor" mechanism(s). The filling of nasal venous sinusoids is regulated by sympathetic vasoconstriction of arteriovenous anastomoses and their dilation by mediators that may include calcitonin-gene-related peptide, histamine, and others (78). The ability of α2-adrenergic agonists to constrict these vessels and reduce the volume of blood in the nasal turbinates and erectile regions of the nasal septum has been used to identify differences between normal and "VMR" subjects. Acoustic rhinometry was used to compare the cross-sectional area of the nostrils and volume of the anterior nasal cavity before and after decongestion (79). Normal subjects had a significant increase in the cross-sectional area for airflow (increase nasal cavity volume). However, "VMR" subjects did not have any change, or, in some cases, actually showed paradoxical decreases in nasal cavity volume. Effects of neuropeptide Y, a second sympathetic neurotransmitter and potent vasoconstrictor, have not been examined in this patient group (80).

One persistently appealing feature of "VMR" is the perceived set of exposures and activities that trigger nasal symptoms. These include odors, perfumes, cigarette smoke, paint fumes, inkjet printer ink, alcoholic beverages, spicy foods, emotions, temperature, barometric pressure changes, and bright lights. However, triggered symptoms also occur in AR (50%) and NARES subjects. Triggers included weather changes (31%), odors (15%), and noxious or irritating substances (12%) in NARES (81). However, these triggers have not been tested for their prevalence in normal and atopic populations. Many represent normal protective oronasal, nasonasal, and bronchonasal reflexes. These include the afferent-parasympathetic cholinergic glandular responses to eating spicy foods (gustatory rhinitis) (82) or exposure to cold temperatures (skier's nose, ski bunny rhinitis) (83). Cold dry air provocations can imitate exposure to cold temperatures and may be able to differentiate hyperresponsive nonallergic from poorly responsive AR subjects (84). However, it is very common to have rhinorrhea when eating spicy foods or hyperventilating in cold dry air (e.g., high altitude skiing). The threshold between hyperreseponsiveness/NAR and a normal response can be difficult to identify.

To evaluate responses to the most commonly cited triggers of NAR/"VMR," we developed an irritant rhinitis score (IRS) questionnaire (6). Subjects scored the severity of their perceived sensations of nasal *Congestion* and *Rhinorrhea* (drip) for the previous six months using 5 point anchored Likert scales graded for no symptom (score = 0), trivial (1), mild (2), moderate (3), and severe (4). The optimal triggers were: (i) weather or humidity changes, (ii) cold air, (iii) air conditioning (A/C), (iv) perfume, (v) strong odors, smells or fumes, (vi) tobacco smoke, (vii) alcoholic beverages, and (viii) stress and emotions (Table 5). Maximum scores were 32 each for *Congestion* and *Rhinorrhea*, and 64 for the IRS. The upper limits of normal, or threshold for abnormally elevated IRS scores, were defined based on the scores from 84 subjects who had no past history of rhinitis or sinusitis. Their upper 95th percentile scores were 11 for *Congestion*, 10 for *Rhinorrhea*, and 16 for *IRS*.

TABLE 5 Scoring for Irritant Rhinitis Score

Severity:	Congestion					Rhinorrhea ("drip")				
	None	Trivial	Mild	Moderate	Severe	None	Trivial	Mild	Moderate	Severe
1. Weather or humidity changes	0	1	2	3	4	0	1	2	3	4
2. Cold air	0	1	2	3	4	0	1	2	3	4
3. Air conditioning	0	1	2	3	4	0	1	2	3	4
4. Perfume	0	1	2	3	4	0	1	2	3	4
5. Strong odors, smells or fumes	0	1	2	3	4	0	1	2	3	4
6. Tobacco smoke	0	1	2	3	4	0	1	2	3	4
7. Alcoholic beverages	0	1	2	3	4	0	1	2	3	4
8. Stress and emotions	0	1	2	3	4	0	1	2	3	4
	Congestion score					Rhinorrhea score				

Sum of Congestion + Rhinorrhea Scores = Irritant Rhinitis Score

Note: The severity and score values are, None, 0; Trivial, 1; Mild, 2; Moderate, 3; Severe, 4.
Abbreviations: IRS, irritant rhinitis score; A/C, air conditioning.

Scores were considered elevated at and above these limits. This retrospective scoring scale may be limited by the recall bias of the subjects.

Data are shown for 168 subjects. Their rhinitis status was defined based on skin tests and symptom severity (6,46,85). First, AST status was defined as positive (≥ 2 positive tests out of 16 geographically relevant aeroallergens) or negative. Second, they scored their recalled level of nasal complaints for the previous six months using the same anchored, 5 point Likert scale (0–4 as above). The 10 symptoms were: (i) itchy nose, (ii) sneezing, (iii) drip, runny nose, (iv) fullness, congestion, (v) generalized headache, (vi) pain in face, (vii) blowing out thick mucus, (viii) postnasal drip in the back of the throat, (ix) throat clearing, and (x) hoarse voice. The sum of the severity scores was the rhinitis score (RhSc) (Table 6). The maximum score was 40. A positive score had been previously defined as greater than or equal to 13. Finally, the qualitative results were assessed in 2 × 2 factorial fashion to define NAR (NAR; positive RhSc and negative AST), AR (AR; positive RhSc and AST), potential atopy (potAt; negative RhSc and positive AST), and no rhinitis (NoRh; negative RhSc and AST).

Congestion and Rhinorrhea scores (mean; 95% C.I.) were determined for each of the eight triggers (6). Scores were plotted for the NAR ($n = 24$), AR ($n = 42$), potAt ($n = 46$), and NoRh ($n = 24$) groups (Figs. 1–3). In general, Congestion scores were about 1 point higher than Rhinorrhea scores for the NAR and AR groups. Weather and humidity changes had slightly higher scores than tobacco. Both had significantly higher scores for several of the other triggers than the potAt and NoRh groups. The latter were equivalent.

Positive IRS were found in 63% of the NAR, 48% of the AR, 15% of the potAt, and 5% of the NoRh groups. Significantly, more NAR and AR subjects had qualitatively positive scores than the other two groups ($p < 0.0001$ by Fisher's Exact tests). Qualitatively, positive Congestion and Rhinorrhea scores gave roughly the same distributions and significant differences.

These results have several implications. NAR cannot be "defined" solely by sensitivity to a battery of irritant triggers and negative allergy tests. As predicted from epidemiology studies, about half of the AR group had positive IRS. The Congestion and Rhinorrhea scores could not separate "runners" from "blockers" in the NAR group.

TABLE 6 Scoring for Rhinitis Score

Severity:	None	Trivial	Mild	Moderate	Severe
1. Itchy nose	0	1	2	3	4
2. Sneezing	0	1	2	3	4
3. Drip	0	1	2	3	4
4. Fullness, congestion	0	1	2	3	4
5. Generalized headache	0	1	2	3	4
6. Pain in face	0	1	2	3	4
7. Blowing out thick mucus	0	1	2	3	4
8. Postnasal drip in the back of the throat	0	1	2	3	4
9. Throat clearing	0	1	2	3	4
10. Hoarse voice	0	1	2	3	4

Sum = Rhinitis Score

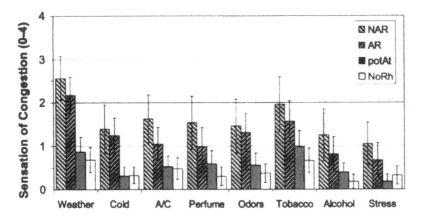

FIGURE 1 Quantitative Congestion Scores for the nonallergic rhinitis group (first column per cluster, *leftward black diagonal stripes*) were equivalent to the allergic rhinitis group (second column, *rightward grey diagonal stripes*), and significantly higher than the potential atopy (potAt; *grey*) and no rhinitis (NoRh; *white*) groups (mean; 95% CI) for each trigger (ANOVA followed by unpaired Student's *t*-tests with Bonferroni corrections; $p \leq 0.05$). Scores for allergic rhinitis were significantly higher than potAt for weather and humidity changes, cold air, and strong odors. They were significantly greater than NoRh for weather, cold air, perfume, strong odors, tobacco, and alcohol. Scores for potAt and NoRh were equivalent. *Abbreviations:* NAR, nonallergic rhinitis; AR, allergic rhinitis.

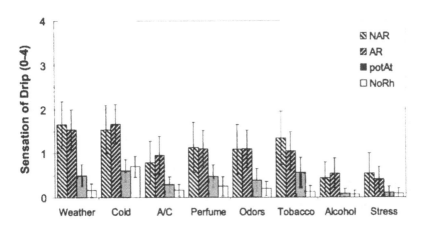

FIGURE 2 Rhinorrhea Scores were lower than the Congestion Scores. Scores for the nonallergic rhinitis (NAR) group (first column per cluster, *leftward diagonal stripes*) were equivalent to the allergic rhinitis (AR) group (second column, *rightward diagonal stripes*), and significantly higher than the potential atopy (potAt; *grey*) and no rhinitis (NoRh; *white*) groups (mean; 95% CI) for weather and cold air (ANOVA followed by unpaired Student's *t*-tests with Bonferroni corrections; $p \leq 0.05$). Scores for NAR were also significantly greater than NoRh for A/C, perfume, strong odors, and tobacco. Scores for the AR group were significantly higher than potAt and NoRh for weather, cold air, air conditioning, and strong odors. They were also significantly higher than NoRh for perfume and alcohol. Scores for potAt and NoRh were equivalent.

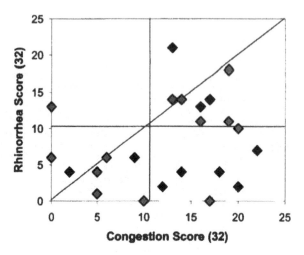

FIGURE 3 The Rhinorrhea Score was plotted against the Congestion Score for the nonallergic rhinitis (NAR) group (*diamonds*). The upper limits of the normal ranges for each score divide the figure into quadrants. The diagonal line is the line of identity. The right lower quadrant represents subjects with greater complaints of congestion than discharge. If so, they may represent the "blocker" subgroup of NAR. There were no comparable subjects in the upper left hand quadrant to represent the "runners." Instead, "runners" may be represented by the presence of both congestion and rhinorrhea (upper right quadrant), but with the complaint of rhinorrhea predominating and causing the sensation of blockage (congestion) of their noses. The NAR subjects in the lower left quadrant had Congestion and Rhinorrhea Scores in the normal ranges. This suggested that other symptoms from the Rhinitis Score were their major complaints. The drip and congestion in these NAR were triggered by the eight conditions listed in the Irritant Rhinitis Score.

IDIOPATHIC RHINITIS

The World Health Organization's initiative of "Allergic Rhinitis and its Impact on Asthma" (ARIA) (86), proposed that the term "VMR" be abolished and replaced by "idiopathic rhinitis" (IR) (Table 4). However, the syndrome remained one of exclusion, which likely explains the continued, interchangeable use of "VMR" (87). We propose that specific neural defects contribute to the diverse symptomatology of "VMR," and that identification of these mechanisms will permit more specific disease categorization and appropriately targeted therapies.

IRRITANT RHINITIS SCORING CARDS

van Rijswijk, Blom, and Fokkens have made progress in reversing the trend of relying on specific inclusion and exclusion criteria to describe IR (15). The inflammatory, infectious, allergic, hormonal, medication, and smoking-related syndromes should be excluded by a thorough history. Nasal endoscopy should be performed to exclude significant anatomical abnormalities. CT scan of the sinuses may be considered if this is a clinical possibility, but it is not obligatory. The pattern of persistent, reproducible symptoms must be documented. These symptoms were based on the work of Mygind and Weeke (88). The patient must fill out a Daily Rhinitis Chart and have their symptom severity, frequency, and duration determined (Table 7). These charts define IR if the affected patient has periods of nasal

TABLE 7 Prototypic Idiopathic Rhinitis Scoring Card for One Day

Symptom	0	1	2	3	Daily score
Nasal blockage (unable to breathe freely through nose)	Absent	Between 0 and 1 hr/ half day	Between 1 and 2 hr/half day	More than 2 hr/ half day	0–6
Runny nose (clear nasal discharge)	Absent	Between 0 and 1 hr/ half day	Between 1 and 2 hr/half day	More than 2 hr/ half day	0–6
Sneezing	Absent	<5 periods/ half day	Between 5 and 10 periods/half day	More than 10 periods/half day	0–6
Coughing	Absent	<5 periods/ half day	Between 5 and 10 periods/half day	More than 10 periods/half day	0–6
Green/yellow mucus production	Absent	Present			0–4

discharge, blockage, and/or sneezing that persist for an average of at least one hour per day on at least five days during a 14-day period. Information on coughing and the color of the discharge are also collected, but not included in the IR criteria. One limitation is the absence of a predefined set of standards for the amount of discharge, blockage, and discoloration. This has proven important in dealing with patients who claim to have profuse rhinorrhea and acute sinusitis based on the later (e.g., day 5) symptoms of a common cold associated with nasal irritation and blowing out of a crust of dried, green mucus. These patients are often taken aback when asked how many "cups of mucus" they are blowing out per day. Generally, the symptoms clear over the next few days as they ponder this question.

Cough is of interest because of the perception that postnasal drainage of mucus may lead to this laryngo-systemic reflex. This syndrome has been called postnasal drip syndrome (PNDS)-induced cough, but has been renamed upper airway cough syndrome (UACS) (89). The differential diagnosis of UACS includes AR, perennial NAR, postinfectious rhinitis, bacterial sinusitis, allergic fungal sinusitis, rhinitis due to anatomic abnormalities, rhinitis due to physical or chemical irritants, occupational rhinitis, rhinitis medicamentosa, and rhinitis of pregnancy. Gastroesophageal reflux disease is associated with a high prevalence of upper respiratory symptoms (90), and can mimic UACS. A crucial unanswered question is whether the conditions listed above actually produce cough through a final common pathway of postnasal drip or whether direct irritation or inflammation of upper airway structures can directly stimulate cough receptors. If so, the produced cough may be generated independently of, or in addition to, that associated with postnasal drip. This issue is discussed in more detail elsewhere in this book.

CONCLUSION

The pathogenic dissection of NAR is intended to provoke creative criticism and debate about the diverse mechanisms and potential categorizations for this condition. The overlap of some syndromes such as eosinophilic rhinitis suggest a progressive worsening from NARES to the Triad syndrome. The dissimilar conditions of NARES, occupational irritant, smoking-induced rhinitis, and "VMR" are all grouped under general category of NANIPER or IR. The authors propose that these "subsyndromes" be separately and properly classified, and that the neurological syndrome of "VMR" be replaced by the redefined term "IR." This retooling must be considered a work with slow progress as will be seen from the various perspectives taken by the authors of the other chapters.

ACKNOWLEDGMENTS

The authors encourage your feedback regarding this NAR classification scheme (baraniuj@georgetown.edu). Supported by Public Health Service Award RO1 AI42403.

REFERENCES

1. Settipane RA, Lieberman P. Update on nonallergic rhinitis. Ann Allergy Asthma Immunol 2001; 86:494–507.
2. Baraniuk JN, Staevska M. Perennial nonallergic rhinitis. In: Lichtenstein LM, Busse WW, Geha RS, eds. Current Therapy in Allergy Immunology and Rheumatology. 6th ed. Mosby Philadelphia, 2004:17–24.
3. Lal D, Corey JP. Vasomotor rhinitis update. Curr Opin Otolaryngol Head Neck Surg 2004; 12:243–247.
4. Litvyakova L, Baraniuk JN. Human nasal allergen provocation for determination of true allergic rhinitis: methods for clinicians. Curr Allergy Asthma Rep 2002; 2:194–202.
5. Malm L, Gerth van Wijk R, Bachert C. Guidelines for nasal provocations with aspects on nasal patency, airflow, and airflow resistance. International committee on objective assessment of the nasal airways, international rhinologic society. Rhinology 2000; 38(1):1–6.
6. Baraniuk JN, Naranch K, Maibach H, Clauw D. Irritant rhinitis in allergic, nonallergic, control and chronic fatigue syndrome populations. J CFS 2000; 7:3–31.
7. Meltzer EO, Hamilos DL, Hadley JA, Lanza DC, Marple BF, Nicklas RA. Rhinosinusitis: establishing definitions for clinical research and patient care. J Allergy Clin Immunol 2004; 114:S156–S212.
8. Meltzer EO, Hamilos DL, Hadley JA, Lanza DC, Marple BF, Nicklas RA. Rhinosinusitis: establishing definitions for clinical research and patient care. Otolaryngol–Head Neck Surg 2004; 131:S1–S62.
9. Rasp G, Thomas PA, Bujia J. Eosinophil inflammation of the nasal mucosa in allergic and non-allergic rhinitis measured by eosinophil cationic protein levels in native nasal fluid and serum. Clin Exp Allergy 1994; 24:1151–1156.
10. Sobol SE, Christodoulopoulos P, Hamid QA. Inflammatory patterns of allergic and nonallergic rhinitis. Allergy Asthma Rep 2001; 1:193–201.
11. Hauser R, Elreedy S, Hoppin JA, Christiani DC. Upper airway response in workers exposed to fuel oil ash: nasal lavage analysis. Occup Environ Med 1995; 52:353–358.
12. Montnemery P, Svensson C, Adelroth E, et al. Prevalence of nasal symptoms and their relation to self-reported asthma and chronic bronchitis/emphysema. Eur Respir J 2001; 17:596–603.
13. Roberts NJ, Lloyd-Owen SJ, Rapado F, et al. Relationship between chronic nasal and respiratory symptoms in patient with COPD. Respir Med 2003; 97:909–914.
14. Hamilton TD, Roe JM, Hayes CM, Jones P, Pearson GR, Webster AJ. Contributory and exacerbating roles of gaseous ammonia and organic dust in the etiology of atrophic rhinitis. Clin Diagn Lab Immunol 1999; 6:199–203.
15. van Rijswijk JB, Blom HM, Fokkens WJ. Idiopathic rhinitis, the ongoing quest. Allergy 2005; 60:1471–1481.
16. Vinke JG, KleinJan A, Severijnen LW, Fokkens WJ. Passive smoking causes an "allergic" cell infiltrate in the nasal mucosa of non-atopic children. Int J Pediatr Otorhinolaryngol 1999; 52:73–81.

17. Villar MT, Holgate ST. IgE, smoking and lung function. Clin Exp Allergy 1995; 25:206–209.
18. Rennard SI, Umino T, Millatmal T, et al. Evaluation of subclinical respiratory tract inflammation in heavy smokers who switch to a cigarette-like nicotine delivery device that primarily heats tobacco. Nicotine Tob Res 2002; 4:467–476.
19. Huggins KG, Brostoff J. Local production of specific IgE antibodies in allergic rhinitis patients with negative skin tests. Lancet 1975; 2:148–150.
20. Merret TG, Houri M, Mayer AL, Merrett J. Measurement of specific IgE antibodies in nasal secretion—evidence for local production. Clin Allergy 1976; 6:69–73.
21. Platts-Mills TA. Local production of IgG, IgA and IgE antibodies in grass pollen hay fever. J Immunol 1979; 122:2218–2225.
22. Ganzer U, Bachert C. Localization of IgE synthesis in immediate-type allergy of the upper respiratory tract. J Otorhinolaryngol Relat Spec 1988; 50:257–264.
23. Durham SR, Gould HJ, Thienes CP, et al. Expression of epsilon germ-line gene transcripts and mRNA for the epsilon heavy chain of IgE in nasal B cells and the effects of topical corticosteroid. Eur J Immunol 1997; 27:2899–2906.
24. KleinJan A, Vinke JG, Severijnen LW, Fokkens WJ. Local production and detection of (specific) IgE in nasal B-cells and plasma cells of allergic rhinitis patients. Eur Respir J 2000; 15(3):491–497.
25. Powe DG, Huskisson RS, Carney AS, Jenkins D, Jones NS. Evidence for an inflammatory pathophysiology in idiopathic rhinitis. Clin Exp Allergy 2001; 31:864–872.
26. Bachert C, Gevaert P, van Cauwenberge P. Nasal polyposis – a new concept on the formation of polyps. ACI Int 1999; 11:130–135.
27. Bachert C, Gevaert P, Holtappels G, Cuvelier C, van Cauwenberge P. Nasal polyposis: from cytokines to growth. Am J Rhinol 2000; 14:279–290.
28. Balaban N, Rasooly A. Staphylococcal enterotoxins. Int J Food Microbiol 2000; 61:1–10.
29. Li H, Llera A, Malchiodi EL, Mariuzza RA. The structural basis of T-cell activation by superantigens. Ann Rev Immunol 1999; 17:435–466.
30. Mollick JA, McMasters RL, Grossmann D, Rich RR. Localization of a site on bacterial superantigens that determines T-cell receptor beta chain specificity. J Exp Med 1993; 177:283–293.
31. Hong SC, Waterbury G, Janeway CA Jr. Different superantigens interact with distinct sites in the Vbeta domain of a single T-cell receptor. J Exp Med 1996; 183:1437–1446.
32. Jabara HH, Geha RS. The superantigen toxic shock syndrome toxin-1 induces CD40 ligand expression and modulates IgE isotype switching. Int Immunol 1996; 8:1503–1510.
33. Hofer ME, Lester MR, Schlievert PM, Leung DY. Upregulation of IgE synthesis by staphylococcal toxic shock syndrome toxin-1 in peripheral blood mononuclear cells from patients with atopic dermatitis. Clin Exp Allergy 1995; 25:1218–1227.
34. Hofer ME, Harbeck RJ, Schlievert PM, Leung DY. Staphylococcal toxins augment specific IgE responses by atopic patients exposed to allergen. J Invest Dermatol 1999; 112:171–176.
35. Mawhorter SD, Kazura JW, Boom WH. Human eosinophils as antigen-presenting cells: relative efficiency for superantigen- and antigen-induced CD4+ T-cell proliferation. Immunology 1994; 81:584–591.
36. Genovese A, Bouvet JP, Florio G, Lamparter-Schummert B, Bjorck L, Marone G. Bacterial immunoglobulin superantigen proteins A and L activate human heart mast cells by interacting with immunoglobulin E. Infect Immun 2000; 68:5517–5524.
37. Miller EJ, Nagao S, Carr FK, Noble JM, Cohen AB. Interleukin-8 (IL-8) is a major neutrophil chemotaxin from human alveolar macrophages stimulated with staphylococcal enterotoxin A (SEA). Inflamm Res 1996; 45:386–392.
38. Bright JJ, Xin Z, Sriram S. Superantigens augment antigen-specific Th1 responses by inducing IL-12 production in macrophages. J Leukocyte Biol 1999; 65:665–670.
39. Benson M. Pathophysiological effects of glucocorticoids on nasal polyps: an update. Curr Opin Allergy Clin Immunol 2005; 5:31–35.
40. Lavigne F, Nguyen CT, Cameron L, Hamid Q, Renzi PM. Prognosis and prediction of response to surgery in allergic patients with chronic sinusitis. J Allergy Clin Immunol 2000; 105:746–751.

41. Karlsson G, Brandtzaeg P, Hansson G, Petruson B, Bjorkander J, Hanson LA. Humoral immunity in nasal mucosa of patients with common variable immunodeficiency. J Clin Immunol 1987; 7:29–36.

42. May A, Zielen S, von Ilberg C, Weber A. Immunoglobulin deficiency and determination of pneumococcal antibody titers in patients with therapy-refractory recurrent rhinosinusitis. Eur Arch Otorhinolaryngol 1999; 256:445–449.

43. Cooper MD, Lanier LL, Conley ME, Puck JM. Immunodeficiency disorders. Hematology (Am Soc Hematol Educ Program) 2003:314–330.

44. von Bubnoff D, Fimmers R, Bogdanow M, Matz H, Koch S, Bieber T. Asymptomatic atopy is associated with increased indoleamine 2,3-dioxygenase activity and interleukin-10 production during seasonal allergen exposure. Clin Exp Allergy 2004; 34:1056–1063.

45. von Bubnoff D, Scheler M, Hinz T, Matz H, Koch S, Bieber T. Comparative immunophenotyping of monocytes from symptomatic and asymptomatic atopic individuals. Allergy 2004; 59:933–939.

46. Baraniuk JN, Clauw JD, Gaumond E. Rhinitis symptoms in chronic fatigue syndrome. Ann Allergy Asthma Immunol 1998; 81:359–365.

47. Elahi MM, Frenkiel S, Fageeh N. Paraseptal structural changes and chronic sinus disease in relation to the deviated nasal septum. J Otolaryngol 1997; 26:236–240.

48. Patel K, Chavda SV, Violaris N, Pahor AL. Incidental paranasal sinus inflammatory changes in the a British population. J Laryngol Otol 1996; 110:649–651.

49. Maly PV, Sundgren PC. Changes in paranasal sinus abnormalities found incidentally on MRI. Neuroradiology 1995; 37:471–474.

50. Gordts F, Clement PA, Buisseret T. Prevalences of sinusitis signs in a non-ENT population. J Otorhinolaryngol Relat Spec 1996; 58:315–319.

51. Jones NS, Strobl A, Holland I. A study of the CT findings in 100 patients with rhinosinusitis and 100 controls. Clin Otolaryngol 1997; 22:47–51.

52. Reiss M, Reiss G. Rhinitis in old age. Schweiz Rundsch Med Prax 2002; 91:535–359.

53. Schmidt J, Zalewski P, Olszewski J, Olszewska-Ziaber A, Mloczkowski D, Pietkiewicz P. Histopathological verifications clinical indications in the inferior turbinoplasty. Otolaryngol Pol 2001; 55:545–550.

54. Schmidt J, Zalewski P, Olszewski J, Olszewska-Ziaber A. Histopathological verification of clinical indications to partial inferior turbinectomy. Rhinology 2001; 39:147–150.

55. Cusimano MD, Sekhar LN. Pseudo-cerebrospinal fluid rhinorrhea. J Neurosurg 1994; 80:26–30.

56. Gani F, Braida A, Lombardi C, Del Giudice A, Senna GE, Passalacqua G. Rhinitis in pregnancy. Allerg Immunol (Paris) 2003; 35:306.

57. Milosevic D, Janosevic L, Dergenc R, Vasic M. Pathologic conditions associated with drug-induced rhinitis. Srp Arh Celok Lek 2004; 132:14–17.

58. Graf P, Enerdal J, Hallen H. Ten days' use of oxymetazoline nasal spray with or without benzalkonium chloride in patients with vasomotor rhinitis. Arch Otolaryngol Head Neck Surg 1999; 125:1128–1132.

59. Mabry RL. Nasal stuffiness due to systemic medications. Otolaryngol Head Neck Surgery 1982; 91:93–94.

60. Sasaki Y. Possible role of plasminogen activator in the occurrence of profuse watery rhinorrhea after topical application of epinephrine to the nasal mucosa. Rhinology 2001; 39:220–225.

61. Bachert C. Persistent rhinitis - allergic or nonallergic? Allergy 2004; 59(suppl 76): 11–15.

62. Malcomson KG. The vasomotor activities of the nasal mucous membrane. J Laryngol 1959; 73:73–75.

63. Garay R. Mechanisms of vasomotor rhinitis. Allergy 2004; 59(suppl 76):4–9.

64. Jaradeh SS, Smith TL, Torrico L, et al. Autonomic nervous system evaluation of patients with vasomotor rhinitis. Laryngoscope 2000; 110(11):1828–1831.

65. Lazarev VN, Suzdal'tsev AE, Maslov Eiu. Characteristics of autonomic dystonia in children with vasomotor rhinitis. Vestn Otorinolaringol 2002; 3:9–11.

66. Segal S, Shlamkovitch N, Eviatar E, Berenholz L, Sarfaty S, Kessler A. Vasomotor rhinitis following trauma to the nose. Ann Otol Rhinol Laryngol 1999; 108:208–210.

67. Mygind N, Naclerio RM. Allergic and Nonallergic Rhinitis. In: Clinical Aspects. Copenhagen: Munksgaard, 1993:12.
68. Corey JP. Vasomotor rhinitis should not be a wastebasket diagnosis. Arch Otolaryngol Head Neck Surg 2003; 129:588–589.
69. Ledford D. Inadequate diagnosis of nonallergic rhinitis: assessing the damage. Allergy Asthma Proc 2003; 24:155–162.
70. Bagenstose SE, Bernstein JA. Treatment of chronic rhinitis by an allergy specialist improves quality of life outcomes. Ann Allergy Asthma Immunol 1999; 83:524–528.
71. Gadzhimirzaev G. Variants of vasomotor rhinitis in children. Vestn Otorinolaringol 1994; (2):25–27.
72. Anon. Management of allergic and nonallergic rhinitis. Evidence Report/Technical Assessment Number 54. AHRQ Publication No. 02-E024, May 2002. Rockville, MD: Agency for Healthcare Research and Quality, 2002 (http://www.ahrq.gov/clinic/rhininv.htm).
73. Ressel GW. Agency for healthcare research and quality. AHRQ releases review of treatments for allergic and nonallergic rhinitis. Agency for Healthcare Research and Quality. Am Fam Physician 2002; 66(11):2164, 2167.
74. Mygind N, Borum P. Anticholinergic treatment of watery rhinorrhea. Am J Rhinol 1990; 4:1.
75. Stjarne P, Lundblad L, Lundberg JM, Anggard A. Capsaicin and nicotine sensitive afferent neurones and nasal secretion in healthy human volunteers and in patients with vasomotor rhinitis. Br J Pharmacol 1989; 96:693.
76. Mullol J, Baraniuk JN, Logun C, et al. M1 and M3 muscarinic antagonists inhibit human nasal glandular secretion in vitro. J Appl Physiol 1992; 73:2069–2073.
77. Rogers DF. Reflexly runny noses: neurogenic inflammation in the nasal mucosa. Clin Exp Allergy 1996; 26(4):365–367.
78. Baraniuk JN. Mechanisms of rhinitis. In: Lasley MV, Altman LC, eds. Rhinitis Immunology and Allergy Clinics of North America. Philadelphia: W.B. Saunders, 2000; 20:245–264.
79. Papon JF, Brugel-Ribere L, Fodil R, et al. Nasal wall compliance in vasomotor rhinitis. J Appl Physiol 2006; 100:107–111.
80. Cervin A, Onnerfalt J, Edvinsson L, Grundemar L. Functional effects of neuropeptide Y receptors on blood flow and nitric oxide levels in the human nose. Am J Respir Crit Care Med 1999; 160:1724–1728.
81. Jacobs RL, Freedman PM, Boswell RN. Nonallergic rhinitis with eosinophilia (NARES syndrome). Clinical and immunological presentation. J Allergy Clin Immunol 1981; 67:253–262.
82. Raphael GD, Hauptschein-Raphael M, Kaliner M. Gustatory rhinitis: a syndrome of food-induced rhinorrhea. J Allergy Clin Immunol 1989; 83:110–115.
83. Silvers WS. The skier's nose: a model of cold-induced rhinorrhea. Ann Allergy 1991; 67:32–36.
84. Braat JP, Mulder PG, Fokkens WJ, van Wijk RG, Rijntjes E. Intranasal cold dry air is superior to histamine challenge in determining the presence and degree of nasal hyperreactivity in nonallergic noninfectious perennial rhinitis. Am J Respir Crit Care Med 1998; 157:1748–1755.
85. Baraniuk JN, Naranch K, Maibach H, Clauw D. Tobacco sensitivity in chronic fatigue syndrome. J CFS 2000; 7:33–52.
86. Bousquet J, van Cauwenberge P, Khaltaev N. Allergic rhinitis and its impact on asthma (ARIA). J Allergy Clin Immunol 2001; 108:S147–S334.
87. Wheeler PW, Wheeler SF. Vasomotor rhinitis. Am Fam Physician 2005; 72:1057–1062.
88. Mygind N, Weeke B. Allergic and vasomotor rhinitis: clinical aspects. Copenhagen, Denmark: Munksgaard, 1985.
89. Pratter MR. Chronic upper airway cough syndrome secondary to rhinosinus diseases (previously referred to as postnasal drip syndrome): ACCP evidence-based clinical practice guidelines. Chest 2006; 129(suppl 1):63S–71S.
90. Shaker R, Bardan E, Gu C, Kern M, Torrico L, Toohill R. Intrapharyngeal distribution of gastric acid refluxate. Laryngoscope 2003; 113:1182–1191.

4 Questionnaire Diagnosis of Nonallergic Rhinitis

Dominique Brandt and Jonathan A. Bernstein

Department of Internal Medicine, Division of Immunology/Allergy Section, University of Cincinnati College of Medicine, Cincinnati, Ohio, U.S.A.

INTRODUCTION

Chronic rhinitis is an inflammatory disease involving the nasal mucosa and characterized by symptoms of sneezing, itching, rhinorrhea, postnasal discharge, and congestion. Chronic rhinitis is typically classified as follows: (i) allergic rhinitis (AR), if symptoms and triggers correlate with a specific immunoglobulin (Ig)E-mediated response; (ii) non-AR (NAR), if symptoms are induced by irritant triggers in the absence of specific IgE-mediated responses; and (iii) mixed rhinitis (MR), if specific IgE-mediated responses are present in conjunction with symptoms induced by both allergic and nonallergic triggers (1). NAR conditions can be further subcategorized on the basis of the presence or absence of nasal eosinophilia.

Chronic rhinitis is a common primary-care disorder associated with significant comorbidities such as sinusitis, otitis media, and asthma, which impact both work and school performance. AR prevalence has been estimated to range between 5% and 22% in the United States, and its economic impact is estimated to cost the health-care system $2.5 billion annually (1,2). While the prevalence and epidemiology of AR is well defined, only a few studies have investigated the frequency of NAR. In a 1998 report, the Joint Task Force on Practice Parameters in Allergy, Asthma and Immunology estimated that 43% of patients presenting with chronic rhinitis have AR, 34% have MR, and 23% have nonallergic vasomotor rhinitis (VMR) (3–6). Other studies found the prevalence of NAR to range between 17% and 52% (5,7–12). However, these studies did not differentiate between noninflammatory VMR (absence of nasal eosinophils with unique physical triggers) and inflammatory NAR with eosinophilia syndrome (NARES).

Establishing a specific clinical entity in the differential diagnosis of chronic rhinitis is challenging because symptoms are not always useful in differentiating patients with AR, MR, or NAR subtypes (NARES and VMR). A detailed patient and family history in conjunction with skin prick and/or serum-specific IgE testing are necessary for a proper diagnosis. Physical examination is important for excluding structural problems but has very limited utility in differentiating between the different chronic rhinitis conditions. The pathophysiology of NAR is less understood and is likely more complex than AR. Studies implicating a role for neuropeptides upsetting the balance of the parasympathetic and sympathetic nervous system, and differences in inflammatory cell and/or cytokine profiles indicate that multiple mechanisms may be involved. Developing a standardized phenotype for NAR subtypes is necessary for conducting future genotype–phenotype association studies and elucidating the mechanism(s) of this disorder. Disease-specific validated questionnaires are the first step in achieving this objective.

In this chapter, we will review the current literature of rhinitis questionnaires, summarize known characteristics of subjects with NAR, and propose a questionnaire designed specifically for the diagnosis of different forms of rhinitis.

RHINITIS QUESTIONNAIRES

Unlike NAR, AR is well understood and has been extensively studied. Multiple questionnaires designed to characterize AR have been developed and validated and are commonly used for research as well as clinical diagnosis. However, for NAR these instruments are lacking. In discussing rhinitis questionnaires and rhinitis subtypes, investigators have applied different definitions and abbreviations for AR and NAR conditions. Although this can be confusing to the reader, the terminology used by each investigator to describe their populations has been left unchanged in our discussion to further illustrate the need to develop consensus definitions and terminology for chronic rhinitis subtypes.

Definition of a Validated Questionnaire

To be considered valid, a questionnaire must satisfy a series of tests demonstrating that it accurately measures a specific aim, regardless of who responds and when and how it is administered to a subject. Surviving these rigorous criteria indicates that the questionnaire is not only an appropriate and meaningful instrument for capturing the intended information but also reliable and reproducible for repeated use. The initial step in developing a validated questionnaire is to either identify an existing nonvalidated questionnaire, which has been already used and/or develop a new questionnaire based on extensive clinical experience. A newly developed questionnaire that addresses specific issues should be clear, simple, and carefully worded to achieve the subjects' optimal understanding prior to testing. To fully appreciate what steps are involved in developing a validated questionnaire, the clinician should be aware of certain definitions.

Validity is most commonly defined in terms of "content validity," "construct validity," and "criterion validity" (13). In the context of the present discussion, a questionnaire is considered "valid" if questionnaire responses can accurately predict a physician's diagnosis. "Content validity" is the degree to which the questionnaire addresses the biological phenomenon in question. For example, a rhinitis questionnaire should concern the cardinal and derivative symptoms of rhinitis and related disorders, as well as perceived exacerbating factors. "Construct validity" is the degree to which a measurement behaves in its theoretically predicted manner. For example, a rhinitis severity index should increase with number of reported triggers, number of medications required to achieve control, etc. In order to achieve construct validity, factor analysis (14) is frequently used to examine the interrelationship among a set of questionnaire items, in order to identify whether an underlying common linkage exists (15). Establishing "criterion validity" requires comparison of questionnaire responses with a gold standard. For example, the questionnaire should ideally correlate with laboratory or other relevant diagnostic tests. Categorical analysis (e.g., chi-square or logistic regression) is often applied to establish criterion validity, as is generation of receiver–operator curves in the establishment of criterion cutoff values.

A useful diagnostic questionnaire should not only be valid but also reliable. For a questionnaire to be reliable it must have "internal consistency," which measures the statistical relationship among items from a single instrument, and "test–retest" reliability, which measures a subject's score on the same questionnaire at different time points to ensure that the time interval(s) do not impact performance. To satisfy the "internal consistency" criteria, all the items of an instrument (or at least a subscale thereof) must measure the same construct and therefore be strongly correlated. The interitem correlation is commonly reported by Cronbach's alpha (α), which varies between 0 (lowest correlation) and 1 (highest correlation) (15). Scales with Cronbach's α between 0.70 and 0.90 are considered reliable (< 0.70 = poor reliability; 0.7–0.8 = moderate reliability; and > 0.80 = high reliability). As mentioned, the "test–retest" reliability criterion of a questionnaire requires repeated scores from the same questionnaire be highly correlated for it to be reliable. This approach can be potentially biased due to the subject's recall of previous responses or because the testing conditions may have changed.

Validated Rhinitis Questionnaires
There are several well-validated questionnaires for AR. The International Study of Asthma and Allergy in Children (ISAAC) questionnaire was developed to improve epidemiologic research in asthma and AR, and to standardize the methodologies for collecting this information around the world by asking the same questions to each study population. It has been successfully used to identify the prevalence and severity of disease within and among different countries (16). The baseline data collected from these early assessments has been used to compare changes in disease prevalence and severity over time and to develop research hypotheses that have investigated environmental and genetic determinants (16). Studies conducted in a variety of countries and in different languages have demonstrated that this questionnaire survey collects consistent and reproducible epidemiologic information about AR as well as other diseases like asthma and atopic dermatitis (16–18).

Other studies have used AR questionnaires to assess symptoms suggestive of different rhinitis subtypes. Jones et al. distributed a questionnaire that used the core questions in the ISAAC questionnaire pertaining to AR (19). The questionnaires were sent to 1200 households and questionnaires were returned by 2114 individuals older than 14 years of age (y/o). Seventeen percent reported nasal congestion on a daily basis for two weeks in the past year, almost 20% reported symptoms of rhinorrhea and hay fever symptoms during the same period, and 7% reported sneezing. Perennial symptoms without hay fever symptoms, which included perennial AR (PAR) and NAR conditions, were reported by 8.6% of subjects. Using this questionnaire, it was not possible to discriminate between a specific diagnosis of PAR and perennial NAR (PNAR). No attempt was made to correlate questionnaire responses with actual physician diagnosis of a specific rhinitis subtype.

Disease-specific quality of life (QOL) questionnaire studies the best examples of the process required to validate a questionnaire. These questionnaires have been developed for asthma and rhinoconjunctivitis. Juniper developed rhinoconjunctivitis QOL questionnaires (RQLQ) for children of all ages, adolescents, and adults (20). The premise of these questionnaires is that individuals who suffer from rhinitis are severely impaired in their day-to-day physical, emotional, occupational, and social functioning and this causes a significant amount of emotional distress. The original RQLQ was developed based on having the following specifications: (i) measures of both physical and emotional functionality; (ii) questions that reflect functional activities most important to sufferers of rhinoconjunctivitis; (iii) results must be amenable to statistical analysis; (iv) responses must be reliable regardless of whether the individual was clinically symptomatic or not; (v) the questionnaire must be responsive to clinically important changes; and (vi) the questionnaire should be valid in that it actually relates rhinoconjunctivitis-specific impairments to QOL (21). Modifications of this questionnaire to make it shorter and relevant to different age groups have succeeded in attaining the specific aims of the gold standard RQLQ. However, QOL questionnaires totally depend on proper characterization and diagnosis of the patient as an accurate reflection of QOL in AR versus NAR. The questions asked to assess emotional and functional impairment in allergic subjects such as "need to rub nose/eyes," "itchy eyes," "need to blow nose repeatedly," "sneezing," "stuffy blocked nose," "tiredness," "irritable," "watery eyes," and "nocturnal symptoms" are not specific and could just as easily apply to an individual with NAR. In these studies, the subject is first diagnosed with AR and then completes the RQLQ (21).

RQLQ questionnaires have been useful in numerous clinical drug trials in AR patients (22). Most of these studies demonstrated that the specific therapeutic intervention improved total RQLQ scores as well as individual domains. However, the RQLQ has not been effective in differentiating between AR and NAR and therefore has no utility for this purpose.

LIMITATIONS OF QUESTIONNAIRE STUDIES INVESTIGATING NAR

To date, there are no validated questionnaires specifically designed for NAR. Some studies have attempted to compare AR and NAR groups to healthy control subjects. Some investigated individual domains in their combined disorders but a disease-specific questionnaire that differentiates between different chronic rhinitis subtypes is yet to be developed.

Before initiating a questionnaire study to assess clinical characteristics of chronic rhinitis subtypes, a consensus definition for each of the individual rhinitis subtypes must be established. This has been more problematic for NAR subtypes because this diagnosis is dependent on excluding an allergic component and requires that clinicians obtain a nasal smear for eosinophils to differentiate between inflammatory (NARES) and noninflammatory (VMR) NAR subtypes. Several studies that attempted to compare AR and NAR populations have presented confusing results because they uniformly failed to well define different rhinitis subtypes including MR where individuals report allergic and nonallergic triggers (Table 1). Furthermore, all of these studies used different definitions for the chronic rhinitis populations they were evaluating. These factors can result in misleading or even erroneous conclusions.

Only two studies sought to define the true allergic status of the study population by allergen prick/puncture skin testing which could be used to confirm questionnaire findings. Even fewer studies have conducted specific challenges to determine if reported triggers actually cause clinical symptoms. Braat et al. analyzed the real-time effects of pollution and weather changes on NAR subjects compared to healthy controls by monitoring symptom scores and visual analog scales over 218 days (23). They found that environmental changes during periods of low air pollution resulted in increased nasal hyperresponsiveness in the NAR

TABLE 1 Comparison of Rhinitis Observational Questionnaire Studies

References	Ages/number of subjects	Testing	Populations studied	Major findings
Jessen and Janzon (26)	16–82 y/o; N = 1469	No	NAR AR	1. Age: NAR with more nasal complaints between ages 20–30 and 70–80 y/o 2. Triggers: For NAR most common was cold air
Sibbald and Rink (27)	16–65 y/o; N = 2969	Skin prick test with 5 common allergens	SAR and SNAR PAR and PNAR PAR/SAR PNAR/SNAR	1. Age: PAR = PNAR; SAR < SNAR 2. Symptoms: PAR with more wheeze and fewer sinus headaches vs. PNAR; SAR more sneeze, itchy eyes and nose vs. SNAR 3. Triggers: PAR bothered by dust and pollen more often than PNAR; SAR bothered by pollen and animals more often than SNAR; food and colds more frequent in SNAR
Lindberg and Malm (7)	0–80 y/o; N = 678	Skin prick test to 10 common allergens	AR VMR	1. Age: VMR > AR 2. Smoking: AR < VMR 3. Symptoms: Nasal congestion more frequent in VMR vs. AR; rhinorrhea more frequent in AR; AR more symptomatic vs. VMR 4. Triggers: AR bothered by aeroallergens > VMR group; AR and VMR bothered by dust, mold, perfume, and cigarette smoke
Jones et al. (19)	≥14 y/o; N = 2200	No	SR PR	1. Age: seasonal symptoms decrease with age 2. Triggers: seasonal rhinitis subjects more likely to work in a dusty environment in past 2 yr

(Continued)

TABLE 1 Comparison of Rhinitis Observational Questionnaire Studies (*Continued*)

References	Ages/number of subjects	Testing	Populations studied	Major findings
Montnemery et al. (31)	20–59 y/o; N = 12,079	No	AR	1. Triggers: tree and grass pollen, animals, dust, mold, damp/cold air, dry air, tobacco fumes, strong smells, spicy food, red wine, and stress 2. Gender: women more symptomatic
Olsson et al. (25)	19–80 y/o; N = 15,000	No	AR NAR	1. Age: AR decreases with age and NAR increases slightly with age 2. Smoking: NAR higher in smokers; AR higher in nonsmokers
Ryden et al. (29)	Mean age: PAR 31/ PNAR 43; N = 63	Skin prick to dust mites	PAR PNAR	1. Symptoms: sneezing worse in PAR; no difference in nasal congestion 2. Gender: quality of life poorer in women vs. men

Abbreviations: y/o, years of age; NAR, nonallergic rhinitis; AR, allergic rhinitis; SAR, seasonal allergic rhinitis; SNAR, seasonal nonallergic rhinitis; PAR, perennial allergic rhinitis; PNAR, perennial NAR; VMR, vasomotor rhinitis; SR, seasonal rhinitis; PR, perennial rhinitis.

population. In spite of these inherent limitations, some useful information can be extracted from these earlier investigations for comparing results reported by more recent rhinitis questionnaire studies.

Age/Age of Onset

The diagnosis of NAR appears to be more frequently made in older individuals compared to AR. Sanico and Togias performed a chart review of a large patient population fully evaluated in an allergy clinic and found that the diagnosis of AR was made in 95% of patients during the first decade of life whereas the diagnosis of NAR was made in 60% of subjects in their fifth decade of life (24). The authors speculated that either AR decreases with age or NAR manifests at an older age. Questionnaire studies have reported conflicting findings with respect to the age of onset for different rhinitis subtypes. Lindberg and Malm administered a computerized questionnaire to patients during their first visit to an allergist's office and found that median ages for AR and VMR were 26 and 32, respectively (7). A limitation of this study was that there was overlap in triggers for the AR and VMR populations indicating that many of these subjects had MR.

A questionnaire study distributed to 10,670 subjects by Olsson et al. demonstrated a slight increase in NAR but not AR with age among those who responded (25). This is in contrast to an earlier study by Jessen and Janzon who administered a rhinitis questionnaire to 1469 randomly selected individuals (26). They found that the prevalence of NAR peaked between the ages 20 and 30 and again between 70 and 80. According to these authors, there was an increased family history of allergy in the younger age group, suggesting that some of these individuals may have actually been allergic. The results of this study are difficult to interpret in that no further characterization of this population was performed (i.e., prick/puncture skin testing, etc.) and different rhinitis subtypes such as MR were not considered. Sibbald and Rink used a postal questionnaire to screen almost 3000 adults between the ages 16 and 62 who were registered with a London general practice (27). They collected information about age of onset for seasonal rhinitis (SR) and perennial rhinitis (PR). They characterized their populations as having seasonal AR (SAR) or seasonal NAR (SNAR) and PAR or PNAR. They also evaluated groups with PAR/SAR and PNAR/SNAR. They subsequently conducted personal interviews with a representative part of this population and confirmed their allergic status with skin testing. Interestingly, they found that individuals with SAR had an earlier onset of symptoms compared to those with SNAR, PAR, and PNAR. However, they found no difference in age of onset between PAR and PNAR subjects. Nonetheless, it appears that most of these questionnaire studies confirm that NAR begins later in life compared to AR.

Gender

The few epidemiological studies designed to distinguish between different subtypes of chronic rhinitis found differences in the prevalence of NAR in females versus males, with a female : male ratio ranging between 58 and 74% (8,28). These findings have not been generalized to the total population. Neither Jones et al., Lindberg and Malm, nor Olsson et al. found any gender differences in their observational questionnaire studies among the different chronic rhinitis subtype populations they investigated (7,19,25). Interestingly, a comparative study between

PAR and PNAR patients found that women in both groups had a significantly greater impairment in QOL compared to men (29).

Family History of Allergy
Sibbald and Rink found that subjects with SR and/or PR regardless of their atopic status had a higher prevalence of family history for nasal problems other than hay fever compared to healthy controls. However, their small sample size as well as limited skin prick/puncture test panel (five allergens) may have biased their findings. None of the other observational questionnaire studies addressed the importance of family history among the different rhinitis subtypes they evaluated (27).

Symptoms
Lindberg and Malm found there was a significant difference in symptoms between VMR patients who had predominantly nasal congestion, whereas AR patients more often reported wheeze, eye irritation, and rhinorrhea in addition to having more symptomatic acute attacks (7). Ryden et al. found that individuals with PAR and PNAR had a similar degree of nasal blockage, throat irritation, nasal dryness, and headache but those with PAR experienced more sneezing (29). Similarly, Sibbald and Rink reported that (i) SAR subjects had a higher prevalence of sneezing and itchy eyes compared to seasonal NAR; (ii) PAR patients had a higher prevalence of wheeze and a lower prevalence of sinus headache compared to PNAR; and (iii) SAR/PAR patients experienced more frequent sneezing, itchy eyes, and itchy nose than SNAR/PNAR patients (27). These findings contradicted those of Jones et al. who found that younger subjects in their population more often complained of having a blocked nose and rhinorrhea compared to older subjects (19). The conflicting results from these studies indicate that it is very difficult to differentiate between rhinitis subtypes based on symptoms alone.

Triggers
Inasmuch as symptoms do not distinguish between allergic and nonallergic patients, it has been suggested that triggers may better differentiate between these two groups. Kaliner (30) proposed that primary care physicians could use a screening tool designed by Lieberman et al. (2002) for a quick diagnosis of chronic rhinitis without the need for additional testing (30). This instrument categorized triggers as being allergic or nonallergic. Allergic triggers included freshly mowed grass, dead grass, hay, dead leaves, pollen, trees/tree pollen, weeds, molds, house dust, cat/cat hair, dog/dog hair, and feathers whereas nonallergic triggers included strong odors such as smoke, perfumes, cosmetics, cleaning products, paint fumes, hairspray, outside dust, and exhaust and gasoline fumes in addition to environmental triggers such as windy, cold, damp days, humidity/temperature changes, and ingestant triggers (alcoholic beverages and spicy foods). The proposed rule for a correct diagnosis was very simple. If a patient checked off at least one of the allergen triggers and none of the other triggers, AR was the correct diagnosis. If the patient checked off at least one of the nonallergic triggers and none of the allergic triggers, the patient could be diagnosed as having NAR. If triggers were checked off in both categories, the patient could be diagnosed as having MR. At face value, this instrument appears to be a convenient and a rapid diagnostic way to differentiate between AR and NAR disorders when testing for specific IgE (skin or serologic)

is not readily available. However, it has never been validated and the few studies that investigated the relevance of triggers for diagnosing specific subtypes of chronic rhinitis indicated that this approach may be too simplistic and not reliable.

In their computerized questionnaire survey, Lindberg and Malm reported that allergic subjects more frequently experienced symptoms aggravated by exposure to grass, deciduous trees, mugwort, and cats (7). However there was no significant difference between AR and VMR patients with respect to symptoms being aggravated by mold and dust mites and after exposure to irritants like smoke and perfumes. Again, this indicates that a larger portion of their population may have been experiencing MR. A study by Montnemery et al. demonstrated that among those subjects with self-reported AR, 26% roughly reported having symptoms while exposed to scented smells, 22% to tobacco fumes, 15% to dry air, 16% to damp/cold air, 8% to spicy food, 7% after drinking red wine, 16% with mold exposure, and 23% around animals (31). Similar findings were shown for self-reported asthma subjects. Interestingly, these investigators found that in all of their chronic rhinitis subjects with nasal symptoms, exposure to grass, tree pollen, or animal triggers had a spring and summer tendency and factors such as damp/cold air, dry air, tobacco-fumes, and strong-smelling scents had less of a seasonal tendency. Nasal symptoms were more frequent during the spring regardless of exacerbating triggers or allergic status. Jones et al. also showed that both SR and PR were related to environmental exposure (19). However, this study did not differentiate between allergic and nonallergic phenotypes.

Reduced Olfactory Sense
Olsson et al. performed a questionnaire survey of a large sample of subjects and observed an increased prevalence of self-reported reduced olfactory sense among self-declared NAR individuals, in a range of three to four times greater than observed for normal individuals. No difference was found between AR subjects and the normal population (25). Mann et al., utilizing multiple test odorants, compared olfactory status in both AR and NAR patients to normal healthy controls (32). They confirmed that nonallergic subjects had greater loss of smell compared to controls and AR subjects, and that allergic and nonallergic males had an overall greater olfactory loss than females for four out of the five odorants investigated (32). A previous study by Simola and Malmberg, utilizing a commercially available odor test kit, also found that study subjects with NAR had a diminished sense of smell compared to subjects with AR independent of gender (33). Odorant threshold studies have previously demonstrated that olfaction diminishes with age with significant reductions occurring after age 50 (33,34). Therefore, these findings may be age dependent rather than a manifestation of NAR itself.

Smokers/Nonsmokers
A few studies compared the prevalence of rhinitis in smokers versus nonsmokers. Jessen and Janzon found no difference in self-reported nonallergic nasal complaints when comparing smokers to nonsmokers (26). Montnemery et al. reported that smokers had slightly more chronic nasal symptoms consisting of thick yellow nasal discharge and nasal blockage than nonsmokers (31). Olsson et al. showed that active and former smokers exhibited more nonallergic nasal symptoms compared to nonsmokers (25).

Other Observations

Lindberg and Malm reported that patients with AR were more likely to have a history of asthma compared to NAR patients whereas patients with NAR had a more frequent history of recurrent sinusitis (7). Interestingly, NAR patients reported that their symptoms were more often aggravated after an infection (7).

QUESTIONNAIRE DEVELOPMENT FOR DIAGNOSIS OF CHRONIC NAR

Recently, a questionnaire for the diagnosis of NAR has been developed in our institution to assist primary care doctors in differentiating between various chronic rhinitis conditions (35). Initially, a self-administered questionnaire listing symptoms and common allergic and nonallergic triggers was blindly distributed to 100 randomly selected new patients presenting to an allergist's office with chronic rhinitis symptoms from spring 2003 to spring 2004. Patients were asked to check any trigger that aggravated their symptoms. Triggers included cat/cat hair, dog/dog hair, feathers, and other furry pets; symptoms occurring outdoors during the spring, summer, or fall; temperature changes; and diesel/gasoline car exhaust fumes, tobacco smoke, perfumes/fragrances, incense, household cleaning products, newsprint, hairspray, and symptoms after alcoholic beverages, spicy food, or eating (35). Exposures that could represent either an allergic or an irritant-induced trigger such as dust, mold, fresh mowed grass, and starting the furnace, were not included in this analysis in order to eliminate the confounding effect of overlapping diseases. A physician diagnosis was obtained by an allergist based on a physician-administered history, physical examination, nasal smear for eosinophils, prick skin testing, and/or serum-specific IgE to 20 indigenous seasonal and perennial allergens. Specific IgE tests had to correlate with clinical symptoms to establish a diagnosis of AR. A diagnosis of NAR was confirmed by a history of symptoms aggravated by irritant triggers, negative allergy skin and/or serologic tests, and the absence of nasal eosinophilia. The results of this analysis found that subjects who had onset of symptoms later in life (>35 y/o), no family history of allergies, no symptoms around cats or outdoors during the spring but increased symptoms after exposure to perfumes/fragrances had a 96% likelihood of having nonallergic VMR which increased to 98% if the onset of symptoms began after age 45 (35). It is not surprising that the only finding from this study supported by the results of the observational questionnaire studies summarized in Table 1 was age of onset because none of these studies utilized well-defined criteria for establishing their rhinitis subtype populations. Confirmation of Brandt et al.'s findings requires further validation in larger populations by multiple investigators. However, studies designed to identify predictive features of chronic rhinitis subtypes have important ramifications with respect to health-care utilization and pharmacoeconomics, as a more accurate diagnosis of chronic rhinitis will lead to more effective treatment recommendations and better clinical outcomes (36).

CONCLUSIONS

The accurate diagnosis of chronic rhinitis requires a careful medical history to ascertain relevant symptoms, frequency, time of year and aggravating triggers in conjunction with a physical examination and confirmatory prick/puncture skin or serum-specific IgE testing. However, primary-care physicians, who usually are the first to encounter the chronic rhinitis patient, are often unaware of how to differentiate between allergic and nonallergic forms of this disease (37,38). Once seen by a primary care physician, diagnosis is usually based solely on clinical symptoms and family history. Demoly et al. found that only 11% of primary care physicians ordered laboratory tests for patients presenting with chronic rhinitis symptoms, and only 10.3% of these patients were subsequently referred to an allergy specialist (39).

The history provided by patients with chronic rhinitis can be confusing and misleading, especially when one considers that many patients with chronic rhinitis have "mixed" disease triggered by both allergic and nonallergic environmental factors. Therefore, the need to better characterize patients with chronic rhinitis by performing confirmatory skin prick or serum-specific IgE testing is essential. Furthermore, many questions patients are asked to ascertain a diagnosis of AR are often nonspecific. For example, symptoms during the spring, summer or fall are commonly confused with temperature and/or barometric pressure changes. Similarly, symptoms around dust may indicate dust mite sensitization or represent a nonallergic irritation of the nasal passages. In contrast, symptoms in response to cat-, dog-, or other furry animal exposure strongly correlated with a physician diagnosis of AR (35).

Compared to AR, NAR is not as well understood. Validated AR questionnaires have been previously developed. For example QOL and clinical drug trial questionnaires for AR have been extensively used. However, instruments that phrase questions more accurately to correlate with physician diagnosis of AR are still needed.

Very few studies have even attempted to characterize NAR and only one study to date has developed and validated a questionnaire to differentiate AR from NAR patients. The lack of interest in developing questionnaires for assessing NAR and for differentiating between NAR subtypes is perplexing when one takes into consideration how different treatment is for these two disorders.

Clinical characteristics determined to be significant for diagnosis of chronic rhinitis by various investigators are fairly heterogeneous and often are contradictory to one another. This is largely because previous questionnaire studies that have differentiated between AR and NAR did not distinguish between MR and the NAR subtypes, NARES and VMR. Brandt and Bernstein found in their study that certain characteristics should be retained as part of the consensus definition of NAR. These include the absence of positive prick skin or serum-specific IgE tests, late age of symptom onset, the absence of symptoms during the spring or around furry animals and aggravation of symptoms around irritants like perfumes or fragrances. Whether other phenotypic characteristics commonly associated with NAR, such as temperature or barometric pressure changes or response to specific medication(s) should be retained, requires further investigation.

Larger studies using validated questionnaires that include characteristics predictive of NAR patients should be conducted in the primary-care setting to determine whether these instruments actually improve the diagnosis, treatment and clinical outcomes of chronic rhinitis subtypes such as NAR compared to the current empiric/therapeutic approach currently used by most clinicians. These studies should also test the inter-reliability of several doctors diagnosing index patients with NAR subtypes such as VMR. It is essential that if studies of this magnitude are conducted in the future that consensus definitions of chronic rhinitis subtypes be developed at the onset.

In summary, chronic rhinitis is a very prevalent disease that is often trivialized and therefore inaccurately diagnosed, leading to inadequate management and unnecessary health care expenditures. The availability of a well-designed short questionnaire that correlates with physician diagnosis of NAR subtypes may serve to modify the current approach taken by primary-care physicians for evaluating and treating this disorder. The difficulty in reliably diagnosing allergic and MR emphasizes the need for primary-care physicians to work more closely with allergy specialists in order to characterize their patients' atopic status early on, thereby preventing inappropriate health care expenditures and unnecessary comorbidities.

REFERENCES

1. Bellanti JA, Wallerstedt DB. Allergic rhinitis update: epidemiology and natural history. Allergy Asthma Proc 2000; 21(6):367–370.
2. Reed SD, Lee TA, McCrory DC. The economic burden of allergic rhinitis: a critical evaluation of the literature. Pharmacoeconomics 2004; 22(6):345–361.
3. Dykewicz MS, et al. Joint task force algorithm and annotations for diagnosis and management of rhinitis. Ann Allergy Asthma Immunol 1998; 81(5 Pt 2):469–473.
4. Settipane RA, Settipane GA. Nonallergic rhinitis. In: Kaliner MA, ed. Current Review of Rhinitis. Philadelphia, 2002:53–65.
5. Settipane RA. Rhinitis: a dose of epidemiological reality. Allergy Asthma Proc 2003; 24(3):147–154.
6. Dykewicz MS, Fineman S, Skoner DP. Joint task force summary statements on diagnosis and management of rhinitis. Ann Allergy Asthma Immunol 1998; 81(5 Pt 2):474–477.
7. Lindberg S, Malm L. Comparison of allergic rhinitis and vasomotor rhinitis patients on the basis of a computer questionnaire. Allergy 1993; 48(8):602–607.
8. Enberg RN. Perennial nonallergic rhinitis: a retrospective review. Ann Allergy 1989; 63(6 Pt 1):513–516.
9. Mullarkey MF. Eosinophilic nonallergic rhinitis. J Allergy Clin Immunol 1988; 82(5 Pt 2): 941–949.
10. Togias A. Age relationships and clinical features of nonallergic rhinitis. J Allergy Clin Immunol 1990; 85:182.
11. Leynaert B, et al. Perennial rhinitis: an independent risk factor for asthma in nonatopic subjects: results from the European Community Respiratory Health Survey. J Allergy Clin Immunol 1999; 104(2 Pt 1):301–304.
12. Mullarkey MF, Hill JS, Webb DR. Allergic and nonallergic rhinitis: their characterization with attention to the meaning of nasal eosinophilia. J Allergy Clin Immunol 1980; 65(2):122–126.
13. Bryant FB. Assessing the validity of measurement. In: Grimm LG, Yarnold PR, eds. Reading and Understanding More Multivariate Statistics. 1st ed. Washington, D.C.: American Psychological Association, 2000:99–146.
14. Rummel RJ. Applied Factor Analysis. Evanston: Northwestern University Press, 1970.
15. Cronbach LJ. Coefficient alpha and the internal structure of tests. Psychometrika 1951; 16:297–334.
16. Asher MI, Weiland SK. The international study of asthma and allergies in childhood (ISAAC). ISAAC steering committee. Clin Exp Allergy 1998; 28(suppl 5):52–66; discussion 90–91.
17. Keil U, et al. The international study of asthma and allergies in childhood (ISAAC): objectives and methods; results from German ISAAC centres concerning traffic density and wheezing and allergic rhinitis. Toxicol Lett 1996; 86(2–3):99–103.
18. Vanna AT, et al. International study of asthma and allergies in childhood: validation of the rhinitis symptom questionnaire and prevalence of rhinitis in schoolchildren in Sao Paulo, Brazil. Pediatr Allergy Immunol 2001; 12(2):95–101.

19. Jones NS, et al. The prevalence of allergic rhinitis and nasal symptoms in Nottingham. Clin Otolaryngol Allied Sci 1998; 23(6):547–554.
20. Juniper EF. Measuring health-related quality of life in rhinitis. J Allergy Clin Immunol 1997; 99(2):S742–S749.
21. Juniper EF, et al. Development and validation of the mini rhinoconjunctivitis quality of life questionnaire. Clin Exp Allergy 2000; 30(1):132–140.
22. Juniper EF, et al. Clinical outcomes and adverse effect monitoring in allergic rhinitis. J Allergy Clin Immunol 2005; 115(3 Pt 2):S390–S413.
23. Braat JP, et al. Pollutional and meteorological factors are closely related to complaints of non-allergic, non-infectious perennial rhinitis patients: a time series model. Clin Exp Allergy 2002; 32(5):690–697.
24. Sanico A, Togias A. Noninfectious, nonallergic rhinitis (NINAR): considerations on possible mechanisms. Am J Rhinol 1998; 12(1):65–72.
25. Olsson P, et al. Prevalence of self-reported allergic and non-allergic rhinitis symptoms in Stockholm: relation to age, gender, olfactory sense and smoking. Acta Otolaryngol 2003; 123(1):75–80.
26. Jessen M, Janzon L. Prevalence of non-allergic nasal complaints in an urban and a rural population in Sweden. Allergy 1989; 44(8):582–587.
27. Sibbald B, Rink E. Epidemiology of seasonal and perennial rhinitis: clinical presentation and medical history. Thorax 1991; 46(12):895–901.
28. Settipane GA, Klein DE. Non allergic rhinitis: demography of eosinophils in nasal smear, blood total eosinophil counts and IgE levels. N Engl Reg Allergy Proc 1985; 6(4):363–366.
29. Ryden O, Andersson B, Andersson M. Disease perception and social behaviour in persistent rhinitis: a comparison between patients with allergic and nonallergic rhinitis. Allergy 2004; 59(4):461–464.
30. Kaliner M. Progressive management strategies in the treatment of rhinitis. Allergy Asthma Proc 2003; 24(3):163–169.
31. Montnemery P, et al. Prevalence of nasal symptoms and their relation to self-reported asthma and chronic bronchitis/emphysema. Eur Respir J 2001; 17(4):596–603.
32. Mann SS, et al. Assessment of olfactory status in allergic and non-allergic rhinitis patients. Indian J Physiol Pharmacol 2002; 46(2):186–194.
33. Simola M, Malmberg H. Sense of smell in allergic and nonallergic rhinitis. Allergy 1998; 53(2):190–194.
34. Doty RL, et al. Smell identification ability: changes with age. Science 1984; 226(4681):1441–1443.
35. Brandt D, Bernstein JA. Questionnaire evaluation and risk factor identification for non-allergic vasomotor rhinitis. Ann Allergy Asthma Immunol 2006; 96(4):526–553.
36. Wang DY, et al. Rhinitis: do diagnostic criteria affect the prevalence and treatment? Allergy 2002; 57(2):150–154.
37. Wang DY, Chan A, Smith JD. Management of allergic rhinitis: a common part of practice in primary care clinics. Allergy 2004; 59(3):315–319.
38. Wang DY, Raza MT, Gordon BR. Control of nasal obstruction in perennial allergic rhinitis. Curr Opin Allergy Clin Immunol 2004; 4(3):165–170.
39. Demoly P, Allaert FA, Lecasble M. ERASM, a pharmacoepidemiologic survey on management of intermittent allergic rhinitis in every day general medical practice in France. Allergy 2002; 57(6):546–554.

5 Differential Diagnosis of Eosinophilic Chronic Rhinosinusitis

John C. Sok and Berrylin J. Ferguson

Department of Otolaryngology, University of Pittsburgh School of Medicine, Pittsburgh, Pennsylvania, U.S.A.

INTRODUCTION

Chronic rhinosinusitis (CRS) affects over 30 million persons in the United States each year and accounts for 11.6 million visits to physicians' offices (1–3). It is increasingly apparent that CRS represents a variety of subtypes, each of which may differ in severity, associated comorbidities, optimal therapies, and prognosis. Past studies of CRS, which lump all subtypes together provide only limited insight with regard to comorbid associations and the efficacy of various targeted medical or surgical therapies. In 2004, a consensus was reached in defining CRS and recommending research parameters, which was drawn from representatives from the organized academies of general allergy, otolaryngology, otolaryngic allergy, and rhinology (4). A general grouping of CRS into forms with nasal polyps (NPs) and without NPs was proposed. A further subgrouping of CRS into either eosinophilic or noneosinophilic histopathologies was suggested. This strategy could potentially aid in identifying targeted therapies for each subtype of CRS, which might not have been appreciated in studies of a more heterogeneous collection of patients with CRS. The most refractory of the subgroups of CRS are those associated with eosinophilia. This chapter will review the epidemiologic evidence of eosinophilic CRS (ECRS) with regard to severity of disease and prognosis, as well as mechanisms that may account for more extensive disease in the eosinophilic conditions. Finally, potentially different and possibly overlapping mechanisms and associations that might serve as a further subgrouping of ECRS will be discussed, both pathophysiologically and in the context of potential logical targeted therapeutic interventions.

REVIEW OF STUDIES OF CRS AND EOSINOPHILIA

Both associated serum eosinophilia and histologic eosinophilia in patients with CRS is associated with more extensive disease and a decreased likelihood of surgical success. In 1994, Newman et al. (5) reported the first large series of patients with symptoms of CRS, which uncovered the association between eosinophilia and extensive sinus disease. In their landmark study of 98 patients, serum and tissue samples were assayed for various immunologic parameters, including immunoglobulin (Ig) E antibodies and total eosinophil counts, and were compared with radiologic analysis of sinus disease extent by computed tomography (CT). This study found a strong positive correlation between the extent of disease and eosinophilia. Sixty-five percent of those with extensive disease had eosinophilia compared with only 7% of patients with limited disease ($p < 0.001$). In vitro allergy positivity was present in only 19 of 95 patients (20%), whereas 8 of 13 patients (62%) with both extensive disease and serum eosinophilia had negative in vitro allergy tests. Thus, more than half the patients with ECRS did not have evidence of allergy. Although all patients had at least one bacterial organism cultured, the majority were coagulase-negative staphylococci. The significance of this as a pathogen is questioned, because normal subjects and asymptomatic patients have an equal incidence of coagulase-negative staphylococcus presence in cultures from their nose and sinuses (5). This same investigative group reported on additional immunologic parameters in 80 patients with CRS in a subsequent publication, in which 37 (46%) patients demonstrated extensive sinus disease. The peripheral eosinophil count (>200 cells/μL) had the strongest correlation to greater disease as measured by the CT scoring criteria. Eosinophilia was observed in 76% of patients with extensive disease compared to 21% in limited disease. The association of eosinophils with the extent of disease was independent of asthma, atopy, or age. There was no correlation with extent of CT disease and any of the following: IgE, IgA, IgG1, IgG2, and IgG3 (6).

In a study of 48 adult CRS patients, Szucs et al. reported that the intensity of the eosinophilic infiltration in the diseased sinus mucosa correlated significantly with the severity of the mucosal inflammation, independent of atopic status. However, 20% to 40% of the patients with CRS had no eosinophilic inflammation of the mucosa (7). Baroody et al. reported similar results in 34 children with CRS; specifically there were significantly more eosinophils in the lamina propria of CRS sinuses (median 32.8 cells/0.5 mm^2, $p = 0.0004$) than in normal ethmoid sinus mucosa (median 0 cells/0.5 mm^2) (8).

Sobol et al. compared the tissue inflammation in CRS in adults with tissue inflammation in CRS in children and in control subjects. T-lymphocytes, eosinophils, and basophils were higher in subjects with CRS, whether adult or child, than in control subjects. The degree of tissue eosinophilia was significantly greater in adults with CRS than in children with CRS (9). Similarly, Chan et al. also reported that adults had a higher density of submucosal eosinophils than children with CRS (10). In addition, children with CRS had a higher density of submucosal lymphocytes, a thinner and more intact epithelium, a thinner basement membrane, and fewer submucosal mucous glands compared to adult CRS controls. They interpreted the lower eosinophilia and fewer morphologic abnormalities in young children compared to adults as evidence of a greater potential for reversibility of CRS and higher potential for cure in children than in adults (10).

Zadeh et al., in a retrospective review of 620 patients with CRS, found that 31 patients (5%) had elevated serum eosinophilia. Despite this low incidence of peripheral eosinophilia, these patients were significantly more likely to have polyps (77% vs. 15%), allergic fungal sinusitis (AFS; 39% vs. 3%), and asthma (35% vs. 24%), as compared to CRS patients with normal eosinophil counts. Postoperatively, patients with serum eosinophilia were more likely to be diagnosed with recurrent sinus infections (94% vs. 32%), recurrent polyps (35% vs. 3%), and require revision surgery (84% vs. 24%). In summary, presence of increased serum eosinophilia was associated with a worse prognosis in every parameter compared with CRS patients without an increase in serum eosinophilia (11).

Despite the increased awareness of eosinophilia both histologically and serologically as a marker of increased disease and a worse prognosis with regard to surgical intervention in CRS, no study to date has subcategorized patients regarding possible etiologic factors for tissue eosinophilia. Allergy is one cause, but certainly not the only cause of eosinophilia, and, in multiple studies, the correlation of eosinophilia to atopic status is weak or absent.

PATHOPHYSIOLOGIC ROLE OF THE EOSINOPHIL

The eosinophil is a granular, bilobed leukocyte, which comprises approximately 2% to 5% of granulocytes in a nonallergic person. Eosinophil progenitors are released from the blood marrow into the circulation and are chemically attracted to the sites of inflammation by chemotrophic factors. Locally, tissue eosinophilia is induced by three canonical pathways. The dominant pathway is mediated by the TH_2-type immune response, with interleukin (IL)-5 as the major mediator. However, both innate immunity and TH_1 immune response are also capable of inducing tissue eosinophilia in the absence of a TH_2 response (12). Nonetheless, the role of these leukocytes in the context of tissue inflammation remains poorly understood. Eosinophils contain a variety of toxic proinflammatory mediators, including preformed granule proteins [such as the major basic protein, eosinophil cationic protein (ECP), and eosinophil-derived neurotoxin], reactive oxygen species, lipid mediators, and cytokines that could contribute to inflammation (12,13). When these preformed granules are released, the mediators can inflict damage to the surrounding tissue. In the asthma model, the major basic protein antagonizes M2 muscarinic receptors in the airways and contributes to neural mechanisms of airway hyperreactivity. The role of M2 muscarinic antagonism by major basic protein in the upper airway is unexplored.

Eosinophils also are a major source of tissue remodeling factors. A study by Dunnill demonstrated that eosinophil-induced myofibroblast differentiation can be blocked by an antibody against transforming growth factor-β (TGFβ) (14), indicating a crucial role of TGFβ-mediated eosinophilia in tissue remodeling. In addition, the presence of other tissue-remodeling factors such as TGFα, heparin-binding epidermal growth factor, platelet-derived growth factor-β, and vascular endothelial factor have been reported (15). Although eosinophils also produce leukotrienes (LTs), IL-4, IL-5, and eotaxin, far greater amounts of these cytokines are produced by other cells. Further complicating the role of the eosinophil in the pathogenesis of ECRS is the participation of other inflammatory cells, including T-cells, mast cells, and basophils. Biological redundancy is observed as these other inflammatory cells also cause excess mucus secretion, vascular leak, and epithelial injury through higher production of these eosinophil-associated mediators (12,13). Intriguingly, there is a growing body of evidence to suggest that eosinophils also have immune-modulatory effects on the inflammatory response in addition to their established role as toxic effector cells. This modulation is produced through a wide variety of cytokines, including TH_2-type cytokines (IL-4, IL-5, IL-6, and IL-13), TH_1-type cytokines (interferon-γ and IL-12), nonpolarizing cytokines [IL-1, IL-2, IL-3, and IL-16, granulocyte macrophage–colony-stimulating factor (GM-CSF), tumor necrosis factor-α], immunoregulatory cytokines (IL-10 and IL-18), and chemokines (IL-8, regulated upon activation, normal T-cell expressed and secreted, eotaxin, and macrophage inflammatory protein-α) (15). However, because these eosinophil-derived cytokines are ubiquitously produced in greater quantities by the other inflammatory cells, the biological relevance of these cytokines is still unknown and warrants further investigation.

Targeting the eosinophil for ECRS therapy requires the identification of molecular feature(s) that distinguishes the eosinophil from other inflammatory cells. Although intensive efforts have been initiated, such as the international leukocyte typing workshops that assemble large panels of monoclonal antibodies (mAbs) (16) and gene chip cDNA microarray studies (17), it is becoming evident that there is no one single known marker that is uniquely expressed on the surface of eosinophils. Among over 100 candidate cell surface molecules (18), the recently identified surface structures that are currently the object of therapeutic interest include the costimulatory molecules CD28 and CD86, the prostaglandin (PG) D_2 receptor $CRTH_2$, the proapoptotic sialic acid–binding Ig-like lectin 8, and members of the inhibitory and activating leukocyte Ig-like receptor family (LIR1, LIR2, LIR3, and LIR7) (13).

To date, there have been three major approaches to eliminate or significantly reduce the level of circulating eosinophils in order to study its role in the pathogenesis of inflammatory diseases:

1. Targeting IL-5
2. Dual targeting of IL-5 and eotaxin
3. Targeting the eosinophil peroxidase promotor

Within the bone marrow, IL-5 is the major hematopoietin responsible for terminal differentiation of human eosinophils. Using a humanized monoclonal antibody to IL-5 in 24 patients, Leckie et al. reported 80% to 90% reduction in he number of circulating eosinophils as well as sputum eosinophilia. However, the treatment had no impact on asthma or allergen-induced early- or late-phase reactions, raising serious concerns regarding the eosinophil as a therapeutic target (19). Subsequent analysis of this study revealed that it was statistically underpowered to make any conclusion regarding efficacy (20). Moreover, a remarkable observation was made, which demonstrated that human eosinophils entering the airway lose their surface receptors for IL-5, yet display an enhanced level of another eosinophil-activating cytokine, GM-CSF (21). Therefore, subsequent murine models have shown that targeting both IL-5 and eotaxin, an eosinophil-specific C–C chemokine, was required for greater inhibition of eosinophilia and airway hyperreactivity (22). Because IL-5–directed therapies failed to completely eliminate eosinophils, attempts have been made to develop other strategies. More recently, a novel strategy was employed using a transgenic mouse model in order to engineer a true "eosinophil knockout mouse" (23). This approach was based on the lineage-specific expression of a cytocidal protein (diphtheria toxin A) driven by a promoter fragment identified from an eosinophil-specific gene. By cloning the highly expressed eosinophil peroxidase promoter into a cytocidal gene, investigators generated a new strain of mice (PHIL that are specifically devoid of eosinophils, but otherwise have a full complement of hematopoietically derived cells. In this landmark study, the targeted ablation of eosinophils had significant effects on allergen-induced pulmonary pathology. Overall, ovalbumin (OVA)-induced histopathology in PHIL mice was attenuated relative to OVA-treated wild-type littermates, manifested by the reduced airway epithelial hypertrophy and pulmonary mucus accumulation (23). These findings clearly suggest a causative role for eosinophils in allergen-induced pulmonary pathology. Therefore, the development of an eosinophil-deficient mouse now permits an unambiguous assessment of a number of human diseases that have been linked to this granulocyte, including susceptibility to helminthic parasite infections, viral infections, tumorigenesis, and allergic diseases such as allergic rhinitis and ECRS.

PATHOGENESIS-BASED SUBCLASSIFICATION OF ECRS

In this section, we present a clinical subclassification of ECRS based on underlying etiologies of tissue eosinophilia and putative therapeutic interventions. The following distinct and potentially overlapping and cosynergistic mechanisms will be discussed as causes of ECRS: Superantigen-induced ECRS (SAI-ECRS), AFS, nonallergic fungal (NAF)-ECRS, and aspirin-exacerbated (AE)-ECRS (AE-ECRS), which is also known as "aspirin triad."

Superantigen-Induced ECRS

"Superantigens" is the term for a group of polypeptide molecules that are extremely potent in stimulating T-cell activation. Superantigens activate larger subpopulations of the T-lymphocyte pool (5% to 30%) than conventional antigens (<0.01%), by binding to the outside of the major histocompatibility complex class II (MHC II), which is also known as human leukocyte antigen class II (HLA II) on antigen-presenting cells (APCs) and cross-linking the APC to the T-cell by simultaneously binding the T-cell receptor (TCR), in its variable beta (Vβ) portion, also outside the T-cell's antigen-specific peptide groove (Fig. 1). This activation of the T-cell thus occurs without antigen peptide specificity, because the activation merely requires that the superantigen bind to the outside of HLA II molecule and the TCR. The frequency of these binding sites will be greater than the frequency of

T Lymphocyte

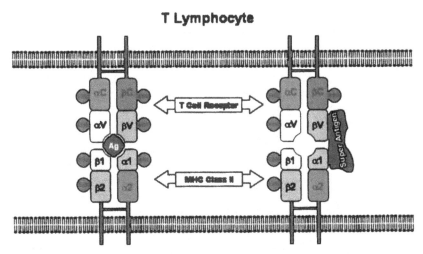

Antigen Presenting Cell

FIGURE 1   Schematic diagram of the conventional antigen ("Ag") presentation by the MHC class II receptor of the antigen presenting cell (*left*) and the presentation of the superantigen by engagement of the α-region of MHC class II to the variable ("V")β region of the T-cell receptor (*left*); "C" represents the constant region; "CHO" represent the glycosylation of the α and β chains. *Abbreviation*: MHC, major histocompatibility complex.

any single antigen fitting the peptide groove, and will differ genetically depending on the MHC II makeup of an individual. For example, a superantigen may be better able to bind to a portion of the APCs of an individual with certain HLA II genetic presence, than to an individual who lacks that particular HLA II molecule. The T-cells activated by superantigen are thus polyclonal with regard to a variety of different antigen specificities based on TCR peptide binding, but which will have a similar Vβ clonality (24). The end result is that conventional antigen specificity is bypassed.

One of the earliest proponents of the superantigen hypothesis is Schubert in 2001 (25), who proposed a unifying model for the creation of chronic eosinophilic–lymphocytic respiratory mucosal disorders by microbial superantigens. By drawing information available from other inflammatory disorders, he proposed that microbial persistence, superantigen production, and host T-lymphocyte response are fundamental components unifying all common chronic severe inflammatory disease. In this model, heterogeneity of immunopathologic signals creates immunopathology, which is amplified through T-cell stimulation by persistent superantigens in the genetically susceptible host, resulting in the chronic inflammatory disorder. The coexisting "immunopathologic" signals include Type I hypersensitivity, cellular antigen-specific immune responses, TH_1/TH_2 dysregulation, and ecosinoid and other cytokine dysregulation; and when combined with superantigen-induced T-lymphocyte activation, they could contribute to the apparent heterogeneity of the disease.

Schubert et al., in support of the concept that disease initiated by superantigen would be more prevalent in certain HLA subpopulations, reported that patients with AFS (66% of 44 patients) were significantly more likely to carry the DQB1*0302 allele than patients with non-AFS but hyperplastic sinus disease (HSD; 50% of 30 patients). Both the AFS groups and the HSD groups were more likely to carry this HLA allele than historical normal controls. DQB1*03 allelic variants did not correlate with allergy skin test results, atopic status, total serum IgE levels, culture results, asthma, or aspirin nonsteroidal anti-inflammatory drug hypersensitivity (26).

Among a broad range of infectious microorganisms that are capable of producing superantigens, the most notorious is *Staphylococcus aureus*. *S. aureus* produces more than a dozen different exotoxins ranging in size between 22 and 30 kD that are capable of eliciting the superantigen response, including toxic shock syndrome toxin 1 (TSST-1) as well as Staphylococcus enterotoxin A (SEA), SEB, SEC, etc. In a recent study of 13 patients with NPs, Bernstein et al. demonstrated the evidence of SEA, SEB, or TSST production in 55% of patients (27). Although seven patients had IgE-mediated allergy, only five of the seven with exotoxin-producing Staphylococcus demonstrated IgE-mediated allergy. Two of four aspirin intolerant/asthmatics had exotoxin-producing *S. aureus* cultured from their polyps. Most telling was the quantitative analysis of the preferential expansion of T-lymphocytes with a distinct Vβ region by flow cytometry, demonstrating Vβ clonal expansion in three patients. The authors termed the resulting histopathology "chronic lymphocytic–eosinophilic nasal mucosal disease." Indeed, the T-cell upregulation would be expected to form lymphocytic aggregates of T-cells and potentially B-cells. The local inflammatory cytokine milieu may induce B-cells to become activated and stimulate isotope class switch to IgE antibodies against the superantigen or any other antigen in proximity. The authors also speculate that these toxins not only lead to T-cell upregulation, but they also may cause epithelial irregularities, leading to the initial event in the development of nasal polyposis (27). In a follow-up article by the same group, similar results were recapitulated in 19 patients with nasal polyposis. Sixty percent of patients demonstrated *S. aureus* with SEA, SEB, or TSST-1 production and clonal proliferation of T-lymphocytes with Vβ expansion of clones 1, 5, and 7 for SEA; 3,12, and 14 for SEB; and β expansion of clone 2 for TSST-1 (28). The study by Seiberling et al. is most recent and the largest study to date (*n* = 29 patients), which identified at least one type of *S. aureus* superantigen detected in 14 of 29 (48%) patients with bilateral nasal polyposis. Moreover, 9 of the 14 patients also had positive findings for additional toxins. Intriguingly, higher mean eosinophil counts were also correlated with the superantigen-positive patients (29).

In an earlier study of patients with nasal polyposis, Bachert et al. indirectly demonstrated the presence of SEA and SEB in 10 of 20 (50%) patients via the upregulation of specific IgE antibodies to these superantigens in homogenized NP tissue (30). In addition, many of the superantigen-positive patients in this study were "nonallergic" on allergy prick testing. This suggests that a local allergic response may be important and provides evidence of a specific IgE-mediated response to the superantigen itself. Thus, superantigens also appear to have the capacity to act as classic antigens in addition to stimulating nonspecific T-cell activation. Interestingly, the latest article by the same research group reports that IgE antibodies to *S. aureus* superantigens were found in the majority of polyp tissues from aspirin-sensitive patients and were associated with a substantial increase in ECP and IL-5 (31). In addition, there is new evidence to suggest that superantigens may also cause downregulation of prostaglandin E2 (PGE2) in airway mucosal tissues, potentially resulting in the development of AE respiratory disease (C. Bachert, personal communication; 11th Congress of the International Rhinologic Society). Noteworthily, this is a paradoxical observation in contrast to other studies with animal models, which demonstrate the upregulation of PGE2 by *S. aureus* superantigens (32,33).

Therapy of SAI-ECRS could, in theory, target the infectious microorganisms responsible for its production. In the majority of cases, this could be *S. aureus*, because this colonizes a third of individuals, and its exotoxin was present in 48% to 60% of patients (27–29). Interestingly, all *S. aureus* produced at least one isoform of the exotoxin in these series. Bernstein et al. advocated the use of a topical antistaphylococcal medication, mupirocin, in these patients (27); however, efficacy for this approach has yet to be seen (30). In addition, vigorous saline nasal washes could wash away proinflammatory cytokines as well as bacteria from the nose. It is possible that exotoxin-producing bacteria could live in biofilms, which would make them resistant to systemic antimicrobials, but amenable to removal with vigorous nasal washings and cleansings, possibly augmented with topical antimicrobials. Other topical agents that inhibit T-cell proliferation via inhibition of calcineurin (e.g., pimecrolimus 1% cream, approved for the treatment of atopic dermatitis) may also have a role in superantigen-induced inflammation of the nose. As in all the ECRS forms, either systemic steroids or topical steroids offer some therapeutic efficacy. Given the recent evidence that SAI-ECRS is also associated with significant upregulation of specific IgE antibodies (30,31), the pathogenesis of SAI-ECRS may be ameliorated by the introduction of anti-IgE antibodies. Recently, a humanized mouse monoclonal antibody that binds specifically to the constant region of the IgE heavy chain has been engineered and has been demonstrated to be effective in the treatment of allergic rhinitis (34,35). Anti-IgE therapy for chronic sinusitis is currently under phase IV clinical trials (Table 1) (36).

TABLE 1 Pathogenesis-Based Subclassification of Eosinophilic Chronic Rhinosinusitis with Therapeutic Interventions by Reported and Therapeutic Efficacy

	Proposed mechanisms	Steroids systemic or topical	Immuno-therapy	Leukotriene modulator	Calcineurin inhibition	Anti-bacterials systemic or topical	Anti-fungals systemic or topical	Anti-IgE	Aspirin desensitization
SAI-ECRS	Superantigen upregulation from bacteria (Staphylococcus) or other microorganisms, i.e., fungus	+++		?	?	++		+	
AFS	IgE-mediated hypersensitivity to fungus growing in mucin	+++	++	+?			++	+	
NAF-ECRS	Non-IgE-mediated hypersensitivity to fungus in nose and mucin	+++		+?			+		
AE-ECRS	Leukotriene overproduction	+++		++				?	++

Abbreviations: ECRS, eosinophilic chronic rhinosinusitis; SAI-ECRS, superantigen-induced ECRS; AFS, allergic fungal sinusitis; NAF-ECRS, nonallergic fungal ECRS; AE-ECRS, aspirin-exacerbated-ECRS.

The evidence to date regarding the role of superantigens in ECRS suggests that this mechanism may potentially come closer than other mechanisms, which will be discussed in unifying ECRS. Bacterial superantigens may act to produce the cytokine milieu of TH_2 dominance that could lead to the expression of IgE-mediated response to fungi present incidentally in the nose. This could lead to the characteristic picture of AFS. Moreover, if superantigens can downregulate PGE2 expression, they may actually cause aspirin hyperreactivity, because a person who has a deficiency in the 5 lipoxygenase enzyme inhibitor, PGE2 would be even less tolerant of further inhibition of PGE2 via a cyclooxygenase 1 inhibitor such as aspirin or other nonsteroidal anti-inflammatories. As of yet, studies of superantigen-induced ECRS are limited, and to date, no study has specifically addressed whether superantigen-targeted therapies such as culture-directed anti-microbials or drugs that inhibit T-cell activation, such as the calcineurin inhibitors, tacrolimus, or pimecrolimus, are effective. One would predict that steroids, which nonspecifically downregulate inflammation, would be effective for superantigen-induced ECRS.

It is possible that there are multiple codependent and interacting causes of ECRS. It is even possible that *S. aureus*–producing superantigens may exist as a biofilm, as has been reported in atopic dermatitis (37). Biofilms are communities of bacteria and or fungi which often coexist and grow on foreign bodies and impaired mucosa. Biofilms are surrounded by a glycocalyx and communicate via quorum sensing. A biofilm would not be expected in and of itself to produce ECRS, but if the biofilm produces substances such as superantigens or provides fungal antigen stimulation to drive AFS, then it is possible that this form of bacterial or fungal growth could be responsible for ECRS. Biofilms are notoriously difficult to cure with antibiotics, although antibiotic therapy may lead to short-term symptom improvement by killing off newly spawned "planktonic bacteria." Biofilms are theoretically an attractive hypothesis to explain the clinical situation in which a patient improves on antibiotics and relapses when antibiotics are withdrawn (38).

Allergic Fungal Sinusitis

First recognized more than 20 years ago because of its histologic similarity to allergic bronchopulmonary aspergillosis, AFS has subsequently come to be recognized as an IgE-mediated response to a variety of fungi, frequently dematiaceous and not usually *Aspergillus*, growing in the eosinophilic mucin of the sinuses. One commonly proposed mechanism is that a patient with an allergic proclivity inhales a fungal spore that, instead of being cleared from the nasal mucosa by normal mucociliary clearance patterns, becomes adherent to the nasal or sinus epithelium long enough to germinate. In the case of the fungus *Alternaria*, this may be less than two hours. The allergic individual secretes eosinophil-rich mucous. The spores and germinated hyphae continue to grow in this allergic mucin, increasing the antigenic stimulation and initiating a positive feedback cycle. The allergy to the germinated hyphae increases the secreted mucous, which allows further growth of the hyphae (39). This theory is supported by the presence of specific IgE to the cultured fungus in a study by Manning et al. (40). Clinically, patients are usually younger, allergic, and mildly asthmatic ($\sim$ one-third), and have unilateral (50%) or bilateral polyps and plugs of sticky eosinophilic translucent green mucin. Sinus CT shows heterogeneity of opacification with the less-intense density of mucosal thickening and the more intense, lighter density of the mucin plugs (39).

Recently, the role of IgE in the etiology of AFS has become more confused. The most stringent requirements for AFS are the presence of specific IgE to the fungus cultured in the eosinophilic mucin, and the demonstration of hyphae in eosinophilic mucin. Most patients have concomitant polyps and characteristic CT changes, neither of which is specific for the diagnosis of AFS. In 2004, Collins et al. in Adelaide, Australia divided patients into four ECRS groups:

1. AFS, i.e., the presence of fungal IgE and fungus in eosinophilic mucin
2. AFS-like, i.e., they had fungal IgE serologically, but no evidence of fungi in the eosinophilic mucin
3. Patients with fungi present in the mucin, but no evidence of fungal IgE serologically, who were termed "nonallergic fungal eosinophilic sinusitis"(NAF-ECRS)
4. Patients with neither IgE to fungus nor fungus in their eosinophilic mucin who were termed "nonallergic nonfungal eosinophilic sinusitis"(NANF-ECRS)

In non allergic rhinitis (NAF)-ECRS and NANF-ECRS, which by definition lacked fungal IgE serologically, they found fungal IgE in the eosinophilic mucin in 19% and 21% of patients in the respective groups. In contrast, in AFS in which all patients had serologic fungal IgE, only 71% had fungal IgE present locally from the sinuses, and only 16% of the AFS-like patients had local fungal IgE (41).

In a follow-up study, Pant described that the only immunologic parameter that separated the above outlined eosinophilic subgroups of Collins (based on fungal presence histologically and serologic IgE to fungus) from non-ECRS patients and allergic patients without sinusitis, was the presence of IgG3 to *Alternaria* (42). In reality, this finding does not negate the significance of IgE in AFS, despite the author's conclusions to the contrary. It has long been appreciated that one may have elevated IgE to fungus in patients with allergic rhinitis who do not develop AFS. The presence of IgE to the fungus may be a necessary but not sufficient condition to develop AFS. In addition to having an allergy to the fungus, the fungus must become lodged in the nose or sinus cavities long enough to germinate and become entrapped in allergic mucin, which the patient is unable to expel. It is assumed that this would occur randomly, with increased occurrence in areas of high mold count or conditions such as the desert or air conditioning, which might cause increased dryness of the nasal mucosa and impair normal mucociliary clearance. Moreover, coimmunologic stimulators such as superantigen presence may be required, and, as already discussed, the susceptibility of individuals to a superantigen will vary with their HLA II genotype. Pant's finding of significantly increased IgG3 to *Alternaria* in the entire group of eosinophilic conditions analyzed compared to non-ECRS and allergic and nonallergic controls speaks to a possible greater fungal exposure or immunologic reaction in patients with ECRS. While the group as a whole demonstrated a mean elevation of IgG3 to *Alternaria*, there were overlapping standard deviations among all subgroups.

The treatment of AFS involves surgical removal of the fungal-infested mucin and polyps; however, recurrence is common. Most clinicians recommend perioperative systemic steroids for several weeks postoperatively, followed by topical steroids. There is one case report of probable efficacy of a LT modulator in AFS (43). Oral and topical antifungal agents may be useful, although only oral itraconazole in the pulmonary form of the disease, allergic bronchopulmonary aspergillosis, has been studied in a randomized, controlled trial and has been shown to be efficacious (44). Vigorous washes of the nose with as much as 20 mL in each nostril of saline with topical steroids and/or antifungal agents may be helpful. Immunotherapy may play a role, although its usefulness has been demonstrated in only retrospective reviews and case–control series. In the most recent retrospective analysis of 60 patients with a diagnosis of AFS, the investigative group at the University of Texas Southwestern, which has been most active in immunotherapy for AFS, reported reoperation rates of 33% in patients not receiving immunotherapy ($n = 24$) compared with 11.1% in those receiving immunotherapy ($n = 36$). Although this is a retrospective comparison, it suggests that immunotherapy is beneficial in reducing recurrence rates in AFS (45). However, with long-term follow-up by this same investigative group, there was found to be no difference in AFS patients treated with immunotherapy and those who were not (Table 1) (46).

Nonallergic Fungal ECRS

In 1999, Ponikau et al. published their review of 99 patients with CRS requiring surgery and noted that almost 90% of them met the criteria for AFS because of the presence of eosinophilic mucin and fungi that could be cultured from the mucous. A smaller number of these patients had hyphae detectable in their histologic specimens. In this series, the authors found that allergy was not detectable in almost half the CRS patients. Therefore, at least half these patients do not have "allergic" fungal sinusitis (47). This finding led to the theory that the response of the eosinophils to the fungi led to the ECRS, and was responsible for most patients' complaints of CRS, primarily by non–IgE-mediated responses. In actuality, in the same paper, the authors studied normal control subjects and found that 100% of them had fungi which could be cultured from their nasal washes (47). This almost ubiquitous finding of a variety of fungi in nasal washes led to the requirement that patients with AFS demonstrate hyphae in the mucin and also an IgE-mediated positivity to the fungus cultured from the mucin. Nevertheless, in some patients, fungi may cause an ECRS independent of IgE-mediated mechanisms. These are the patients who would be designated with the term "nonallergic fungal eosinophilic chronic rhinosinusitis."

Proof of non–IgE-mediated fungal-induced inflammation is supported by in vitro studies of peripheral blood mononuclear cells (PBMCs) from patients with CRS, in which *Alternaria* supernatant can induce IL-5 and IL-13 production from PBMCs from the majority of patients with ECRS, but not in controls. This immune response also occurred when the PBMCs from CRS patients were stimulated with *Aspergillus* (22%) or *Cladosporium* (33%) antigens, but not with *Penicillium*. They also reported no correlation between atopic status and response to fungal supernatants (48).

Other investigators have also noted that, if searched for diligently enough, fungus can be cultured from almost anyone's nose. Stammberger's group found positive cultures in more than 90% of CRS patients, eosinophilic mucin in almost 95%, and fungal elements in 75% on histologic evaluation. Once again, normal control subjects yielded positive fungal cultures in more than 90% of subjects (49). And even with standard laboratory methods, fungus can be cultured from the mucin in 56% of CRS specimens (50). Again, the significance of the presence of fungus is unknown, because it is also present in normal noses.

Ferguson (51), in a review of the literature of AFS compared with eosinophilic mucin rhinosinusitis without fungi, found significant clinical differences between the two groups. Primarily, the AFS patients were less likely to have severe asthma and had unilateral disease approximately 50% of the time, whereas the eosinophilic mucin rhinosinusitis patients virtually always have bilateral disease and more severe asthma, with many of them representing AE-ECRS. It is likely that this non-AFS group represents a number of pathologic mechanisms besides AFS and includes those postulated by Ponikau et al. (52).

Therapy for NAF-ECRS is similar to AFS, with the exception of immunotherapy, which does not have a role in a non–IgE-mediated disease. Topical antifungal washes using 20 mL amphotericin B in distilled water to the nose once or twice a day resulted in symptomatic improvement in 70% of patients (Table 2) (52). Ricchetti et al., in an uncontrolled study utilizing intranasal amphotericin B applied as a 20 mL suspension per nostril twice a day with a bulb syringe for four weeks in patients with NPs, reported disappearance of NPs on endoscopy in 62% of patients with small polyps, and 42% of patients with moderate polyps. None of the patients with obstructing NPs improved, possibly because the very obstruction of the polyps precluded an effective application of the topical amphotericin to the nasal mucosa. Patients who had had prior surgery were significantly more likely to respond, again presumably the surgery allowed better access of the amphotericin to the sinus cavities as well as to the nasal cavities (53). The first double-blind placebo–controlled study of topical amphotericin utilized a smaller dose (200 μL, four times a day in a spray bottle for eight weeks), excluded patients with AFS and enrolled all other CRS patients. The end point for success was set at a 50% reduction in Sinus CT mucosal thickening. No significant differences were noted, although the patients utilizing the amphotericin spray complained significantly more often of nasal blockage and burning. In reality two of the amphotericin spray patients and none of the placebo–controlled patients met the rather rigid requirement of a 50% reduction in sinus CT mucosal thickening, suggesting that possibly a small subgroup of non-AFS, CRS patients may respond to even very small doses of topical amphotericin (54). The delivery method of a bulb syringe, more volume and higher concentrations of amphotericin, would intuitively lead to a higher success rate. In the most recent blind controlled study, the end point set by Ponikau et al. was considerably less rigorous than a 50% improvement in CT scores. After a six-month treatment period of unselected CRS patients with either 20 mL of amphotericin delivered in a manner similar to the initial uncontrolled study or a placebo of colored water, the amphotericin group had a significantly greater reduction in sinus CT mucosal thickening

TABLE 2 Studies on the Effect of Topical Amphotericin B in the Treatment of Chronic Rhinosinusitis

	Entry criteria	Design	Amphotericin B dose	Result
Ponikau, 2002	CRS	NR, NB $n=51$	20 mL b.i.d. 100 μg/ mL × >3 mo	Imp in 75%
Ricchetti, 2002	NPs	NR, NB $n=74$	20 mL b.i.d. 1:1000 × 4 wk	Resolution of polyps in 42% to 62% of moderate and mild NP, 0% severe
Weschta 2004	NP without AFS	R, DB, PC $n=74$	200 μL spray q.i.d. × 8 wk	NS imp
Ponikau, 2005	CRS	R, DB, PC $n=24$	20 mL b.i.d. 100 μg/mL × 6 mo	8% imp in CT

Abbreviations: NR, nonrandomized; NB, nonblinded; R, randomized; DB, double blind; PC, placebo controlled; NP, nasal polyps; CRS, chronic rhinosinusitis; AFS, allergic fungal sinusitis; Ns, No significant; imp = improvement.

compared to controls of an underwhelming 8%. There was no difference in symptom scores between the two groups (55).

Aspirin-Exacerbated ECRS

In 1897, a German chemist named Felix Hoffmann developed aspirin as a treatment to ease his father's rheumatic pains. Since then, aspirin has been widely recognized as one of the safest and most frequently consumed drugs of all times. However, the association of bronchospasm after aspirin ingestion was recognized soon after its introduction; and in 1922, Widal et al. was the first to publish the association of aspirin sensitivity, asthma, and NPs (56). There are multiple terms that have been described for this entity; the most widely accepted terms include "aspirin-exacerbated respiratory disease" (AERD) and "aspirin-induced asthma." However, in the context of ECRS, the most appropriate term is "aspirin-exacerbated disease" ECRS (AE–ECRS).

The incidence of aspirin sensitivity in asthmatic adults is 3% to 5%; however, this percentage can triple when asthmatic patients are challenged with ASA. Recently, this disorder has been extensively reviewed by Szczeklik and Stevenson who are the pioneers of aspirin desensitization therapy and are among the leaders of this field (57). It is now well recognized that the principal mediator of aspirin sensitivity is the overproduction of cysteinyl LTs (Cys-LTs). Cys-LTs are potent bronchoconstrictors, causing airway edema and mucus production. The synthesis of Cys-LTs is catalyzed from arachidonic acid metabolism by the enzyme, 5-lipoxygenase. At homeostasis, the production of Cys-LTs is inhibited by PGE_2, a product of cyclooxygenase oxidation, through the inhibition of 5-lipoxygenase. Aspirin and other nonselective nonsteroidal anti-inflammatory agents such as ibuprofen inhibit cyclooxygenase and downregulate the production of PGE_2. Therefore, aspirin can potentially increase production of Cys-LTs via disinhibition of 5-lipoxygenase through PGE_2 reduction, resulting in increased bronchospasm and mucous secretion (Fig. 2).

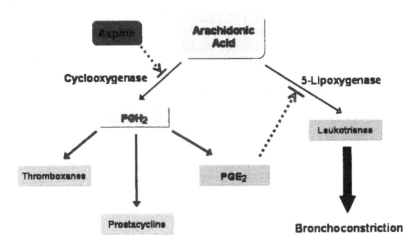

FIGURE 2 Schematic diagram of the pathway leading to the pathophysiologic upregulation of leukotrienes by the irreversible inhibition of the cyclooxygenase enzyme by aspirin. Inhibitory pathways are denoted by dashed arrows.

To date, there are no approved in vitro tests for AE-ECRS, and diagnosis is usually made by medical history or potentially by provocation challenges with aspirin or other nonselective nonsteroidal anti-inflammatory agents. Consequently, this is an area under active investigation. Sousa et al. demonstrated significantly higher number of leukocytes expressing a specific receptor to Cys-LTs (Cys-LT1R) in the aspirin-sensitive patients compared with the non–aspirin-sensitive patients (58). Moreover, their study demonstrated that the application of lysine aspirin (a form of aspirin used in desensitization therapy) resulted in significant downregulation of Cys-LT1R expression when compared with the application of placebo (58). More recently, a study by Kowalski et al. uncovered differential levels of an arachidonic acid metabolite, 15-hydroxyeicosateraenoic acid (15-HETE), between aspirin-sensitive and aspirin-tolerant asthmatics. They reported that incubation of peripheral blood leukocytes with aspirin at $200\,\mu M$ resulted in a significant increase of 15-HETE (mean increase $+421\%$) in aspirin-sensitive asthmatics compared to control subjects, with sensitivity and specificity of 83% and 82%, respectively (59). Although the authors acknowledge that further studies will be needed before 15-HETE testing can be approved for in vitro screening, these results show much promise.

Therapy of AE-ECRS includes the use of systemic and topical steroids, the use of LT modifiers such as the lipoxygenase inhibitor zileuton, and the Cys LT antagonists such as montelukast or zafirlukast. Recurrence of NPs and even return of the sense of smell can occur with aspirin desensitization. Other nonsteroidal anti-inflammatory agents such as ibuprofen, which can provoke the symptoms, are not effective in desensitization. Desensitization can only be accomplished with aspirin or lysine aspirin (Stevenson, personal communication) (57). The authors recommend that nasal polypectomy be performed initially, followed by aspirin desensitization under LT inhibition. Continuation of aspirin desensitization will help prevent recurrence of nasal polypoid disease (57).

CONCLUSION

In summary, four mechanisms which may potentially cause ECRS are SAI-ECRS, AFS, NAF-ECRS, and AE-ECRS. Schubert has speculated that SAI-ECRS may even drive AFS, and Bachert has presented evidence that superantigens may down-regulate PGE2 production and so predispose a patient to AERD. It is clear that patients with ECRS represent the most difficult of an CRS patient. The mechanisms promoting an eosinophilic response are probably diverse and overlapping. While four mechanisms are discussed in this chapter, there may well be many other yet undiscovered mechanisms of ECRS. Convincing proof of the four proposed mechanisms is as of yet lacking; however, the evidence reviewed in this chapter suggests some role for each mechanism discussed. Therapeutic interventions for these theoretically disparate etiologies are also overlapping and are summarized in table form. Animal models are in development and hold promise in the study of the complex, confusing, and refractory entity, ECRS (60,61).

REFERENCES

1. Benninger MS, Ferguson BJ, Hadley JA, et al. Adult chronic rhinosinusitis: definitions, diagnosis, epidemiology, and pathophysiology. Otolaryngol Head Neck Surg 2003; 129(suppl 3):S1–S32.

2. Lethbridge-Cxejku M, Schiller JS, Bernadel L. Summary health statistics for U.S. adults: National Health Interview Survey, 2002. National Center for Health Statistics. Vital Health Stat 2004; 10:222.

3. http://www.emedicine.com/med/topic2556.htm (accessed November 2005).

4. Meltzer EO, Hamilos DL, Hadley JA, et al. Rhinosinusitis: establishing definitions for clinical research and patient care. J Allergy Clin Immunol 2004; 114(suppl 6):155–212.

5. Newman LJ, Platts-Mills TA, Phillips CD, et al. Chronic sinusitis: relationship of computed tomographic findings to allergy, asthma, and eosinophilia. JAMA 1994; 271:363–367.

6. Hoover GE, Newman LJ, Platts-Mills TA, et al. Chronic sinusitis: risk factors for extensive disease. J Allergy Clin Immunol 1997; 100:185–191.

7. Szucs E, Ravandi S, Goossens A, et al. Eosinophilia in the ethmoid mucosa and its relationship to the severity of inflammation in chronic rhinosinusitis. Am J Rhinol 2002; 16(3):131–134.

8. Baroody FM, Hughes CA, McDowell P, et al. Eosinophilia in chronic childhood sinusitis. Arch Otolaryngol Head Neck Surg 1995; 121(12):1396–1402.

9. Sobol SE, Fukakusa M, Christodoulopoulos P, et al. Inflammation and remodeling of the sinus mucosa in children and adults with chronic sinusitis. Laryngoscope 2003; 113(3):410–414.

10. Chan KH, Abzug MJ, Coffinet L, et al. Chronic rhinosinusitis in young children differs from adults: a histopathology study. J Pediatr 2004; 144(2):206–212.

11. Zadeh MH, Banthia V, Anand VK, et al. Significance of eosinophilia in chronic rhinosinusitis. Am J Rhinol 2002; 16(6):313–317.

12. Alam R, Busse WW. The eosinophil—quo vadis? J Allergy Clin Immunol 2004; 113(1):38–42.

13. Bochner BS. Verdict in the case of therapies versus eosinophils: the jury is still out. J Allergy Clin Immunol 2004; 113(1):3–9.

14. Dunnill MS. Pulmonary fibrosis. Histopathology 1990; 16(4):321–329.

15. Weller PF. Human eosinophils. J Allergy Clin Immunol 1997; 100(3):283–287.

16. Ebisawa M, Schleimer RP, Bickel C, et al. Phenotyping of purified human peripheral blood eosinophils using the blind panel mAb. In Schlossman S, Boumsell L, Gilks W, et al., eds. Leukocyte Typing V: White Cell Differentiation Antigens. New York: Oxford University Press, 1995:1036–1038.

17. Temple R, Allen E, Fordham J, et al. Microarray analysis of eosinophils reveals a number of candidate survival and apoptosis genes. Am J Respir Cell Mol Biol 2001; 25(4):425–433.

18. Tachimoto H, Bochner BS. The surface phenotype of human eosinophils. Chem Immunol 2000; 76:45–62.

19. Leckie MJ, Brinke A, Khan J, et al. Effects of an interleukin-5 blocking monoclonal antibody on eosinophils, airway hyper-responsiveness, and the late asthmatic response. Lancet 2000; 356(9248):2144–2148.

20. O'Byrne PM, Inman MD, Parameswaran K. The trials and tribulations of IL-5, eosinophils, and allergic asthma. J Allergy Clin Immunol 2001; 108(4):503–508.

21. Liu LY, Sedgwick JB, Bates ME, et al. Decreased expression of membrane IL-5 receptor alpha on human eosinophils: I. Loss of membrane IL-5 receptor alpha on airway eosinophils and increased soluble IL-5 receptor alpha in the airway after allergen challenge. J Immunol 2002; 169(11):6452–6458.

22. Mattes J, Yang M, Mahalingam S, et al. Intrinsic defect in T cell production of interleukin (IL)-13 in the absence of both IL-5 and eotaxin precludes the development of eosinophilia and airways hyperreactivity in experimental asthma. J Exp Med 2002; 195(11):1433–1444.

23. Lee JJ, Dimina D, Macias MP, et al. Defining a link with asthma in mice congenitally deficient in eosinophils. Science 2004; 305(5691):1773–1776.

24. Irwin MJ, Hudson KR, Fraser JD, et al. Enterotoxin residues determining T-cell receptor V binding specificity. Nature 1992; 359(6398):841–843.

25. Schubert MS. A superantigen hypothesis for the pathogenesis of chronic hypertrophic rhinosinusitis, allergic fungal sinusitis, and related disorders. Ann Allergy Asthma Immunol 2001; 87(3):181–188.

26. Schubert MS, Hutcheson PS, Graff RJ, et al. HLA-DQB1*03 in allergic fungal sinusitis and other chronic hypertrophic rhinosinusitis disorders. J Allergy Clin Immunol 2004; 114(6):1376–1383.

27. Bernstein JM, Ballow M, Schlievert PM, et al. A superantigen hypothesis for the pathogenesis of chronic hyperplastic sinusitis with massive nasal polyposis. Am J Rhinol 2003; 17(6):321–326.

28. Bernstein JM, Kansal R. Superantigen hypothesis for the early development of chronic hyperplastic sinusitis with massive nasal polyposis. Curr Opin Otolaryngol Head Neck Surg 2005; 13(1):39–44.

29. Seiberling KA, Conley DB, Tripathi A, et al. Superantigens and chronic rhinosinusitis: detection of staphylococcal exotoxins in nasal polyps. Laryngoscope 2005; 115(9):1580–1585.

30. Bachert C, Gevaert P, Holtappels G, et al. Total and specific IgE in nasal polyps is related to local eosinophilic inflammation. J Allergy Clin Immunol 2001; 107(4):607–614.

31. Zhang N, Gevaert P, van Zele T, et al. An update on the impact of *Staphylococcus aureus* enterotoxins in chronic sinusitis with nasal polyposis. Rhinology 2005; 43(3):162–168.

32. Hendricks A, Leibold W, Kaever V, et al. Prostaglandin E2 is variably induced by bacterial superantigens in bovine mononuclear cells and has a regulatory role for the T cell proliferative response. Immunobiology 2000; 201(5):493–505.

33. Desouza IA, Franco-Penteado CF, Camargo EA, et al. Inflammatory mechanisms underlying the rat pulmonary neutrophil influx induced by airway exposure to staphylococcal enterotoxin type A. Br J Pharmacol 2005; 146(6):781–791.

34. Casale TB, Condemi J, LaForce C, et al. Effect of omalizumab on symptoms of seasonal allergic rhinitis: a randomized controlled trial. JAMA 2001; 286(23):2956–2967.

35. Chiang DT, Clark J, Casale TB. Omalizumab in asthma: approval and postapproval experience. Clin Rev Allergy Immunol 2005; 29(1):3–16.

36. http://clinicaltrials.gov/show/NCT00117611 (accessed November 2005).

37. Katsuyama M, Ichikawa H, Ogawa S, et al. A novel method to control the balance of skin microflora. Part 1. Attack on biofilm of *Staphylococcus aureus* without antibiotics. J Dermatol Sci 2005; 38(3):197–205.

38. Ferguson BJ, Stolz DB. Demonstration of biofilm in human bacterial chronic rhinosinusitis. Am J Rhinol 2005; 19(5):452–457.

39. Marple BF. Allergic fungal rhinosinusitis: current theories and management strategies. Laryngoscope 2001; 111(6):1006–1019.

40. Manning S, Mabry R, Schaefer S, et al. Evidence of IgE-mediated hypersensitivity in allergic fungal sinusitis. Laryngoscope 1993; 103(7):717–721.

41. Collins M, Nair S, Smith W, et al. Role of local immunoglobulin E production in the pathophysiology of noninvasive fungal sinusitis. Laryngoscope 2004; 114(7):1242–1246.

42. Pant H, Kette FE, Smith WB, et al. Fungal-specific humoral response in eosinophilic mucus chronic rhinosinusitis. Laryngoscope 2005; 115(4):601–606.

43. Schubert MS. Antileukotriene therapy for allergic fungal sinusitis. J Allergy Clin Immunol 2001; 108(3):466–467.

44. Stevens DA, Schwartz HJ, Lee JY, et al. A randomized trial of itraconazole in allergic bronchopulmonary aspergillosis. N Engl J Med 2000; 342(11):756–762.

45. Bassichis BA, Marple BF, Mabry RL, et al. Use of immunotherapy and previously treated patients with allergic fungal sinusitis. Otolaryngol Head Neck Surg 2001; 125(5):487–490.

46. Marple B, Newcomer M, Schwade N, et al. Natural history of allergic fungal rhinosinusitis: a 4- to 10-year follow-up. Otolaryngol Head Neck Surg 2002; 127(5):361–366.

47. Ponikau JU, Sherris DA, Kern EB, et al. The diagnosis and incidence of allergic fungal sinusitis. Mayo Clin Proc 1999; 515:18–21.

48. Shin SH, Ponikau JU, Sherris DA, et al. Chronic rhinosinusitis: an enhanced immune response to ubiquitous airborne fungi. J Allergy Clin Immunol 2004; 114(6):1369–1375.

49. Braun H, Buzina W, Freudenschuss K, et al. Eosinophilic fungal rhinosinusitis: a common disorder in Europe? Laryngoscope 2003; 113(2):264–269.

50. Lebowitz RA, Waltzman MN, Jacobs J, et al. Isolation of fungi by standard laboratory methods in patients with chronic rhinosinusitis. Laryngoscope 2002; 112(12):2189–2191.

51. Ferguson BJ. Eosinophilic mucin rhinosinusitis—a distinctive clinicopathological entity. Laryngoscope 2000; 110:799–813.
52. Ponikau J, Sherris D, Kita H, et al. Intranasal antifungal treatment in 51 patients with chronic rhinosinusitis. J Allergy Clin Immunol 2002; 110(6):862–866.
53. Ricchetti A, Landis BN, Maffioli A, et al. Effect of anti-fungal nasal lavage with amphotericin B on nasal polyposis. J Laryngol Otol 2002; 116(4):261–263.
54. Weschta M, Rimek D, Formanek M, et al. Topical antifungal treatment of chronic rhinosinusitis with nasal polyps: a randomized, double-blind clinical trial. J allergy Clin Immunol 2004; 113(6):1122–1128.
55. Ponikau JU, Sherris DA, Weaver A, et al. Treatment of chronic rhinosinusitis with intranasal amphotericin B: a randomized, placebo-controlled, double-blinded pilot trial. J Allergy Clin Immunol 2005; 115(1):125–131.
56. Widal MF, Abrani P, Lermoyez J. Anaphylaxie et idiosyncrasie. Presse Med 1922; 30:189–192.
57. Szczeklik A, Stevenson DD. Aspirin-induced asthma: advances in pathogenesis, diagnosis, and management. J Allergy Clin Immunol 2003; 111(5):913–921.
58. Sousa AR, Parikh A, Scadding G, et al. Leukotriene-receptor expression on nasal mucosal inflammatory cells in aspirin-sensitive rhinosinusitis. N Engl J Med 2002; 347(19):1493–1499.
59. Kowalski ML, Ptasinska A, Jedrzejczak M, et al. Aspirin-triggered 15-HETE generation in peripheral blood leukocytes is a specific and sensitive aspirin-sensitive patients identification test (ASPITest). Allergy 2005; 60(9):1139–1145.
60. Lindsay RW, Slaughter T, Britton-Webb J, et al. The development of a murine model of chronic rhinosinusitis. Oto HNS. 2006; 134:724–730.
61. Ferguson BJ. Commentary: The development of a murine model of chronic rhinosinusitis. Oto HNS. 2006; 134:731–732.

6 Nonallergic Rhinitis with Eosinophilia Syndrome and Related Disorders

Anne K. Ellis and Paul K. Keith

Department of Medicine, Division of Clinical Immunology and Allergy, McMaster University, Hamilton, Ontario, Canada

INTRODUCTION

The most recent classification and differential diagnosis of rhinitis (rhinosinusitis), as described in previous chapters, are outlined in the allergic rhinitis (AR) and its impact on asthma document (Table 1) (1). Non-AR can be further classified into perennial or persistent non-AR, noninfectious non-AR, and six structurally related syndromes as outlined in Table 2. This chapter will concentrate on a few of the perennial causes of non-AR: the non-AR with eosinophilia syndrome (NARES) and the related entities of blood eosinophilia non-AR syndrome (BENARS) and metachromatic non-AR.

NONALLERGIC RHINITIS WITH EOSINOPHILIA SYNDROME

Historical Background

NARES was first described in 1981 by Jacobs et al. (3). They presented a series of 52 patients with perennial symptoms of sneezing paroxysms, profuse watery rhinorrhea, and nasal pruritus of the nasopharyngeal mucosa in an "on-again-off-again" symptomatic pattern. Historically, age at onset of symptoms showed equal distribution from the first through the fifth decades. Trigger factors associated with the 52 patients with the acute onset of nasal symptoms were none or unknown in 22 (42%), weather changes in 16 (31%), odors in eight (15%), and noxious or irritating substances in six (12%). No patients had a history or physical examination consistent with nasal polyposis, bronchial asthma, current sinusitis, or otitis media. Fifty percent had a negative family history for either chronic rhinitis or bronchial asthma. Nasal secretion smears revealed marked eosinophilia during symptomatic periods. Intradermal skin tests were negative in most (49 of 52) patients. Mean total eosinophil count was 218/mm^3. Neither elevated total immunoglobulin E (IgE) nor evidence of specific IgE was found in the study patients' nasal secretions. Nasal smears showed marked eosinophilia, but relevant allergic triggers could not be identified by skin testing or by Radioallergosorbant test (RAST). The authors concluded that a characteristic pattern of symptomatic presentation and a paucity of in vivo and in vitro findings associated with IgE-dependent nasal disease distinguished this homogeneous disorder from perennial AR (PAR).

Clinical Features and Diagnosis

The condition "NARES" was originally characterized, as described above, on the basis of a nonatopic patient (by allergen skin testing) with perennial sneezing

TABLE 1 Classification of Rhinitis According to the Allergic Rhinitis and Its Impact on Asthma Document

---

Infectious
  Viral
  Bacterial
  Other infective agents
Allergic
  Intermittent
  Persistent
Occupational (allergic/nonallergic)
  Intermittent
  Persistent
Drug-induced
  Aspirin
  Other medications
Hormonal
Other causes
  Nonallergic rhinitis with eosinophilia syndrome
  Irritants
  Food
  Emotional
  Atrophic
  Gastroesophageal reflux
Idiopathic

Source: From Ref. 1.

attacks, a profuse watery rhinorrhea, nasal pruritis, nasal obstruction, and occasional loss of smell with greater than 20% of the cells in nasal smears being eosinophils. Most authors still support the use of a 20% diagnostic cutoff (2–5); however, the lower limit of nasal eosinophilia varies according to different authors

TABLE 2 Classification of Nonallergic Rhinitis (Based on Immunologic and Nasal Cytologic Features)

Perennial Non-AR (Inflammatory)	Noninflammatory, nonallergic rhinitis	Structurally related rhinitis
Eosinophilic nasal disease (NARES, BENARS)	Rhinitis medicamentosa	Septal deviation, turbinate deformation, nasal valve dysfunction
Basophilic/ metachromatic nasal disease	Reflex-induced rhinitis (bright light or other physical modalities	Neoplastic and non-neoplastic tumors
Infectious	Vasomotor rhinitis Irritant rhinitis Cold air rhinitis Gustatory rhinitis	Miscellaneous (choanal atresia, trauma, foreign body, malformation, cleft palate, adenoid hypertrophy
Nasal polyps	Rhinitis sicca	
Atrophic rhinitis	Metabolic (estrogen related or hypothyroidism)	
Immunologic nasal disease (non-IgE mediated)		

Abbreviations: NARES, nonallergic rhinitis with eosinophilia syndrome; BENARS, blood eosinophilia nonallergic rhinitis syndrome.
Source: From Ref. 2.

from 5% to 25% (6–9). As mentioned, a marked feature of NARES was the lack of evidence of allergy, as indicated by negative skin prick tests and/or absence of serum IgE antibodies to specific allergens.

NARES patients tend to have more intense nasal symptoms than patients with either vasomotor rhinitis (VMR) or AR (10). Additionally, the presence of anosmia is common (3,11), a feature not usually associated with other, more common, rhinitis conditions, with the exception of nasal polyposis.

A recent evaluation of patients with NARES demonstrated that all patients had impaired polysomnographic parameters (hypopnea index, apnea-hypopnea index, and mean and minimal oxygen saturation) compared with patients without nasal inflammation (12). Thus, NARES patients are at higher risk of developing obstructive sleep apnea, and may have clinical signs and symptoms consistent with this diagnosis.

Evaluating Nasal Cytology
The nasal cytology of NARES is characterized by an increased number of eosinophils, which may range from mild to massive, and is frequently associated with increased basophilic/metachromatic cells (13). Given that the accurate diagnosis of NARES requires, by definition, an evaluation of nasal cytology for eosinophils, a discussion regarding the various methodologies for completing such an evaluation is given.

Several methods of collecting nasal secretions have been described. The patient can blow secretions into wax paper or Saran wrap, which is the simplest way of collecting a sample. By collecting secretions by this technique, less cellular material may be collected (14). Alternative, but also simple methods for collecting nasal samples include using a cytology brush, cotton swab, or a Rhinoprobe (Synbiotics Corporation, San Diego, California, U.S.A.). Drawbacks of these methods include the increased risk of sampling error because the area scraped may not represent the entire surface area and the possibility of not obtaining any cellular material, thus potentially prohibiting useful analysis.

More reliable assessments of nasal cytology are obtained using nasal lavage. Because nasal lavage dilutes the specimen, cytospins are made and the eosinophils counted are compared to the total number of cells retrieved. It is minimally invasive but reflects an anatomically wider sample of nasal cells (15). The most commonly used techniques of nasal lavage are that described by Naclerio et al. (16) and by Greiff et al. (17), which were later modified by Grunberg et al. (18) by using a Foley's catheter to instill saline solution into the nostril.

Nasal lavage by the modified Grunberg et al. (18) method is performed using a 14 G all-silicone Foley catheter. The tip of the catheter is cut just distal to the balloon while keeping the balloon intact and introduced about 1.5 cm into the frontal nasal chamber (not against the nasal septum) with the subject holding it in place. With the subject in a writing position, the balloon is inflated and 10 mL of isotonic saline (0.9%) is instilled using a syringe attached to the other end of the catheter trimmed to fit the syringe snugly. After five minutes, the mixture of saline and mucus is recovered into the syringe. The balloon is then deflated and the procedure repeated on the other nostril.

Nasal lavage by the Naclerio method (16) is performed with the subject seated with the neck extended approximately 30° from the vertical. Five milliliters of isotonic saline (0.9%) at room temperature are instilled into one nostril with a syringe. The subject is instructed not to breathe or swallow. After 10 seconds, the subject flexes the neck and expels the sample of mucus and saline into a container. The procedure is then repeated in the other nostril. Alternatively both nostrils can be flushed at the same time (19).

A direct comparison of these two methods to evaluate reliability and reproducibility has been performed by Belda et al. (19). Both methods were able to discriminate between healthy and rhinitic subjects, and in subjects with rhinitis, the repeatability of eosinophil counts is similar in both methods, although the modified Greiff/Grunberg method gave more reproducible eosinophilic cationic protein (ECP) measurements.

Once the sample is collected (and, in the case of nasal lavage, centrifuged), it is fixed by cytofixation or heat fixation, and then stained. Hansel stain is often used to identify eosinophils, or the modified Wright's stain can be used as an alternative (19).

EPIDEMIOLOGY

The prevalence of NARES has been shown to range between 13% and 33% in patients with non-AR (8,10). An evaluation by Schiavano et al. demonstrated that 26% of 81 patients with chronic non-AR met the diagnostic criteria for NARES (5). In these patients, NARES usually occurred as an isolated disorder. However, it may be associated with non–IgE-dependent asthma, aspirin intolerance, and nasal polyps. In another study of 78 consecutive patients with non-AR (Table 3), NARES was found in 33% (8). The syndrome appears to have a female predominance (10,20,21). Indeed, gender may be a risk factor for the development of non-AR in general. In the series of Settipane and Klein, 58% of the non-AR patients were female (8). Enberg found 74% of non-AR patients to be female (22). However, these two studies lacked a control group. The National Rhinitis Classification Task Force study found that 71% of patients with non-AR were female compared with 55% in the AR group (23).

Although the specific etiology of NARES is not clear, in view of the features shared by this syndrome and the aspirin (ASA) triad (nasal polyposis, intrinsic asthma, and intolerance to aspirin) and because NARES patients frequently develop nasal polyps and asthma later on in life, it has been suggested that NARES may be an early expression of the triad (10). Indeed, in about 50% of NARES patients without a history of respiratory symptoms, bronchial hyperresponsiveness is

TABLE 3 Diagnosis of 78 Patients with Nonallergic Rhinitis

Diagnosis	Patients (N)	Patients considered (N)	Percentage of patients
Vasomotor rhinitis	44	72	61
NARES	25	75	33
Sinusitis[a]	11	68	16
Possible allergy[b]	9	76	12
BENARS	3	76	4
Hypothyroidism	1	68	2

[a]Overlapping diagnosis present.
[b]Based on elevated serum immunoglobulin E levels.
Abbreviations: NARES, nonallergic rhinitis with eosinophilia syndrome; BENARS, blood eosinophilia nonallergic rhinitis syndrome.
Source: From Ref. 8.

associated with an increase in the number of sputum eosinophils, but there is no correlation with the number of nasal eosinophils (24). Some investigators have suggested that NARES is a variant of VMR, and referred to the condition as "perennial intrinsic rhinitis" (25). Most, however, restrict the diagnosis of VMR to those without significant nasal eosinophilia.

PATHOPHYSIOLOGY

The pathophysiology of NARES is not yet fully elucidated, but a chronic, nonspecific liberation of histamine and a self-perpetuating, chronic eosinophilic nasal inflammation are suggested as the pathogenic factors of the disease. An evaluation of 20 patients with NARES was able to demonstrate a three-staged process in the evolution of the disease: (i) migration of eosinophils from the vessels into nasal secretions; (ii) retention of eosinophils in the mucosae, which might be linked to activation of unknown origin; and (iii) development of nasal micropolyposis and polyposis (11). While this activated eosinophilic infiltrate is likely an essential component, recent studies suggest mast cells are important as well.

Activation of resident mast cells is well described in the pathophysiology of AR, but it has been reported to play a relevant role in nasal polyposis as well (26). Tryptase, a major protein component of human mast cells, is found in both connective tissue and mucosal mast cells (27). It is found in negligible amounts in basophils, but not in other human cell types (28). Tryptase is a neutral serine protease, located in the secretory granules of mast cells and is released together with histamine during degranulation (29). The physiologic role of nasal tryptase is not yet clear. Among its effects, it cleaves C3 into the anaphylatoxin C3a, increasing vascular permeability and causing bronchospasm (30).

Eosinophils are pivotal in the pathophysiology of most studied forms of chronic nasal inflammation (the exception being VMR). There is strong evidence for the crucial role of eosinophils in ongoing inflammation and tissue damage (31). Granules of eosinophils contain toxic basic proteins. The major part of these proteins constitutes ECP (32). Experimental studies on eosinophil function have shown cytotoxic effects on airway epithelium (33) resulting in ciliostasis and lysis of epithelium (34). ECP constitutes a well-described and standardized marker for tissue eosinophilia and activation (35). ECP levels in nasal secretions can be used to monitor eosinophilic inflammation in different kinds of rhinitis with eosinophilic involvement, and they constitute an indicator of the efficacy of treatment (35).

A recent study by Kramer et al. (36) was able to show significant differences in the markers of mast cell and eosinophil presence and activation between patients with NARES and controls, as well as elucidate differences between NARES and other forms of chronic nasal inflammation, namely sinusitis, polyposis, and AR (both perennial and seasonal).

Nasal tryptase was significantly elevated in polyposis, NARES, and in AR compared with controls (Fig. 1A). The highest concentration was found in polyposis. Nasal ECP was significantly increased in all studied forms of chronic nasal inflammation with excessive amounts in NARES (Fig. 1B).

Intergroup comparison revealed elevated concentrations of nasal tryptase for polyposis ($p < 0.001$), for NARES ($p < 0.01$), and for AR ($p < 0.05$) when compared with sinusitis. Significantly elevated concentrations were observed in polyposis ($p < 0.05$), perennial AR ($p < 0.05$), and perennial and seasonal AR ($p < 0.05$) when compared with NARES.

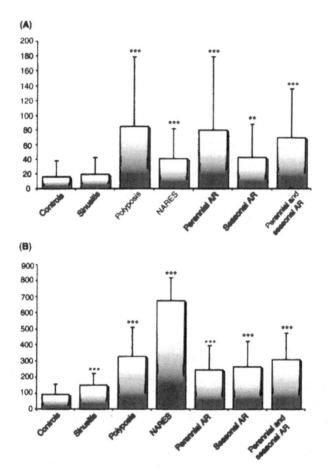

FIGURE 1 Differences between nonallergic rhinitis with eosinophilia syndrome and other forms of chronic nasal inflammation, namely sinusitis, polyposis, and allergic rhinitis in tryptase (**A**), and eosinophilic cationic protein **P < 0.01 (B)**, and eosinophils ***P < 0.001. *Abbreviations*: NARES, nonallergic rhinitis with eosinophilia syndrome; AR, allergic rhinitis. *Source*: From Ref. 36.

Intergroup comparisons revealed significantly elevated concentrations of nasal ECP for all studied diseases when compared with sinusitis. Compared with isolated perennial AR, they observed elevated levels of ECP in NARES and polyposis. ECP concentrations in NARES were still significantly elevated when compared with that of polyposis (Figs. 1A–B).

Given that excessive eosinophilia in nasal secretions is pathognomonic for this disease, this eosinophilia may well contribute to nasal mucosal dysfunction. This may occur as a result of the release of toxic substances such as major basic protein and ECP contained in eosinophil granules. These toxic proteins may damage nasal ciliated epithelium and prolong mucociliary clearance (37–42). Davidson et al. (43) reported on 56 non-AR patients and found a significant correlation between nasal eosinophilia and prolonged nasal ciliary clearance time. Delayed mucociliary clearance may result in an increased propensity toward infection. Recurrent infections may be a factor predisposing to the development of nasal polyps. Because nasal polyps are frequently associated with nasal eosinophils, there is some concern that nasal eosinophilia may be a precursor for nasal polyps or aspirin intolerance (10). In cases where aspirin intolerance exists, it is believed this intolerance is not the cause of the eosinophilic rhinosinusitis, but rather a marker of the severity of the NARES that is often associated with asthma, sinusitis, and nasal polyps.

The role of eicosanoids in the inflammatory process of NARES has been evaluated as well. Shahab et al. measured levels of prostaglandins (PG) E2, PGD2 and of leukotrienes (LT) E4 and LTB4 in nasal biopsies from the inferior turbinates of 101 patients suffering from perennial rhinitis and a control group (44). Rhinitis patients were classified into PAR, NARES, and noneosinophilic non-AR on the basis of symptoms, nasal secretion eosinophilia, nasal resistance, and allergy testing. Patients with rhinitis were randomized into two groups. One received fluticasone propionate aqueous nasal spray (FPANS) and the other a placebo over a period of six weeks prior to repeat biopsies. The control group consisted of 21 patients with no evidence of rhinitis but with nasal obstruction due to septal deviation. Untreated rhinitics had significantly lower levels of PGE2, PGD2 and LTE4 than nonrhinitic controls. Six weeks of treatment with FPANS decreased the numbers of eosinophils but increased the levels of those eicosanoids in patients with PAR and NARES, but they were still significantly below that of controls who did not have eosinophils. Levels of LTB4 in all three rhinitis groups were not significantly different from controls and treatment with topical steroids had no effect. Their findings are contrary to current thinking that increased levels of eicosanoids, in particular cysteinyl LTs, play an important role in the pathogenesis of chronic, noninfective upper airway inflammation (44).

Nasal neural dysfunction likely also contributes to the symptomatology present in NARES, because nasal hyperresponsiveness has been shown to develop in the setting of inflamed nasal passages (45). Hyperresponsive nasal tissue shows increased blockage and drip after "nonspecific" nonimmune stimulants such as bradykinin, endothelin, and methacholine (46–48). In some cases, it might result from an imbalance between the nasal sympathetic and parasympathetic nervous system (49). In general, autonomic stimuli such as exercise or changes in temperature have a greater effect on patients with non-AR than with AR. In addition, the inflammatory process in NARES has been associated with increased bronchial hyperresponsiveness in a significant number of patients, despite a lack of respiratory symptoms (24). As mentioned earlier, this hyperresponsiveness is associated with an increased number of eosinophils in induced sputum, but there is no correlation with the number of eosinophils in nasal secretions.

The role of staphylococcal superantigens in other atopic diseases has recently been recognized, and new evidence suggests that similar mechanisms might be relevant in allergic and non-AR. In recent studies, it has been suggested that there is an association between increased levels of eosinophilic inflammation in nasal polyps and the presence of specific IgE to *Staphylococcus aureus* enterotoxin A and *S. aureus* enterotoxin B, pointing to a possible role of bacterial superantigens in this disease (50,51).

Other evaluations have been completed with histologic examinations. Full thickness turbinate biopsies from patients with well-defined non-AR were compared with AR turbinates and with those from normal control individuals (52). The epithelium revealed mast cells and IgE-positive cells in both the nonallergic and the allergic groups, but not in normal individuals without rhinitis. Nasal challenge studies were abnormal in one half of the non-AR patients, with definite positive responses in 27%. These results echo those of Romero and Scadding (53) who examined skin prick test positivity and nasal eosinophilia and nasal allergen challenge results and found that a proportion of skin prick test negative patients show nasal eosinophils and are positive on nasal allergen challenge.

The hypothesis of an allergic Th2 disease pathway localized in the nasal mucosa of "nonallergic" rhinitis subjects despite an absence of atopic responses has been furthered by Powe et al. (54). The presence of house dust mite and grass pollen-specific IgE antibodies was investigated in nonatopic ($n = 10$) and atopic ($n = 11$) subjects with persistent rhinitis and compared to normal ($n = 12$) control subjects. Grass pollen allergen binding was detected in the nasal mucosa of 3 out of 10 nonatopic rhinitis subjects but, in contrast, dust mite-specific antibodies were not detected. Specific antibodies were present in a total of 8 out of 11 mucosal samples from the allergic group, but none were detected in normal control tissues; their findings support the concept of localized nasal allergy in "nonatopic" rhinitis subjects (54). Huggins and Brostoff (55) also showed positive nasal allergen challenges in skin prick test negative patients. Finally, a study by Carney et al. (52) found that a significant proportion (62%) of patients with idiopathic rhinitis have positive nasal challenges, the vast majority to house dust mite allergen. Their findings add to the weight of evidence that suggests "localized allergy" may exist in the absence of systemic atopic markers. Thus, the diagnosis of nasal allergy is no longer simple, and skin prick test negative patients with nasal eosinophilia may require allergen challenge before they can be reliably ascribed to the non-AR group (Fig. 2) (56). A parallel finding has been previously reviewed in nasal polyposis with local IgE production in nasal tissue in the absence of positive skin tests (57).

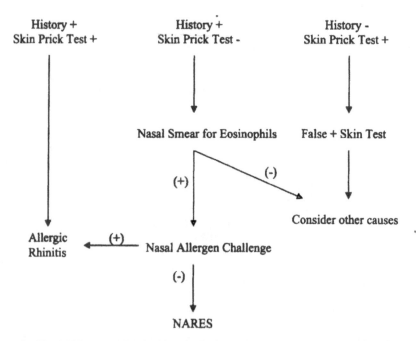

FIGURE 2 Diagnosis of distinct types of allergy, but with negative skin prick tests, further tests looking for evidence of local allergy should be undertaken in the form of nasal smears for eosinophils and nasal challenge with likely allergens. The results will categorize the patient into one of three groups: local allergic rhinitis, nonallergic rhinitis with eosinophilia syndrome, or nonallergic rhinitis. *Abbreviation:* NARES, nonallergic rhinitis with eosinophilia syndrome. *Source:* From Ref. 57.

BLOOD EOSINOPHILIA NONALLERGIC RHINITIS SYNDROME

BENARS is a subtype of NARES (8). It differs from NARES in that BENARS has markedly elevated blood eosinophilia and often no associated sinusitis. It is similar to NARES in that it is associated with negative allergy skin tests, normal serum IgE, and increased eosinophils in nasal secretions (8). In a study of 78 consecutive patients with non-AR (Table 3), BENARS was found in 4% (8). These patients with BENARS had an average elevation in blood eosinophil counts of $957/mm^3$ (normal range $100–600/mm^3$). A parallel disorder is seen as a subtype of AR, in that often some AR patients will have blood eosinophilia as well [dubbed blood eosinophilia with AR syndrome (BEARS)].

Nasal ciliary beat frequency is inhibited in patients with BENARS, which may predispose the nasal mucosa to infections and increased risk for developing nasal polyps. Indeed, nasal polyps are frequently associated with this condition (58).

METACHROMATIC NONALLERGIC RHINITIS

Metachromatic cells from nasal mucosae include large mast cells, atypical mast cells, and basophils. Basophilic/metachromatic cell nasal disease, or nasal masto-cytosis, is a subcategory of non-AR that, along with NARES, is a histologic diagnosis (59,60). A small number of patients with non-AR have an increased number of these metachromatic cells without a similar increase in nasal eosinophilia and thus are felt to represent a clinically distinct, albeit rare, nonallergic rhinitic syndrome. These patients similarly share the increased risk of nasal polyposis associated with NARES and BENARS. Mast cell infiltration (frequently >2000/ mm^3) without nasal eosinophilia is the hallmark of this syndrome (3). Nasal symptoms are more likely to be secretion/rhinorrhea and congestion/blockage without significant sneezing/pruritus. Physical examination reveals an especially pale nasal mucosa.

A study by Ruhno et al. examined epithelial scrapings of the inferior turbinates in polyp patients who were allergic, polyp patients who were not allergic, and non-allergic normal control subjects looking for metachromasia (61). Metachromatic cell counts in epithelial scrapings obtained in vivo from nasal polyps of allergic patients were lower than from polyps of nonallergic patients; it was concluded that the number of metachromatic cells in the epithelium of nasal polyps and the adjacent nasal mucosa is elevated compared with normal nasal epithelium and the increased number does not depend upon allergy as defined by a positive skin test to a panel of inhalant allergens (61).

The pathophysiology of metachromatic non-AR has not been evaluated in humans. Animal models of AR provide evidence, however, that inflammation of nasal mucosa and nasal hyperreactivity can occur in the absence of eosinophils, even in interleukin-5 knockout mice, suggesting that basophils and other meta-chromatic cells can drive a nonallergic rhinitic process without the contribution of eosinophils (62).

OTHER DIAGNOSTIC CONSIDERATIONS

Very rare nonallergic disorders associated with nasal eosinophilia include phaeo-hyphomycosis of the maxilloethmoid sinus (63) (a soft-tissue infection with dematiacious septate fungi), and Churg–Strauss syndrome (64) (a small vessel eosinophilic vasculitis seen in patients who often are atopic and have asthma).

TREATMENT

The treatment of non-AR is covered extensively in subsequent chapters; thus we will discuss treatment of NARES only briefly.

Intranasal corticosteroids are the mainstay of treatment for NARES, with many studies showing clinical improvement with this treatment (65,66). Indeed, the presence of nasal eosinophilia in patients with non-AR is generally regarded as a good prognostic indicator for response to treatment with topical steroid therapy (3). These topically applied drugs, studied in many controlled trials, reduce rhinitis symptoms, improve nasal breathing, reduce the size of polyps and their recurrence, but have a poor effect on the sense of smell (67). Systemic steroids, less well studied, appear to have an effect on all types of symptoms and pathology, the sense of smell included, particularly if there are concomitant polyps (67,68). Occasionally, intermittent use of oral glucocorticoid may be required to control symptomology (3). Administration of antihistamines in combination with corticosteroids may be clinically effective because of the different mechanism of action of the two drugs (69,70).

Specific evaluations of various treatments for NARES are uncommon, but those controlled trials that have been completed are summarized here.

Two studies have shown the benefit of adding loratadine, a second-generation H1 antihistamine, to an intranasal corticosteroid treatment regimen (70,71) in the management of NARES. The combination of loratadine and intranasal corticosteroid performed better than either drug alone. Additionally, nedocromil sodium preparations have been shown to be of benefit in the treatment of this syndrome (72).

Given the proven benefit of LT receptor antagonists in the treatment of AR (73), aspirin sensitive asthma (74) and nasal polyposis (75,76), and the concomitant reduction in eosinophils with treatment (77), these agents may have similar benefit in the NARES syndrome, but they have not been formally studied.

SUMMARY

NARES is a clinical syndrome consisting of symptoms consistent with AR in which an absence of atopy has been demonstrated by allergen skin testing, with nasal cytology analysis showing greater than 20% eosinophils. Anosmia is a prominent feature not shared with AR. The pathophysiology of NARES is poorly understood, but a key component involves a self-perpetuating, chronic eosinophilic nasal inflammation with development of nasal micropolyposis and polyposis. Mast cells likely play an important role as well. NARES is a risk factor for the development of nasal polyposis and aspirin sensitivity, as well as obstructive sleep apnea. Treatment consists mainly of intranasal corticosteroids with or without the addition of second-generation antihistamines and/or LT receptor antagonists as an adjuvant.

REFERENCES

1. Bousquet J, van Cauwenberge P. World Health Organisation Initiative, allergic rhinitis and its impact on Asthma (ARIA). Geneva: WHO, 2000.
2. Settipane RA, Lieberman P. Update on nonallergic rhinitis. Ann Allergy Asthma Immunol 2001; 86:494–507.

3. Jacobs RL, Freedman PM, Boswell RN. Nonallergic rhinitis with eosinophilia (NARES syndrome). Clinical and immunologic presentation. J Allergy Clin Immunol 1981; 67:253–262.
4. van Cauwenberge P, Wang DY, Ingels KJAO, Bachert C. Rhinitis: the spectrum of the disease. In: Busse WW, Holgate ST, eds. Asthma and Rhinitis. 2nd ed. Oxford: Blackwell Science Ltd., 2000:6–13.
5. Schiavano D, Nucera E, Milani A, et al. Nasal lavage cytometry in the diagnosis of nonallergic rhinitis with eosinophilia syndrome (NARES). Allergy Asthma Proc 1997; 18:363–366.
6. Mygind N, Dirkasen A, Johnsen NJ, Weeke B. Perennial rhinitis; an analysis of skin testing, serum IgE and blood and smear eosinophilia in 201 patients. Clin Otolaryngol 1978; 3:189–196.
7. Mullarkey MF, Hill JS, Webb DR. Allergic and nonallergic rhinitis: their characterization with attention to the meaning of nasal eosinophilia. J Allergy Clin Immunol 1980; 65:122–126.
8. Settipane GA, Klein DE. Nonallergic rhinitis: demography of eosinophils in nasal smear, blood total eosinophil counts, and IgE levels. N Engl Reg Allergy Proc 1985; 6:363–366.
9. Crobach M, Hermans J, Kaptein A, Ridderikhoff J, Mulder J. Nasal smear eosinophilia for the diagnosis of allergic rhinitis and eosinophilic nonallergic rhinitis. Scand J Prim Health Care 1996; 14:116–121.
10. Moneret-Vautrin DA, Hsieh V, Wayoff M, et al. Nonallergic rhinitis with eosinophilia syndrome a precursor of the triad: nasal polyposis, intrinsic asthma, and intolerance to aspirin. Ann Allergy 1990; 64:513–518.
11. Moneret-Vautrin DA, Jankowski R, Wayoff M. Clinical and pathogenic aspects of NARES (nonallergic rhinitis with eosinophilic syndrome). Rev Laryngol Otol Rhinol (Bord) 1991; 112:41–44.
12. Kramer MF, de la Chaux R, Fintelmann R, Rasp G. NARES: a risk factor for obstructive sleep apnea? Am J Otolaryngol 2004; 25:173–177.
13. Zeiger RS. Differential diagnosis and classification of rhinosinusitis. In Schatz M, Zeiger RS, Settipane GA, eds. Nasal Manifestations of Systemic Diseases. Providence, Rhode Island: OceanSide Publications, 1991.
14. Lara Becerra A, Gonzalez Diaz SN, Gonzalez Morales JE, Canseco Gonzalez C. Determination of the eosinophil count in nasal mucus. Comparison of two techniques. Rev Alerg Mex 1990; 37:123–126.
15. Kohler C, Stringini R, Moneret-Vautrin DA, Grignon G. Study of cells harvested in nasal secretions after lavage. Improvement of the cytologic technique and application to ORL and bronchial pathology. Bull Assoc Anat 1992; 76:43–46.
16. Naclerio RM, Meier HL, Kagey-Sobotka A, et al. Mediator release after nasal airway challenge with allergen. Am Rev Respir Dis 1983; 597–602.
17. Greiff L, Pipkorn U, Alkner U, Persson CGA. The 'nasal pool' device applied controlled concentrations of solutes on human nasal airway mucosa and samples its surface exudations/secretions. Clin Exp Allergy 1990; 20:253–259.
18. Grunberg K, Timmers MC, Smits HH, et al. Effect of experimental rhinovirus 16 colds on airway responsiveness to histamine and interleukin-8 in nasal lavage in asthmatic subjects in vivo. Clin Exp Allergy 1997; 27:36–45.
19. Belda J, Parameswaran K, Keith PK, Hargreave FE. Repeatability and validity of cell and fluid-phase measurements in nasal fluid: a comparison of two methods of nasal lavage. Clin Exp Allergy 2001; 31:1111–1115.
20. Bousquet J, van Cauwenberge P, Khaltaev N. Allergic rhinitis and its impact on asthma. J Allergy Clin Immunol 2001; 108:S147–S334.
21. Fokkens WJ. Thoughts on the pathophysiology of nonallergic rhinitis. Curr Allergy Asthma Rep 2002; 2:203–209.
22. Enberg RN. Perennial nonallergic rhinitis: a retrospective review. Ann Allergy 1989; 63:513–516.
23. National Allergy Advisory Council Meeting (NAAC). The broad spectrum of rhinitis: etiology, diagnosis, and advances in treatment, St. Thomas, U.S. Virgin Islands, Oct 16, 1999.

24. Leone C, Teodoro C, Pelucchi A, et al. Bronchial responsiveness and airway inflammation in patients with nonallergic rhinitis with eosinophilia syndrome. J Allergy Clin Immunol 1997; 100:775–780.

25. Marshall KG, Attia EL, Danoff D. Vasomotor rhinitis. In: Marshall KG, Attia EL, eds. Disorders of the Nose, Paranasal Sinuses. Littleton: PSG Publishing, 1987:195–203.

26. Di Lorenzo G, Drago A, Pellitteri ME, et al. Measurement of inflammatory mediators of mast cells and eosinophils in native nasal lavage fluid in nasal polyposis. Int Arch Allergy Immunol 2001; 125:164–175.

27. Craig SS, Schwartz LB. Tryptase and chymase, markers of distinct types of human mast cells. Immunol Res 1989; 8:130–138.

28. Castells MC, Irani AM, chwartz LB. Evaluation of human peripheral blood leukocytes for mast cell tryptase. J Immunol 1987; 138:2184–2189.

29. Schwartz LB, Austen KF. The mast cell and mediators of immediate hypersensitivity. In: Samter M, Talmage DW, Frank MM, Claman HN, eds. Immunological Diseases. Boston: Little Brown & Co., 1988:157.

30. Schwartz LB, Kawahara MS, Hugli TE, Vik D, Fearon DT, Austen KF. Generation of C3a anaphylatoxin from human C3 by human mast cell tryptase. J Immunol 1983; 130: 1891–1895.

31. Togias A, Naclerio RM, Proud D, et al. Studies on the allergic and nonallergic nasal inflammation. J Allergy Clin Immunol 1988; 81:782–790.

32. Gleich GA, Loegering DA, Maldonado JE. Identification of a major basic protein in guinea pig eosinophil granules. J Exp Med 1973; 137:1459–1471.

33. Motojima S, Frigas E, Loegering DA, Gleich GJ. Toxicity of eosinophil cationic proteins for guinea tracheal epithelium in vitro. Am Rev Respir Dis 1988; 139:801–805.

34. Kramer MF, Rasp G. Nasal polyposis: eosinophils and interleukin-5. Allergy 1999; 54:669–680.

35. Klimek L, Rasp G. Norm values for eosinophil cationic protein in nasal secretions: influence of specimen collection. Clin Exp Allergy 1999; 29:367–374.

36. Kramer MF, Burow G, Pfrogner E, Rasp G. In vitro diagnosis of chronic nasal inflammation. Clin Exp Allergy 2004; 34:1086–1092.

37. Bousquet J, Chanez P, Lacoste JY, et al. Eosinophilic inflammation in asthma. N Engl J Med 1990; 333:1033–1039.

38. Hastie AT, Loegering DA, Gleich GJ, Kueppers F. The effect of purified human eosinophil major basic protein on mammalian ciliary activity. Am Rev Respir Dis 1987; 135:848–853.

39. Flavahan NA, Slifman NR, Gleich GJ, Vanhoutte PM. Human eosinophil major basic protein causes hyperreactivity of respiratory smooth muscle. Am Rev Respir Dis 1988; 138:685–688.

40. Venge P, Dahl R, Fredens K, Peterson CG. Epithelial injury by human eosinophils. Am Rev Respir Dis 1988; 138:S54–S57.

41. Spector SL, English G, Jones L. Clinical and nasal biopsy response to treatment of perennial rhinitis. J Allergy Clin Immunol 1980; 66:129–137.

42. Ayars GH, Altman LC, McManus MM, et al. Injurious effect of the eosinophil peroxide-hydrogen peroxide-halide system and major basic protein on human nasal epithelium in vitro. Am Rev Respir Dis 1989; 140:125–131.

43. Davidson AE, Miller SD, Settipane RJ, Ricci AR, Klein DE, Settipane GA. Delayed nasal mucociliary clearance in patients with nonallergic rhinitis and nasal eosinophilia. Allergy Proc 1992; 13:81–84.

44. Shahab R, Phillips DE, Jones AS. Prostaglandins, leukotrienes and perennial rhinitis. J Laryngol Otol 2004; 118:500–507.

45. Baraniuk J. Neuroregulation. Proceedings of the St. Thomas Aventis Meeting, 1–14, 2000.

46. Baraniuk J, Silver PB, Kaliner MA, Barnes PJ. Perennial rhinitis subjects have altered vascular, glandular, and neural responses to bradykinin nasal provocation. Int Arch Allergy Immunol 2005; 103:202–208.

47. Ricchio MM, Reynolds CJ, Hay DW, Proud D. Effects of intranasal administration of endothelin-1 to allergic and non-allergic individuals. Am J Respir Crit Care Med 1995; 152:1757–1764.

48. Ricchio MM, Proud D. Evidence that enhanced neural reactivity to bradykinin in patients with symptomatic allergy is mediated by neural reflexes. J Allergy Clin Immunol 1996; 97:1252–1253.
49. Wilde AD, Cook JA, Jones AS. The nasal response to isometric exercise in non-eosinophilic intrinsic rhinitis. Clin Otolaryngol 1996; 21:84–86.
50. Bachert C, Gevaert P, Holtappels G, Johansson SG, van Cauwenberge P. Total and specific IgE in nasal polyps is related to local eosinophilic inflammation. J Allergy Clin Immunol 2001; 107:607–614.
51. Suh YJ, Yoon SH, Sampson AP, et al. Specific immunoglobulin E for staphylococcal enterotoxins in nasal polyps from patients with aspirin-intolerant asthma. Clin Exp Allergy 2004; 34:1270–1275.
52. Carney AS, Powe DG, Huskisson RS, Jones NS. Atypical nasal challenges in patients with idiopathic rhinitis: more evidence for the existence of allergy in the absence of atopy? Clin Exp Allergy 2002; 32:1436–1440.
53. Romero JN, Scadding GK. Eosinophilia in nasal secretions compared to skin prick test and nasal challenge test in the diagnosis of nasal allergy. Rhinology 1992; 30:169–175.
54. Powe DG, Jagger C, Kleinjan A, Carney AS, Jenkins D, Jones NS. 'Entopy': localized mucosal allergic disease in the absence of systemic responses for atopy. Clin Exp Allergy 2003; 33:1374–1379.
55. Huggins KG, Brostoff J. Local production of specific IgE antibodies in allergic-rhinitis patients with negative skin prick tests. Lancet 1976; 7926:148–150.
56. Scadding GK. Nonallergic rhinitis: diagnosis and management. Curr Opin Allergy Clin Immunol 2001; 1:15–20.
57. Keith P, Dolovich J. Allergy and nasal polyposis. In: Mygind N, Lildholdt T, eds. Nasal Polyposis—An Inflammatory Disease and Its Treatment. Copenhagen: Munksgaard, 1997:68–77.
58. Settipane GA. Nasal polyps and immunoglobulin E (IgE). Allergy Asthma Proc 1996; 17:269–273.
59. Connell JT. Nasal mastocytosis. J Allergy 1969; 43:182.
60. McKenna EL. Nasal mastocytosis. Laryngoscope 1974; 84:112–115.
61. Ruhno J, Howie K, Anderson M, et al. The increased number of epithelial mast cells in nasal polyps and adjacent turbinates is not allergy-dependent. Allergy 1990; 45: 370–374.
62. Saito H, Matsumoto K, Denburg AE, et al. Pathogenesis of murine experimental allergic rhinitis: a study of local and systemic consequences of IL-5 deficiency. J Immunol 2002; 168:3017–3023.
63. Sobol SM, Love RG, Stutman HR, Pysher TJ. Phaeohyphomycosis of the maxilloethmoid sinus caused by *Drechslera spicifera*: a new fungal pathogen. Laryngoscope 1984; 94:620–627.
64. Olsen KD, Neel HB, DeRemee RA, Weiland LH: Nasal manifestations of allergic granulomatosis and angiitis (Churg–Strauss syndrome). Otolaryngol Head Neck Surg 1980; 88:85–89.
65. Swierczynska M, Strek P, Skladzien J, Nizankowska-Mogilnicka E, Szczeklik A. Nonallergic rhinitis with eosinophilia syndrome: state of knowledge. Otolaryngol Pol. 2003; 57:81–84.
66. Webb DR, Meltzer EO, Finn AF Jr., et al. Intranasal fluticasone propionate is effective for perennial nonallergic rhinitis with or without eosinophilia. Ann Allergy Asthma Immunol 2002; 88:385–390.
67. Mygind N. Effects of corticosteroid therapy in non-allergic rhinosinusitis. Acta Otolaryngol 1996; 116:164–166.
68. Mygind N, Lildholdt T. Nasal polyps treatment: medical management. Allergy Asthma Proc 1996; 17:275–282.
69. Cipolla C, Lugo G, Tartari F, Giannini A, Monterastelli G, D'Antuono G. Clinical, diagnostic and therapeutic aspects of non-allergic forms of rhinitis: non-allergic rhinitis with eosinophilia syndrome and vasomotor rhinitis. Minerva Med 1986; 77:145–148.
70. Kunkel G, Baumgarten C, Jablonski K. Loratadine (L) added to intranasal Beclomethasone (BDP) is more effective than BDP alone. Allergy 1993; 48(37):1246.

71. Purello-D'Ambrosio F, Isola S, Ricciardi L, Gangemi S, Barresi L, Bagnato GF. A controlled study on the effectiveness of loratadine in combination with flunisolide in the treatment of nonallergic rhinitis with eosinophilia (NARES). Clin Exp Allergy 1999; 29:1143–1147.

72. Nelson BL, Jacobs RL. Response of nonallergic rhinitis with eosinophilia (NARES) syndrome to 4% cromolyn sodium nasal solution. J Allergy Clin Immunol 1982; 70:125–128.

73. Peters-Golden M, Henderson WR Jr. The role of leukotrienes in allergic rhinitis. Ann Allergy Asthma Immunol 2005; 94:609–618.

74. Berges-Gimeno MP, Simon RA, Stevenson DD. The effect of leukotriene-modifier drugs on aspirin-induced asthma and rhinitis reactions. Clin Exp Allergy 2002; 32:1491–1496.

75. Ragab S, Parikh A, Darby YC, Scadding GK. An open audit of montelukast, a leukotriene receptor antagonist, in nasal polyposis associated with asthma. Clin Exp Allergy 2001; 31:1385–1391.

76. Bachert C, Watelet JB, Gevaert P, Van Cauwenberge P. Pharmacological management of nasal polyposis. Drugs 2005; 65:1537–1552.

77. Saito H, Morikawa H, Howie K, et al. Effects of a cysteinyl leukotriene receptor antagonist on eosinophil recruitment in experimental allergic rhinitis. Immunology 2004; 113:246–252.

Relationship Between Nonallergic Upper Airway Disease and Asthma

Jonathan Corren and Rita Kachru

Department of Medicine, University of California, Los Angeles, California, U.S.A.

INTRODUCTION

During the past century, practicing clinicians have frequently observed that chronic rhinitis, sinusitis, and asthma coexist in the same patients. Despite a wealth of data supporting an association between the upper and lower airways, not until recently has strong data emerged which suggests that the pathogenesis of the three conditions is quite similar, and that treatment of upper airway disorders may lead to improvements in asthma. Although much of the emphasis in the experimental literature has been directed toward atopic airway disease, there is now a growing realization that nonallergic rhinitis, sinusitis, and asthma are causes of considerable morbidity and deserve clinical investigation. In this chapter, data from a variety of epidemiologic, laboratory, and clinical studies will be highlighted to help clarify our understanding of this complex and important relationship.

EPIDEMIOLOGIC STUDIES

Nonallergic Nasal Symptoms and Asthma

As has been carefully outlined in other sections of this book, chronic nonallergic rhinitis is a descriptive term that encompasses several different nasal syndromes. Primary nonallergic rhinitis may occur in two predominant and distinct forms based upon the nature and degree of mucosal inflammation: nonallergic rhinitis without eosinophilia (previously referred to as "vasomotor rhinitis") and nonallergic rhinitis with eosinophilia (NARES). Unfortunately, epidemiologic studies of airway disease have not generally obtained nasal cytologic specimens for characterization of inflammation. However, there are data suggesting that nasal eosinophilia is universally identified in the nasal secretions of nonallergic patients with asthma, even in the absence of nasal symptoms (1). This important finding suggests that in nonallergic patients with asthma, chronic rhinitis is usually characterized by eosinophilic inflammation.

Another important issue in categorizing patients with nonallergic nasal symptoms is the determination of whether patients have isolated rhinitis or whether they have concomitant paranasal sinus involvement. In a study of 20 patients with NARES (nasal eosinophils >20% of total cells), Jankowski performed sinus computed tomography (CT) scans and demonstrated that 87% of patients had some degree of opacification of the ethmoid air cells, along with variable thickening of the other sinuses (maxillary 75%; frontal 46%; sphenoid 31%) (2). Although this data has not been confirmed in larger case series, it does suggest that the majority of patients with NARES have some degree of sinus mucosal involvement.

Surveys have revealed some general observations regarding the demographic characteristics of patients with nonatopic rhinitis and asthma. Both nonallergic rhinitis and nonallergic asthma are significantly more common in female than male patients, occur more frequently in adults than children, and are more likely to have year-round symptoms (3).

A limited number of cross-sectional epidemiologic studies have sought to establish the concordance of rhinitis and asthma in nonatopic patients. In a survey of patients attending an allergy specialty clinic, those with nonatopic asthma had a very high prevalence of chronic rhinitis (80%), nearly equaling that in patients with allergic asthma (4). In an analysis of the European Community Respiratory Health Survey database, Leynaert carefully assessed a large group of randomly selected adults using a questionnaire, measurement of total and specific immunoglobulin (Ig)E, allergy skin-prick tests, and bronchoprovocation challenges with methacholine (5). As expected, the frequency of asthma was higher in subjects with rhinitis (16.2%) versus those without (1%). Furthermore, asthma was strongly associated with both allergic [odds ratio (OR) = 8.1] as well as nonallergic rhinitis (OR = 11.6). This association remained highly significant when the analysis was restricted to nonatopic subjects with relatively low IgE levels (IgE < 80 kIU/L: OR = 13.3). In a later study designed to elucidate the most critical cofactors in the relationship between rhinitis and asthma, Leynaert et al. again demonstrated that asthma and bronchial hyperreactivity were significantly more common in subjects with rhinitis than in those without (OR = 6.63 and 3.02, respectively) (6). Although the association between rhinitis and asthma was higher in allergic compared with nonallergic subjects, the association was still highly significant after adjustment for markers of atopy, including sensitization to specific allergens, total IgE, and parental history of allergy. These findings suggest that atopy did not fully explain the strong coexistence of rhinitis and asthma.

Even though cross-sectional surveys are helpful in establishing the concordance of nonallergic rhinitis and asthma, longitudinal studies are required to define whether rhinitis is a risk factor for developing asthma. Plaschke et al. examined a cohort of Swedish adults over a period of three years in order to evaluate potential risk factors for developing asthma (7). Rhinitis strongly predicted the development of asthma in both allergic and nonallergic patients (OR = 5.7 and 3.5, respectively). Interestingly, the risk of developing asthma in patients with nonallergic rhinitis was enhanced in chronic smokers compared with nonsmokers (OR = 5.7). Guerra et al. similarly sought to establish risk factors for adult-onset asthma as part of the Tuscon Epidemiology Study of Obstructive Lung Diseases (8). One hundred and seventy-three patients above the age of 20 who had a new physician-confirmed diagnosis of asthma during the study period were compared to 2177 control subjects who reported no prior physician diagnosis of asthma or asthma symptoms during the interval of study. Rhinitis was found to be a significant risk factor for asthma, even after adjustment for atopic status. In both allergic and nonallergic patients, rhinitis increased the risk for developing asthma approximately threefold.

Chronic Rhinosinusitis and Asthma

Chronic rhinosinusitis (CRS) has been difficult to define, as the symptoms are quite heterogeneous in nature and strict criteria have been difficult to devise (9).

However, most experts would agree that radiographic abnormalities are universal, and grading schemes have been proposed and standardized (10). In addition, the histopathology of CRS is usually characterized by eosinophilic inflammation, particularly in patients with asthma (9). Inclusion of CRS is keenly relevant to this chapter, as roughly one-quarter of patients with sinus disease are nonatopic (11). Unfortunately, most studies examining the relationship between rhinosinusitis and asthma do not include any measures of atopy; therefore, much of the data presented is based upon a mixed population of rhinosinusitis patients who are both atopic and nonatopic.

Clinicians have noted a relationship between CRS and asthma since early in the 20th century, and more recent analyzes have confirmed the high prevalence of sinus disease in asthmatics. A large cross-sectional study established that upwards of 75% of asthmatics have chronic symptoms of rhinosinusitis, irrespective of asthma severity (12). Perhaps even more importantly, evidence of sinusitis assessed by CT is present in up to 84% of severe asthmatics (13). In addition, in patients with severe asthma, significant correlations have been noted between sinus CT scores and indicators of bronchial inflammation, including sputum eosinophilia and exhaled nitric oxide (13). Conversely, asthma is very common in patients with CRS. In patients seeking care in an otolaryngologic clinic, patients with CRS have a 20% prevalence of asthma, compared to 3% to 5% prevalence in the general population (14). In patients with refractory rhinosinusitis undergoing sinus surgery, the prevalence of asthma increases to 42% (15).

Nasal Polyposis and Asthma

Nasal polyps represent outgrowths of inflamed sinus mucosa into the nasal airway, and polyps are identified endoscopically in approximately 20% of patients with CRS (16). Conversely, virtually all patients with polyps have significant radiographic evidence of sinusitis (9). Similar to the above data regarding CRS, inclusion of nasal polyp patients is pertinent to our discussion, as approximately one-third of patients with polyps are nonallergic (17). However, existing clinical data sources do not differentiate between atopic and nonatopic patients, thereby limiting conclusions that can be drawn from these studies.

The prevalence of nasal polyps in a general population of asthmatics is approximately 4%; however, it increases to 13% to 15% in patients with nonatopic asthma (18,19). Conversely, studies of patients presenting with nasal polyposis have estimated that up to 50% had a history of asthmatic symptoms (16). The prevalence of polyp disease rises dramatically in patients with aspirin-exacerbated respiratory disease. In a European study of 500 patients with aspirin-induced asthma, radiographic evidence of severe hyperplastic sinusitis was detected in 75% of patients and approximately 60% of the group was diagnosed with nasal polyposis (20).

In summary, epidemiologic studies do suggest that nonallergic nasal symptoms and asthma frequently occur together, and that nonallergic rhinitis is a significant risk factor for developing asthma. CRS, both with and without nasal polyposis, is also strongly associated with asthma, although most data include patients who are both atopic and nonatopic. At the present time, prospective, longitudinal studies of patients with CRS, both with and without nasal polyposis, are lacking.

COMPARATIVE PATHOGENESIS OF UPPER AND LOWER NONALLERGIC AIRWAY DISEASE

Pathogenetic Aspects of Allergic Airway Disease

Before exploring the histopathology of nonallergic airway disease, it is appropriate to first review what has been learned from work performed on allergic patients. During the past decade, a large number of experimental studies have established the striking similarities between the nose and lungs in atopic airway disease. Both allergic rhinitis and allergic asthma demonstrate chronic infiltration of CD4+ T-lymphocytes and eosinophils (21,22). In addition, tissue mast cells, an important source of inflammatory mediators, are increased in both allergic rhinitis and asthma (23,24). A number of Th2-derived cytokines, including IL-4, IL-5, and IL-13 (25,26), along with chemokines, such as regulated on activation, normal T expressed and secreted (27,28) and eotaxin (29,30), have been identified in both conditions. Endothelial adhesion molecules, particularly vascular cell adhesion molecule-1 (VCAM-1), have also been shown to assist in the recruitment of eosinophils into the mucosa in both allergic rhinitis and asthma (31,32).

Even though similarities abound between the upper and lower airways, it is also important to comment upon two areas in which there are histopathologic differences: epithelial desquamation and basement membrane thickening. Although the bronchial epithelium has been shown to separate from the underlying basement membrane in asthma (33), this phenomenon has not been demonstrated in allergic rhinitis (34). Basement membrane thickening has also been shown to be a universal finding in allergic asthma (35), but has not been shown to occur consistently in allergic rhinitis (36).

Along with the largely analogous tissue pathology in allergic rhinitis and asthma, allergen provocation of the upper and lower airways results in similar physiologic sequelae, with early and late phase responses characterized by reduced airflow (37,38). Taken together, these shared features have fostered the notion of allergic airway disease as a "united airway disease," which has led to a renewed outlook on how to treat these conditions.

Cellular Inflammation in Nonallergic Airway Disease

Even though not studied to nearly the same extent, nonallergic eosinophilic nasal disorders also share a number of key features with nonallergic asthma. NARES and chronic sinusitis (both with and without nasal polyposis) demonstrate marked mucosal eosinophilia (9). Of note, patients with chronic sinusitis but without polyps have far fewer eosinophils present than those with nasal polyposis (39), suggesting potential differences in pathophysiology of these two conditions. As noted above, although allergic rhinitis does not appear to result in either epithelial shedding or basement membrane thickening of the nasal mucosa, both of these histologic findings have been shown to be present in patients with chronic sinusitis (40). These data may reflect the intensity and chronicity of mucosal inflammation in chronic sinusitis.

As noted for nonallergic nasal and sinus disease, airway infiltration with eosinophils has been found to be a characteristic feature of nonallergic asthma (22). However, with regard to T-lymphocytes, although allergic asthmatics manifest predominantly CD4+ cells in bronchoalveolar lavage fluid, nonallergic patients have been shown to have both CD4+ and CD8+ T-cells (41).

Cytokines and Mediators in Nonallergic Airway Disease

Most of the available data regarding cytokine production in nonallergic upper airway disease comes from studies of CRS with nasal polyps. Although a number of cytokines have been identified in various groups of polyp patients, including IL-4, IL-5, granuclocyte macrophage colony simulating factor, and transforming growth factor-beta, IL-5 has been most consistently identified in patients with both allergic and nonallergic disease (42). The key role of IL-5 was supported by the finding that in vitro treatment of eosinophil-infiltrated polyp tissue with neutralizing anti–IL-5 monoclonal antibody resulted in eosinophil apoptosis and decreased tissue eosinophilia (43). Even though some studies have demonstrated a difference in the profile of cytokines released by allergic versus nonallergic patients, with greater IL-4 production in the allergic group and more TNF-alpha in the nonallergic patients (44), other investigators have not demonstrated these findings (45). Interestingly, the highest levels of IL-5 have been identified in the mucosal tissue of nonallergic patients with aspirin intolerance (46). With regard to asthma, allergic asthmatics have been shown to have increased levels of IL-4 and IL-5, whereas nonallergic asthmatics have elevated levels of IL-5 and IL-2 (41). In both types of asthma, the close correlation of IL-5 levels with bronchial eosinophilia suggests that IL-5 is primarily responsible for the characteristic eosinophilic infiltrate of asthma (41).

A variety of inflammatory mediators have also been shown to be present in both allergic and nonallergic rhinitis and asthma, particularly cysteinyl leukotrienes. Increased levels of leukotrienes, including LTC4, LTD4, and LTE4, have been identified in sinus washings taken from patients with chronic sinusitis (47) and appear to be related to the presence of eosinophilic infiltration (48). These mediators have also been identified as playing a critical role in bronchial asthma, as they contribute significantly to resting bronchial smooth muscle and mucus secretion (49).

Local IgE in Nonallergic Airway Disease

Although IgE serves as a critical component in allergic airway pathogenesis, some investigators have proposed that nonallergic rhinitis may represent a "localized" IgE-mediated inflammatory response. Powe et al. tested this hypothesis with a four-year prospective study that evaluated the nasal mucosa of patients with allergic or nonallergic rhinitis compared with normal controls (50). They reported an increase in IgE+ cells, the majority being mast cells, in the nasal mucosa of patients with both allergic and nonallergic rhinitis, although the number of cells were higher in the allergic patients. In a follow-up study, they reported grass pollen–specific IgE antibodies in 3 out of 10 nonatopic rhinitis subjects (51). The reproducibility and relevance of these findings in larger groups of patients will require future study.

PATHOPHYSIOLOGIC MECHANISMS CONNECTING NONALLERGIC UPPER AIRWAY DISEASE AND ASTHMA

Upper Airway Reflexes

Dating back to the early 20th century, physicians have suspected the existence of a nasal–bronchial reflex, in which trigeminal afferent nerves originating in the nose result in efferent bronchoconstriction. Early mechanistic studies investigated the effects of several mucosal irritants on lower airway function in normal human subjects. In 1969, Kaufman and Wright applied silica particles onto the nasal mucosa of individuals without lower airway disease and noted significant, immediate increases in lower airway resistance (52). Bronchospasm induced by nasal silica was blocked by both resection of the trigeminal nerve and systemic administration of atropine (53). More recently, Fontanari et al. reevaluated the possibility of a neural connection between the upper and lower airways by using cold, dry air as the nasal stimulus (54). These investigators demonstrated that nasal exposure to very cold air caused an immediate and profound increase in pulmonary resistance that was prevented by both topical nasal anesthesia and cholinergic blockade induced by inhalation of ipratropium bromide. Both these studies strongly suggested the presence of a reflex involving irritant receptors in the upper airway (afferent limb) and cholinergic nerves in the lower airway (efferent limb).

Other studies have utilized provocative substances that may have more relevance to the endogenous effects of chronic, nonallergic nasal inflammation upon the lower airway. Yan and Salome performed nasal histamine challenges in subjects with perennial rhinitis and stable asthma, and observed that forced expiratory volume in one second was reduced by 10% or more immediately after provocation in 8 of 12 subjects (55). Importantly, radiolabeling studies were performed as part of this study, which demonstrated that histamine was not deposited into the lower airway. Similarly, in patients with chronic rhinitis and asthma, capsaicin challenge of the nose (known to release endogenous substance-P) has been shown to cause acute reductions in airflow that resolve within one minute (56).

Another reflex, which may originate in the upper airway and alter lower airway function, is the possibility of a pharyngobronchial reflex. Such a reflex might begin with the drainage of secretions from the nose and sinuses into the hypopharynx, resulting first in irritation of sensory nerve fibers, then induction of pharyngeal constriction, and ultimately bronchoconstriction. Experimental support for such a pharyngobronchial reflex comes from observation of pulmonary function measurements in patients with exacerbations of chronic sinusitis (57). In these patients, maximal midinspiratory flow rate, MIF_{50}, which is an indicator of upper airway narrowing, is reduced during recurrent bouts of sinusitis, and is also significantly associated with increases in bronchial hyperresponsiveness.

Mouth Breathing Caused by Nasal Obstruction

Nasal blockage resulting from tissue swelling and secretions may cause a shift from the normal pattern of nasal breathing to predominantly mouth breathing. Speizer and Frank evaluated the role of nasal filtration by having a group of patients inhale sulfur dioxide for 10 minutes, either through the nose or mouth, while monitoring their lower respiratory function (58). Pulmonary resistance increased more during oral than nasal administration of the sulfur dioxide, suggesting that nasal filtration may have played an important . role in reducing sulfur dioxide deposition into the lungs. Other investigators have shown that mouth breathing associated with nasal obstruction resulted in worsening of exercise-induced bronchospasm, whereas exclusive nasal breathing significantly reduced asthma after exercise (59). Improvements in asthma associated with nasal breathing may be the result of superior humidification and warming of inspired air before it reaches the lower airway (60).

Aspiration of Upper Airway Secretions

Aspiration of nasal and sinus secretions has long been implicated as a possible factor in bronchial asthma, and one favored empirically by many practicing clinicians. Early studies from the 1920s and 1930s demonstrated that material from the upper respiratory tract was recoverable from the tracheobronchial tree (61). Huxley et al. studied pharyngeal aspirations during sleep in normal volunteers and patients with depressed consciousness by delivering intermittent boluses of a radiolabeled tracer into the nasopharynx (62). Although nearly half of the normal subjects demonstrated pulmonary aspiration, this method of bolus delivery may have overcome natural defense mechanisms. In a more recent study, Bardin et al. have investigated 13 patients with chronic sinusitis, of which nine had asthma. After placement of radionuclide into maxillary sinus, radioactivity was detected in the sinus, nasopharynx, and esophagus of all patients during 24 hours of follow-up. Pulmonary deposition of radionuclide, however, was not demonstrated in any patient, suggesting that there was no significant pulmonary aspiration of sinus contents (63).

As a final note regarding aspiration, a rabbit model was recently developed to determine the mechanisms by which sinusitis might affect asthma (64). A sterile inflammatory rhinosinusitis was produced by injection of C5desArg into the maxillary sinuses, which resulted in increased lower airway responsiveness to inhaled histamine. However, if upper airway secretions were prevented from entering the lower airway either by placing the animals in a head-down position or by inflation of a tracheal cuff, lower airway reactivity remained unchanged. Although the relevance of this animal model to humans is questionable, these experimental findings are intriguing and suggest that further research in humans is warranted.

Systemic Connections Between the Upper and Lower Airways

It has also been suggested that inflammatory products from the upper airway may reach the lungs via the systemic circulation. Studies have demonstrated that CD34+ eosinophil–basophil progenitor cells are identified in the blood of atopic patients, including those with allergic rhinitis and asthma, and increase during seasonal allergen exposure (65). Importantly, these allergic progenitor cells express the IL-5 receptor, allowing them to potentially respond to systemic signals released during allergic reactions.

Recent allergen challenge studies have sought to further define the systemic link between the upper and lower airways. Braunstahl et al. performed segmental bronchial provocation with allergen in a group of patients with allergic rhinitis (66). Twenty-four hours after challenge, eosinophilic infiltration was observed in bronchial mucosa, blood, and nasal tissue, and levels of IL-5 were elevated. In a subsequent study, this same group of investigators performed nasal allergen challenge in patients with rhinitis alone, and 24 hours later noted increased numbers of eosinophils along with increased staining of vascular endothelium for the adhesion molecules intercellular adhesion molecule-1, VCAM-1, and E-selectin on both nasal and bronchial tissue (67). As observed in the bronchial challenge study, IL-5 was again elevated. These findings in allergic patients suggest that a localized allergic stimulus in one part of the respiratory tree releases a systemic proinflammatory signal, which is capable of inducing inflammation in another site remote to the original stimulus, and that this systemic pathway is a "two-way street."

Although it is attractive to apply this same reasoning to patients with nonallergic disease, the evidence for such a relationship in this group of patients is less

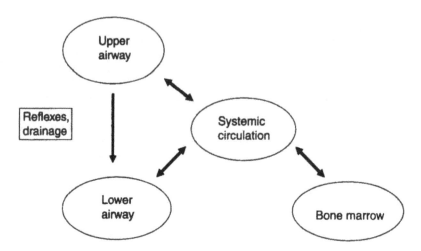

FIGURE 1 Inflammation in the two compartments of the airway may amplify inflammation in another compartment via the release of progenitor inflammatory cells from the bone marrow and movement of inflammatory cells in and out of the systemic circulation. Nasal– and pharyngeal–bronchial reflexes as well as aspiration of inflammatory cells and mediators may also play roles in modulation of lower airway inflammation and/or responsiveness by the upper airway.

direct and more speculative. Toward this end, a small number of studies have examined the relationship between sinus mucosal thickening (as measured by CT scan) and markers of asthma severity. Newman et al. surveyed a group of 104 patients undergoing sinus surgery for chronic sinusitis (68). They found that extensive sinus disease was present in 39% of the group and was strongly associated with asthma and peripheral blood eosinophilia. In a later study, Brinke et al. noted a significant correlation between the degree of mucosal thickening on sinus CT scans and blood eosinophil numbers, sputum eosinophilia, and exhaled nitric oxide (13). Much like the allergen challenge studies by Braunstahl, these two investigations suggest that the degree of eosinophilic inflammation in one compartment of the respiratory tree (paranasal sinuses) is reflected in the systemic circulation, which may subsequently influence the degree of inflammation and clinical disease in another portion of the respiratory tract (bronchi) (Fig. 1).

Role of Staphylococcus Enterotoxins

Staphylococcus aureus–derived enterotoxins are a family of proteins that act as potent superantigens in that they have the ability to cross-link the V-beta chain of the T-cell receptor with major histocompatibility complex class II molecules and, thereby, stimulate these cells. In one study, approximately 50% of nasal polyps demonstrated IgE antibodies directed against *S. aureus* enterotoxin A or B (69). The presence of these antienterotoxin IgE was correlated to higher levels of eosinophilic inflammation and proinflammatory cytokines and mediators (e.g., IL-5, cysteinyl leukotrienes). In the same study, those patients most likely to have these antienterotoxin IgE antibodies had aspirin-exacerbated respiratory disease (69).

There is corresponding evidence that these staphylococcal enterotoxins may also trigger T-cell activation in the lower airway. Hauk et al. demonstrated that there is increased expression of the T-cell receptor V-beta-8 on T-lymphocytes taken from bronchoalveolar lavage fluid of patients with poorly controlled asthma (70). Similarly, antienterotoxin IgE levels have been shown to be higher in patients with severe, chronic asthma compared with a group of controls (71). Given this data derived from patients with upper and lower airway disease, one can speculate that *S. aureus* colonization or infection of the paranasal sinuses leads to an immune response, which induces or aggravates asthma. Future work in this area will hopefully clarify the pathogenetic role of *S. aureus* in patients with chronic sinusitis and asthma and potentially assist in devising therapeutic strategies.

EFFECTS OF TREATMENT OF UPPER AIRWAY DISEASE ON ASTHMA

Another line of evidence supporting the link between disorders of the upper airway and asthma comes from studies demonstrating that treatment of rhinitis or sinusitis improves asthma. A large number of trials have examined the effect of local and systemic treatment of allergic rhinitis upon asthma, and found variable degrees of improvement (72). To date, however, similar studies have not yet been conducted in patients with nonallergic rhinitis and concomitant asthma. Most relevant to this chapter, therefore, are studies examining the effect of sinus therapy (including patients with both allergic and nonallergic disease) upon the clinical severity of asthma.

Medical Treatment

During the past 25 years, multiple investigators have studied the effect of medical therapy for rhinosinusitis on asthma symptoms, primarily in children. In 1981, Businco et al. reported that 10 of 12 children with chronic asthma had an improvement in lower airway symptoms after medical therapy but no objective measures of pulmonary function were performed (73). In 1983, Cummings et al. performed a double-blind, placebo-controlled study of sinus therapy in asthma (74). Active treatment (antibiotics, nasal steroids, and oral decongestants) of children with opacification or marked thickening of the maxillary sinuses resulted in significantly fewer asthma symptoms and a reduced requirement of inhaled bronchodilator and oral steroid therapy. Neither pulmonary function results nor measures of bronchial reactivity were significantly improved with active treatment. In 1984, Rachelefsky et al. studied 48 children with a three-month or longer history of sinusitis and wheezing (75). After two to four weeks of antibiotics with or without antral lavage, 38 of the patients were able to discontinue daily bronchodilator therapy, and 20 out of 30 demonstrated normalization of pulmonary function tests. During that same year, Friedman et al. studied eight children experiencing asthma exacerbations associated with sinusitis. After two to four weeks of antimicrobial therapy, seven of eight patients reported improvement in lower airway symptoms. Although baseline indices of pulmonary function were not changed after the completion of antibiotics, there was a mean twofold improvement in FEV_1 following inhaled bronchodilator (76). Although these generally positive results from pediatric studies are encouraging, only one of these studies was blinded, and a full report has never been published. In addition, it is not clear that these results are applicable to adult patients with CRS, as chronic sinus disease in adults does not appear to be nearly as amenable to antibacterial therapy (9).

Surgical Treatment

Early in the 20th century, physicians observed that surgical treatment of rhinosinu-sitis and nasal polyposis resulted in variable improvements in asthma symptoms. Beginning in the 1930s and extending into the 1990s, a number of reports emerged which employed older methods of sinus surgery (e.g., Caldwell-Luc) and sug-gested that these techniques resulted in an overall improvement in many patients with asthma. More recent clinical series have included patients under-going functional endoscopic sinus surgery (FESS), and many have reported significant lasting improvements in asthma severity (77). However, few of these published reports included any type of control group, or used objective parameters (e.g., pulmonary function) to assess clinical status of asthma. In addition, it is not clear from most of these observational studies whether patients were atopic or nonatopic. In a group of 15 asthmatic patients undergoing sinus surgery, Palmer et al. compared medication requirements during the one-year period preceding surgery with the postoperative period (78). One significant finding from this report was the 25% reduction of prednisone treatment (84 days pre-op, 63 days post-op, $p < 0.0001$). In a long-term study, a large group of adult patients with CRS and asthma was observed for an average of 6.5 years following FESS (15). Ninety percent of the group stated that their asthma was less severe, two-thirds of the patients were able to reduce their dose of oral corticosteroids, and there was an overall reduction in the number of asthma exacerbations and medications required to control their asthma. Although studies such as this are promising, other data have not shown the same degree of improvement. Goldstein et al. assessed asthma outcomes in 13 patients undergoing FESS, comparing pre- and postoperative asthma symptom scores, medication use, pulmonary function test results and emergency department visits, and hospital admissions for asthma (79). Following FESS, there was no statistically significant change in any of these parameters. In another study of 13 patients who underwent FESS for massive nasal polyposis, Uri et al. reported that seven had minimal improvement of their asthma and six showed definite signs of worsening (80). In addition, as some older data do indicate that asthma symptoms may improve spontaneously in the absence of sinus surgery, it is impossible to estimate the true benefit of surgical intervention (81). Therefore, it will be paramount to perform large, well-controlled clinical trials of both medical and surgical therapy for chronic sinusitis in patients with asthma.

SUMMARY

A growing body of scientific evidence supports the link between nonallergic upper airway disorders and asthma. Multiple studies have demonstrated that most patients with nonallergic asthma have chronic nasal symptoms as well as radio-graphic evidence of sinus mucosal disease. Equally important, preexisting symptoms of rhinitis place nonallergic patients at higher risk for developing asthma. Experimental studies demonstrate that the upper and lower airways may be connected via a number of paths, and that the systemic circulation may play a key role in amplifying inflammation in other portions of the respiratory tract. Finally, given this complex relationship between localized and systemic inflammation, it behooves all physicians to assess and treat rhinitis and sinusitis when they are present in patients with asthma.

REFERENCES

1. Gaga M, Lambrou P, Papageorgiou N, et al. Eosinophils are a feature of upper and lower airway pathology in non-atopic asthma, irrespective of the presence of rhinitis. Clin Exp Allergy 2000; 30(5):663–669.
2. Moneret-Vautrin DA, Jankowski R, Bene MC, et al. NARES: a model of inflammation caused by activated eosinophils? Rhinology 1992; 30(3):161–168.
3. Settipane RA, Lieberman P. Update on nonallergic rhinitis. Ann Allergy Asthma Immunol 2001; 86(5):494–507.
4. Kapsali T, Horowitz E, Diemer F, et al. Rhinitis is ubiquitous in allergic asthmatics. J Allergy Clin Immunol 1997; 99(556):S138.
5. Leynaert B, Bousquet J, Neukirch C, et al. Perennial rhinitis: an independent risk factor for asthma in nonatopic subjects: results from the European Community Respiratory Health Survey. J Allergy Clin Immunol 1999; 104:301–304.
6. Leynaert B, Neukirch C, Kony S, et al. Association between asthma and rhinitis according to atopic sensitization in a population-based study. J Allergy Clin Immunol 2004; 113:86–93.
7. Plaschke P, Janson C, Norrman E, et al. Onset and remission of allergic rhinitis and asthma and the relationship with atopic sensitization and smoking. Am J Respir Crit Care Med 2000; 162:920–924.
8. Guerra A, Sherrill D, Martinez F, et al. Rhinitis as an independent risk factor for adult onset asthma. J Allergy Clin Immunol 2002; 109:419–425.
9. Meltzer EO, Hamilos DL, Hadley JA, et al. Rhinosinusitis: establishing definitions for clinical research and patient care. J Allergy Clin Immunol 2004; 114(suppl 6):155–212.
10. Metson R, Gliklich RE, Stankiewicz JA, et al. Comparison of sinus computed tomography staging systems. Otolaryngol Head Neck Surg 1997; 117(4):372–379.
11. Karlsson G, Holmberg K. Does allergic rhinitis predispose to sinusitis? Acta Otolaryngol Suppl 1994; 515:26–29.
12. Bresciani M, Paradis L, Des Roches A, et al. Rhinosinusitis in severe asthma. J Allergy Clin Immunol 2001; 107(1):73–80.
13. Brinke A, Grootendorst DC, Schmidt JT, et al. Chronic sinusitis in severe asthma is related to sputum eosinophilia. J Allergy Clin Immunol 2002; 109(4):621–626.
14. Hamilos DL. Chronic sinusitis. J Allergy Clin Immunol 2000; 106(2):213–227.
15. Senior BA, Kennedy DW, Tanabodee J, et al. Long-term impact of functional endoscopic sinus surgery on asthma. Otolaryngol Head Neck Surg 1999; 121(1):66–68.
16. Settipane G. Epidemiology of nasal polyps. Allergy Asthma Proc 1996; 17(5):231–236.
17. Wong D, Dolovich J. Blood eosinophilia and nasal polyps. Am J Rhinol 1992; 6:195–198.
18. Grigoreas C, Vourdas D, Petalas K, Simeonidis G, Demeroutis I, Tsioulos T. Nasal polyps in patients with rhinitis and asthma. Allergy Asthma Proc 2002; 23(3):169–174.
19. Kanani AS, Broder I, Greene JM, Tarlo SM. Correlation between nasal symptoms and asthma severity in patients with atopic and nonatopic asthma. Ann Allergy Asthma Immunol 2005; 94(3):341–347.
20. Szczeklik A, Stevenson DD. Aspirin-induced asthma: advances in pathogenesis and management. J Allergy Clin Immunol 1999; 104(1):5–13.
21. Varney VA, Jacobson MR, Sudderick RM, et al. Immunohistology of the nasal mucosa following allergen-induced rhinitis: identification of activated T-lymphocytes, eosinophils, and neutrophils. Am Rev Respir Dis 1992; 146(1):170–176.
22. Busse WW, Horwitz RJ, Reed CE. Asthma: definition and pathogenesis. In: Middelton E Jr., Reed CE, Ellis EF, et al., eds. Allergy: Principles and Practice. St. Louis, MO: Mosby, 1998.
23. Skoner DP. Allergic rhinitis: definition, epidemiology, pathophysiology, detection and diagnosis. J Allergy Clin Immunol 2001; 108:S2–S8.
24. Fokkens WF, Godthelp T, Holm AF, et al. Dynamics of mast cells in the nasal mucosa of patients with allergic rhinitis and non-allergic controls: a biopsy study. Clin Exp Allergy 1992; 22:701–710.
25. Ghaffar O, Laberge S, Jacobson MR, et al. IL-13 mRNA and immunoreactivity in allergen-induced rhinitis: comparison with IL-4 expression and modulation by topical glucocorticoid therapy. Am J Respir Cell Mol Biol 1997; 17(1):17–24.

26. Robinson DS, Hamid Q, Ying S, et al. Predominant TH2 like bronchoalveolar T-lymphocyte population in atopic asthma. N Engl J Med 1992; 326:298–304.
27. Lee CH, Lee KS, Rhee CS, Lee SO, Min YG. Distribution of RANTES and interleukin-5 in allergic nasal mucosa and nasal polyps. Ann Otol Rhinol Laryngol 1999; 108(6):594–598.
28. Conti P, DiGioacchino M. MCP-1 and RANTES are mediators of acute and chronic inflammation. Allergy Asthma Proc 2001; 22:133–137.
29. Busse WW, Calhoun WF, Sedgwick JD. Mechanism of airway inflammation in asthma. Am Rev Respir Dis 1993; 147:S20–S24.
30. Bousquet J, Chanez P, Lacoste Y, et al. Eosinophilic inflammation in asthma. N Engl J Med 1990; 323:1033–1039.
31. Lee BJ, Naclerio RM, Bochner BS, Taylor RM, Lim MC, Baroody FM. Nasal challenge with allergen upregulates the local expression of vascular endothelial adhesion molecules. J Allergy Clin Immunol 1994; 94:1006–1016.
32. Gaurus SN, Liu MC, Newman W, Beall LD, Stealey BA, Bochner BS. Altered adhesion molecule expression and endothelial cell activation accompany the recruitment of human granulocytes to the lung after segmental allergen challenge. Am J Respir Cell Mol Biol 1992; 7:261–269.
33. Montefort S, Roche WR, Holgate ST. Bronchial epithelial shedding in asthmatics and non-asthmatics. Respir Med 1993; 87:9–11.
34. Braunstahl GJ, Fokkens WJ, Overbeek SE, KleinJan A, Hoogsteden HC, Prins JB. Mucosal and systemic inflammatory changes in allergic rhinitis and asthma; a comparison between upper and lower airways. Clin Exp Allergy 2003; 33(5):579–587.
35. Roche WR, Beasley R, Williams JH, Holgate ST. Subepithelial fibrosis in the bronchi of asthmatics. Lancet 1989; 1:520–524.
36. Chanez P, Vignola AM, Vic F, et al. Comparison between nasal and bronchial inflammation in asthmatic and control subjects. Am J Resp Crit Care Med 1999; 159:588–595.
37. Del Prete GF, De Carli M, D'Elios MM, et al. Allergen exposure induces the activation of allergen-specific Th2 cells in the airway mucosa of patients with allergic respiratory disorders. Eur J Immunol 1993; 23:1445–1449.
38. Baggiolini M. Chemokines and leukocyte traffic. Nature 1998; 392:565–568.
39. Jankowski R, Bouchoua F, Coffinet L, et al. Clinical factors influencing the eosinophil infiltration of nasal polyps. Rhinology 2002; 40(4):173–178.
40. Ponikau JU, Sherris DA, Kephart GM, et al. Features of airway remodeling and eosinophilic inflammation in chronic rhinosinusitis: is the histopathology similar to asthma? J Allergy Clin Immunol 2003; 112:877–882.
41. Walker C, Bode E, Boer L, et al. Allergic and nonallergic asthmatics have distinct patterns of T-cell activation and cytokine production in peripheral blood and bronchoalveolar lavage. Am Rev Respir Dis 1991; 146(1):109–115.
42. Bachert C, Wagenmann M, Rudack C, et al. The role of cytokines in infectious sinusitis and nasal polyposis. Allergy 1998; 53(1):2–13.
43. Simon HU, Yousefi S, Schranz C, et al. Direct demonstration of delayed eosinophil apoptosis as a mechanism causing eosinophilia. J Immunol 1997; 158(8):3902–3908.
44. Hamilos DL, Leung DY, Wood R, et al. Evidence for distinct cytokine expression in allergic versus nonallergic chronic sinusitis. J Allergy Clin Immunol 1995; 96(4):537–544.
45. Lee CH, Rhee CS, Min TG. Cytokine gene expression in nasal polyps. Ann Otol Rhinol Laryngol 1998; 107(8):665–670.
46. Kowalski ML, Grzegorezyk J, Pawliczak R, et al. Decreased apoptosis and distinct profile of infiltrating cells in the nasal polyps of patients with aspirin hypersensitivity. Allergy 2002; 57(6):493–500.
47. Georgitis JW, Matthews BL, Stone B. Chronic sinusitis: characterization of cellular influx and inflammatory mediators in sinus lavage fluid. Int Arch Allergy Immunol 1995; 106(4):416–421.
48. Steinke JW, Bradley D, Arango P, et al. Cysteinyl leukotriene expression in chronic hyperplastic sinusitis-nasal polyposis: importance to eosinophilia and asthma. J Allergy Clin Immunol 2003; 111(2):342–349.
49. Spector SL. Leukotriene activity: modulation in asthma. Drugs 1997; 54(3):588–595.

50. Powe DG, Hiskisson RS, Carney AS, Jenkins D, Jones NS. Idiopathic and allergic rhinitis show a similar inflammatory response. Clin Otolaryngol Allied Sci 2000; 25(6):570–576.
51. Powe DG, Jagger C, Kleinjan A, Carney AS, Jenkins D, Jones NS. 'Entopy': localized mucosal allergic disease in the absence of systemic responses for atopy. Clin Exp Allergy 2003; 33(10):1374–1379.
52. Kaufman J, Wright GW. The effect of nasal and nasopharyngeal irritation on airway resistance in man. Am Rev Respir Dis 1969; 100:626–630.
53. Kaufman J, Chen JC, Wright GW. The effect of trigeminal resection on reflex broncho-constriction after nasal and nasopharyngeal irritation in man. Am Rev Respir Dis 1970; 101:768–769.
54. Fontanari P, Burnet H, Zattara-Harmann MC, Jammes Y. Changes in airway resistance induced by nasal inhalation of cold dry, dry, or moist air in normal individuals. J Appl Physiol 1996; 81:1739–1743.
55. Yan K, Salome C. The response of the airways to nasal stimulation in asthmatics with rhinitis. Eur J Respir Dis 1983; 64:105–108.
56. Togias A. Mechanisms of nose-lung interaction. Allergy 1999; 54(suppl 57):94–105.
57. Bucca C, Rolla G, Scappaticci E, et al. Extrathoracic and intrathoracic airway responsive-ness in sinusitis. J Allergy Clin Immunol 1995; 95(1):52–59.
58. Speizer FE, Frank NR. A comparison of changes in pulmonary flow resistance in healthy volunteers acutely exposed to SO_2 by mouth and by nose. Br J Ind Med 1966; 23:75.
59. Shturman-Ellstein R, Zeballos RJ, Buckley JM, Souhrada JF. The beneficial effect of nasal breathing on exercise-induced bronchoconstriction. Am Rev Respir Dis 1978; 118:65–73.
60. Griffin MP, McFadden ER, Ingram RH. Airway cooling in asthmatic and nonasthmatic subjects during nasal and oral breathing. J Allergy Clin Immunol 1982; 69:354–359.
61. McLaurin JG. Chest complications of sinus disease. Ann Otol Rhinol Laryngol 1932; 41:780.
62. Huxley EJ, Viroslav J, Gray WR, Pierce AK. Pharyngeal aspiration in normal adults and patients with depressed consciousness. Am J Med 1978; 64:564–568.
63. Bardin PG, Van Heerden BB, Joubert JR. Absence of pulmonary aspiration of sinus con-tents in patients with asthma and sinusitis. J Allergy Clin Immunol 1990; 86:82–88.
64. Brugman SM, Larsen GL, Henson PM, et al. Increased lower airways responsiveness associated with sinusitis in a rabbit model. Am Rev Respir Dis 1993; 147(2):314–320.
65. Denburg JA, Inman MD, Leber B, et al. The role of the bone marrow in allergy and asthma. Allergy 1996; 51(3):141–148.
66. Braunstahl GJ, Kleinjan A, Overbeek SE, et al. Segmental bronchial provocation induces nasal inflammation in allergic rhinitis patients. Am J Respir Crit Care Med 2000; 161(6):2051–2057.
67. Braunstahl GJ, Overbeek SE, Kleinjan A, et al. Nasal allergen provocation induces adhesion molecule expression and tissue eosinophilia in upper and lower airways. J Allergy Clin Immunol 2001; 10(3):469–476.
68. Newman LJ, Platts-Mills TA, Phillips CD, Hazen KC, Gross CW. Chronic sinusitis. Relationship of computed tomographic findings to allergy, asthma, and eosinophilia. JAMA 1994; 271(5):363–367.
69. Bachert C, Bevaert P, Holtappels G, et al. Total and specific IgE in nasal polyps is related to local eosinophilic inflammation. J Allergy Clin Immunol 2001; 107(4):607–614.
70. Hauk PJ, Wenzel SE, Trumble AE, et al. Increased T-cell receptor V-beta-8+ T-cells in bronchoalveolar lavage fluid of subjects with poorly controlled asthma: a potential role for microbial superantigens. J Allergy Clin Immunol 1999; 104(1):37–45.
71. Bachert C, Gevaert P, van Cauwenberge P. *Staphylococcus aureus* enterotoxins: a key in airway disease? Allergy 2002; 57(6):480–487.
72. Corren J. Allergic rhinitis and asthma: how important is the link? J Allergy Clin Immu-nol 1997; 99(2):S781–S786.
73. Businco L, Fiore L, Frediani T, et al. Clinical and therapeutic aspects of sinusitis in chil-dren with bronchial asthma. Int J Pediatr Otorhinolaryngol 1981; 3:287.
74. Cummings NP, Wood RW, Lere JL, et al. Effect of treatment of rhinitis/sinusitis on asthma: results of a double-blind study. Pediatr Res 1983; 17:373.

75. Rachelefsky GS, Katz RM, Siegel SC. Chronic sinus disease with associated reactive airway disease in children. Pediatrics 1984; 73:525.
76. Friedman R, Ackerman M, Wald E, et al. Asthma and bacterial sinusitis in children. J Allergy Clin Immunol 1984; 74:185.
77. Lund VJ. The effect of sinonasal surgery on asthma. Allergy 1999; 54(suppl 57):141–145.
78. Palmer JN, Conley DB, Dong RG, et al. Efficacy of endoscopic sinus surgery in the management of patients with asthma and chronic sinusitis. Am J Rhinol 2001; 15(1):49–53.
79. Goldstein MF, Grundfast SK, Dunsky EH, et al. Effect of functional endoscopic sinus surgery on bronchial asthma outcomes. Acta Otolaryngol Head Neck Surg 1999; 125(3):314–319.
80. Uri N, Cohen-Kerem R, Barzilai G, et al. Functional endoscopic sinus surgery in the treatment of massive polyposis in asthmatic patients. J Laryngol Otol 2002; 116(3):185–189.
81. Weille FL. Studies in asthma: nose and throat in 500 cases of asthma. N Engl J Med 1936; 215:235.

8 | Differentiating Osteomeatal Complex Disease and Chronic Rhinosinusitis from Nonallergic Rhinitis

James N. Baraniuk

Department of Medicine, Division of Rheumatology, Immunology and Allergy, and Georgetown University Proteomics Laboratory, Georgetown University Medical Center, Washington, D.C., U.S.A.

Begona Casado

Georgetown University Proteomics Laboratory, Georgetown University Medical Center, Washington, D.C., U.S.A.

Sonya Malekzadeh

Department of Otolaryngology, Head and Neck Surgery, Georgetown University Medical Center, Washington, D.C., U.S.A.

INTRODUCTION

We have determined that chronic rhinosinusitis (CRS) can be divided into two mutually exclusive histological subtypes based on the presence of polyps or glandular hypertrophy (1). CRS with nasal polyps (CRSwNP) destroy the full thickness and organs of normal nasal mucosa and replace it with an edematous, generally eosinophilic, epithelium-coated "bag" of interstitial matrix "ground substance." This macromolecular content has not been fully characterized. The other histological finding has been designated "hyperplastic rhinosinusitis" or CRS without nasal polyps (CRSsNP). We have demonstrated that glandular hypertrophy is responsible for the thickening of the mucosa in this syndrome (1–4). The typical mucosal structures of subbasement membrane superficial vasculature, submucosal glands, nerves, and deep venous sinusoids are maintained. However, there is a transition away from the usual mixed leukocytic infiltrate found in normal inferior turbinates with an expansion of the mucosal area containing submucosal serous and mucous cells. Examination of patterns of mRNA (5,6) and protein (7,8) expression has begun to accelerate our understanding of potential mechanisms that may explain these two distinct pathological processes. This histopathological distinction is clinically important because CRS is truly a chronic disorder that persists for over 20 years of follow-up despite current surgical and topical glucocorticoid treatment (9). Different treatments may be required for each phenotype. In the early stages of CRS, there may be discriminate complaints of idiopathic rhinitis, other forms of nonallergic rhinitis (NAR), CRSwNP (small polyps or limited to very early middle turbinate changes), and CRS with mucosal thickening due to glandular hypertrophy. The clinical diagnosis of "turbinate hypertrophy" may represent one aspect of this overlapping spectrum of illnesses.

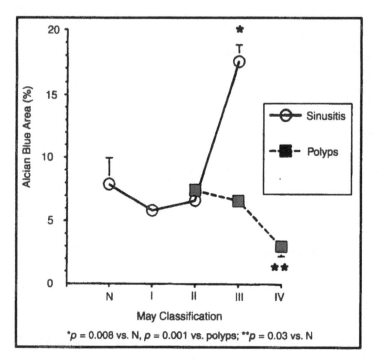

FIGURE 1 Percent Alcian Blue–stained area versus May computed tomography scan class. Histopathology worsened with sinusitis severity. Histology was normal in normal (Class 0), mild sinusitis (Classes 1 and 2) except for one Class 2 subject with polypoid changes. Significant glandular hypertrophy (percent Alcian Blue–stained mucus cell area > 11.5%) occurred in Class 3. Nasal polyps were identified visually and by microscopy in Class 2, 3, and all Class 4 subjects. By definition, there was no histological overlap between polyps and glandular hypertrophy. Therefore, distinct pathogenic mechanisms were responsible for the two subtypes. *Source:* Courtesy of J.N. Baraniuk, M.D.

NASAL POLYPS VS. NONPOLYPOID, GLANDULAR HYPERTROPHY IN CRS

Evidence for dimorphic histopathology was provided by staining surgically removed middle turbinate biopsies stained for mucous cells using Alcian Blue (1). The results were stratified by computerized tomography (CT) scan severity using the May CT scan classification system (10). The ratio of Alcian Blue–staining glands to total mucosal area was $6.88\% \pm 0.48\%$ (mean $\pm$ SEM, $n = 22$) in normal (May CT scan Class 0), symptomatic May Class 1 [osteomeatal complex disease (OMC)], and 2 (mild ethmoid disease) subjects (Figs. 1 and 2) (1–4). The upper 95th percentile ($\geq 11.5\%$) was set as a threshold for gland hypertrophy. The threshold was exceeded in four of seven Class 3 (moderate bilateral disease) subjects ($17.7\% \pm 1.4\%$, $p < 0.0001$). The other three of seven Class 3 subjects had visual and histological evidence of eosinophilic, edematous polyps that replaced the normal nasal mucosa. The ratio was reduced in pansinusitis (May Class 4, $n = 6/6$) to $3.0\% \pm 0.8\%$ ($p < 0.001$) with polypoid degeneration of the full thickness of the mucosa. There were clear associations between (i) pansinusitis and polyposis (May Class 4), (ii) multisinus mucosal thickening (May Class 3) with either, *but*

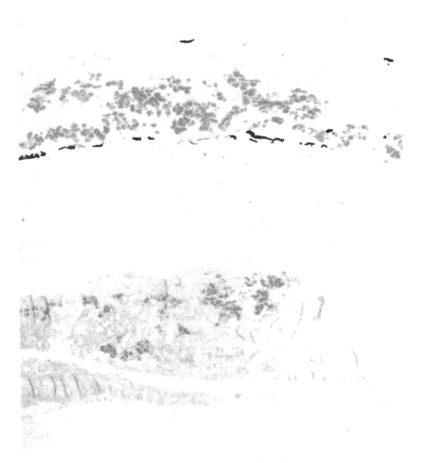

FIGURE 2 Alcian Blue–stained middle turbinate. (*Top*) Glandular hypertrophy in May computed tomography Class 3. Alcian Blue–staining mucous cells (*dark*) were increased in area indicating submucosal gland hypertrophy. Normal superficial vessels and deep venous sinusoids were present in the lamina propria (*lower*) and periostial (*upper*) regions. (*Bottom*) May Grade 2 sinusitis. Normal mucous and serous cells were seen in the glands. The superficial and deep venous sinusoids were normal. Polyps (see preliminary data) have few glands or vessels, but many eosinophils in an edematous tissue matrix. *Source*: Courtesy of J.N. Baraniuk, M.D.

never both, gland hypertrophy or polyposis, (iii) early polyp changes in some Class 2 subjects, and (iv) minimal CT scans changes (May Classes 0–2; no polyps) with minimal histological changes. Our work has been confirmed (11), and is consistent with Eichel's radiological classification of hyperplastic rhinosinusitis ± nasal polyps (12), and distinct mRNA patterns for "edematous" and "glandular" polyps by genomic microarray studies (6). The nature of "glandular polyps" is controversial in the absence of systematic investigations.

PATHOGENESIS OF NASAL POLYPOSIS

The early vestiges of polyposis may not be evident without rhinoscopy and middle turbinate biopsy. Nasal complaints at this stage may be nonspecific, and attributed to allergic rhinitis in skin test–positive subjects, or NAR in skin test–negative subjects. Associated pathological features of nasal polyposis (13–15) such as nasal eosinophilic diseases including nonallergic rhinitis with eosinophilia syndrome (NARES), "triad CRSwNP and asthma," and aspirin sensitivity are discussed elsewhere in this chapter.

This overlap of syndromes makes it critical to reinforce the distinction between CRS with and without nasal polyposis. In a retrospective analysis, we found that polyp and nonpolyp groups were best discriminated by FEV_1/FVC (66.7% ± 4.7 vs. 80.7% ± 4.0, respectively; mean ± 95% C.I.; $p = 0.0002$ by two-tailed unpaired t-tests with Bonferroni corrections for multiple comparisons); total lung capacity (TLC) (111.1% ± 5.9 vs. 96.1 ± 8.1; $p = 0.006$); and $FEF_{25\%-75\%}$ (52.2% ± 11.0 vs. 70.4 ± 12.2; $p < 0.05$) (16). Clinical asthma was equally prevalent, but the polyp group had more severe disease. Aspirin sensitivity was the next discriminator, and was present in 11 of 33 polyp and 1 of 41 (urticaria only) nonpolyp subjects. These findings reinforce the concept that distinct mechanisms are responsible for polypoid and nonpolypoid CRS. The importance of the mechanism(s) of aspirin sensitivity is clear given the increased severity of the "systemic" upper and lower airway disease in "Triad CRS." Mechanisms of polyposis stand in sharp contrast to those responsible for nonpolypoid CRS.

Bachert et al. have demonstrated very early polypoid changes in the middle turbinate (medial wall of the OMC). A "cap" of eosinophils was found under the epithelial basement membrane (Fig. 3) (17,18). The cause of the primary influx of eosinophils and other polyp-related cells is the fundamental issue underlying polyp pathogenesis. Chronic epithelial cell activation by adenovirus or other pathogens has been proposed by Hogg and coworkers in chronic bronchitis (19). Similar mechanisms may lead to the predominantly ethmoid–OMC region origin of polyps. This region is also the area of highest deposition of toxic inhalants, particularly water-soluble chemical toxins (e.g., aldehydes) and particulate (e.g., diesel particles, pollen grains, and fungal spores) (20,21). It would be anticipated that the general population is exposed to a similar pattern of toxicants, but clinical practice demonstrates that only a small proportion develops CRS. This suggests underlying comorbid factors including genetic predispositions.

Once activated, epithelial, antigen-presenting, mast or other sentinel cells can generate chemoattractant factors such as RANTES (22–26), eotaxin (2 > 1,3) (27,28), and monocyte chemotactic proteins (MCP)-3 and MCP-4 (26,29). These will promote the influx of eosinophils. Newly arrived, differentiating, and activated mucosal eosinophils may promote their own survival and further cellular influx by autocrine and paracrine release of GM-CSF (22,30,31), interleukin (IL)-5 (22,28,32), eotaxin (2 > 1,3) (26,27), RANTES (22–26), transforming growth factor (TGF)-β (24,33–35), and platelet-derived growth factor (PDGF)-B (36). Continued epithelial and potentially mast cell and lymphocyte mediators may add to this eosinophilic milieu.

Tissue destruction by the alkaline eosinophilic proteins (37) and halide-free radicals may destroy normal tissue elements such as vessels and glands. LTC4/D4/E4 (38) may promote vascular leak that generates an albumin and fibronectin pseudocyst under the eosinophil cap (13). We propose that evaporation of water from the surface of the polyp generates an osmotic and capillary pressure gradient that will "wick" ever greater amounts of plasma ultrafiltrate from adjacent normal mucosa through the polyp. Water influx and evaporation will increase the concentration of salts and other nonvolatile plasma components within the polyp matrix.

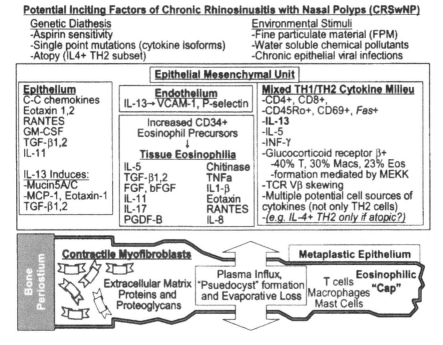

Potential Inciting Factors of Chronic Rhinosinusitis with Nasal Polyps (CRSwNP)

Genetic Diathesis
-Aspirin sensitivity
-Single point mutations (cytokine isoforms)
-Atopy (IL4+ TH2 subset)

Environmental Stimuli
-Fine particulate material (FPM)
-Water soluble chemical pollutants
-Chronic epithelial viral infections

FIGURE 3   Chronic rhinosinusitis with nasal polyps (CRSwNP). We propose that specific environmental and microbial stimuli acting in a host with the appropriate genetic diathesis will lead to CRSwNP (*upper panel*). Regional epithelial activation leads to local dysregulation of the epithelial-mechenchymal unit (*middle panel*). The cellular influx of eosinophils, mast cells, and different types of T cells generates a mixed "TH1/TH2" cytokine mileu. Atopic subjects also express IL-4. The distinct polyp histology will result from the constrained pattern of cytokine secretion, eosinophil chemoattraction and juxtacrine inflammation, plasma flux into the polypoid pseudocyst, differentiation and contraction of myofibroblasts (*lower panel*). This process has many parallels with bronchial and bronchiolar remodeling in asthma. *Source*: Courtesy of J.N. Baraniuk, M.D. *Abbreviation*: IL, interleukin.

These will contribute to the osmotic gradient and provide a continuous "sink" that induces additional plasma transudation (39).

Myofibroblasts (40) differentiate from tissue fibroblasts beneath the pseudocyst. Eosinophilic and other cell cytokines such as TGF-β2 (>-β1, -β3) (23–25,32,33), PDGF-A > PDGF-B (36), basic fibroblast growth factor (41), insulin-like growth factor-1 (42), endothelin-1 (43), IL-11 (44), and keratinocyte growth factor (45–49) are likely of importance. Contraction of myofibroblast α-1-smooth muscle actin (50) may extrude the pseudocyst gel into the airway lumen (33,36,50,51). Polyp pathology extends deep to the periostium with the loss of glands, vessels, and nerves (52). Denervation may enhance fibrosis (53,54).

Total immunoglobulin (Ig) E concentrations were significantly higher in polyps than in nonpolyp tissues, and correlated significantly with those of IL-5, eosinophil cationic protein (ECP), LTC4/D4/E4, sCD23 (sFcεRII), and eosinophil density. Eotaxin and collagen types I and III were also increased (18,27,34). Mast cells may be activated by IgE (allergic) or anaphylactoid histamine–releasing factors (e.g., not IgE-mediated, cytokines, and C3a). Multilogistic modeling demonstrated that nasal lavage fluid tryptase, histamine, and ECP levels were most predictive of polyposis (55,56). This model has not been examined prospectively. Macrophage, TH1, and natural killer (NK) cell function may be dysregulated because interferon (INF)-γ and IL-12 can be elevated in both allergic and nonallergic CRSwNP (57–59).

Several polyp classification systems have been proposed based on the predominance of eosinophils or neutrophils (60), or more complex mechanisms and comorbid asthma (1,18,44). Neutrophils predominate in children, and in particular those with cystic fibrosis where *Pseudomonas* and *Staphylococcus* sp. are important pathogens. The factors that lead to predominantly neutrophilic polyploid infiltrates (60) may include the neutrophil chemoattractants IL-8, C3b (immune complex activation), and LTB4. However, the relevance and preeminence of these potential mechanisms are poorly understood.

An alternative system is based on the concomitant IgE response in CRS (18).

1. Nonatopic polyploid asthmatics have aspirin sensitivity [Widel's syndrome (61); Samter's syndrome (62)] and high cysteinyl leukotriene 2 receptor expression (63), but no specific IgE.
2. Subjects with polyps, allergic rhinitis, and asthma have IgE to dust mites, molds, and other perennial aeroallergens, and may be more susceptible to allergic fungal sinusitis (64).
3. Hyper-IgE asthmatics have multiclonal, antigen-specific IgE to *Staphylococcus aureus* enterotoxins A and B superantigens (17). As yet unknown, precipitating insults or innate immunity deficiencies may permit *S. aureus* colonization and successful evasion of the adaptive immune system. *S. aureus* colonizes the nares of 33% to 50% of chronic sinusitis subjects compared to 22% to 33% of nonsinusitis controls (65,66).

PATHOGENESIS OF GLANDULAR HYPERTROPHY

Factors responsible for glandular hypertrophy and dysfunction in CRS (67) have just begun to be investigated. In part, this is because the histological similarities to normal inferior turbinates have led to its designation as "hyperplastic" or "hypertrophic" sinusitis (68). The latter designation is still clinical, and without a clearly defined mechanism. Glandular hypertrophy may have been mistaken in the past for microglandular adenosis analogous to tubular carcinoma of the breast (69), seromucous maxillary sinusitis (70), or the elongated epithelial invaginations within polyps (10,11). "Glandular polyps" with an increased area of submucosal glands (6,71–73) have been differentiated from "edematous polyps" (74). However, there has been no data to define these putative phenotypes of "polyps," nor long-term follow-up studies to determine if "early" glandular polyps (6) eventually generated macroscopic "edematous" polyps. In fact, microscopic edema and eosinophilia may appear in the middle turbinate in the earliest stages of polyposis (13). This lack of informed opinion occurred despite the millions of sinus operations that have had "routine" histological examinations. Detailed analysis of glandular hypertrophy began with the systematic analyses provided by Biedlingmaier and Trifillis (75), Malekzadeh et al. (1–3), and Sakakura and coworkers (76). Majima et al. demonstrated that submucosal gland density in inferior turbinates of chronic sinusitis subjects was increased compared to nonrhinitic controls (76). Goblet cell density was not different.

Quantitative histochemical assessments have been coupled with demographic and clinical analysis in larger populations to identify multiple CRS subtypes. Multifactorial analysis identified distinct phenotypes with aspirin sensitivity and asthma, frontal sinus disease, and glandular hypertrophy (77). Principal components analysis of CT scan for extent of disease and symptoms permitted classification of 474 patients with chronic perennial and persistent rhinosinusitis (78). A chronic rhinitis group shared nasal obstruction, anterior and posterior nasal discharge, sneezing, and facial congestion with the other groups, but did not have sinus involvement on CT scan. This group may have a component of neural hyperalgesia and allodynia that heightens their symptomatic perceptions from this visceral mucosa (79–82). A second group had localized anterior ethmoid sinusitis and complained of cacosmia (pain in the nasal cavity). Those with sinusitis localized to other regions tended to have more severe, chronic facial pain. Subjects with diffuse rhinosinusitis due to nasal polyposis had anosmia and loss of taste. These studies reinforce the hypothesis that separate pathophysiological mechanisms lead to distinct phenotypes of CRS.

Mucous Cells

Malekzadeh et al. (1) demonstrated a relationship between the percent area of Alcian Blue–staining mucous material in submucosal glands and the extent of maxillary and other large sinus disease detected by CT scan. Their tissue was obtained from the lateral middle turbinate that forms the medial wall of the osteomeatal complex. The data indicated hypertrophy of the mucin-secreting mucous cells in comparison to both normal middle turbinate mucosa and nasal polyps (Fig. 1). The degree of glandular hypertrophy increased in proportion to the extent of the sinusitis (May CT scan grade).

Alcian Blue at pH 2.5 stains the carboxylic acid side chains of sialic acid (neuraminic acid) (Fig. 2) (83,84). Sialic acid groups terminate the highly branched O-linked glycoconjugate side chains of "acidic" mucins. These carboxylate groups are oriented away from the glycoconjugate and so greatly increase the size of the mucin hydration shell and electrostatic interactions between these tenaciously adherent glycoproteins and particulate, microbial, or cellular materials. Very highly acidic, sulfated mucins stain with pH 1.0 Alcian Blue.

Mucins

Mucins are long chain proteins that may (i) be anchored in the membrane (transmembrane mucins 1, 3A, 3B, 4, 8, 12, and 17), (ii) be secreted into the gel or sol phases, or (iii) have been cloned but remain poorly characterized in airways (mucins 9, 13, 15, 16, I, TBM). The transmembrane mucins are important for intercellular and matrix interactions. *Muc4* mRNA may be a marker of ciliated cells (85) or an indicator of epithelial regeneration after acute injury (86). The acidic, gel-forming mucin genes map to 11p5.5, and are differentially expressed in goblet (*muc5A/C, muc2*) and glandular mucous (*muc5B*) cells (87). *Muc6* mRNA has not been detected in airways. *Muc7* is probably a "neutral mucin" secreted from serous cells into the sol phase (88). These mucins are of great functional importance for airway epithelial-lining fluid rheology, humidification, lubrication, particle adhesion, and host defense. They form "gel rafts" that are pulled along by ciliary motion. The secreted mucins have multiple cysteine residues in their N- and C-terminal regions. These form disulfide links to create the gel phase of mucus. The middle region of the polypeptide contains multiple, repeated sequences rich in serine and threonine repeats. These amino acids are the sites for O-glycosylation. The cysteine-rich, cross-linking areas may become cleaved from the adhesive carbohydrate-rich domain and so release the "sticky sponge" into the freely mobile phase of epithelial-lining fluid mucus (85). The mucin fragment and any adherent foreign material may be removed from mucoclots and expelled or carried posteriorly and digested in the stomach. The material may also become phagocytosed by macrophages or other dedicated mucosal antigen-presenting cells and localized, tissue-specific immune responses generated against the ensnared foreign antigens.

Mucins in CRS express more sialic acid, SO_4, and galactose, and less mannose in their polysaccharide side chains (89). Sialylation may be regulated by tumor necrosis factor (TNF)-α (90). Proteomic methods demonstrated the induction of glycosyl sulfotransferase in acute sinusitis subjects after one week of treatment (7). This finding suggested that further acidification of mucous cell acidic mucins was a host response to viral, bacterial, and potentially other mucosal injury. It may also be an indication of mucous and goblet cell hyperplasia and/or hypertrophy in both acute sinusitis and CRS.

We propose that acidic mucin hypersecretion in CRS with glandular hypertrophy plays an unintended role in pathogenesis. The tightly cross-linked mucins may congeal with fibrinogen, albumin, lysozyme, DNA, and other materials to form indigestible barriers, or mucoclots that are intended to prevent microbial spread and repair mucosal epithelial and basement membrane lesions. They may become irreversibly attached to the sinus mucosa, and eventually become buried under newly generated basement membranes and epithelium during remission and convalescence. We propose that these form the cores of postinfectious mucocoeles. The mucocoagulant may also become the substrate for microbial growth and formation of biofilms. If so, these "protective barriers" would be subverted to protect the colonizing microbes rather than the host.

Muc5A/C and *muc5B* mRNAs are most significantly upregulated in CRSsNP (91). *Muc4*, *muc7*, and *muc8* are upregulated in chronic ethmoid sinusitis in a process that may require retinoic acid (92). However, IL-4 and IL-13 may downregulate *muc5A/C* and upregulate *muc8* mRNA expression in nasal polyps (93). Mucin expression has been assessed in idiopathic nonallergic rhinitis ("vasomotor rhinitis"). The only difference from normal turbinate mucosa was a slightly lower in situ hybridization signal for *muc1* mRNA in nonallergic rhinitis (94). As we have discussed in this text, the criteria for vasomotor rhinitis may have been negative allergy skin tests without consideration for other syndromes of the differential diagnosis.

NFκB is a key mucin transcriptional regulator (95). PKC, cGMP-dependent phosphokinase, and myristoylated alanine-rich C kinase substrate mediate mucin granule exocytosis (95). Rodent mucous cell proliferation and mucin gene expression are upregulated by epithelial growth factor (EGF) (96–100), TNF-α (101), IL-9 (102,103), IL-4 (104,105), and IL-13 (106–108). IL-9 expression is strongly linked to expression of the calcium-activated chloride channel and mucus production in bronchial epithelium from asthmatics (109). EGF may also regulate goblet cell proliferation (97).

Serous Cells

About one-third of the total nasal lavage protein is synthesized by submucosal gland serous cells in normal nasal mucosa. These antimicrobial proteins

(83,87,88,110,111) include lysozyme (~14% of total nasal protein) (112), lactoferrin, secretory leukocyte protease inhibitor (113), and proteases. The latter include neutral endopeptidase, which degrades neuropeptides and bradykinin (114), membrane-bound puromycin-resistant aminopeptidase M (115), and secreted glandular kallikrein that cleaves plasma kininogen to release bradykinin (116).

A major task of glandular serous cells is the secretion of antigen-specific IgA (15% of nasal mucus total protein). IgA-producing plasma cells express CCR10 (117). In the lactating breast, these cells migrate toward the CCL28 chemokine that is upregulated on secretory mammary gland epithelium. The IgA is secreted as a dimer ($[IgA]_2$-joining chain) that diffuses to the interstitial side of the epithelium, and binds to the polymeric immunoglobulin receptor (poly IgR) expressed on this surface. TNF-α upregulates expression of poly IgR (118). The complex is translocated to the luminal side of the acinar cell, and then exocytosed as secretory IgA [sIgA: J-$(IgA)_2$-poly IgR] (119,120). We propose that CCL28 and CCR10 may be responsible for the close proximity of IgA-producing plasma cells to submucosal gland serous cells in human nasal mucosa and in CRS with glandular hypertrophy.

The lipocalin (LC) superfamily of lipid-binding proteins is a very important component of the innate immune system (121). LC1 is secreted from glands. LC2, or neutrophil gelatinase–associated lipocalin (NGAL), is packaged with elastase in neutrophil secretory granules. The Palate, Lung, Upper airway, Nasal Clone (PLUNC) proteins are a subfamily of LC's. The PLUNC family is well represented in glandular cells (8,121,122). There are two general forms with a lipid-binding domain ± a cell-binding domain. The "short PLUNCs" such as SPLUNC1 (the "classic" PLUNC) (8,122) have only the lipid-binding, eight-fold β-barrel domain. LUNX is a purported lung cancer marker that differs from SPLUNC1 by one amino acid. It may represent a polymorphism of this gene. SPLUNC proteins may sequester lipopolysaccharide (LPS) or other microbial lipids to protect against cellular overactivation by long PLUNCs (LPLUNCs) or CD14 (123) that activate toll-like receptor (TLR)-4 (124). TLR-2 and TLR-4 mRNA expression were not significantly different between normal and sinusitis tissues (125). SPLUNC2 and SPLUNC3 mRNA were detected in human nasal mucosa (121), but their proteins were not (7,8,122). Related families of odorant-binding proteins are released into the mucus of the olfactory region. These proteins are distinct from the odorant receptors on olfactory nerves. The odorant-binding proteins may bind excessive amounts of inhaled odorants so that a lower concentration of odorant can interact with olfactory nerve receptors without causing neural desensitization and tachyphylaxis (126).

The LPLUNC1 (von Ebner's gland protein), bacteriocidal/permeability inhibitory protein (LPLUNC2), and LPS-binding protein (127,128) have two domains. When lipids slide into the LP pocket of one domain, the second domain is released. This domain may bind to uncharacterized cellular proinflammatory receptors. The polypeptide that tethers between the domains may be cleaved by elastase or other proteases to release the ligand domain so it can diffuse and activate its receptors, while the first domain and its captured lipid are expelled, or swallowed and destroyed in the gastrointestinal tract.

The cationic antimicrobial factor human β-defensin (HBD) 1 may be constitutively expressed by normal nasal epithelium and glands (129). Nasal polyp epithelium expressed HBD2 mRNA and immunoreactive material, indicating upregulation during inflammation (130). HBD3 had negligible expression in nasal and sinusitis tissue (125).

GENOMICS AND PROTEOMICS: TRANSCRIPTOMES AND PROTEOMES IN CRS

Genomics

Genomic methods of Northern blotting and in situ hybridization assess mRNA expression one gene at a time. They have now been augmented by more extensive screening by mRNA microarray analysis and other advanced methods that assess expression patterns from the entire genome (131).

Fritz et al. studied nasal mucosal biopsies from allergic rhinitis subjects with ($n = 3$) and without ($n = 4$) nasal polyps (5). Apparently, polyp tissue was not examined. mRNAs that showed more than twofold difference in expression (fluorescence intensity) and $p < 0.05$ between the two groups were considered significant. As a result, their transcriptome (list of significantly altered mRNAs) reflected the influence of polyp-forming mechanisms in subjects with allergic rhinitis, but not the changes occurring inside nasal polyps. Mammoglobin was the most highly increased mRNA in the polyp group. It was localized to the cytoplasm of distal serous demilunes in submucosal glands. This raises the possibility that glandular hypertrophy was surveyed in this study. Fos was elevated as has been shown previously (132). Lipophilin B, tryptase beta 1, kallikrein 8, glutathione S-transferase theta 2, purinergic receptor P2Y, pyrimidinergic receptor P2Y, retinoblastoma-binding protein 8, allograft inflammatory factor 1, prostaglandin D2 synthase, and cystatin S were among the significantly increased mRNAs. mRNAs that were decreased by more than threefold were butyrophilin 3, prostate stem cell antigen, proplatelet basic protein, T-cell receptor gamma constant 2, myosin light polypeptide 4, and soluble acid phosphatase 1.

Nasal polyp tissue expressed different mRNAs. Lui et al. compared nasal polyps to normal nasal turbinate tissue to define the differentially expressed polypoid transcriptome (6). They found 192 mRNAs that were upregulated and 156 that were downregulated in polyps. Thirty-nine were more than fivefold higher, but only 10 were more than fivefold lower, in polyps than in normal tissue. The highest fold-changes were confirmed by quantitative RT-PCR. Histological analysis of the lamina propria divided the polyps into edematous, eosinophilic, and glandular subtypes. The "glandular polyps" had more glands than normal turbinates. This conformed to the findings of Malekzadeh et al. (1). The mRNAs showing the largest differences were from the glandular polyp set and included deleted in malignant brain tumor 1 (DMBT1), lactoferrin, prolactin-induced protein (PIP), and stratherin. Immunohistochemistry localized lactoferrin, PIP, and stratherin to the serous cells of submucosal glands. Stratherin may maintain oral mineral homeostasis. PIP may have many functions, including fibronectin-specific aspartyl protease activity. Lactoferrin is an avid iron-sequestering molecule. DMBT1 may have been present in either serous or mucous cells of glands. DMBT1 is a member of the multiple scavenger receptor cysteine-rich superfamily. DMBT1 or its splice variant gp340 may bind serous and epithelial cell trefoil proteins 1 and 3 (133), *Streptococcus mutans*, and influenza virions. Clara cell protein 10 (CC10, CC16, and uteroglobin) was the most downregulated mRNA. It was identified only in normal epithelial cells, but not in sinusitis.

Proteomics

Proteomics is the general title for broad-spectrum identification of the list of proteins that are unique to a given tissue or that may be differentially altered under distinct experimental conditions (134,135). A simple example is the differences in protein concentrations or immunohistochemical analysis by protein expression. More advanced methods employ a two-stage process. First, a sample is fractionated. Methods include two-dimensional gel electrophoresis and liquid chromatography. Second, mass spectrometry is used to identify the mass/charge ratio for all proteins or trypsin-digested peptides from a gel peak or chromatography fraction. Matrix-assisted laser desorption ionization–time-of-flight (MALDI–ToF) is an example of one-dimensional mass spectrometry. More elaborate two-dimensional mass spectrometry methods permit peptide sequencing. These sequences are used for precise identification of the protein and any polymorphisms, splice variants, or posttranslational modifications that may be present. Most results are qualitative, and should be considered an indication of the detectability of a given protein. Detectability is determined by the relative abundance of a protein in a mixture compared to the high abundance proteins such as albumin and immunoglobulins, the protein's susceptibility to trypsin (or other endoprotease) digestion (no digestion = no peptides for sequencing), and the chemical properties of the peptides that enable chromatographic and mass spectrometric separation and sequencing.

Proteomics and genomics assess different aspects of tissues, and have a poor concordance. For example, the proteome and transcriptome specific for LPS–stimulated neutrophils had a concordance of only 28% (136). Further analysis was more disconcerting. The neutrophils expressed 923 genes, with 100 increasing threefold and 56 decreasing threefold after four hours of LPS. Two-dimensional gel electrophoresis revealed about 1200 "protein spots," but comparison of 12 replicate runs identified only 125 reproducible spots. Spot intensity increased by 1.5-fold for an average of 24 spots (19%), and decreased 1.5-fold in 22 spots (17%) per replicate. These "significantly altered" protein spots were sequenced by MALDI–ToF and then compared to the Affymetrix 7070 chip results. Only 18 proteins and mRNAs matched. Of these, 2 showed concordant increases and 3 showed concordant decreases for both protein and mRNA (5 of 18, 28% concordance). When placed in the perspective of the 156 significantly altered mRNAs and 46 protein spots, these 5 concordant results may have occurred as a result of chance (probability of 5 of 46 potential mRNA-protein matches = 0.11 = $p > 0.05$, not significant). In contrast, two new proteins were identified by proteomics that were not present on the Affymetrix 7070 chip. This is a limitation of presumptively assuming that these chips can detect all gene transcripts. In a simpler case, platelets have 2928 mRNAs (microarray result) that can be translated into 82 proteins (proteomic result) (137). However, only 57 of the proteins matched the mRNA results.

The proteins expressed in acute sinusitis and acute exacerbations of CRS (7) have been compared to those expressed in nasal secretions from healthy subjects (Tables 1–4) (8). As expected (138), plasma contributed albumin, immunoglobulins, transferrin, plasminogen, haptoglobin, C3 complement factor, apolipoprotein A1, α-1-antitrypsin, and other antiproteases (detected in more than 30% of samples) (8). Submucosal gland serous cell products (112) were abundant including poly IgR, IgA, lysozyme, lactoferrin, LPLUNC1, LPLUNC2 (bacterial/permeability-increasing protein-like 1), SPLUNC1, LC1, proline rich protein 4, PIP, and mammoglobin. Mucous cell MUC5A/C and MUC5B were also detected.

These acute sinusitis nasal lavage fluid proteins were similar to those in normal lavage fluid, but many were present in more samples (e.g., serous cell proteins). This suggested that higher concentrations of some proteins may have

TABLE 1 Plasma Proteins in Human Nasal Lavage Fluid

Protein identification number	Plasma proteins	Percentage of 20 samples
1	Albumin	100
2	α1-Antitrypsin	95
3	Apolipoprotein A-I	45
4	Apolipoprotein J precursor ("clusterin")[a]	30
5	Apolipoprotein D	20
6	Complement component 3 precursor	35
7	Complement component 4, gene 4A	20
8	β-Fibrinogen	20
9	Haptoglobin	75
10	Hemoglobin β chain	25
11	Hemoglobin α chain	25
12	Ig α1[b]	100
13	Ig α2[b]	70
14	Ig γ1	100
15	Ig γ2	70
16	Ig γ heavy chain regions[c]	55
17	Ig μ	50
18	Ig κ	100
19	Ig λ	50
20	Immunoglobulin variable (VDJ) regions	100
21	α2-Macroglobulin	50
22	β2-Microglobulin	30
23	Plasminogen	60
24	Transferrin	95
25	Zn-α2-Glycoprotein	60

Note: Proteins were suspended, digested with trypsin, then analyzed by capillary bore liquid chromatography–electrospray–tandem mass spectrometry. The percentages of the 20 samples that contained evidence of each protein are shown.
[a]Not previously identified by proteomic methods in nasal lavage fluid.
[b]Most of the IgA is synthesized as secretory IgA in the nasal mucosa.
[c]Ig γ heavy chain regions shared by all 4 γ chains.
Abbreviation: Ig, immunoglobulin.

been present in sinusitis (7). Conversely, immunoglobulins and mucins were detected less frequently in sinusitis. This was surprising because these components would have been expected to increase as part of the mucopurulent drainage.

Many proteins such as plasma-derived fibrinogen-β and -γ were detected only on the day of initial presentation. IL-17E was detected only in sinusitis (7). IL-17E can activate NFκB and stimulate secretion of IL-8 in vitro (139). Over-expression of IL-17E in a murine model led to high serum levels of IL-2, IL-4, IL-5, granulocyte colony-stimulating factor, eotaxin, and INF-γ (140). Eosinophilia and B-lymphocyte hyperplasia resulted. The B-cell lymphocytosis was associated with significant elevations of serum IgM, IgG, and IgE. However, antigen challenge caused antigen-specific IgA and IgE, but not IgG, production. Matrix metallopro-tease-27 (MMP-27) (141), which has also been associated with B-lymphocytes (142), was detected acutely (7). S100 calcium–binding proteins A12 (S100A12; EN-RAGE or the extracellular receptor for advanced glycation end products; cal-granulin C) and S100A9 (calgranulin B) were other markers of inflammation in sinusitis (143). 5-Lipoxygenase, LC2 (NGAL), and myeloperoxidase were consist-ent with an influx of neutrophils. The concentration of autocrine neutrophil

TABLE 2 Proteins with Glandular or Epithelial Origin

Protein identification number	Glandular proteins	Percentage of 20 samples
	Glands: serous cells	
26	Lactoferrin precursor	90
27	Similar to common salivary protein 1	80
28	Poly-Ig receptor	80
29	Lacrimal proline rich protein	25
30	Lipocalin 1	80
31	Lysozyme	60
32	SPLUNC1 ("PLUNC")	85
33	Bacterial/permeability-increasing protein-like 1[a]	45
34	LPLUNC1 (Von Ebner minor salivary protein)	95
35	Secretoglobin family 2A (mammoglobin)	15
36	Prolactin-induced protein	45
	Glands: mucous cells	
37	Deleted in malignant brain tumors 1 isoform, a precursor[a]	60
38	Mucin 5B precursor[a]	60
39	MUC5AC protein[a]	45

[a]Not previously identified by proteomic methods in nasal lavage fluid.
Abbreviations: SPLUNC, short palate, lung, upper airway, nasal clone; LPLUNC, long palate, lung, upper airway, nasal clone; PLUNC, palate, lung, upper airway, nasal clone.

TABLE 3 Cytoskeletal Proteins Identified by Proteomics

Protein identification number	Cytoskeletal proteins	Percentage of 20 samples
40	Actin α-1 prepeptide	30
41	Actin α-2[a]	25
42	Actin β (cytoplasmic and mutant isoforms)[a]	100
43	Annexin A2[a]	20
44	Glial fibrillary acidic protein[a]	20
45	Keratin 1	45
46	Keratin 2a[a]	30
47	Keratin 3[a]	25
48	Keratin 4[a]	25
49	Keratin 5	15
50	Keratin 6A	30
51	Keratin 6B[a]	10
52	Keratin 6F	30
53	Keratin 6L[a]	25
54	Keratin 7[a]	20
55	Keratin 8[a]	40
56	Keratin 9[a]	30
57	Keratin 10	25
58	Keratin 12[a]	10
59	Keratin 14[a]	25
60	Keratin 16[a]	20
61	Keratin 19[a]	25
62	Keratin 25D, type I inner root sheath[a]	25
63	Nesprin-1[a]	20
64	Squamous cell carcinoma antigen[a]	30
65	τ-Tubulin kinase[a]	10

[a]Not previously identified by proteomic methods in nasal lavage fluid.

TABLE 4 Other Cellular Proteins

Protein identification number	Other cellular proteins	Percentage of 20 samples
66	Aldehyde dehydrogenase[a]	10
67	Apoptosis-inducing factor-homologous mitochondrion associated induced of death[a]	20
68	Carbonic anhydrase form B[a]	5
69	Histone H2B	25
70	Histone H4	15
71	Nasopharyngeal carcinoma-associated proline rich 4[a]	15
72	Neutrophil gelatinase-associated lipocalin (LC2)[a]	10
73	Phospholipase c-like 2[a]	10
74	RBBP8 protein[a]	10
75	Thiol-specific antioxidant protein[a]	5
76	TCN1 (transcobalamin I) protein[a]	10
77	Hypothetical protein KIAA0133	20
78	Similar to RIKEN cDNA 2310057J18	30

[a]Not previously identified by proteomic methods in nasal lavage fluid.

chemokine IL-8 increased in acute sinusitis, but was too low for detection by mass spectrometry (47). Curiously, α-1B adrenergic receptors were detected in acute sinusitis. This suggested that inflammation- or stressor-activated mechanisms may release catecholamines from adrenal or sympathetic sources. The site of receptor expression has not been identified as yet. Glycosylsulphotransferase was detected only on Day 6 indicating the long-duration conversion to secretion to highly acidified mucins.

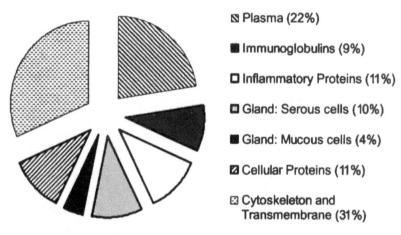

N Plasma (22%)

■ Immunoglobulins (9%)

□ Inflammatory Proteins (11%)

▫ Gland: Serous cells (10%)

■ Gland: Mucous cells (4%)

▨ Cellular Proteins (11%)

▨ Cytoskeleton and Transmembrane (31%)

FIGURE 4 Diversity of origins for the combined nasal and sinusitis lavage fluid proteome. Plasma and immunoglobulins, and cytoskeletal and transmembrane proteins each contributed about one-third of the total proteins detected in this proteome. Inflammatory proteins were only found on the day of presentation with acute sinusitis. The number of serous and mucous cell proteins was relatively small, but they were present in high concentrations and detected in most samples. *Source:* Courtesy of J.N. Baraniuk, M.D.

SERPINB (squamous cell carcinoma antigen 2) protein was also detected more readily in the sinusitis group. SERPINB inhibits dust mite proteases and may protect against other microbial serine proteases (144). SERPINB mRNA is highly upregulated by IL-4 and IL-13 (145). The recurring association of IL-4, IL-9, and IL-13 implies roles for TH2 lymphocytes (107), mast cells, and eosinophils in sinusitis as have been shown for allergic rhinitis and asthma. IL-4 also causes the dose-limiting sensation of nasal congestion when administered parenterally to humans (146). The mechanism does not appear to involve changes in vascular permeability or parasympathetic cholinergic glandular secretory reflexes. Activation of a specific set of "congestion" neurons is one possible explanation.

The sources of the proteins contained within the combined nasal and sinusitis proteome are depicted in Figure 4. Plasma plus the immunoglobulins accounted for 31% of the different types of proteins in the lavage fluids. Cytoskeletal, transmembrane, and cell surface proteins contributed an equal proportion. The final third were secreted from submucosal glands and epithelium (10% from serous and 4% from mucous cells), present in the nucleus and other cellular sites (11%), and inflammatory proteins that were detected only in acute sinusitis (11%).

CELL, CYTOKINES, AND CRS WITH GLANDULAR HYPERTROPHY

The presence of IL-4, IL-5, IL-9, IL-13, and other cytokines suggests that TH2-IgE-mast cell-eosinophil mechanisms of atopy have a strong influence on the development of CRS. However, many studies have been performed without stratification of patients by the clinical expression of atopic disease or histological diagnosis. Neither the detection of "TH2 cytokines" nor eosinophils is proof positive that atopy initiates or accentuates the development of any of the phenotypes of sinusitis that have been discussed. Allergic rhinitis has been diagnosed based on positive allergy skin tests or RAST results in 84% of endoscopic sinus surgery patients (147), 54% of CRS outpatients (148), and 37% of children with sinusitis (149). Perennial allergic rhinitis may be more closely linked to sinusitis (150). In retrospect, these studies were flawed by their simplicity. It is now necessary to stratify patients according to the presence of nasal polyps and atopy that specifically affects the target organ (i.e., allergic rhinitis) as opposed to other sites (skin as in eczema or the gastrointestinal tract as in food allergy), or even the presence of potentially suppressed, asymptomatic allergy (151,152).

Atopy may modify glandular cytokine production. Methacholine nasal provocation in house-dust mite–allergic rhinitis subjects caused a significant increase in IL-6 concentration in mucus, indicating its release from glands (153). Both IL-6 and IL-8 were immunolocalized to glands, the apical portions of epithelial cells, and cells in the lamina propria (154). GM-CSF–immunoreactive material was more strongly localized to the basal part of epithelial cells, basement membrane, glandular ducts, and leukocytes. If atopy can augment cytokine production in allergic rhinitis, then it would be anticipated to have similar effects in CRS with glandular hypertrophy. An increased prevalence of atopy is predicted in the glandular hypertrophy phenotype.

Serous cells of glands synthesize IL-17, macrophage migration inhibitory factor (155), EGF, the EGF-receptor, and other EGF-R ligands (Fig. 5) (96–100,156). EGF and nerve growth factor (NGF) were increased in salivary gland secretions during oral inflammation suggesting that EGF and NGF secretion in mucus may be upregulated in CRS with glandular hypertrophy (157). Glands and epithelium

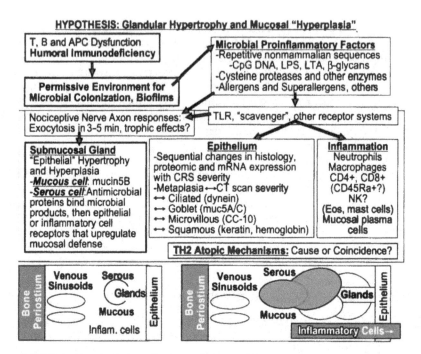

FIGURE 5 Hypothetical mechanisms of chronic rhinosinusitis rhinitis with glandular hypertrophy. Humoral immunodeficiency plays a permissive role in the colonization and infection of the sinuses (*upper left*). Microbial factors may stimulate glandular hypertrophy by several pathways (*middle panel*). We propose that microbial virulence factors activate epithelial cells either directly via *toll*-like or other receptor systems. Secreted innate immune proteins such as lipocalins that bind lipopolysaccharide and related materials may serve as sentinels to detect colonization, and activate epithelial and inflammatory pathways. Neutrophils become activated as indicated by our proteomic data. Acquired immune cell mechanisms may be activated, but not eliminate the microbial colonization. The inflammatory milieu of acidosis and hypoxia will depolarize specific subsets of nociceptive nerves. We have shown that their activation leads to rapid glandular exocytosis (three to five minutes) by the axon response mechanism. Exocytosis of mucin, antimicrobial innate immune proteins, and secretory IgA will attempt to eliminate the microbes, but may only provide a substrate for biofilm formation. This chronic process will lead to epithelial metaplasia (e.g., loss of cilia proteins and increased inflammatory keratins), neutrophil and mononuclear inflammation, and serous and mucous cell hypertrophy with mucosal thickening (*bottom*). *Source*: Courtesy of J.N. Baraniuk, M.D.

synthesize and store IL-16 that is secreted after stimulation by IL-9 (158). These mechanisms may be greatly magnified in the presence of glandular hypertrophy in CRS. ECP, IL-1β, TNF-α, and GM-CSF stimulated glandular exocytosis from human turbinate explants, suggesting that they may play similar roles in vivo (159). Corticosteroids significantly reduced the cytokine-induced glandular output.

A role for TGF-β1 was inferred by the detection of actin-γ1 and -γ2 that are regulated by this cytokine, and TGF-β II receptor (7) in acute sinusitis (160). These proteins and α2-smooth muscle actin may be markers of myofibroblast differentiation. TGF-β1 protein ($p = 0.0008$) and mRNA ($p = 0.025$) levels were significantly higher in nonpolypoid CRS than in nasal polyp samples (72). Extensive TGF-β1–immunoreactive material was found in the fibrotic extracellular matrix of nonpolypoid CRS tissues. In contrast, no TGF-β1 staining was found in the pseudocyst region of nasal polyps. Watelet et al. proposed that TGF-β1 expression linked to fibrosis may differentiate nonpolypoid CRS from nasal polyposis (72).

The cellular infiltrates in CRS with and without nasal polyps are distinct. When nasal polyps were absent, CD38+ lymphocytes and elastase-staining neutrophils were the predominant leukocytes in the tissue (161). Polyps also contained neutrophils, but had higher tissue concentrations of albumin and IL-5, and high densities of ECP-staining eosinophils.

A role for macrophages in CRS with and without nasal polyposis has been based on the detection of IL-12 mRNA (162). This has suggested analogies to smokers with chronic bronchitis, because CD68+ macrophages and CD8+ lymphocytes that lacked IL-4 and IL-5 ("T_{C1}" lymphocytes) were the predominant epithelial inflammatory cells in that disorder (163–165). These cells and their cytokines were not associated with glands. This finding suggests that gland hypertrophy may be stimulated by alternative pathways that do not involve "TH2" cytokines. For example, salivary glands in Sjogren's syndrome are surrounded by mononuclear cells. They appear to secrete INF-γ that induces interferon-inducible T-cell α chemoattractant (I-TAC or CXCL11) from the ductal epithelium (166). CXCL11 is absent from normal salivary glands. This TH1 mechanism may be active in autoimmune or vasculitic nasal disorders (167). We predict that upregulation of CXCL11 in CRS with glandular hypertrophy will provide indirect support for mechanisms involving INF-γ and its potential sources of CD4+ TH1, CD8+ Tc1-like, or NK cells in this subset of CRS. CXCL11 is not anticipated in nasal polyposis because of its reduced glandular volume, and the supposition that most of the "glandular" material represents invagination of surface epithelium during polyp formation (13).

INF-γ–induced activation of ductal epithelium may also increase arachidonic acid metabolism in CRS with glandular hypertrophy. Cycloxygenase (Cox)-1 and Cox-2 immunoreactive materials were detected in the ductal epithelium of submucosal glands. More intense Cox-1 staining was present in the epithelial lining in sinusitis compared to normal turbinate tissue (168). The exact prostaglandin, thromboxane, and other products are yet to be established. The pattern of Cox expression may be different from aspirin sensitivity in polyposis.

CRS with and without polyposis also differ in the expression of MMPs (169). Nasal polyps demonstrate MMP-9–positive inflammatory cells in pseudocysts, more intense MMP-9– and MMP-7–immunoreactive material in blood vessels, and higher tissue concentrations of MMP-7 compared to control turbinates and nonpolypoid CRS. In contrast, the concentrations of tissue MMP-9 and tissue inhibitor of metalloproteinase-1 protein were equally elevated in both types of CRS compared to control tissue. We suggest that differences in the regulation of enzyme expression and activities account for the distinct patterns of tissue remodeling observed in polypoid and nonpolypoid CRS.

HYPOTHESIS: HUMORAL IMMUNE DEFECTS LEAD TO GLANDULAR HYPERTROPHY IN CRS

We hypothesize that humoral immunodeficiencies are one of the fundamental factors underlying CRS with glandular hypertrophy (Fig. 5). In a retrospective analysis, we assessed the frequencies of low immunoglobulin isotype levels in CRS with and without nasal polyp subjects (Table 5) (170). Absence of IgE has been

TABLE 5 Frequencies (%) of Qualitatively Low Antibody Levels for the CRSwNP and CRSsNP[a] Groups

Serum concentration below normal	CRSwNP	CRSsNP	ANOVA
Number per group	39	36	–
IgE < 10 IU/mL	3	21	0.000003
IgG1	8	21	0.0020
IgG2	2	5	0.2
IgG3	4	11	0.028
IgG4	2	7	0.058
IgA	3	6	0.2
IgM	3	9	0.042

Note: The lower limits of normal established by each of the clinical laboratories were used for this qualitative analysis.
[a]Presumed glandular hypertrophy.
Abbreviations: CRSwNP, chronic rhinosinusitis with nasal polyps; CRSsNP, chronic rhinosinusitis without nasal polyps; Ig, immunoglobulin.

associated with CRS (171). Because there is no consensus for a lower limit of normal, we assumed that IgE < 10 IU/mL was indicative of a dysfunctional capacity to synthesize antigen-specific IgE. The lower limits of normal established by clinical laboratories were used to qualitatively define immune deficits for the other immunoglobulin isotypes. The CRSsNP group had significantly more subjects with IgE < 10 IU/mL and low IgG1, IgG3, and IgM. These frequencies were much higher than previously reported. However, previous reports did not stratify CRS subjects according to presumed histological subtype as done here.

Immunodeficiencies are more prevalent in CRS than control populations (172–174). Reduced total IgG was found in 18%, and IgA in 17% (174). Anergy to delayed type hypersensitivity skin tests was detected in 40%. Common variable hypogammaglobulinemia was diagnosed in 10%. These findings suggest dysfunction of antigen presentation, T-cell help, and/or B-cell heavy chain switching and immunoglobulin secretion. We hypothesize that the humoral deficits play a "permissive" role by allowing novel and increasingly aggressive, virulent pathogens to occupy "unprotected" mucosal ecological niches in the nasal recesses and sinuses (Fig. 5) Specific types of microbes may take advantage of the loss of sIgA, or IgG1- and IgG3-mediated immune complex, complement activation, and Fcγ-receptor–mediated opsonization (175). Dysfunctional host defense mechanisms in IgE deficiency are unclear (171) but could involve low occupancy of FCεR-II on eosinophils and macrophages (176).

We hypothesize that the colonizing microbes shed LPS, lipotechoic acids, β-glucans, CpG-rich DNA, and other products that are bound by the PLUNC and other families of innate immune proteins (120–124,126,127). These proteins then activate leukocytes and epithelial cells via TLRs and other mechanisms. This may lead to paracrine release of cytokines and other innate immune biological response modifiers that initiate and promulgate glandular hypertrophy.

Epithelial Metaplasia in Chronic Rhinosinusitis
Evidence to support the changing ecological niches has been provided by the correlation between CT scan severity and epithelial metaplasia documented by

scanning electron microscopy (75). Normal epithelium is dominated by ciliated cells. Narrowing of the osteomeatal complex (May Class 1) was associated with the replacement of ciliated cells by goblet cells. The result was epithelial mucin hypersecretion with decreased mucociliary activity. These findings may occur in some other NAR subtypes as well. Progression to May Class 3 was associated with differentiation to microvillous cells. In pansinusitis (May Class 4), there was squamous metaplasia with denuded basement membranes and local hemorrhage. We propose that gram-negative and anaerobic microbes that become bacteremic during brushing of the teeth and bowel movements may gain access to the sinuses through the injured mucosa.

Subsequent Progression to Glandular Hypertrophy

We hypothesize that activation of innate immune proteins by microbial factors is the first active step leading to epithelial metaplasia and glandular hypertrophy. These microbial factors may stimulate TLR and other mechanisms leading to epithelial chemokine release and the influx of leukocytes. Any of a series of dysfunctional TH1, TH2, CD8, NK, B, or antigen-presenting cell activities could play permissive roles for microbial colonization. Recruitment of cells possessing dysfunctional mechanisms of action, or of secondary, but less-effective immune mechanisms may accentuate the local immune deficit. The consequences may be an exuberant immune response, but one that is inappropriate or unable to eliminate the colonizing microbes. This situation may be analogous to that of leprosy (177). Tuberculoid leprosy is the better-contained form of *Mycobacterium leprae* infection. It is characterized by appropriate TH1 and granulomatous macrophage responses that stop the spread of the organism. In contrast, the absence of effective TH1 defenses with recruitment of TH2-like responses occurs in lepromatous leprosy. Hypergammaglobulinemia and eosinophilia lead to ineffective killing of this intraphagolysozomal parasite. The ensuing attempts to eliminate the mycobacterium lead to tissue necrosis without limiting the spread of the microbe. *Mycobacterium avium-intracellulare* may be another model (178). Defects in INF-γ and IL-12 signaling pathways lead to ineffective TH1 responses. The absence of protective immunity may lead to the default recruitment of other, less-effective antimicrobial mechanisms that lead to disease progression. In each of these situations, and in CRS in particular, it is probable that the recruitment and activation of macrophages, neutrophils, eosinophils, endothelium, glands, and fibroblasts would lead to novel combinations of cytokines and other regulatory molecules that further stimulate the innate immune system. Glandular hypertrophy that maximizes exocytosis of mucins and serous cell antimicrobial proteins and cytokines may represent one stereotyped mucosal-defensive response.

DIFFERENTIATING NAR FROM CRS

This information suggests that the early stages of many of the syndromes of nonallergic rhinitis are difficult to differentiate. Methods to discriminate precise pathological mechanisms in these early stages are largely lacking. If allergy skin tests are negative, a diagnosis of nonallergic rhinitis may be made. Only more intensive analysis with a search for specific pathogenic mechanisms, responses to therapy, and perhaps the passage of time with increasing symptom severity will lead to a clear diagnosis.

An algorithm for the investigation of CRS has been proposed that includes an analysis of the concomitant syndromes associated with CRS limited to the nasal cavity, i.e., OMC (179). This model was based on patient stratification and factor analyses of 99 retrospectively assessed CRS subjects. A series of decision points were identified that predicted a series of comorbid underlying conditions (Table 6). The order of decisions was based on the frequency of each variable and their ability to define subgroups based on potential pathogenic mechanisms.

The 1st decision regarded polyps. Their presence or absence divided the CRS group in half.

The 2nd decision was whether there was a strong history or evidence from provocation testing of aspirin or other nonsteroidal anti-inflammatory drug sensitivity with airway obstruction. Positive subjects represented the nasal polyps with aspirin sensitivity category (NPasa). Other causes must have predominated in the other nasal polyp subjects (NPother). Angioedema did not discriminate between groups.

The 3rd decision was based on a CT scan that showed sinus mucosal thickening more than 5 mm or more extensive and severe abnormalities (May Classes 2, 3, and 4). This extent of disease in the absence of polyps defined the CRSsNP group. The OMC group (May Class 1) was limited to nasal disease, and so entered the differential diagnosis of nonallergic rhinitis.

These three decisions defined our four major categories of CRS.

The 4th decision was based on pulmonary function. The NPasa group had significantly worse airway function than the other groups. The qualitative reduction of FEV_1/FVC ratio to below 0.70 was the single most significant discriminating variable. Small airways function was present in 91% of NPasa, and near 50% in the other three groups. Independent polypoid and atopic mechanisms may contribute to the links between CRS and asthma in the four categories.

The 5th decision was to determine if the peripheral blood eosinophil count was more than 4%. Other thresholds such as absolute cell counts may be more sensitive, but were not examined here. Eosinophilia was associated with asthma and negative skin tests in 47% of the NPasa group. By contrast, 21% of the NPother and CRSsNP groups had eosinophilia and asthma with positive skin tests (atopic asthma). Tissue eosinophilia may have been an even more discriminating marker (60).

The 6th decision was immune status. IgE was less than 10 IU/mL in 44% of the nonpolypoid CRS subgroup, compared to 21% when polyps were present ($p = 0.015$ by Fisher's Exact test). The small number of subjects per group meant that statistical significance was lost when each CRS group was compared. Groups of at least 30 subjects each should facilitate investigation of this finding. The combination of low IgE plus either low IgG1 or IgG3 was more prevalent in the CRSsNP group.

The 7th decision was based on skin test reactivity. Positive skin tests to allergens associated with persistent allergic rhinitis in temperate, seasonal climates (dust mites, cat, and fungi) dominated with only 4% of CRS subjects having solely seasonal patterns (trees, grasses, and weeds). Based on the extrapolations of Table 6, the allergic contingents within the NPother and CRSsNP categories accounted for 43% of the CRS population, and contributed 12.7 excess cases of atopy per 100 subjects compared to a separate, normal reference population. The majority was sensitized to dust mites.

The low rating for this 7th decision should be cautionary. The NPother and CRSsNP groups were almost identical in their patterns of allergic sensitization.

TABLE 6 Proposed Algorithm for the Classification of CRS and Its Overlap with Nonallergic Rhinitis

	CRS (n = 100)				N
	CRSwNP Present: N = 50.5		CRSsNP	CRSsNP Absent: N = 49.4	
	NPasa	NPOther	CRSsNP	OMC	
1st decision: polyps					50.5
2nd decision: aspirin sensitivity	17.1 (airways)	0	3.6 (urticaria)	4.8 (urticaria)	—
	17.1	33.3	28.3	21.2 (normal sinuses)	25.5
3rd decision: sinus mucosal thickening					78.7
4th decision					
$FEV_1/FVC < 70\%$	12.8 (75%)	13.7 (41%)	5.9 (21%)	3.0 (14%)	35.4
$FEF_{25\%-75\%} < 70\%$	15.6 (91%)	18.3 (55%)	8.2 (29%)	9.1 (43%)	51.2
5th decision					
Peripheral eosinophils >4% Eos + asthma	11.1 (65%)	13.1 (39%)	9.4 (33%)	4.0 (19%)	37.6
Atopic	3.0 (18%)	6.9 (21%)	5.9 (21%)	0.0 (0%)	15.8
Nonatopic	8.0 (47%)	3.0 (9%)	2.0 (7%)	2.0 (9%)	15.0
Eos/no asthma	0.0 (0%)	3.0 (9%)	1.0 (4%)	2.0 (9%)	6.0
6th decision					
IgE < 10 IU/mL	4.9 (29%)	5.5 (17%)	12.5 (44%)	9.5 (45%)	32.4
Low IgE + low IgG1 or IgG3	2.4 (14%)	1.4 (4%)	9.0 (32%)	2.1 (10%)	14.9
7th decision					
Positive allergy skin tests	7.5 (44%)	23.6 (71%)	19.2 (68%)	8.7 (41%)	59.0
Seasonal only	1.0 (6%)	1.0 (3%)	2.0 (7%)	0 (0%)	4.0
Persistent	6.5 (38%)	22.6 (68%)	17.3 (61%)	8.7 (41%)	55.1
Negative	9.6 (56%)	9.7 (29%)	9.1 (32%)	12.5 (59%)	40.9
Excess atopy cases per group	−0.3 (−2%)	7.9 (24%)	7.1 (25%)	−2.0 (−9%)	12.7
Total per group	17.1 (100%)	33.3 (100%)	28.3 (100%)	21.2 (100%)	99.9

Note: The numbers of subjects in each category and for each variable were extrapolated to a sample size of 100. The 4 categories (columns) were generated from the 1st, 2nd, and 3rd decisions. The numbers of putative subjects per category (and percent per category) were shown in each column. The far right column gives the sum for each variable per 100 CRS subjects.

Abbreviations: CRS, chronic rhinosinusitis; OMC, osteomeatal complex disease; CRSwNP, CRS with nasal polyps; CRSsNP, CRS without nasal polyps; NPasa, NP with aspirin sensitivity; NP other, NP with other features.

Source: Courtesy of J.N. Baraniuk, M.D.

However, these similarities do not explain why half develops polyps, while the other half does not. It may be that the mucosal microenvironment promotes TH2 reactivity and atopic sensitization to persistent allergens. Additional environmental, genetic, and molecular influences that remain to be discovered may force the inflammatory cascade to diverge into the mutually exclusive polypoid and glandular hypertrophy histological subtypes of CRS (5,18). The perplexing prevalence of low IgE in the otherwise highly allergic CRSsNP group was distinctly different from the NPother group. It suggests that immune dysregulation may contribute to CRSsNP pathophysiology.

OMC may represent a hybrid group that could progress to polypoid or glandular hypertrophy pathologies, develop allergic rhinitis alone, or regress. It would be necessary to perform middle turbinate biopsies with longitudinal follow-up to answer this question of disease progression. Subjects with OMC narrowing represent a legitimate category of CRS (82,180–184). Structural causes include concha bullosa (92%), Haller's cells (33%), alterations in the uncinate process (25%), and ethmoid bulla (5%) (May Grade 1) (185,186). Mucosal contact (39%) may be the cause of the rhinitis symptoms. If significant nasal septal deviation is excluded, then 86% of subjects with OMC narrowing by rhinoscopy will have anterior ethmoid mucosal disease on CT scan (May Grade 2). The ipsilateral maxillary sinus mucosa may be thickened in up to 46%. These findings demonstrate the subtle mucosal changes that occur during the progression of nasal cavity OMC disease into ethmoid and maxillary sinus involvement.

It is important to remember that these radiological findings are not diagnostic for OMC. Up to 32% of MRI and CT scans performed to assess headache, orbital, and intracranial disease have incidental abnormalities (187–190). These range from mucosal thickening to polyps, air–fluid levels, and pansinusitis. Even the common cold can lead to a sterile pansinusitis that clears spontaneously (unless a secondary bacterial infection ensues). When similar radiological studies were performed along with a rhinitis and headache questionnaire, it was found that nasal blockage was the only item to be significantly associated with the abnormal sinus scans (191). The patients' explanation of their sensations of blockage was not refined enough to evaluate potential patholophysiological mechanisms. "Blockage" has also been associated with persistent allergic rhinitis, although "sneezing and running" were more typical of intermittent allergic rhinitis where histaminergic mechanisms may predominate (192). These findings illustrate the need to use multiple, rigorously defined historical, physical examination, questionnaire, radiological, and other criteria for evaluating the early stages of CRS where the physical signs are limited to intranasal findings of OMC narrowing.

CONCLUSION

This review identified a number of observations that may generate a multifactorial definition of CRS with glandular hypertrophy. Increased tissue area devoted to Alcian Blue–staining mucous (>11.5% of area) and serous cells (threshold not established) represent the cornerstone for this diagnosis. Products of glandular exocytosis would be anticipated to be higher in this subtype compared to nasal polyposis. Polyps are associated with a 10-fold increase in albumin transudation compared to normal (39). If the glands are capable of responding to secretagogues such as methacholine (67) or hypertonic saline (80), then provocations with these agents may lead to glandular exocytosis in nonpolypoid CRS and negligible responses from polyps that lack glands, nerves, and vessels. The specificity and sensitivity of indices of macrophage, neutrophil, eosinophil, and myofibroblast proliferation are not resolved, but may offer logical histochemical tools to distinguish glandular hypertrophy from polyposis. Immunohistochemical detection of TGF-β1 and associated fibrosis may be another marker of glandular hypertrophy (72). Immunodeficiency and atopy must be used to stratify subjects into potentially more homogenous subsets so that common mechanisms of CRS pathology can be identified. Multivariate and principal component analysis will be extremely valuable tools for dissecting and organizing the genomic, proteomic, histological, cytokine, atopy, immunodeficiency, asthmatic, and other clinical data (77,78). The advanced methods discussed above require that investigators consider the multifactorial causes of CRS in much more sophisticated and nuanced fashion. The result will be a set of better defined disorders that can be classified by pathophysiological mechanism, and be approached in a more individualized and targeted manner than is currently the case.

ACKNOWLEDGMENTS

Supported by Public Health Service Award RO1 AI42403 and 1 M01-RR13297–01A1 from the General Clinical Research Center Program of the National Center for Research Resources, National Institutes of Health.

REFERENCES

1. Malekzadeh S, Hamburger MD, Whelan PJ, Biedlingmaier JF, Baraniuk JN. Density of middle turbinate subepithelial mucous glands in patients with chronic rhinosinusitis. Otolaryngol Head Neck Surg 2002; 127:190–195.
2. Malekzadeh S, Hamburger M, Biedlingmaier JF, Baraniuk JN. Density of middle turbinate subepithelial mucous glands in patients with chronic sinusitis and polyposis. Otolaryngology Society, Southern meeting, 1997.
3. Malekzadeh S, Hamburger M, Biedlingmaier JF, Trifillis A, Baraniuk JN. Epithelial and glandular metaplasia in the middle turbinates of chronic sinusitis patients correlate with CT scan severity (May classification). J Allergy Clin Immunol 1998; 101:S250.
4. Malekzadeh S, McGuire JF. The new histologic classification of chronic rhinosinusitis. Curr Allergy Asthma Rep 2003; 3:221–226.
5. Fritz SB, Terrell JE, Conner ER, Kukowska-Latallo JF, Baker JR. Nasal mucosal gene expression in patients with allergic rhinitis with and without nasal polyps. J Allergy Clin Immunol 2003; 112:1057–1063.
6. Liu Z, Kim J, Sypek JP, Wang IM, Horton H, Oppenheim FG, Bochner BS. Gene expression profiles in human nasal polyp tissues studied by means of DNA microarray. J Allergy Clin Immunol 2004; 114:783–790.
7. Casado B, Pannell LK, Viglio S, Iadarola P, Baraniuk JN. Analysis of the sinusitis nasal lavage fluid proteome using capillary liquid chromatography interfaced to electrospray ionization quadrupole-time of flight tandem mass spectrometry. Electrophoresis 2004; 25:1386–1393.
8. Casado B, Pannell KL, Iadarola P, Baraniuk J. Identification of human nasal mucous proteins using proteomics. Proteomics 2005; 5:2949–2959.
9. Vento SI, Ertama LO, Hytonen ML, Wolff CH, Malmberg CH. Nasal polyposis: clinical course during 20 years. Ann Allergy Asthma Immunol 2000; 85:209–214.
10. May M, Levine HL. Endoscopic Sinus Surgery. York: Thiem Medical Publishing, 1993:105–125.
11. Cousin JN, Har-El G, Li J. Is there a correlation between radiographic and histologic findings in chronic sinusitis? J Otolaryngol 2000; 29:170–173.

12. Eichel BS. A proposal for a staging system for hyperplastic rhinosinusitis based on the presence or absence of intranasal polyposis. ENT J 1999; 78:262–268.
13. Mygind N, Lildholdt T. Nasal Polyposis. In: An Inflammatory Disease and Its Treatment. Copenhagen: Munksgaard, 1997:1–183.
14. Settipane GA, Lund VJ, Bernstein JM, Tos M. Nasal Polyps: Epidemiology, Pathogenesis and Treatment. Providence, RI: OceanSide Publications, 1997:1–189.
15. Lennard CM, Mann EA, Sun LL, Chang AS, Bolger WE. Interleukin-1 beta, interleukin-5, interleukin-6, interleukin-8, and tumor necrosis factor-alpha in chronic sinusitis: response to systemic corticosteroids. Am J Rhinol 2000; 14(6):367–373.
16. White K, Baraniuk JN. Chronic sinusitis subtypes and airway function. J Allergy Clin Imunol 2004; 113:S203.
17. Bachert C, Gevaert P, van Cauwenberge P. Nasal polyposis—a new concept on the formation of polyps. ACI Int 1999; 11:130–135.
18. Bachert C, Gevaert P, Holtappels G, Cuvelier C, van Cauwenberge P. Nasal polyposis: from cytokines to growth. Am J Rhinol 2000; 14:279–290.
19. Ogawa E, Elliott WM, Hughes F, Eichholtz TJ, Hogg JC, Hayashi S. Latent adenoviral infection induces production of growth factors relevant to airway remodeling in COPD. Am J Physiol Lung Cell Mol Physiol 2004; 286(1):L189–L197.
20. Shusterman D. Toxicology of nasal irritants. Curr Allergy Asthma Rep 2003; 3(3): 258–265.
21. Saijo R, Majima Y, Hyo N, Takano H. Particle deposition of therapeutic aerosols in the nose and paranasal sinuses after transnasal sinus surgery: a cast model study. Am J Rhinol 2004; 18(1):1–7.
22. Hamilos DL, Leung DY, Huston DP, Kamil A, Wood R, Hamid Q. GM-CSF, IL-5 and RANTES immunoreactivity and mRNA expression in chronic hyperplastic sinusitis with nasal polyposis (NP). Clin Exp Allergy 1998; 28:1145–1152.
23. Fakhri S, Frenkiel S, Hamid QA. Current views on the molecular biology of chronic sinusitis. J Otolaryngol 2002; 31(suppl 1):S2–S9.
24. Lee CH, Lee KS, Rhee CS, Lee SO, Min YG. Distribution of RANTES and interleukin-5 in allergic nasal mucosa and nasal polyps. Ann Otol Rhinol Laryngol 1999; 108: 594–598.
25. Allen JS, Eisma R, LaFreniere D, Leonard G, Kreutzer D. Characterization of the eosinophil chemokine RANTES in nasal polyps. Ann Otol Rhinol Laryngol 1998; 107:416–420.
26. Bartels J, Maune S, Meyer JE, et al. Increased eotaxin-mRNA expression in non-atopic and atopic nasal polyps: comparison to RANTES and MCP-3 expression. Rhinology 1997; 35:171–174.
27. Minshall EM, Cameron L, Lavigne F, et al. Eotaxin mRNA and protein expression in chronic sinusitis and allergen-induced nasal responses in seasonal allergic rhinitis. Am J Respir Cell Mol Biol 1997; 17:683–690.
28. Kamil A, Ghaffar O, Lavigne F, Taha R, Renzi PM, Hamid Q. Comparison of inflammatory cell profile and Th2 cytokine expression in the ethmoid sinuses, maxillary sinuses, and turbinates of atopic subjects with chronic sinusitis. Otolaryngol Head Neck Surg 1998; 118:804–809.
29. Wright ED, Frenkiel S, Ghaffar O, et al. Monocyte chemotactic protein expression in allergy and non-allergy-associated chronic sinusitis. J Otolaryngol 1998; 27:281–287.
30. Hamilos DL, Leung DL, Wood R, et al. Chronic hyperplastic sinusitis: association of tissue eosinophilia with mRNA expression of granulocyte-macrophage colony-stimulating factor and interleukin-3. J Allergy Clin Immunol 1993; 92:39–48.
31. Ohno I, Lea R, Finotto S, et al. Granulocyte/macrophage colony-stimulating factor (GM-CSF) gene expression by eosonophils in nasal polyposis. Am J Respir Cell Mol Biol 1991; 5:505–510.
32. Hamilos DL, Leung DY, Wood R, et al. Evidence for distinct cytokine expression in allergic versus nonallergic chronic sinusitis. J Allergy Clin Immunol 1995; 96:537–544.
33. Montesano R, Orci L. Transforming growth factor-b stimulates collagen-matrix contraction by fibroblasts: implications for wound healing. Proc Natl Acad Sci USA 1988; 85:4894–4897.

34. Coste A, Lefaucher JP, Wang QP, et al. Expression of the transforming growth factor beta isoforms in inflammatory cells of nasal polyps. Arch Otol Head Neck Surg 1998; 124:1361–1366.
35. Eisma RJ, Allen JS, LaFreniere D, Leonard G, Kreutzer DL. Eosinophil expression of transforming growth factor-beta and its receptors in nasal polyposis: role of the cytokines in this disease process. Am J Otolaryngol 1997; 18:405–411.
36. Clark RAF, Folkvord JM, Hart CE, Murray MJ, McPherson JM. Platelet isoforms of platelet-derived growth factor stimulate fibroblasts to contract collagen matrices. J Clin Invest 1989; 84:1036–1040.
37. Rasp G, Thomas PA, Bujia J. Eosinophil inflammation of the nasal mucosa in allergic and non-allergic rhinitis measured by eosinophil cationic protein levels in native nasal fluid and serum. Clin Exp Allergy 1994; 24:1151–1156.
38. Georgitis JW, Matthews BL, Stone B. Chronic sinusitis: characterization of cellular influx and inflammatory mediators in sinus lavage fluid. Int Arch Allergy Immunol 1995; 106:416–421.
39. Biewenga J, Stoop AE, van der Heijden HA, van der Baan S, van Kamp GJ. Albumin and immunoglobulin levels in nasal secretions of patients with nasal polyps treated with endoscopic sinus surgery and topical corticosteroids. J Allergy Clin Immunol 1995; 96:334–340.
40. Gabbiani G. Evolution and clinical implications of the myofibroblast concept. Cardiovasc Res 1998; 38:545–548.
41. Powers MR, Qu Z, LaGesse PC, Liebler JM, Wall MA, Rosenbaum JT. Expression of basic fibroblast growth factor in nasal polyps. Ann Otol Rhinol Laryngol 1998; 107:891–897.
42. Petruson B, Hansson HA, Petrusson K. Insulin-like growth factor I immunoreactivity in nasal polyps. Arch Otolaryngol Head Neck Surg 1988; 114(11):1272–1275.
43. Zhang S, Smartt H, Holgate ST, Roche WR. Growth factors secreted by bronchial epithelial cells control myofibroblast proliferation: an in vitro co-culture model of airway remodeling in asthma. Lab Invest 1999; 79(4):395–405.
44. Tang W, Geba GP, Zheng T, et al. Targeted expression of IL-11 in the murine airway causes lymphocytic inflammation, bronchial remodeling, and airways obstruction. J Clin Invest 1996; 98:2845–2853.
45. Ishibashi T, Tanaka T, Nibu K, Ishimoto S, Kaga K. Keratinocyte growth factor and its receptor messenger RNA expression in nasal mucosa and nasal polyps. Ann Otol Rhinol Laryngol 1998; 107:885–890.
46. Ghaffar O, Lavigne F, Kamil A, Renzi P, Hamid Q. Interleukin-6 expression in chronic sinusitis: colocalization of gene transcripts to eosinophils, macrophages, T Lymphocytes, and mast cells. Otolaryngol Head Neck Surg 1998; 118(4):504–511.
47. Rudack C, Stoll W, Bachert C. Cytokines in nasal polyposis, acute and chronic sinusitis. Am J Rhino 1998; 12(6):383–388.
48. Zhang S, Howarth PH, Roche WR. Cytokine production by cell cultures from bronchial subepithelial myofibroblasts. J Pathol 1996; 180(1):95–101.
49. Mullol J, Xaubet A, Gaya A, et al. Cytokine gene expression and release from epithelial cells. A comparison study between healthy nasal mucosa and nasal polyps. Clin Exp Allergy 1995; 25(7):607–615.
50. Singer AJ, Clark RAF. Cutaneous wound healing. N Engl J Med 1999; 341:738–746.
51. Schiro JA, Chan BM, Roswit WT, et al. Integrin a2b1 (VLA-2) mediates reorganization and contraction of collagen matrices by human cells. Cell 1999; 67:403–410.
52. Gungor A, Baroody FM, Naclerio RM, White SR, Corey JP. Decreased neuropeptide release may play a role in the pathogenesis of nasal polyps. Otolaryngol Head Neck Surg 1999; 121(5):585–590.
53. Norlander T, Bolger WE, Stierna P, Uddman R, Carlsoo B. A comparison of morphological effects on the rabbit nasal and sinus mucosa after surgical denervation and topical capsaicin application. Eur Arch Otorhinolaryngol 1996; 253:205–213.
54. Carver TW Jr., Srinathan SK, Velloff CR, Perez Fontan JJ. Increased type I procollagen mRNA in airways and pulmonary vessels after vagal denervation in rats. Am J Respir Cell Mol Biol 1997; 17:691–701.

55. Di Lorenzo G, Drago A, Esposito Pellitteri M, et al. Measurement of inflammatory mediators of mast cells and eosinophils in native nasal lavage fluid in nasal polyposis. Int Arch Allergy Immunol 2001; 125:164–175.
56. Bhattacharyya N, Vyas DK, Fechner FP, Gliklich RE, Metson R. Tissue eosinophilia in chronic sinusitis: quantification techniques. Arch Otolaryngol Head Neck Surg 2001; 127:1102–1105.
57. Kassim SK, Elbeigermy M, Nasr GF, Khalil R, Nassar M. The role of interleukin-12, and tissue antioxidants in chronic sinusitis. Clin Biochem 2002; 35:369–375.
58. Wright ED, Christodoulopoulos P, Frenkiel S, Hamid Q. Expression of interleukin (IL)-12 (p40) and IL-12 (beta 2) receptors in allergic rhinitis and chronic sinusitis. Clin Exp Allergy 1999; 29:1320–1325.
59. Jyonouchi H, Sun S, Le H, Rimell FL. Evidence of dysregulated cytokine production by sinus lavage and peripheral blood mononuclear cells in patients with treatment-resistant chronic rhinosinusitis. Arch Otolaryngol Head Neck Surg 2001; 127: 1488–1494.
60. Kountakis SE, Arango P, Bradley D, Wade ZK, Borish L. Molecular and cellular staging for the severity of chronic rhinosinusitis. Laryngoscope 2004; 114:1895–1905.
61. Widel F, Abrami P, Lermoyez J. Anaphylaxie et idiosyncrasie. Presse Medicale 1922; 30:189–193.
62. Samter M, Beers RF. Intolerance to aspirin: clinical studies and consideration of its pathogenesis. Ann Int Med 1968; 68:975–983.
63. Sousa AR, Parikh A, Scadding G, Corrigan CJ, Lee TK. Leukotriene receptor expression on nasal mucosal inflammatory cells in aspirin-sensitive rhinosinusitis. N Engl J Med 2002; 347:1493–1499.
64. Marple BF. Allergic fungal rhinosinusitis: current theories and management strategies. Laryngoscope 2001; 111:1006–1019.
65. Kremer B, Jacobs JA, Soudijn ER, van der Ven AJ. Clinical value of bacteriological examinations of nasal and paranasal mucosa in patients with chronic sinusitis. Eur Arch Otorhinolaryngol 2001; 258:220–225.
66. Perl TM, Cullen JJ, Wenzel RP, et al. Mupirocin and the Risk of *Staphylococcus aureus* Study Team. Intranasal mupirocin to prevent postoperative *Staphylococcus aureus* infections. N Engl J Med 2002; 346:1871–1877.
67. Raphael GD, Meredith SD, Kaliner MA. Abnormal cholinergic parasympathetic responsiveness in the nasal mucosa of patients with recurrent sinusitis. J Allergy Clin Immunol 1990; 86:10–18.
68. Larsen PL, Tos M, Mogensen C. Nasal glands and goblet cells in chronic hypertrophic rhinitis. Am J Otolaryngol 1986; 7:28–33.
69. Eusebi VV. Microglandular adenosis arising in a chronic paranasal sinusitis. Histopathology 2000; 37:474.
70. Assimakopoulos D, Danielides V, Kontogiannis N, Skevas A, Evangelou A, Van Cauwenberge P. Seromucous maxillary sinusitis (SMMS): a clinicophysiological approach. Acta Otorhinolaryngol Belg 2001; 55:65–69.
71. Kakoi H, Hiraide F. A histological study of formation and growth of nasal polyps. Acta Otolaryngol 1987; 103:137–144.
72. Watelet JB, Claeys C, Perez-Novo C, Gevaert P, Van Cauwenberge P, Bachert C. Transforming growth factor beta1 in nasal remodeling: differences between chronic rhinosinusitis and nasal polyposis. Am J Rhinol 2004; 18:267–272.
73. Caye-Thomasen P, Hermansson A, Tos M, Prellner K. Polyps pathogenesis—a histopathological study in experimental otitis media. Acta Otolaryngol 1995; 115:76–82.
74. Leprini S, Garaventa G, Pallestrini R, Leprini E, Pallestrini EA. Analysis of the cellular infiltrate and epithelial class I and II molecular expression in edematous type nasal polyps. Allergy 2004; 59:54–60.
75. Biedlingmaier JF, Trifillis A. Comparison of CT scan and electron microscopic findings on endoscopically harvested middle turbinates. Otolaryngol Head Neck Surg 1998; 118:165–173.
76. Majima Y, Masuda S, Sakakura Y. Quantitative study of nasal secretory cells in normal subjects and patients with chronic sinusitis. Laryngoscope 1997; 107:1515–1518.

77. Facon F, Paris J, Guisiano B, Dessi P. Multifactorial analysis of preoperative functional symptoms in nasal polyposis (report of 403 patients). Rev Laryngol Otol Rhinol (Bord) 2003; 124:151–159.
78. Bonfils P, Halimi P, Le Bihan C, Nores JM, Avan P, Landais P. Correlation between nasosinusal symptoms and topographic diagnosis in chronic rhinosinusitis. Ann Otol Rhinol Laryngol 2005; 114:74–83.
79. Adam G. Visceral Perception: Understanding Internal Organs. New York: Plenum Press, 1998.
80. Baraniuk JN, Petrie KN, Le U, et al. Neuropathology in rhinosinusitis. Am J Respir Crit Care Med 2005; 171:5–11.
81. Naranch K, Park YJ, Repka-Ramirez SM, Velarde A, Clauw D, Baraniuk JN. A tender sinus does not always mean sinusitis. Otolaryngol Head Neck Surg 2002; 127:387–397.
82. Acquardo MA, Montgomery WW. Treatment of chronic paranasal sinus pain with minimal sinus CT changes. Ann Otol Rhinol Laryngol 1996; 105:607–614.
83. Ali M, Maniscalco J, Baraniuk JN. Spontaneous release of submucosal gland serous and mucous cell macromolecules from human nasal explants in vitro. Am J Physiol 1996; 270(4 Pt 1):L595–L600.
84. Pon DJ, van Staden CJ, Rodger IW. Hypertrophic and hyperplastic changes of mucus-secreting epithelial cells in rat airways: assessment using a novel, rapid, and simple technique. Am J Respir Cell Mol Biol 1994; 10:625–634.
85. Davies JR, Herrmann A, Russell W, Svitacheva N, Wickstrom C, Carlstedt I. Respiratory tract mucins: structure and expression patterns. Novartis Found Symp 2002; 248:76–88.
86. Bhattacharyya SN, Dubick MA, Yantis LD, et al. In vivo effect of wood smoke on the expression of two mucin genes in rat airways. Inflammation 2004; 28:67–76.
87. Copin MC, Buisine MP, Devisme L, et al. Normal respiratory mucosa, precursor lesions and lung carcinomas: differential expression of human mucin genes. Front Biosci 2001; 6:D1264–D1275.
88. Sharma P, Dudus L, Nielsen PA, et al. MUC5B and MUC7 are differentially expressed in mucous and serous cells of submucosal glands in human bronchial airways. Am J Respir Cell Mol Biol 1998; 19:30–37.
89. Kaneko T, Komiyama K, Horie N, Tsuchiya M, Moro I, Shimoyama T. A histochemical study of inflammatory lesions of the maxillary sinus mucosa using biotinylated lectins. J Oral Sci 2000; 42:87–91.
90. Delmotte P, Degroote S, Merten MD, et al. Influence of TNF-alpha on the sialylation of mucins produced by a transformed cell line MM-39 derived from human tracheal gland cells. Glycoconj J 2001; 18:487–497.
91. Kim DH, Chu HS, Lee JY, Hwang SJ, Lee SH, Lee HM. Up-regulation of MUC5AC and MUC5B mucin genes in chronic rhinosinusitis. Arch Otolaryngol Head Neck Surg 2004; 130:747–752.
92. Jung HH, Lee JH, Kim YT, Lee SD, Park JH. Expression of mucin genes in chronic ethmoiditis. Am J Rhinol 2000; 14:163–170.
93. Seong JK, Koo JS, Lee WJ, et al. Upregulation of MUC8 and downregulation of MUC5AC by inflammatory mediators in human nasal polyps and cultured nasal epithelium. Acta Otolaryngol 2002; 122:401–407.
94. Aust MR, Madsen CS, Jennings A, Kasperbauer JL, Gendler SJ. Mucin mRNA expression in normal and vasomotor inferior turbinates. Am J Rhinol 1997; 11:293–302.
95. Rogers DF. The airway goblet cell. Int J Biochem Cell Biol 2003; 35:1–6.
96. Takeyama K, Fahy JV, Nadel JA. Relationship of epidermal growth factor receptors to goblet cell production in human bronchi. Am J Respir Crit Care Med 2001; 163:511–516.
97. Burgel PR, Escudier E, Coste A, et al. Relation of epidermal growth factor receptor expression to goblet cell hyperplasia in nasal polyps. J Allergy Clin Immunol 2000; 106(4):705–712.
98. Reindel JF, Gough AW, Pilcher GD, Bobrowski WF, Sobocinski GP, de la Iglesia FA. Systemic proliferative changes and clinical signs in cynomolgus monkeys administered a recombinant derivative of human epidermal growth factor. Toxicol Pathol 2001; 29(2):159–173.

99. Takeyama K, Dabbagh K, Lee HM, et al. Epidermal growth factor system regulates mucin production in airways. Proc Natl Acad Sci USA 1999; 16:3081–3086.
100. Amishima M, Munakata M, Nasuhara Y, et al. Expression of epidermal growth factor and epidermal growth factor receptor immunoreactivity in the asthmatic human airway. Am J Respir Crit Care Med 1998; 157:1907–1912.
101. Levine SJ, Larivee P, Logun C, Angus CW, Ognibene FP, Shelhammer JH. Tumor necrosis factor-alpha induces mucin hypersecretion and MUC-2 gene expression by human airway epithelial cells. Am J Respir Cell Mol Biol 1995; 12:196–204.
102. Louahed J, Toda M, Jen J, et al. Interleukin-9 upregulates mucus expression in the airways. Am J Respir Cell Mol Biol 2000; 22:649–656.
103. Longphre M, Li D, Gallup M, et al. Allergen-induced IL-9 directly stimulates mucin transcription in respiratory epithelial cells. J Clin Invest 1999; 104:1375–1382.
104. Dabbagh K, Takeyama K, Lee HM, Ueki IF, Lausier JA, Nadel JA. IL-4 induces mucin gene expression and goblet cell metaplasia in vitro and in vivo. J Immunol 1999; 162:6233–6237.
105. Temann UA, Prasad B, Gallup MW, et al. A novel role for murine IL-4 expression and mucin hypersecretion. Am J Respir Cell Mol Biol 1997; 16:471–478.
106. Wills-Karp M, Luyimbazi J, Xu X, et al. Interleukin-13: central mediator of allergic asthma. Science 1999; 282:2258–2261.
107. Whittaker L, Niu N, Temann UA, et al. Interleukin-13 mediates a fundamental pathway for airway epithelial mucus induced by CD4 T cells and interleukin-9. Am J Respir Cell Mol Biol 2002; 27:593–602.
108. Cohn L, Whittaker L, Niu N, Homer RJ. Cytokine regulation of mucus production in a model of allergic asthma. Novartis Found Symp 2002; 248:201–213 (discussion 213–220, 277–282).
109. Toda M, Tulic MK, Levitt RC, Hamid Q. A calcium-activated chloride channel (HCLCA1) is strongly related to IL-9 expression and mucus production in bronchial epithelium of patients with asthma. J Allergy Clin Immunol 2002; 109:246–250.
110. Wickstrom C, Davies JR, Eriksen GV, Veerman EC, Carlstedt I. MUC5B is a major gel-forming, oligomeric mucin from human salivary gland, respiratory tract and endocervix: identification of glycoforms and C-terminal cleavage. Biochem J 1998; 334:685–693.
111. Kim CH, Song KS, Kim SS, Kim HU, Seong JK, Yoon JH. Expression of MUC5AC mRNA in the goblet cells of human nasal mucosa. Laryngoscope 2000; 110:2110–2113.
112. Raphael GD, Jeney EV, Baraniuk JN, Kim I, Meredith SD, Kaliner MA. The pathophysiology of rhinitis: lactoferrin and lysozyme in nasal secretions. J Clin Invest 1989; 84:1528–1535.
113. Lee CH, Igarashi Y, Hohman RJ, Kaulbach H, White MV, Kaliner MA. Distribution of secretory leukoprotease inhibitor in the human nasal airway. Am Rev Respir Dis 1993; 147:710–716.
114. Baraniuk JN, Ohkubo K, Kwon OJ, et al. Localization of neutral endopeptidase mRNA in human nasal mucosa. J Appl Physiol 1993; 74:272–279.
115. Ohkubo K, Baraniuk JN, Hohman R, Merida M, Hersh LB, Kaliner MA. Aminopeptidase activity in human nasal mucosa. J Allergy Clin Immunol 1998; 102:741–750.
116. Hamaguchi Y, Ohi M, Sakakura Y, Miyoshi Y. Purification of glandular kallikrein in maxillary mucosa from humans suffering from chronic inflammation. Enzyme 1985; 33(1):41–48.
117. Wilson E, Butcher CE. CCL28 controls immunoglobulin (Ig)A plasma cell accumulation in the lactating mammary gland and IgA antibody transfer to the neonate. J Exp Med 2004; 200:805–809.
118. Kvale D, Lovhaug D, Sollid LM, Brandtzaeg P. Tumor necrosis factor-alpha up-regulates expression of secretory component, the epithelial receptor for polymeric Ig. J Immunol 1988; 140:3086–3089.
119. Brandtzaeg P. Immunocompetent cells of the upper airway: functions in normal and diseased mucosa. Eur Arch Otorhinolaryngol 1995; 252(suppl 1):S8–S21.
120. Meredith SD, Raphael GD, Baraniuk JN, Banks SM, Kaliner MA. The pathophysiology of rhinitis. III. The control of IgG secretion. J Allergy Clin Immunol 1989; 84:920–930.

121. Bingle CD, Craven L. Characterisation of the human plunc gene, a gene product with an upper airways and nasopharyngeal restricted expression pattern. Biochim Biophys Acta 2000; 1493:363–367.
122. Casado B, Pannell L, Iadarola P, Baraniuk J. Identification of lipocalin family proteins in nasal secretions. Exp Lung Res 2003; 29(suppl):93–121.
123. Koppelman GH, Postma DS. The genetics of CD14 in allergic disease. Curr Opin Allergy Clin Immunol 2003; 3:347–352.
124. Dabbagh K, Lewis DB. Toll-like receptors and T-helper-1/T-helper-2 responses. Curr Opin Infect Dis 2003; 16:199–204.
125. Claeys S, de Belder T, Holtappels G, et al. Human beta-defensins and toll-like receptors in the upper airway. Allergy 2003; 58:748–753.
126. Pelosi P. Odorant-binding proteins. Crit Rev Biochem Mol Biol 1994; 29:199–228.
127. Weber JR, Freyer D, Alexander C, et al. Recognition of pneumococcal peptidoglycan: an expanded, pivotal role for LPS binding protein. Immunity 2003; 19:269–279.
128. Weiss J. Bactericidal/permeability-increasing protein (BPI) and lipopolysaccharide-binding protein (LBP): structure, function and regulation in host defence against Gram-negative bacteria. Biochem Soc Trans 2003; 31:785–790.
129. Lee SH, Lim HH, Lee HM, Choi JO. Expression of human beta-defensin 1 mRNA in human nasal mucosa. Acta Otolaryngol 2000; 120:58–61.
130. Chen PH, Fang SY. Expression of human beta-defensin 2 in human nasal mucosa. Eur Arch Otorhinolaryngol 2004; 261:238–241.
131. Saito H, Abe J, Matsumoto K. Allergy-related genes in microarray: an update review. J Allergy Clin Immunol 2005; 116:56–59.
132. Baraniuk JN, Wong G, Ali M, Sabol M, Troost T. Glucocorticoids decrease c-fos expression in human nasal polyps in vivo. Thorax 1998; 53:577–582.
133. Lee SH, Lee SH, Oh BH, Lee HM, Choi JO, Jung KY. Expression of mRNA of trefoil factor peptides in human nasal mucosa. Acta Otolaryngol 2001; 121:849–853.
134. Yates JR III. Mass spectrometry from genomics to proteomics. TIG 2000; 16:5–8.
135. Patterson SD, Aebersold RH. Proteomics: the first decade and beyond. Nat Genet 2003; 33(suppl):311–323.
136. Fessler MB, Malcolm KC, Duncan MW, Worthen GS. A genomic and proteomic analysis of activation of the human neutrophil by lipopolysaccharide and its mediation by p38 mitogen-activated protein kinase. J Biol Chem 2002; 277:31291–31302.
137. McRedmond JP, Park SD, Reilly DF, et al. Integration of proteomics and genomics in platelets: a profile of platelet proteins and platelet-specific genes. Mol Cell Proteomics 2004; 3:133–144.
138. Rapheal GD, Meredith SD, Baraniuk JN, Druce HM, Banks SM, Kaliner MA. The pathophysiology of rhinitis. II. Assessment of the sources of protein in histamine-induced nasal secretions. Am Rev Respir Dis 1989; 139:791–800.
139. Kempuraj D, Frydas S, Conti P, et al. Interleukin-25 (or IL-17E): a new IL-17 family member with growth factor/inflammatory actions. Int J Immunopathol Pharmacol 2003; 16:185–188.
140. Kim MR, Manoukian R, Yeh R, et al. Transgenic overexpression of human IL-17E results in eosinophilia, B-lymphocyte hyperplasia, and altered antibody production. Blood 2002; 100:2330–2340.
141. Clark HF, Gurney AL, Abaya E, et al. The secreted protein discovery initiative (SPDI), a large-scale effort to identify novel human secreted and transmembrane proteins: a bioinformatics assessment. Genome Res 2003; 13:2265–2270.
142. Bar-Or A, Nuttall RK, Duddy M, et al. Analyses of all matrix metalloproteinase members in leukocytes emphasize monocytes as major inflammatory mediators in multiple sclerosis. Brain 2003; 126:2738–2749.
143. Kosaki A, Hasegawa T, Kimura T, et al. Increased plasma S100A12 (EN-RAGE) levels in patients with type 2 diabetes. J Clin Endocrinol Metab 2004; 89:5423–5428.
144. Sakata Y, Arima K, Takai T, et al. The squamous cell carcinoma antigen 2 inhibits the cysteine proteinase activity of a major mite allergen, Der p 1. J Biol Chem 2004; 279:5081–5087.

145. Yuyama N, Davies DE, Akaiwa M, et al. Analysis of novel disease-related genes in bronchial asthma. Cytokine 2002; 19:287–296.

146. Emery BE, White MV, Igarashi Y, et al. The effect of IL-4 on human nasal mucosal responses. J Allergy Clin Immunol 1992; 90:772–781.

147. Emanuel IA, Shah SB. Chronic rhinosinusitis: allergy and sinus computed tomography relationships. Otolaryngol Head Neck Surg 2000; 123:687–691.

148. Benninger MS. Rhinitis, sinusitis, and their relationships to allergies. Am J Rhinol 1992; 6:37–43.

149. Rachelefsky GS. Chronic sinusitis. The disease of all ages. Am J Dis Child 1989; 143:886–888.

150. Kalfa VC, Spector SL, Ganz T, Cole AM. Lysozyme levels in the nasal secretions of patients with perennial allergic rhinitis and recurrent sinusitis. Ann Allergy Asthma Immunol 2004; 93(3):288–292.

151. von Bubnoff D, Fimmers R, Bogdanow M, Matz H, Koch S, Bieber T. Asymptomatic atopy is associated with increased indoleamine 2,3-dioxygenase activity and interleukin-10 production during seasonal allergen exposure. Clin Exp Allergy 2004; 34: 1056–1063.

152. von Bubnoff D, Hanau D, Wenzel J, et al. Indoleamine 2,3-dioxygenase-expressing antigen-presenting cells and peripheral T-cell tolerance: another piece to the atopic puzzle? J Allergy Clin Immunol 2003; 112:854–860.

153. Ohkubo K, Ikeda M, Pawankar R, Gotoh M, Yagi T, Okuda M. Mechanisms of IL-6, IL-8, and GM-CSF release in nasal secretions of allergic patients after nasal challenge. Rhinology 1998; 36:156–161.

154. Tabary O, Zahm JM, Hinnrasky J, et al. Selective up-regulation of chemokine IL-8 expression in cystic fibrosis bronchial gland cells in vivo and in vitro. Am J Pathol 1998; 153:921–930.

155. Delbrouck C, Gabius HJ, Vandenhoven G, Kiss R, Hassid S. Budesonide-dependent modulation of expression of macrophage migration inhibitory factor in a polyposis model: evidence for differential regulation in surface and glandular epithelia. Ann Otol Rhinol Laryngol 2004; 113:544–551.

156. Lee HM, Choi JH, Chae SW, Hwang SJ, Lee SH. Expression of epidermal growth factor receptor and its ligands in chronic sinusitis. Ann Otol Rhinol Laryngol 2003; 112: 132–138.

157. Ruhl S, Hamberger S, Betz R, et al. Salivary proteins and cytokines in drug-induced gingival overgrowth. J Dent Res 2004; 83:322–326.

158. Little FF, Cruikshank WW, Center DM. IL-9 stimulates release of chemotactic factors from human bronchial epithelial cells. Am J Respir Cell Mol Biol 2001; 25:347–352.

159. Roca-Ferrer J, Mullol J, Xaubet A, et al. Proinflammatory cytokines and eosinophil cationic protein on glandular secretion from human nasal mucosa: regulation by corticosteroids. J Allergy Clin Immunol 2001; 108:87–93.

160. Untergasser G, Gander R, Lilg C, Lepperdinger G, Plas E, Berger P. Profiling molecular targets of TGF-beta1 in prostate fibroblast-to-myofibroblast transdifferentiation. Mech Ageing Dev 2005; 126:59–69.

161. Rudack C, Sachse F, Alberty J. Chronic rhinosinusitis—need for further classification? Inflamm Res 2004; 53:111–117.

162. Davidsson A, Danielsen A, Viale G, et al. Positive identification in situ of mRNA expression of IL-6, and IL-12, and the chemotactic cytokine RANTES in patients with chronic sinusitis and polypoid disease. Clinical relevance and relation to allergy. Acta Otolaryngol 1996; 116:604–610.

163. Jeffery PK. Comparison of the structural and inflammatory features of COPD and asthma. Giles F. Filley Lecture. Chest 2000; 117(5 suppl 1):251S–260S.

164. Jeffery PK. Differences and similarities between chronic obstructive pulmonary disease and asthma. Clin Exp Allergy 1999; 29(suppl 2):14–26.

165. Zhu J, Majumdar S, Oui Y, et al. Interleukin-4 and interleukin-5 gene expression and inflammation in the mucus-secreting glands and subepithelial tissue of smokers with chronic bronchitis. Lack of relationship with CD8(+) cells. Am J Respir Crit Care Med 2001; 164:2220–2228.

166. Ogawa N, Kawanami T, Shimoyama K, Ping L, Sugai S. Expression of interferon-inducible T cell alpha chemoattractant (CXCL11) in the salivary glands of patients with Sjogren's syndrome. Clin Immunol 2004; 112:235–238.
167. Rotondi M, Lazzeri E, Romagnani P, Serio M. Role for interferon-gamma inducible chemokines in endocrine autoimmunity: an expanding field. J Endocrinol Invest 2003; 26:177–180.
168. Gosepath J, Brieger J, Gletsou E, Mann WJ. Expression and localization of cyclooxigenases (Cox-1 and Cox-2) in nasal respiratory mucosa. Does Cox-2 play a key role in the immunology of nasal polyps? J Investig Allergol Clin Immunol 2004; 14:114–118.
169. Watelet JB, Bachert C, Claeys C, Van Cauwenberge P. Matrix metalloproteinases MMP-7, MMP-9 and their tissue inhibitor TIMP-1: expression in chronic sinusitis vs. nasal polyposis. Allergy 2004; 59:54–60.
170. Baraniuk, JN, White K. Immunodeficiency in subtypes of chronic sinusitis. J Allergy Clin Imunol 2004; 113:S203.
171. Smith JK, Krishnaswamy GH, Dykes R, Reynolds S, Berk SL. Clinical manifestations of IgE hypogammaglobulinemia. Ann Allergy Asthma Immunol 1997; 78:313–318.
172. Finocchi A, Angelini F, Chini L, et al. Evaluation of the relevance of humoral immunodeficiencies in a pediatric population affected by recurrent infections. Pediatr Allergy Immunol 2002; 13(6):443–447.
173. Litzman J, Sevcikova I, Stikarovska D, Pikulova Z, Pazdirkova A, Lokaj J. IgA deficiency in Czech healthy individuals and selected patient groups. Int Arch Allergy Immunol 2000; 123:177–180.
174. Chee L, Graham SM, Carothers DG, Ballas ZK. Immune dysfunction in refractory sinusitis in a tertiary care setting. Laryngoscope 2001; 111:233–235.
175. Lund VJ, Scadding GK. Immunologic aspects of chronic sinusitis. J Otolaryngol 1991; 20:379–381.
176. Abdelilah SG, Bouchaib L, Morita M, et al. Molecular characterization of the low-affinity IgE receptor Fc epsilonRII/CD23 expressed by human eosinophils. Int Immunol 1998; 10:395–404.
177. Modlin RL. Learning from leprosy: insights into contemporary immunology from an ancient disease. Skin Pharmacol Appl Skin Physiol 2002; 15:1–6.
178. Cosma CL, Sherman DR, Ramakrishnan L. The secret lives of the pathogenic mycobacteria. Annu Rev Microbiol 2003; 57:641–676.
179. Baraniuk JN, Maibach H. Pathophysiological classification of chronic rhinosinusitis. BMC Respir Res 2005; 6:149.
180. Stewart MG, Donovan DT, Parke RB Jr., Bautista MH. Does the severity of sinus computed tomography findings predict outcome in chronic sinusitis? Otolaryngol Head Neck Surg 2000; 123:81–84.
181. Bhattacharyya T, Piccirillo J, Wippold FJ. Relationship between patient-based descriptions of sinusitis and paranasal sinus CT. Arch Otolaryngol Head Neck Surg 1997; 123:1189–1192.
182. Steward MG, Sicard MW, Piccirillo JF, Diaz-Marchan PJ. Severity staging in chronic sinusitis: are CT scan findings related to patient symptoms? Am J Rhinol 1999; 13:161–167.
183. Tarabichi M. Characteristics of sinus-related pain. Otolaryngol Head Neck Surg 2000; 122:842–847.
184. West B, Jones NS. Endoscopy-negative, computed tomography-negative facial pain in a nasal clinic. Laryngoscope 2001; 111:581–586.
185. Scribano E, Ascenti G, Loria G, Cascio F, Gaeta M. The role of the ostiomeatal unit anatomic variations in inflammatory disease of the maxillary sinuses. Eur J Radiol 1997; 24:172–174.
186. Dunham ME. Evaluating the limited sinus computed tomography scan in children. Laryngoscope 1997; 107:402–404.
187. Patel K, Chavda SV, Violaris N, Pahor AL. Incidental paranasal sinus inflammatory changes in the a British population. J Laryngol Otol 1996; 110:649–651.
188. Maly PV, Sundgren PC. Changes in paranasal sinus abnormalities found incidentally on MRI. Neuroradiology 1995; 37:471–474.

189. Gordts F, Clement PA, Buisseret T. Prevalences of sinusitis signs in a non-ENT popu-
     lation. ORL J Otorhinolaryngol Relat Spec 1996; 58:315–319.
190. Jones NS, Strobl A, Holland I. A study of the CT findings in 100 patients with rhino-
     sinusitis and 100 controls. Clin Otolaryngol 1997; 22:47–51.
191. Tarp B, Fiirgaard B, Christensen T, Jensen JJ, Black FT. The prevalence and significance
     of incidental paranasal sinus abnormalities on MRI. Rhinology 2000; 38:33–38.
192. Khanna P, Shah A. Categorization of patients with allergic rhinitis: a comparative pro-
     file of "sneezers and runners" and "blockers." Ann Allergy Asthma Immunol 2005;
     94:60–64.

9 | Aspirin-Sensitive Rhinosinusitis and Asthma

Marek L. Kowalski

Department of Immunology, Rheumatology and Allergy, Faculty of Medicine, Medical University of Łódź, Łódź, Poland

INTRODUCTION

A subpopulation of asthmatic patients reacts to aspirin with an acute dyspnea, usually accompanied by nasal symptoms (rhinorrhea/nasal congestion) within two hours after ingestion of aspirin. These patients present a typical "aspirin triad," which involves chronic rhinosinusitis complicated by polyp formation, severe bronchial asthma, and hypersensitivity reactions in response to aspirin and also other cross-reacting nonsteroidal anti-inflammatory drugs (NSAIDs). The first case of a hypersensitivity reaction to aspirin manifesting as dyspnea and angioedema was described in 1902 (two years after aspirin was marketed) by Hirschberg from Poznań in western Poland (1). The association of aspirin hypersensitivity, nasal polyposis, and asthma was noticed by Widal et al. (2) and the syndrome was characterized in a larger group of patients by Samter and Beers (3). Since that time, several various terms have been used to describe respiratory reactions to NSAIDs: aspirin sensitivity, pseudoallergy, idiosyncrasy, or intolerance (4). Having in mind the nonimmunological mechanism of respiratory reactions to aspirin and other NSAIDs, the term "hypersensitivity" seems to be the most appropriate and in agreement with current recommendations for nomenclature (5). The coexistence of aspirin hypersensitivity with upper airway (rhinosinusitis/nasal polyps) and lower airway (asthma) inflammatory disease was referred to as aspirin triad, asthma triad, Samter's syndrome, aspirin-induced asthma, and aspirin-sensitive rhinosinusitis/asthma syndrome. More recently, the term "aspirin-exacerbated respiratory disease" (AERD) was proposed stressing the fact that the core issue in these patients is not acetylsalicylic acid (ASA) hypersensitivity but the underlying chronic inflammatory respiratory disease only occasionally exacerbated by aspirin or other NSAIDs (6). A subgroup of ASA-hypersensitive patients manifests a reaction exclusively in the upper respiratory tract; they do not have asthma, but the clinical picture of the nasal disease in these patients (hyperplastic rhinosinusitis with polyps) is similar to that observed in patients with ASA triad (7). Because the mechanism of the disease seems to be the same and some patients will evolve with time into full aspirin triad including bronchial asthma, it seems practical to discuss both subpopulations together as patients with AERD.

Several other types of hypersensitivity to ASA and NSAIDs have been also described including NSAIDs-induced urticaria/angioedema, and anaphylaxis (8). Although some patients with aspirin-induced rhinosinusitis/asthma may present cutaneous symptoms after exposure to NSAIDs, this subtype of hypersensitivity will not be discussed in this chapter.

EPIDEMIOLOGY

The real prevalence of hypersensitivity to aspirin has been difficult to assess because it varies depending on method of detection, gender, and age of patients, as well as the other characteristics of the population studied. In general adult populations the prevalence of aspirin-induced shortness of breath or asthmatic attack has been estimated to be around 1.2% but was significantly higher in patients with doctor-diagnosed asthma (8.8%; RR = 11.4) (9). The overall incidence of ASA hypersensitivity among adult asthmatics, if assessed by history alone, varies from 4.3% to 12% in various populations (10,11). However, determination of aspirin hypersensitivity by oral provocation increases the overall incidence to 21.1% in recent systematic review of reported studies (12). In patients with severe asthma (e.g., those admitted to the ICU with asthmatic attack) the prevalence of ASA-sensitivity may be as high as 14% to 24% (13,14). The presence of chronic rhinosinusitis and/or nasal polyps in asthmatics further increases the prevalence of aspirin hypersensitivity from 30% to 40% (15,16). Prevalence of aspirin hypersensitivity in children with asthma is less common than in adults and varies from 1% to 3%; when determined by history alone, it is close to 5% in asthmatic children subjected to oral provocation. The presence of allergic rhinitis is also associated with increased risk of hypersensitivity to aspirin as compared to subjects without rhinitis (2.6% vs. 0.3%; RR = 7.7; 95% CI: 3.0–19.7). Gender seems to be also a predisposing factor because the condition affects more women than men by a ratio 3:2 in most populations.

It is generally believed that aspirin hypersensitivity in asthmatics remains widely undiagnosed because, for example 15% of asthmatic patients with positive bronchial reaction to aspirin during the challenge were unaware of aspirin hypersensitivity before the provocation (17).

CLINICAL CHARACTERISTICS OF ASPIRIN TRIAD

In a sensitive patient ingestion of aspirin or other NSAID induces 30 to 120 minutes nasal congestion, watery rhinorrhea followed by shortness of breath and rapidly progressing respiratory distress. In some more sensitive patients with unstable asthma exposed to a therapeutic dose of aspirin, the reaction may appear as early as five minutes after ingestion, leading to severe bronchospasm and even to death in some severe cases (18). Bronchoconstriction is usually also accompanied by extrabronchial symptoms including ocular, cutaneous (flushing, urticaria, and/or angioedema), or gastric symptoms. The threshold dose of aspirin defined as the smallest dose evoking significant fall in FEV_1 seems to be an individual feature of a patient and varies from 10 mg up to 600 mg of ASA. Some patients with a history of asthma induced by aspirin may react to ingestion of lower doses of aspirin only with upper airway symptoms, but increasing the dose may induce both upper and lower airway symptoms (19,20).

Natural History

The typical patient with AERD is a 30- to 40-year-old woman with a history of chronic rhinosinusitis and/or asthma that usually precede the development of hypersensitivity to aspirin. Some patients associate the beginning of the disease with flu-like infection, which is followed by development of chronic intractable rhinosinusitis; already at this stage nasal polyps are frequently detected. Asthma is usually the second component of the triad precipitated in almost half of patients by upper respiratory tract infection—in the AIANE study aspirin or NSAID were factors precipitating the first asthmatic attack only in 14% of patients (17). Asthma once developed runs a protracted course, which is independent of avoidance of aspirin and other NSAIDs.

According to earlier reports, ASA-hypersensitive asthmatics have been traditionally considered to have an "intrinsic" (i.e., nonallergic) type of asthma. More recent studies show that most of them have a history of inhalant allergy and the frequency of positive skin test results in common inhalant allergens is not lower than in patients with aspirin-tolerant asthma (21). In a study from Venezuela, positive prick tests to inhalant allergens were found in 86.6% of patients with aspirin hypersensitivity as compared to 29.1% in ASA-tolerant asthmatics and a similar high frequency of atopy was found in surveys from Turkey and Poland (22–24). Thus, presence of atopy seems to be a significant risk factor for presence of hypersensitivity to aspirin and analgesics among asthmatic patients. This shift from earlier studies presenting ASA-hypersensitive asthmatics as nonatopic to more recent ones indicating an high prevalence of atopy seems to reflect an increase in the prevalence of allergic sensitization in the general population rather than any type of causal relationship between IgE-mediated respiratory disease and hypersensitivity to aspirin. Interestingly, aspirin sensitivity is also associated with higher prevalence of food intolerance and antibiotic allergy (25).

Rhinosinusitis and Nasal Polyps

In the majority of aspirin-hypersensitive asthmatics signs and symptoms of chronic rhinitis and sinusitis are present. Although patients report nasal symptoms typical for nonallergic rhinitis, exacerbations of symptoms on exposure to both seasonal and perennial inhalant allergens are reported by a significant proportion of patients. Rhinosinusitis has a usually protracted course and in most cases is complicated by mucosal hypertrophy and polyp formation. In the AIANE study including 500 ASA-sensitive patients collected from 14 centers, the prevalence of nasal polyposis was 60% in most cases diagnosed by rhinoscopy. However, on computer tomography mucosal hypertrophy is present in up to 100% of patients and the frequency of nasal polyps may be as high as 90% (26). Polypoid hypertrophy of the mucosa is not limited to the nasal cavity but usually involves all sinuses and is more extensive in ASA-sensitive as compared to ASA-tolerant patients with nasal polyposis. Nasal polyposis has a high tendency to recurrence after surgery; the recurrence rate in ASA-sensitive patients is almost three times higher than in intrinsic asthmatics and seven times higher than in atopic asthmatics (27). There is also clinical evidence that uncontrolled chronic rhinosinusitis often aggravates the course of asthma in ASA-sensitive patients (28).

A subgroup of ASA-sensitive patients manifests a reaction exclusively in the upper respiratory tract; they do not have asthma, but the clinical picture of the nasal disease (hypertrophic rhinosinusitis) in these patients is similar to that observed in patients with ASA triad. Although some of these patients may evolve with time to a full aspirin triad, their risk of developing asthma in the future is not known.

Bronchial Asthma

Patients hypersensitive to aspirin suffer from persistent asthma of greater than average severity and of higher than ordinary medication requirements, including dependence on steroids. Unusual severity of bronchial asthma in patients with coexisting hypersensitivity to aspirin is not a novel finding and was noticed as early as in 1922 (29). In the AIANE study, chronic treatment with moderate to high doses of inhaled glucocorticosteroids was used in 80% of aspirin-hypersensitive asthmatics and oral steroids were necessary to control asthma in up to 50% of these patients. In the TENOR study, ASA-sensitive asthmatics were more likely to have severe asthma as assessed by physicians (66% vs. 49%), to have been intubated (20% vs. 11%), to have a steroid burst in the previous three months (56% vs. 46%), and to have required high doses of inhaled steroids (34% vs. 26%) or use of leukotrienes modifiers (67% vs. 57%) (30). Furthermore, these patients had a significantly lower postbronchodilator increase in FEV_1 as compared with subjects with aspirin-tolerant asthma, suggesting the presence of irreversible airway obstruction related to the airway remodeling.

Although ingestion of aspirin or other NSAIDs may aggravate respiratory symptoms in hypersensitive patients, both lower and upper airway disease persist and have a protracted course even in the absence of exposure to ASA/NSAIDs. Aspirin hypersensitivity is not only a significant risk factor for development of severe chronic asthma (OR = 5.44) but is also strongly associated with near-fatal asthma, and fatal outcome of asthma occurs more often than in asthmatics without the triad (31). A recent study from Japan confirmed that the history of aspirin hypersensitivity had been a significant indicator of potential near fatal-asthma, suggesting the importance of education for prevention of near-fatal asthma exacerbations (32).

PATHOMECHANISM OF ASA-HYPERSENSITIVITY

The mechanism of aspirin hypersensitivity in asthmatic patients is not immunological because the presence of specific immunoglobulins or sensitized T-cells has been never documented. Immunological mechanisms can be also ruled out based on the observation that aspirin cross-reacts with other nonsteroidal anti-inflammatory compounds with completely different chemical structure. Original observations of Szczeklik et al. (33) attributed the mechanism of hypersensitivity to ASA and other NSAIDs to their pharmacological properties documenting only those NSAIDs that are strong or at least moderate inhibitors of prostaglandin synthesis that can evoke reaction in ASA-hypersensitive patients. Later on, they proposed that ASA-induced reaction is the result of inhibition of cyclooxygenase, an enzyme that metabolizes arachidonic acid to prostaglandins, thromboxanes, and prostacyclin. Classical NSAIDs demonstrate a range of cyclooxygenase (prostaglandin synthesis) inhibitory activity in vitro that correlates with the potency of these drugs to induce adverse reactions. Discovery of two prostaglandin synthase isoforms designated cyclooxygenase-1 (COX-1) and cyclooxygenase-2 (COX-2) led to the development of COX-2 selective NSAIDs which are better tolerated by gastrointestinal mucosa. Aspirin (ASA), a prototypic prostaglandin synthesis inhibitor, is a preferential COX-1 inhibitor with potency toward this enzyme over 160 times than toward COX-2. Other NSAIDs such as indomethacin, naproxen, or ibuprofen are considered to be strong cyclooxygenase inhibitors with dominant preferential activity toward COX-1 (34). These NSAIDs precipitate adverse symptoms in a significant (ranging from 30% to 80%) proportion of ASA-hypersensitive patients. On the other hand, weak COX-1 inhibitors, e.g., salicylic acid or acetaminophen and selective COX-2 inhibitors are usually well tolerated by these patients (Table 1).

TABLE 1 Cyclooxygenase-1/Cyclooxygenase-2 Inhibitory Ratio and
Selectivity of Nonsteroidal Anti-inflammatory Drugs for Cyclooxygenases

Generic name	IC50 COX-2/COX-1	Selectivity
Aspirin	166	COX-1 > COX-2
Indomethacin	60	
Ibuprofen	15	
Sodium Salicylate	2.8	COX-1 = COX-2
Flurbiprofen	1.3	
Naproxen	0.6	COX-1 < COX-2
Meloxicam	0.3	
Celecoxib		COX-1 <<< COX-2
Rofecoxib		

IC50-concentration of a drug inducing 50% inhibition of cyclooxygenase activity.
Abbreviation: COX, cyclooxygenase.
Source: From Ref. 34.

Cyclooxygenase Hypothesis

According to the "cyclooxygenase" hypothesis, the mechanism of hypersensitivity
to aspirin and other NSAIDs is related to arachidonic acid metabolism (Fig. 1)
because inhibition of COX-1 by ASA or other NSAIDs triggers a mechanism leading to asthmatic attack and/or nasal symptoms (35). However, the chain of
biochemical events linking COX-1 inhibition and the release of mediators responsible for development of symptoms is not known and can only be a matter of
speculation. It has been proposed that in ASA-sensitive patients, but not in ASA-
tolerant patients, prostaglandin E_2 (PGE_2), generated by the COX-1 pathway, may
have a key role in stabilizing inflammatory cells by the deprivation of PGE_2 may
lead to activation of inflammatory pathways. Accordingly, inhalation of PGE_2 or

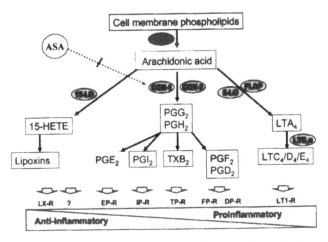

FIGURE 1 Pathways of arachidonic acid metabolism related to the pathogenesis of aspirin-
exacerbated respiratory disease. Eicosanoid mediators activating specific receptors may induce
either anti-inflammatory (cell stabilizing) or proinflammatory activity. In patients with hypersensitivity
to aspirin, even at baseline, this balance is probably shifted toward proinflammatory eicosanoids.
Aspirin or other nonsteroidal anti-inflammatory drugs by inhibition of cyclooxygenase-1 may further
enhance proinflammatory mechanisms.

oral pretreatment with misoprostol (a synthetic PGE_2 analogue) prevents ASA-induced bronchoconstriction (36–38). It has been proposed that local deficiency in PGE_2 synthesis that was found in nasal polyp epithelial cells and bronchial fibroblasts from ASA-hypersensitive patients may reflect decreased regulatory capacity of these molecules more prone to inhibition by NSAIDs (39,40). And although PGE_2 has well-documented inhibitory effects on inflammatory mechanisms and may prevent activation of mast cells and eosinophils, there is no direct evidence that this mechanism operates differentially in ASA-sensitive patients. Szczeklik et al. (41) reported an increased susceptibility of nasal polyp cells from ASA-sensitive patients to inhibitory action of aspirin, but this observation has never been reproduced. On the contrary, several studies documented that ASA and NSAIDs inhibit cyclooxygenase activity and generation of prostaglandins to the same degree in airway cells and peripheral blood leukocytes from ASA-sensitive and tolerant patients (42). Although a decreased expression of COX-2 mRNA was found in nasal polyps of ASA-sensitive patients, the relevance of these findings to the pathomechanism of acute reaction is not clear because COX-1 and not COX-2 inhibition is prerequisite for acute hypersensitivity reaction to occur (43). Discovery of several splice variants of COX-1 and COX-2 and an acetominophen sensitive COX-3 isoform have prompt sensitive to acetominophen cyclooxygenase isoform COX-3 prompt further investigations in this area to better understand the role of cyclooxygenase in triggering the reaction. Because aspirin-induced reaction is associated with increased generation of cysteinyl leukotrienes, it has been postulated that inhibition of cyclooxygenase pathways by ASA could result in "a shunt" of arachidonic acid to alternative lipoxygenase pathways and generation of leukotrienes. However, this explanation is not feasible because both COX and LOX have completely different intracellular pools of arachidonic acid available for their activity. PGE_2 is capable of reducing biosynthesis of cysteinyl leukotrienes through inhibition of lipoxygenase. Thus deprivation of PGE by aspirin could directly stimulate leukotriene synthesis in ASA-sensitive patients (44). However, no specific defect of lipoxygenase regulation has ever been detected in ASA-sensitive patients and leukotrienes are not the only mediators triggered during ASA-induced reactions (45,46).

Mediators Involved in Aspirin-Induced Reaction

The chain of events linking inhibition of COX-1 by aspirin and subsequent development of symptoms is not known (Fig. 2). The ASA-induced reaction involves release of both mast cell (tryptase, histamine) and eosinophil (ECP)-specific mediators into nasal washes and/or bronchial lavages, clearly indicating activation of both types of cells (47–49). Concentrations of PGD_2 stable metabolite and mast cell tryptase increase also in blood plasma after inhaled aspirin challenge (50). The reaction is accompanied by release of cysteinyl leukotrienes into nasal secretions (51,52) or induced sputum (53), and leukotriene metabolites into urine (54,55). The cellular source of cysteinyl leukotrienes has not been determined and may include both mast cells and eosinophils as well as other inflammatory cells present in the airway mucosa. Although leukotrienes are considered as typical mediators of ASA-evoked response, an increased cysteinyl leukotriene generation is not specific for ASA-induced reaction. Cysteinyl leukotrienes are also released into nasal and bronchial fluid during IgE-mediated reaction to allergen, and following non-immunologically mediated reaction to hypertonic saline. Furthermore, leukotriene LT1 receptor antagonists only partially prevent ASA-induced reactions

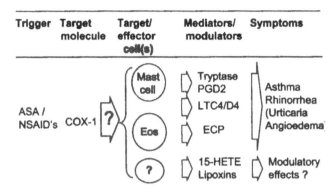

Trigger	Target molecule	Target/ effector cell(s)	Mediators/ modulators	Symptoms

FIGURE 2 Pathomechanism of acetylsalicylic acid–induced hypersensitivity reactions. The key mechanism (?) linking cycloxygenase-1 inhibition by aspirin and subsequent activation of inflammatory cells leading to development of symptoms remains an enigma.

and these preventive effects may be overcome with increased period doses of ASA, questioning the pivotal role of these mediators during ASA-induced reactions (56–58). Other AA-derived mediators have been also associated with hypersensitivity reactions: 8-isoprostanes are increased in expired breath are condensate cysteinyl leukotrienes, and LTB4 glucuronide are released into urine following aspirin-induced bronchial reactions (59,60).

More recently, in vitro studies of nasal polyp epithelial cells and peripheral blood leukocytes demonstrated that in sensitive patients aspirin triggers specifically 15-hydroxyeicosatetraenoic (15-HETE) generation, suggesting the presence in these patients of a specific abnormality in the 15-LO pathway (61). 15-HETE has multiple potential proinflammatory activities including stimulation of the release of mediators from mast cells (62), induction of the release of mucous glycoprotein from human airways in vitro (63), and contraction of human bronchial smooth muscle in vitro (64). These data suggest that 15-HETE could be regarded as a trigger or mediator of asthmatic and inflammatory reactions in the airways of ASA-hypersensitive asthmatics. However, 15-HETE may also have an anti-inflammatory activity, being capable of inhibiting 5-lipoxygenase and LTB_4 generation in leukocytes (65,66). Thus, it is also possible that triggering by aspirin of 15-HETE production may represent a regulatory mechanism, secondary to still unknown mechanisms responsible for evoking symptoms of ASA-sensitivity. Furthermore, conversion of 15-HETE to lipoxins seems to represent a novel and potent regulatory mechanism by which LXA_4 and 15-epi-LXA_4 may down-regulate leukocyte trafficking and activation (67). Aspirin-triggered 15-HETE release from PBL mimicked hypersensitivity reactions to aspirin observed in vivo. Release of 15-HETE could be also triggered by another nonselective cyclooxygenase inhibitor naproxen, but COX-2-selective NSAIDs did not affect the release. Furthermore, misoprostol, a synthetic PGE analogue, which was shown to prevent aspirin-induced asthmatic reactions, inhibited 15-HETE generation triggered by aspirin in vitro.

The enzymatic source and mechanism leading to increased generation of 15-HETE following in vitro incubation with aspirin is not known. In addition to 15-lipoxygenase, both COX-1 (PGH synthase-1) and COX-2 (PGHsynthase-2) are capable of synthesizing 15-HETE. Aspirin treatment inhibits prostaglandin generation, and stimulates formation of 15-HETE by COX-2 but not by COX-1 (68,69). 15(R)-HETE produced by ASA-treated COX-2 has a configuration at C15 opposite to 15(S)-HETE produced by 15-lipoxygenase, thus allowing for identification of the source of the 15-HETE. 15-HETE release upon aspirin challenge by PBL from ASA-sensitive patients had 15(S)-HETE configuration and the reaction was inhibited by caffeic acid, a 15-LO inhibitor, suggesting that 15-LO and not COX-2 was the source of ASA-induced 15-HETE in this reaction (Jedrzejczak M, Kowalski ML, Ptasinska A, et al. Regulation of arachidonic acid metabolism in ASA-sensitive asthmatics and aspirin-tolerant patients. In preparation). One may speculate that the activity of 15-LO in ASA-sensitive patients is controlled by endogenous COX-1-derived PGE_2, and removal of PGE_2 production by aspirin results in activation of 15-LO and 15-HETE production. It is not clear, however, if this quite specific increase in 15-HETE generation is causally related to a hypersensitivity reaction or merely reflects a bystander phenomenon.

PATHOGENESIS OF CHRONIC INFLAMMATION IN THE AIRWAYS

Chronic eosinophilic inflammation of higher than usual severity is a typical feature of airway mucosa in ASA-hypersensitive patients. Etiopathogenesis of persistent eosinophilic inflammation of the airway mucosa and nasal polyps in these patients do not seem to be related to intake of aspirin or other NSAIDs—even complete avoidance of NSAIDs does not lead to clinical improvement (Fig. 3). Moreover in most patients the presence of chronic eosinophilic inflammation in the upper

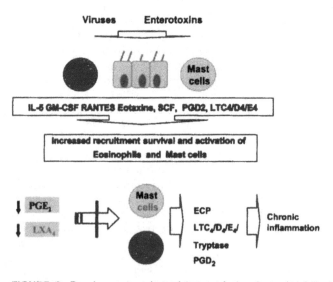

FIGURE 3 Development and persistence of chronic eosinophilic inflammation in the airway mucosa of acetylsalicylic acid (ASA)-hypersensitive subjects. Hypothetical triggers (viruses, enterotoxins?) may activate structural and inflammatory cells to increase recruitment of eosinophils and mast cells involving mechanisms similar to those operating in patients without hypersensitivity. However, once initiated, inflammation is further exacerbated in ASA-hypersensitive patients due to impaired regulatory mechanisms related to local deficiency in prostaglandin E2 and lipoxin production and leading to, e.g., upregulation of cysteinyl-leukotrienes and their receptors.

or lower airways can precede the, development of hypersensitivity to aspirin by several years. Observations that respiratory cross-reactive type of hypersensitivity to aspirin does not occur in healthy persons without rhinosinusitis/asthma (i.e., without underlying airway inflammation) suggest that the presence of chronic inflammation may be prerequisite for hypersensitivity to occur. Putative viral factors have been proposed as primary triggers of aspirin hypersensitivity but also as a cause of underlying chronic inflammation in the airways of ASA-sensitive patients (70). Latent viral infection could trigger immunological response to infectious agents (potentially T-cell–mediated) involving cytotoxic leukocytes and leading to persistent mucosal inflammation, although there is no direct evidence for the presence of latent viral infections in the airways. Alternatively, transient acute viral infection, which often precedes development of hypersensitivity, could induce autoimmune response to unknown antigens. Some data suggest that autoimmunity may play a role in the pathogenesis of inflammation in hypersensitivity: autoimmune response markers have been found in ASA-sensitive patients (71,72) and expression of specific HLA-DR antigens has been associated with aspirin hypersensitivity (73).

The role of bacterial infection as a trigger of immunological response in the airways of hypersensitive patients has been also proposed. Bachert et al. (74) demonstrated that IgE antibodies to Staphylococcal enterotoxins (SAEs) were present in nasal polyp tissue and their concentration correlated with the levels of ECP, eotaxin, and IL-5. These relations seemed to be particularly evident in ASA-sensitive patients, suggesting that an increased expression of IL-5 and ECP in polyp tissue from ASA-sensitive patients may be related to the presence of SAE that can exert direct effects on eosinophil proliferation and survival or may act as superantigen to trigger T-cell–mediated inflammatory reaction (75,76).

On the other hand, it should be stressed that a significant proportion of aspirin-hypersensitive patients (30–70%) demonstrate atopic sensitization to inhalant allergens, thus IgE-mediated mechanisms may also contribute to the chronicity of inflammation in some patients with AERD.

Inflammatory Cells and Cytokine Profile

Several microscopical, biochemical molecular observations suggest that the pathomechanism underlying airway inflammation in aspirin-hypersensitive may be different from that present in aspirin-tolerant patients (28). The higher severity of asthma, rhinosinusitis, and nasal polyposis in ASA-hypersensitive patients seems to reflect by characteristic cellular profile. A high degree of tissue eosinophilia is a prominent feature in the mucosal inflammation in the bronchi and nasal mucosa. Significantly more information is available concerning immunomorphology of the nasal mucosa and nasal polyp tissue as compared to the bronchial mucosa because of better accessibility to the upper airways (77,78). Prominent eosinophilia has been documented in nasal polyps of aspirin-sensitive patients and both nonstimulated and stimulated nasal polyp dispersed cells from ASA-sensitive patients were shown to release significantly more ECP as compared to polyps from ASA-tolerant subjects (79). An increased number of eosinophils in the tissue has been linked to distinctive profiles of cytokine expression with upregulation of several cytokines related to eosinophil activation and survival (e.g., IL-5, GMC-SF, RANTES, eotaxins) both in upper and lower airway mucosa (80–83). It has been proposed that overproduction of IL-5 might be a major factor responsible for an increased survival of eosinophils in the nasal polyps, resulting in increased intensity of the eosinophilic inflammation particularly in aspirin-sensitive patients (84). This hypothesis has been supported recently by observation of significant differences in the intensity of local apoptosis and immunological profile of inflammation in nasal polyps from ASA-hypersensitive and ASA-tolerant patients (85). Decreased apoptosis in polyps from aspirin-sensitive patients, and increased infiltration with eosinophils were associated with prominent expression of CD45RO+ activated/memory cells. This cellular pattern was related to clinical features of rhinosinusitis. Mast cells are abundant in the upper and lower airway tissue of ASA-sensitive patients (86). Serum baseline levels of mast cell–derived mediators (tryptase and PGD_2 stable metabolite) are elevated. In the nasal polyp tissue, the density of mast cells was correlated with the number of polypectomies, implicating an important role for these cells in the pathogenesis of nasal polyposis (19). Stem cell factor (SCF), also called c-kit ligand, is a cytokine critical for differentiation, survival, chemotaxis, and activation of human mast cells. SCF expression was found to be increased in nasal polyp epithelial cells from aspirin-hypersensitive asthmatics and correlated closely with the density of mast cells and number of polypectomies (87). The mechanism responsible for increased expression of SCF in nasal polyps epithelium of ASA-sensitive patients is not known, although one may speculate that viral infections associated with the onset of nasal polyposis and aspirin sensitivity may be responsible for activation of epithelial cells to release several cytokines including SCF.

Mononuclear cells may also be involved in the development and control of inflammation in the airway mucosa. Hamilos et al. (81,88) found a distinct profile of cytokine expression in a group of patients with nonallergic (presumably ASA-sensitive) polyps, and Bachert et al. (89) demonstrated elevated IL-5 protein concentrations in polyps from ASA-hypersensitive patients. The disproportionate increase in IL-5 mRNA as compared to IL-4 mRNA positive cells was also found in nonpolyposis nasal mucosa, suggesting that other than classical "allergic" mechanisms may be important in the disease. Nasal polyps from ASA-sensitive subjects contain a significantly greater number of CD45RO+ cells which are considered to be activated T-cells (both CD4 and CD8 cells may express CD45 RO phenotype) with memory or effector function (90). Prominent expression of CD45RO+ cells was associated with decreased apoptosis, and increased infiltration by eosinophils reflecting a distinct pattern of immunologic cell activation. These phenomena were also related to clinical features of rhinosinusitis. These observations suggest an important role for activated T-cells in perpetuating the inflammatory response in ASA-sensitive patients. Whether similar distinct patterns of T-cell and cytokines are present in the lower airways of aspirin-hypersensitive subjects is to be investigated.

Arachidonic Acid Metabolites

PGE$_2$ Deficiency
Another distinctive feature of the airways inflammation in aspirin-hypersensitive patients is the presence of several abnormalities of arachidonic acid metabolism. A significantly lower generation of PGE_2 by nasal polyps and nasal polyp epithelial cells as well as bronchial fibroblasts, has been documented. COX-2 mRNA expression is decreased in nasal polyps of these patients. Low expression of

COX-2 mRNA in nasal polyps was in turn linked to a down regulation of NF-κB activity and to abnormal regulation of COX-2 expression at the transcriptional level (91,92). Because PGE_2 has significant anti-inflammatory activity, including inhibitory effects on eosinophil chemotaxis and activation, it may be speculated that an intrinsic defect in local generation of PGE_2 could contribute to development of more severe eosinophilic inflammation in aspirin-sensitive patients.

Overproduction of Leukotrienes

Cysteinyl leukotrienes may also be important mediators of persistent airway inflammation because basal levels of leukotriene metabolites in the urine of ASA-sensitive patients are elevated as compared to ASA-tolerant asthmatics, even in the absence of aspirin challenge (93,94). However, the differences in basal levels of LTs in the airways of ASA-hypersensitive and ASA-tolerant patients are less consistently observed. Concentrations of cysteinyl leukotrienes were similar in the bronchoalveolar fluid of ASA-sensitive and ASA-tolerant subjects (95,96) but significantly higher in induced sputum of ASA-hypersensitive asthmatics (53). In exhaled expiratory breath condensate cysteinyls-leukotrienes were found to be increased in one study and not different in both groups in the other. An increased number of cells expressing LTC4 synthase, an enzyme involved in transformation of arachidonic acid to cysteinyl leukotrienes, were found in the bronchi of ASA-hypertensive asthmatics with significantly higher LTC4S expression levels in mast cells than in eosinophils (97,98). Data concerning basal leukotriene levels in the upper airways of aspirin hypersensitive patients are also inconclusive. Although earlier studies demonstrated an increased production of cysteinyl leukotrienes in nasal polyps of ASA-sensitive asthmatics as compared to aspirin-tolerant patients in vitro (99,100), these observations could not be reproduced in vivo when nasal washes were analyzed (51,52). Both basal and stimulated release of LTC4 were found to be similar in nasal polyp dispersed cells from ASA-sensitive and ASA-tolerant patients (79). Perez-Novo et al. (101) found an increased generation of LTC4/D4/E4 and overexpression of enzymes involved in the production of leukotrienes (5-LOX and LTC4 synthase) in nasal polyp tissue from ASA-sensitive patients. Production of cysteinyl leukotrienes correlated with tissue concentration of ECP in both ASA-sensitive and ASA-tolerant polyps. These observations suggest that increased basal levels of cysteinyl leukotrienes may be linked to increased tissue eosinophil (and possibly mast cell) numbers (a feature typical for aspirin-hypersensitive patients) rather than to basic mechanisms of chronic inflammation. Along these lines, increased leukotrienuria has been associated with the presence and intensity of chronic hyperplastic rhinosinusitis and polyposis in both ASA-sensitive and ASA-tolerant patients (102). A significant decrease in urinary leukotrienes that was observed following nasal sinus surgery indicate that urinary leukotrienes may reflect an overall increase in number of leukotriene-producing cells (mostly eosinophils) in different tissues rather than overproduction per cell within target organs. On the other hand, in support of the special role of leukotriene pathways in patients with AERD, increased expression of leukotriene LT1 receptors was found in the nasal mucosa of ASA-sensitive patients, suggesting local hyperresponsiveness to leukotrienes (103). If similar overexpression of LT1 receptors is found in the lower airways it could explain selective bronchial hyperresponsiveness to LTE4 observed in aspirin-sensitive asthmatics (104). The role of cysteinyl leukotrienes and their receptors in the pathogenesis of chronic mucosal inflammation in ASA-sensitive patients needs further investigation because chronic treatment with LT1 receptor antagonists do not demonstrate better effectiveness in relieving nasal and bronchial symptoms or reducing polyp size in ASA-hypersensitive as compared to ASA-tolerant patients (105,106).

15-Lipoxygenase Pathways

More recently, other arachidonic acid metabolites generated by the 15-LOX pathway have been associated with chronic inflammation in ASA-sensitive patients. Lipoxins are anti-inflammatory derivates of AA generated by transcellular metabolism, which involves cooperation of at least two lipoxygenases (5-LO and 15-LO). LXA_4 synthesized by isolated phagocytic cells such as human alveolar macrophages and neutrophils is detected in vivo in bronchoalveolar lavage fluid and may inhibit polymorphonuclear neutrophil (PMN) and eosinophil chemotaxis and PMN transmigration into inflammatory tissues (107). Sanak et al. (108) observed a significantly lower production of LXA_4 in PBLs from ASA-sensitive asthmatics, which was also evident in our study. Upregulation of 15-lipoxygenase and decreased production of anti-inflammatory 15-LO metabolite lipoxin A4 found in nasal polyp tissue from ASA-sensitive patients is further evidence of a distinctive but not yet understood role for 15-LO metabolites in patients with AERD.

Taken together these data implicate a role for eicosanoids in the pathogenesis of chronic eosinophilia in the lower and upper airways of patients with AERD. However, specificity of these abnormalities in arachidonic metabolism for ASA-sensitivity remains to be established. The differences in cellular and mediator profiles between tissue from ASA-sensitive and ASA-tolerant patients seem to be more quantitative than qualitative and one cannot exclude that they are secondary to the intensity of local inflammatory reactions rather than true pathophysiological abnormalities in ASA-hypersensitive patients.

Genetics of ASA Triad

Several single nucleotide polymorphisms in candidate genes coding molecules related mainly to the arachidonic acid metabolic pathway were found to be associated with ASA hypersensitivity including LTC4 synthase (109), 5-LOX (110), thromboxane A2 receptor (111), and prostaglandin EP2 receptor (112). However, most studies indicating a potential genetic component in the pathogenesis of the disease were reported by single centers and not yet reproduced by others. The importance of reproducing genotyping findings is exemplified by experience with LTC4 synthase-444 promotor polymorphism, which was associated with aspirin-hypersensitivity in one population of patients (113) and could not be reproduced by a series of other studies (114). Interestingly, LTC4S synthase-444 promoter polymorphism has been associated with other related phenotypes of asthma as severity or clinical response to LT1 receptor antagonists (115). Similarly, different HLA-DR/DQ antigens were associated in different populations with aspirin hypersensitivity probably reflecting ethnic differences in HLA antigen distribution (73,116,117). The weakness of association studies in patients with AERD is also related to the fact that we are dealing not with a single well-defined disease but rather with a syndrome, which includes several not always well-defined but overlapping phenotypes (hypersensitivity to ASA, asthma, rhinosinusitis, nasal polyps). Each phenotype may be coded by separate genes and thus one cannot be sure if association with a polymorphism is related to the mechanism of hypersensitivity to aspirin or to other phenotypic features of the aspirin triad related to an increased severity of inflammation.

DIAGNOSIS OF ASA-SENSITIVITY

In most clinical circumstances the diagnosis of ASA hypersensitivity is based on a history of adverse reaction precipitated by ASA or other NSAIDs. In ASA-hypersensitive patients with a convincing history of repeated drug-induced adverse reactions, confirmation of hypersensitivity by challenge test is not necessary. On the other hand, negative history does not exclude the possibility of adverse reaction on exposure, because up to 15% of asthmatic patients with a negative history may reveal hypersensitivity reactions when challenged with aspirin. In asthmatic patients with a negative history and/or those who have never been exposed to NSAIDs but have additional risk factors (rhinosinusitis, nasal polyposis, history of near fatal reactions), the risk of adverse reaction is further increased and provocation testing may be required. Thus, it is up to the clinician to consider in every individual case if circumstances justify diagnostic provocatic testing before treatment with NSAIDs is implemented in a patient with asthma (Table 5).

Although in the United States only oral ASA provocation challenges are performed because of unavailability of a soluble aspirin (Lysin-aspirin), in most countries inhaled, intranasal, and even intravenous routes of challenge are employed for routine diagnosis (118).

Oral Provocation

Oral challenge is the reference standard for the diagnosis of hypersensitivity to aspirin and other NSAIDs. Although several protocols for oral aspirin provocation have been developed and described, a uniformly accepted protocol has not been devised (15,119,120) (Table 2). Before the challenge, the patient should have well-controlled asthma, FEV_1 should exceed 70% of predicted values, and anti-inflammatory treatment should not be interrupted. On the first day, placebo is administered in a way identical to the following aspirin challenge. On the second day, the patient receives initially 10 to 30 mg of aspirin and the dose is doubled in two- to three-hour intervals until a positive reaction occurs. The reaction is considered positive if FEV_1 falls by $\geq 20\%$ and/or extrabronchial symptoms appear. The reaction usually begins within 20 to 90 minutes and then should be treated with nebulization of albuterol, intravenous antihistamine (clemastine), and oral or intravenous glucocorticosteroids to prevent development of delayed symptoms. If 600 to 650 mg of aspirin is ingested and well tolerated the patient is considered to be aspirin tolerant.

TABLE 2 Oral Acetylsalicylic Acid Challenge Protocol in an Outpatient Setting Used in Allergy and Asthma Center in Lodz

Time	Day 1	Day 2 (aspirin)	Day 3 (aspirin)
8:00 A.M.	Placebo	10–20 mg	160 mg
10:30 A.M.	Placebo	40 mg	320 mg
13:00 P.M.	Placebo	80 mg	600 mg
15:00 P.M.	Patient discharged	Patient discharged	Patient discharged

The negative challenge results in patients with suspected aspirin hypersensitivity is 16% and may reflect lack of sensitivity ("silent desensitization") or to a lesser extent blocking effects of medications used to control chronic inflammatory diseases (121). The use of asthma controller therapy (not particularly antileukotrienes but also long acting beta-2 agonists and inhaled steroids) may alleviate the reaction and shift the response during aspirin challenge from bronchial (asthmatic symptoms and fall in FEV_1) to nasocular reactions (58). Similarly, the use of antihistamines may significantly decrease development not only of cutaneous but also respiratory symptoms, thus increasing the rate of false negative aspirin challenge results. On the other hand, systemic steroids do not seem to affect the response to aspirin challenge in sensitive patients. Although potential blocking effects of some medications have to be borne in mind, it is not advisable to discontinue controller medications before aspirin challenge in patients with suspected ASA hypersensitivity because it may increase the risk of severe reactions. Oral challenge tests, although a gold standard for diagnosis of ASA-sensitivity, is a time-consuming procedure bearing a risk of severe systemic reaction, thus requiring well-experienced personnel and close availability of emergency facilities.

Bronchial Provocation

Inhalation challenge with lysine-aspirin (a soluble form of ASA) was introduced by Bianco et al. in 1977 (122); and in Europe is currently considered the test of choice to confirm/exclude aspirin sensitivity in patients with bronchial asthma. According to a standard protocol following inhalation of diluent, increasing doses of L-aspirin are inhaled by means of a dosimeter in 30-minute intervals, allowing completion of the procedure in an outpatient setting in less than five hours (123). Inhalation testing is faster and safer to perform than oral challenge (the reaction is usually easily reversible by nebulized beta-2 agonists) and both tests have similar sensitivity and specificity (124,125). Inhalation challenge in some patients induces extrabronchial symptoms, which are related to systemic recruitment of inflammatory cell progenitors from bone marrow (126). A severe generalized reaction to lysine-aspirin was reported, indicating that even inhalation challenge is associated with a potential risk of severe reaction and should be performed by experienced centers with proper emergency assistance (127).

Nasal Provocation

Nasal provocation testing with lysine-aspirin is also a reliable tool to diagnose hypersensitivity to aspirin, providing that the clinical symptoms are combined with the objective and standardized technique of airflow measurement for assessment of the results (128). The test is rapid and safe and can be performed in an outpatient setting even in asthmatic patients with low pulmonary function not suitable for bronchial provocation. In experienced hands, the sensitivity of intranasal aspirin provocation may exceed 80% and specificity is close to 95%, thus approaching performance of bronchial challenge (129–131). Some limitations of this route of challenge are related to patients with significant nasal obstruction, turbulent nasal flow, or unspecific nasal responsiveness.

In Vitro Tests

Platelet activation tests, histamine release assay, or earlier versions of basophil activation test were unreliable to distinguish aspirin/NSAIDs sensitive from insensitive individuals (132–134). More recently, three in vitro tests measuring aspirin-specific peripheral blood leukocytes activation have been proposed for the diagnosis of aspirin sensitivity.

Sulfidoleukotrienes Release Assay

Release of leukotrienes from PBL upon stimulation with aspirin have been measured employing commercially available assay (CAST-ELISA) in which leukocytes are primed with IL-3. Although several studies demonstrated that aspirin may trigger release of LTC4 from peripheral blood leukocytes, the differences between ASA-hypersensitive asthmatics and ASA-tolerant subjects have only been quantitative and the results (mostly due to the small number of patients) usually were not expressed in terms of sensitivity and specificity (135–138). In other studies, even in highly selected patient populations, the sensitivity was usually low (20–50%) although specificity could reach 100% (139,140). The performance of sulfidoleukotriene tests could be further improved if in addition to aspirin other NSAIDs were tested and the combined results analyzed. However, completely negative studies showing mostly nonspecific release of leukotrienes from PBL upon stimulation with aspirin in vitro were also reported (141). Taken together at present, measurement of aspirin-induced sulfidofleukotrienes release from PBL cannot be recommended as a reliable tool for the routine diagnosis of ASA sensitivity.

Basophil Activation Test

Cytofluorimetric measurement of cell surface molecule CD63 expression upon in vitro challenge has been proposed for diagnosis of various hypersensitivities including hypersensitivity to aspirin (142). In a study by Sanz et al., the commercially available test (Flow Cast; Buhlmann) resulted in a sensitivity of 41% and specificity of 100% with positive and negative predictive values approaching 100%. However, a quite heterogenous population of patients was included for analysis (both respiratory and cutaneous type of hypersensitivity to different NSAIDs) and the control population was not clinically characterized. Further studies in larger and more clearly defined patient populations are necessary to estimate the real performance of this test in aspirin-hypersensitive asthmatics.

15-HETE Generation Assay

More recently, we described Aspirin-Sensitive Patient Identification Test (ASPITest[R]) based on measurement of 15-HETE release from PBL. Aspirin could trigger in vitro generation of arachidonic acid metabolite (15-HETE) from nasal polyp epithelial cells, and peripheral blood leukocytes from ASA-sensitive patients but not ASA-tolerant asthmatics or healthy subjects. In contrast to other in vitro tests, ASPITest within the range of aspirin concentrations tested demonstrated mostly qualitative and not only quantitative differences between ASA-sensitive and ASA-tolerant asthmatics. Aspirin-triggered 15-HETE release from PBL mimicked to some extent sensitivity reaction to aspirin observed in vivo: in some patients release of 15-HETE could be triggered by other nonselective cyclooxygenase inhibitors naproxen or ibuprofen, but COX-2 selective NSAID celecoxib did not affect the release. When the test was probed in a relatively large population of patients to confirm the diagnosis, the sensitivity was 82% and the specificity was 83% with negative and positive predictive values 0.79 and 0.86, respectively (61). These data indicate that ASPITest based on 15-HETE release measurement from PBL may be useful for detection of ASA hypersensitivity in asthmatic patients.

The overall performance of different methods for the diagnosis of aspirin hypersensitivity in patients with AERD is presented in (Table 3).

Although a combination of a positive history and placebo-controlled aspirin challenge by oral, bronchial, or nasal route still remains the standard for the diagnosis of ASA-hypersensitivity, the newly developed in vitro tests (FLOW CAST and ASPITest) seem to demonstrate promising performance and after further investigation and validation could become valuable tools for confirming the presence of aspirin hypersensitivity.

MANAGEMENT OF A PATIENT WITH ASPIRIN TRIAD

Although aspirin is only one of the many triggers exacerbating symptoms of rhinosinusitis and asthma in patients with AERD, the presence of aspirin sensitivity heralds severe and protracted disease of the respiratory tract, requiring comprehensive management of all components of the syndrome. Observations that atopic sensitization is at least as common among ASA-hypersensitive patients as in ASA-tolerant patients, asthmatics have practical implications and should prompt a physician to carry out comprehensive allergic investigations in patients with ASA hypersensitivity and to consider, if necessary, implementing full antiallergic treatment. Although management of asthma and rhinosinusitis in ASA-hypersensitive patients should follow general guidelines, there are several important, specific for AERD points that have to be taken into account.

Avoidance of NSAIDs and Use of Alternative Analgesics

Patient education and careful avoidance of ASA and other NSAIDs in sensitive patients seem to be of high importance, because aspirin may be a cause of severe asthmatic attack in a significant proportion of patients admitted to the intensive care unit (Table 4). However, before any avoidance and alternative treatment are recommended the patient requires comprehensive investigation and diagnosis. The type of reaction (asthmatic, cutaneous, and anaphylactic) has to be determined and, if possible, the presence of true hypersensitivity confirmed by the challenge test. Although 0% to 16% patients with AERD may have respiratory reaction on

TABLE 3 Overall Performance of Methods for the Diagnosis of Aspirin Hypersensitivity in Patients with Asthma

Method	Sensitivity (%)	Specificity (%)	References
Bronchial	90	100	Dahlen-idem Nizankowska-idem
Nasal	73–86.7	84–95.7	Casadevall-idem Milewski-idem AlonzoLlamares
CAST-ELISA	20–72	83–100	May-idem Sanz[a]-idem
BASo	41.7	100	Sanz[a]-idem
ASPITest	82	83	Kowalski-idem

[a]Populations studied included patients with both respiratory and cutaneous type of hypersensitivity.
Abbreviation: ASPITest, aspirin-sensitive patient identification test.

TABLE 4 Nonsteroidal Anti-inflammatory Drugs Cross-Reacting in Majority of Patients with Aspirin Exacerbated Respiratory Disease

Ibuprofen	Etodolac
Indomethacin	Diclofenac
Sulindac	Ketoprofen
Naproxen	Flurbiprofen
Fenoprofen	Piroxicam
Meclofenamate	Nabumetone
Ketorolac	Mefanamic acid

oral challenge with acetaminophen, in most patients acetaminophen in low or moderate doses (below 1000 mg) can be recommended as an alternative antipyretic or analgesic drug (143). Preferential COX-2 inhibitors (nimesulide and meloxicam) are also tolerated by the majority of, but not all, hypersensitive patients and can be recommended in an individual patient after tolerability is proved by oral challenged (144–146). Selective COX-2 inhibitors (celecoxib and withdrawn from the market rofecoxib) are well tolerated by aspirin-sensitive asthmatics and could be an ideal alternative NSAID for patients with aspirin triad (147–149). However, recent reports including randomized, controlled trials demonstrated that significant cardiovascular toxicity is associated with rofecoxib celecoxib, valdecoxib, and parecoxib, suggesting that this is a class effect of COX-2 selective NSAIDs (150,151). This information seems to significantly limit the use of COX-2 selective NSAIDs prompting a physician to investigate other available options before deciding to treat an ASA-hypersensitive patient with COX-2. If a COX-2 inhibitor is necessary, the patient should be informed of the potential risk and the lowest possible dose should be used for the shortest possible time. In conclusion, although for a majority of patients with hypersensitivity to aspirin an alternative anti-inflammatory drug can be found, in each individual case a physician must carefully consider the choice of an alternative drug (152).

Management of Chronic Rhinosinusitis and Nasal Polyposis
Management of chronic rhinosinusitis is essential and may be prerequisite for the improvement of bronchial symptoms. Traditional medicines, nasal decongestants and antihistamines, give limited relief in these patients, but topical steroids seem to be quite effective in controlling symptoms of rhinitis and may slow down recurrence of nasal polyps (153). Antibiotics should be used whenever an infectious

TABLE 5 Indications for Aspirin Desensitization in Aspirin-Hypersensitive Asthmatics

Need for improvement in control of asthma/ rhinosinusitis
  Patients with hypersensitivity to aspirin and with aggressive nasal polyposis not responding to pharmacological treatment
  At risk of significant corticosteroid-induced side effects
Need for chronic prevention of cardiovascular events
  Coronary heart disease
Need for chronic anti-inflammatory treatment
  Rheumatoid arthritis
  Osteoarthrosis

component is evident. Preliminary observations suggest that antileukotriene drugs may also alleviate symptoms of chronic rhinosinusitis and improve nasal patency in ASA-hypersensitive patients. However, they do not seem to be more effective than in ASA-tolerant patients (106). Treatment with zileuton, a 5-LOX inhibitor, resulted in remarkable return of smell, less rhinorrhea, but only a trend for less stuffiness and higher nasal inspiratory flow (105).

In many patients, various nasal surgical procedures are needed to relieve chronic rhinosinusitis, and to remove nasal polyps. Employing computed tomography imaging for assessment of the extent of the sinus disease seems to be of exceptional value. Depending on the stage of the disease, surgery consists of polypectomy, functional endoscopic sinus surgery or ethmoidectomy in resistant cases (154). Assessment of the outcome of endoscopic surgery in ASA-sensitive patients with chronic rhinosinusitis and ASA-tolerant controls revealed that patients with ASA triad responded less well to surgical intervention (155,156). Sinus surgery performed in patients with ASA triad resulted in significant improvement in asthma symptoms and decreased dosing of oral and inhaled steroids (157). One year after surgery, an improvement in pulmonary function as compared to the preoperative period was also observed. Because surgery does not affect the underlying inflammatory component of rhinosinusitis, medical treatment with topical steroids is also necessary postsurgery. Antileukotrienes and/or chronic oral aspirin after desensitization may also be considered as the follow-up treatment after surgery.

Management of Bronchial Asthma

Inhaled glucocorticosteroids, often in combination with long-acting beta-2 agonists are the most effective drugs for controlling asthmatic inflammation and asthma symptoms in aspirin-sensitive patients. In some patients either an occasional burst of oral corticosteroids or chronic treatment with oral prednisone is necessary to control the disease. Leukotriene receptor antagonists and synthesis inhibitors have been shown to be of clinical benefit in patients with ASA-sensitive asthma. Addition of a leukotriene receptor antagonist such as montelukast to standard anti-inflammatory therapy (inhaled glucocorticosteroids, theophylline, short-acting beta-2 agonists) improved respiratory function and alleviated clinical symptoms over a four-week treatment period in a group of aspirin-sensitive asthmatics (158). However, in this study, none of the patients used long-acting beta-2 agonists, thus not allowing for the assessment of ALD efficacy over standard combination therapy. Six weeks of treatment with zileuton in ASA-hypersensitive asthmatics resulted in improvement in pulmonary function despite less use of a rescue bronchodilator with zileuton—the magnitude of improvement did not seem to exceed that observed in ASA-tolerant patients in other studies (159).

The statement that antileukotrienes are drugs of choice in the treatment of asthmatic patients with aspirin hypersensitivity has notoriously been repeated in the literature without any support by data showing superior efficacy in this subpopulation of asthmatics. To the contrary, available data indicate that although ALD may be effective in relieving symptoms and improving respiratory function in some ASA-sensitive asthmatics, the degree of improvement is similar in sensitive and tolerant asthmatics [160; Kowalski ML, Bieńkiewicz B, Ptasińska A, DuBuske L. Enhanced generation of LTC4 by polymorphonuclear blood leukocytes (PBL) from asthmatic patients during treatment with zafirlukast (Accolate). In preparation]. However, a significant individual heterogeneity of response to antileukotrienes that have been observed may be determined by genetic polymorphisms. Patients with hypersensitivity to aspirin bearing variant C allele of LTS4 synthase and HLA DRB1∗301 allele respond better to antileukotrienes, thus pointing to the importance of a pharmacogenetic approach to treatment of this apparently heterogenous population of asthmatic patients (117).

Desensitization to Aspirin—An Alternative Approach to a Hypersensitive Patient

A more specific approach to ASA-hypersensitive rhinosinusitis/asthma is aspirin given orally after desensitization. Most aspirin-hypersensitive asthmatics can be desensitized after repeated challenges with aspirin; following the initial adverse reaction, repeating of the dose is tolerated by more than 50% of patients and further incremental aspirin challenges lead to a tolerance (Fig. 4) (161). A patient who tolerates 600 mg of aspirin is considered "desensitized" and then can take aspirin on a daily basis, indefinitely without further adverse respiratory reactions. In most patients desensitization can be also achieved silently i.e., without evoking initial adverse reaction providing the challenge starts with a subthreshold dose and then the dose is slowly increased in appropriate intervals (162). In order to maintain the tolerance a patient has to ingest aspirin on a regular, usually daily basis—the tolerance state disappears after two to five days without aspirin with the full hypersensitivity returning after seven days (163). During the ASA-refractory period, patients may also tolerate other previously cross-reacting NSAIDs.

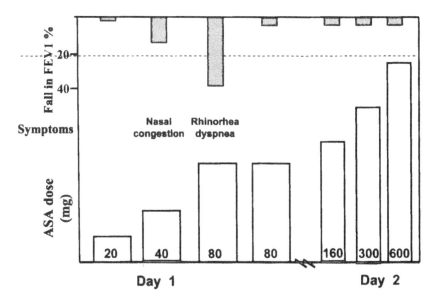

FIGURE 4 Aspirin desensitization in an acetylsalicylic acid–sensitive patient (a.c.). On day 0 (not shown) the patient was challenged with repeated doses of placebo every two hours without any reaction. On day 1 second dose of aspirin (40 mg) induced only nasal symptoms, but next dose (80 mg) triggered full nasal and bronchial reaction (rhinorrhea, dyspnea, and fall in FEV$_1$). Dose of 80 mg repeated two hours later was well tolerated and on the day 2 patient could take with impunity up to 600 mg of aspirin. *Abbreviation:* ASA, acetylsalicylic acid.

Several protocols of desensitization have been proposed allowing for completing the procedure usually within three to five days. The standard protocol of desensitization is an extension of the oral aspirin challenge protocol and all the safety precautions recommended for the challenge should be employed. Although several biochemical events occur directly after achieving aspirin desensitization (e.g., downregulation of arachidonic acid metabolism, decreased inflammatory cell activation, or downregulation in leukotriene LT1 receptor expression), the real mechanism of aspirin desensitization is not known and may be only the matter of speculation (164).

It has been documented that in a subgroup of hypersensitive patients ingestion of aspirin after desensitization results in alleviation of chronic upper and lower airway symptoms (165,166). When the patients were treated with aspirin for six months to six years a significant reduction in hospitalization, emergency room visits, outpatient visits, and need for nasal/sinus surgery were observed; and in some patients a reduction in daily oral prednisone doses could be achieved (167–169). Usually daily aspirin was efficacious within the first six months of treatment after desensitization and continued to be effective for up to five years of follow-up. In patients with rhinosinusitis but without asthma aspirin given after desensitization significantly reduced symptoms of hypertrophic rhinitis and decreased recurrence of nasal polyps (7). Interestingly, even treatment with a low dose of aspirin (100 mg daily) for one to three years may provide benefit with respect to the recurrence rate of nasal polyps, severity of bronchial asthma, and sense of smell in desensitized patients with AERD (170). However, some patients report a relief in nasal obstruction immediately after desensitization and overall improvement can be seen in the majority of patients within the first week of treatment. We have observed that two-thirds of patients receiving 600 mg of aspirin after desensitization experienced significant improvement in nasal symptoms score and 50% of them experienced reduction in asthma score within the first four weeks of treatment with aspirin (171). Similar observation of early clinical effects of desensitization have been reported recently in a group of 38 patients taking 650 mg of aspirin twice daily after desensitization. In addition, 8 of 15 patients taking oral prednisone reduced their doses by 50% or more and two of five patients who had been taking doses every other day discontinued this treatment after four weeks.

The potential effect of aspirin desensitization and treatment may be limited because: (i) not all patients can be desensitized because of the severity or nonstability of underlying asthma; (ii) desensitization is contraindicated because of concomitant gastric/peptic ulcer disease; (iii) patient dropout related to gastric intolerance of aspirin; (iv) clinical improvement can be achieved in some but not all patients. Considering these limitations, only a fraction of patients with AERD will benefit from aspirin desensitization and at present it is not possible to identify these patients before the procedure is implemented (172). Aspirin given after desensitization may also be a valuable solution for ASA-hypersensitive patients requiring chronic treatment with aspirin for rheumatoid diseases or coronary heart disease (173). Table 5 summarizes indications for ASA-desensitization in patients with asthma and hypersensitivity to NSAIDs.

Desensitization can also be achieved after repeated intranasal application of lysine aspirin (174). It has been reported, that intranasal desensitization and prolonged treatment with soluble intranasal aspirin (Lysine-aspirin) has a beneficial effect on CRS, reducing recurrency rate for nasal polyps in ASA-treated groups as compared to placebo-treated patients (175,176). However, such beneficial effects of the nasal route were not confirmed by other studies and similar improvement in nasal symptoms after intranasal aspirin could be obtained in ASA-tolerant patients with nasal polyps, questioning specificity of these approaches for patients with AERD.

REFERENCES

1. Hirschberg. Mitheilung uber einenfall von nebenwirkung des aspirin. Deutsch Med Wschr 1902; 416:1902.
2. Widal MF, Abrami P, Lenmoyes J. Anaphylaxie et idiosyncrasie. Presse Med 1922; 30:189–192.
3. Samter M, Beers RF. Intolerance to aspirin: clinical studies and consideration of its pathogenesis. Ann Intern Med 1968; 68:875–883.
4. Szczeklik A, Stevenson DD. Aspirin-induced asthma: advances in pathogenesis, diagnosis, and management. J Allergy Clin Immunol 2003; 111(5):913–921.
5. Johansson SG, Bieber T, Dahl R, et al. Revised nomenclature for allergy for global use: report of the Nomenclature Review Committee of the World Allergy Organization, October 2003. J Allergy Clin Immunol 2004; 113(5):832–836.
6. Berges-Gimeno MP, Simon RA, Stevenson DD. The natural history and clinical characteristics of aspirin exacerbated respiratory disease. Ann Allergy Asthma Immunol 2002; 89:474–478.
7. Lumry WR, Curd JG, Zeiger RS. Aspirin-sensitive rhinosinusitis: the clinical syndrome and effects of aspirin administration. J Allergy Clin Immunol 1983; 71:580–587.
8. Stevenson DD, Sanchez-Borges M, Szczeklik A. Classification of allergic and pseudoallergic reactions to drugs that inhibit cyclooxygenase enzymes. Ann Allergy Asthma Immunol 2001; 87(3):177–180.
9. Hedman J, Kaprio J, Poussa T, Nieminen M. Prevalence of asthma, aspirin intolerance, nasal polyposis and chronic obstructive pulmonary disease in a population-based study. Int J Epidemiol 1999; 28:717–722.
10. Kasper L, Sladek K, Duplaga M, et al. Prevalence of asthma with aspirin hypersensitivity in the adult population of Poland. Allergy 2003; 58(10):1064–1066.
11. Vally H, Taylor ML, Thompson PJ. The prevalence of aspirin intolerant asthma (AIA) in Australian asthmatic patients. Thorax 2002; 57(7):569–574.
12. Jenkins C, Costello J, Hodge L. Systematic review of prevalence of aspirin induced asthma and its implications for clinical practice. BMJ 2004; 328(7437):43.
13. Castillo J, Picado C. Prevalence of aspirin intolerance in asthmatics treated in a hospital. Respiration 1986; 50:153–157.
14. Marquette CH, Saulnier F, Leroy O, et al. Long-term prognosis of near-fatal asthma. A 6-year follow-up study of 145 asthmatic patients who underwent mechanical ventilation for a near-fatal attack of asthma. Am Rev Respir Dis 1992; 146(1):76–81.
15. McDonald JR, Mathison DA, Stevenson DD. Aspirin intolerance in asthma. Detection by oral challenge. J Allergy Clin Immunol 1972; 50(4):198–207.
16. Settipane GA. Nasal polyps: epidemiology, pathology, immunology, and treatment. Am J Rhinol 1987; 1:119–126.
17. Szczeklik A, Nizankowska E, Duplaga M. Natural history of aspirin-induced asthma. AIANE Investigators. European Network on Aspirin-Induced Asthma. Eur Respir J 2000; 16(3):432–436.
18. Kuehm SL, Doyle MJ. Medication errors: 1977 to 1988. Experience in medical malpractice claims. N J Med 1990; 87(1):27–34.
19. Grzelewska-Rzymowska I, Rożniecki J, Szmidt M, Kowalski ML. Asthma with aspirin intolerance. Clinical entity or coincidence of nonspecific bronchial hyperreactivity and aspirin intolerance. Allergol Immunopathol 1981; 9:533–541.
20. Pleskow WW, Stevenson DD, Mathison DA, Simon RA, Schatz M, Zeiger RS. Aspirin-sensitive rhinosinusitis/asthma: spectrum of adverse reactions to aspirin. J Allergy Clin Immunol 1983; 71(6):574–579.
21. Bochenek G, Nizankowska E, Szczeklik A. The atopy trait in hypersensitivity to nonsteroidal anti-inflammatory drugs. Allergy 1996; 51(1):16–23.

22. Sanchez-Borges M, Capriles-Hulett A. Atopy is a risk factor for non-steroidal anti-inflammatory drug sensitivity. Ann Allergy Asthma Immunol 2000; 84(1): 101–106.
23. Kalyoncu AF, Karakaya G, Sahin AA, Baris YI. Occurrence of allergic conditions in asthmatics with analgesic intolerance. Allergy 1999; 54(5):428–435.
24. Kupczyk M, Kuprys I, Gorski P, Kuna P. Aspirin intolerance and allergy to house dust mites: important factors associated with development of severe asthma. Ann Allergy Asthma Immunol 2004; 92(4):453–458.
25. Karakaya G, Demir AU, Kalyoncu AF. Related articles, links is there an association between bronchial asthma, food allergy/intolerance and analgesic intolerance? Eur Respir J 1999; 13(1):227–228.
26. Kowalski ML, Bienkiewicz B, Kordek P, et al. Nasal polyposis in aspirin-hypersensitive patients with asthma (aspirin triad) and aspirin-tolerant patients. Allergy Clin Immunol Int – J World Allergy Org 2003; 6:246–250.
27. Jantti-Alanko S, Holopainen E, Malmberg H. Recurrence of nasal polyps after surgical treatment. Rhinology 1989; 8:59–64.
28. Kowalski ML. Rhinosinusitis and nasal polyps in aspirin-sensitive and aspirin-tolerant patients: are they different? Thorax 2000; 55(2):S84–S86.
29. Wierzuchowski M. Dozylne stosowanie peptonu w dychawicy oskrzelowej. Pol Arch Med Wewn 1925; 2:42–76.
30. Mascia K, Haselkorn T, Deniz YM, et al. TENOR Study Group. Aspirin sensitivity and severity of asthma: evidence for irreversible airway obstruction in patients with severe or difficult-to-treat asthma. J Allergy Clin Immunol 2005; 116(5):970–975.
31. Plaza V, Serrano J, Picado C, Sanchis J High Risk Asthma Research Group. Frequency and clinical characteristics of rapid-onset fatal and near-fatal asthma. Eur Respir J 2002; 19(5):846–852.
32. Yoshimine F, Hasegawa T, Suzuki E, et al. Contribution of aspirin-intolerant asthma to near fatal asthma based on a questionnaire survey in Niigata Prefecture, Japan. Respirology 2005; 10(4):477–484.
33. Szczeklik A, Gryglewski RJ, Czerniawska-Mysik G. Relationship of inhibition of prostaglandins biosynthesis by analgesics to asthma attacks in aspirins-sensitive patients. Br Med J 1975; 1:67–69.
34. Warner TD, Giuliano F, Vojnovic I, Bukasa A, Mitchell JA, Vane JR. Nonsteroid drug selectivities for cyclo-oxygenase-1 rather than cyclo-oxygenase-2 are associated with human gastrointestinal toxicity: a full in vitro analysis. Proc Natl Acad Sci USA 1999; 96(13):7563–7568.
35. Szczeklik A. Mechanism of aspirin-induced asthma. Allergy 1997; 52:613–619.
36. Szczeklik A et al. Protective and bronchodilator effects of PGE and salbutamol in aspirin –induced asthma. Am J Respir Crit Care Med 1996; 153:567–571.
37. Szmidt M, Wasiak W. The influence of misoprostol (synthetic analogue of prostaglandin E1) on aspirin-induced bronchoconstriction in aspirin-sensitive asthma. J Invest Allergol Clin Immunol 1996; 6(2):121–125.
38. Sestini P, Armetti L, Gambaro G, et al. Inhaled PGE2 prevents aspirin-induced bronchoconstriction and urinary LTE4 excretion in aspirin-sensitive asthma. Am J Respir Crit Care Med 1996; 153(2):572–575.
39. Pierzchalska M, Szabo Z, Sanak M, Soja J, Szczeklik A. Deficient prostaglandin E2 production by bronchial fibroblasts of asthmatic patients, with special reference to aspirin-induced asthma. J Allergy Clin Immunol 2003; 111(5):1041–1048.
40. Kowalski ML, Pawliczak R, Woźniak J, et al. Differential metabolism of arachidonic acid in nasal polyp epithelial cells cultured from aspirin-sensitive and aspirin-tolerant patients. Am J Respir Crit Care Med 2000; 161:391–398.
41. Szczeklik A, Gryglewski RJ, Olszewski E, et al. Aspirin-sensitive asthma: the effect of aspirin on the release of prostaglandins from nasal polyps. Pharmacol Res Commun 1977; 9:415–425.
42. Gray PA, Warner TD, Vojnovic I, et al. Effects of non-steroidal anti-inflammatory drugs on cyclo-oxygenase and lipoxygenase activity in whole blood from aspirin-sensitive asthmatics versus healthy donors. Br J Pharmacol 2002; 137(7):1031–1038.

43. Picado C, Fernandez-Morata JC, Juan M, et al. Cyclooxygenase-2 mRNA is down-expressed in nasal polyps from aspirin-sensitive asthmatics. Am J Respir Crit Care Med 1999; 160:291–296.
44. Christman BW, Christman JW, Dworski R, Blair IA, Prakash C. Prostaglandin E2 limits arachidonic acid availability and inhibits leukotriene B4 synthesis in rat alveolar macrophages by a nonphospholipase A2 mechanism. J Immunol 1993; 151(4): 2096–2104.
45. Kowalski ML, Ptasinska A, Bienkiewicz B, et al. Differential effects of aspirin and misoprostol on 15-hydroxyeicosatetraenoic acid generation by leukocytes from aspirin-sensitive asthmatic patients. J Allergy Clin Immunol 2003; 112:505–512.
46. Sanak M, Kielbasa B, Bochenek G, Szczeklik A. Related articles, links exhaled eicosanoids following oral aspirin challenge in asthmatic patients. Clin Exp Allergy 2004; 34(12):1899–1904.
47. Fischer AR, Rosenberg MA, Lilly CM. Direct evidence for role of the mast cell in the nasal response to aspirin in aspirin-sensitive asthma. J Allergy Clin Immunol 1994; 94:1046–1056.
48. Nasser S, Christie PE, Pfister R, et al. Effect of endobronchial aspirin challenge on inflammatory cells in bronchial biopsy samples from aspirin-sensitive asthmatic subjects. Thorax 1996 Jan; 51(1):64–70.
49. Kowalski ML, Grzegorczyk J, Wojciechowska B, Poniatowska M. Intranasal challenge with aspirin induces cell influx and activation of eosinophils and mast cells in nasal secretions of ASA-sensitive patients. Clin Exp Allergy 1996; 26:807–814.
50. Bochenek G, Nagraba K, Nizankowska E, Szczeklik A. Related articles, links a controlled study of 9alpha,11beta-PGF2 (a prostaglandin D2 metabolite) in plasma and urine of patients with bronchial asthma and healthy controls after aspirin challenge. J Allergy Clin Immunol 2003; 111(4):743–749.
51. Picado C, Ramis I, Rosello, et al. Release of peptide leukotrienes into nasal secretions after local instillation of aspirin in sensitive asthmatic patients. Am Rev Respir Dis 1992; 145:65–69.
52. Kowalski ML, Sliwinska-Kowalska M, Igarashi Y, et al. Nasal secretions in response to acetylsalicylic acid. J Allergy Clin Immunol 1993; 91(2):580–598.
53. Obase Y, Shimoda T, Tomari SY, et al. Effects of pranlukast on chemical mediators in induced sputum on provocation tests in atopic and aspirin-intolerant asthmatic patients. Chest 2002; 121(1):143–150.
54. Christie PE, Tagari P, Ford-Hutchinson AW, et al. Urinary leukotriene E4 concentrations increase after aspirin challenge in aspirin-sensitive asthmatic subjects. Am Rev Respir Dis 1991; 143(5 Pt 1):1025–1029.
55. Mita H, Endoh S, Kudoh M, et al. Possible involvement of mast-cell activation in aspirin provocation of aspirin-induced asthma. Allergy 2001; 56(11):1061–1067.
56. Christie PE, Smith CM, Lee TH. The potent and selective sulfidopeptide leukotriene antagonist, SK&F 104353, inhibits aspirin-induced asthma. Am Rev Respir Dis 1991; 144(4):957–958.
57. Broadfoot A, Gillis D, Heddle R, Smith W, Kette F. Failure of montelukast to prevent aspirin-induced asthma. Intern Med J 2002; 32(5–6):271–272.
58. White AA, Stevenson DD, Simon RA. The blocking effect of essential controller medications during aspirin challenges in patients with aspirin-exacerbated respiratory disease. Ann Allergy Asthma Immunol 2005; 95(4):330–335.
59. Antczak A, Montuschi P, Kharitonov S, Gorski P, Barnes PJ. Increased exhaled cysteinyl-leukotrienes and 8-isoprostane in aspirin-induced asthma. Am J Respir Crit Care Med 2002; 166(3):301–306.
60. Mita H, Higashi N, Taniguchi M, Higashi A, Akiyama K. Related articles, links increase in urinary leukotriene B4 glucuronide concentration in patients with aspirin-intolerant asthma after intravenous aspirin challenge. Clin Exp Allergy 2004; 34(8):1262–1269.
61. Kowalski ML, Ptasinska A, Jedrzejczak M, et al. Aspirin-triggered 15-HETE generation in peripheral blood leukocytes is a specific and sensitive Aspirin-Sensitive Patients Identification Test (ASPITest). Allergy 2005; 60:1139–1145.

62. Goetzl EJ, Phillips MJ, Gold WM. Stimulus specificity of the generation of leukotrienes by dog mastocytoma cells. J Exp Med 1983; 158:731–737.

63. Marom Z, Shelhamer JH, Kaliner M. Effects of arachidonic acid, monohydroxyeicosatetraenoic acid and prostaglandins on the release of mucous glycoproteins from human airways in vitro. J Clin Invest 1981; 67:1695–1702.

64. Salari H, Schellenberg RR. Stimulation of human airway epithelial cells by platelet activating factor (PAF) and arachidonic acid produces 15-hydroxyeicosatetraenoic acid (15-HETE) capable of contracting bronchial smooth muscle. Pulm Pharmacol 1991; 4:1–7.

65. Schewe T, Petrich K, Ludwig P, Kuhn H, Nigam S. Effect of 15-HETE on the 5-lipoxygenase pathway in neutrophils. Genuine inhibitor or alternative substrate? Adv Exp Med Biol 1999; 447:95–105.

66. Profita M, Sala A, Riccobono L, et al. 15(S)-HETE modulates LTB(4) production and neutrophil chemotaxis in chronic bronchitis. Am J Physiol Cell Physiol 2000; 279:C1249–C1258.

67. Bandeira-Melo C, Bozza PT, Diaz BL, et al. Cutting edge: lipoxin (LX) A4 and aspirin-triggered 15-epi-LXA4 block allergen-induced eosinophil trafficking. J Immunol 2000; 164:2267–2271.

68. Holtzman MJ, Turk J, Shornick LP. Identification of a pharmacologically distinct prostaglandin H synthase in cultured epithelial cells and save. J Biol Chem 1992; 267: 21438–21445.

69. Lecomte M, Laneuville O, Ji C, DeWitt DL, Smith WL. Acetylation of human prostaglandin endoperoxide synthase-2 (cyclooxygenase-2) by aspirin. J Biol Chem 1994; 269:13207–13215.

70. Szczeklik A. Aspirin-induced asthma as a viral disease. Clin Allergy 1988; 18:15–20.

71. Szczeklik A, Nizankowska E, Serafin A, Dyczek A, Duplaga M, Musial J. Autoimmune phenomena in bronchial asthma with special reference to aspirin intolerance. Am J Respir Crit Care Med 1995; 152(6 Pt 1):1753–1756.

72. Szczeklik A, Musial J, Pulka G. Related articles, links autoimmune vasculitis and aortic stenosis in aspirin-induced asthma (AIA). Allergy 1997; 52(3):352–354 (no abstract available).

73. Dekker JW, Nizankowska E, Schmitz-Schumann M, et al. Aspirin-induced asthma and HLA-DRB1 and HLA-DPB1 genotypes. Clin Exp Allergy 1997; 27(5):574–577.

74. Bachert C, Gevaert P, Holtappels G, Johansson SG, Van Cauwenberge P. Total and specific IgE in nasal polyps is related to local eosinophilic inflammation. J Allergy Clin Immunol 2001; 107:607–614.

75. Perez-Novo CA, Kowalski ML, Kuma P, et al. Aspirin sensitivity and IgE antibodies to *Staphylococcus aureus* enterotoxins in nasal polyposis: studies on the relationship. Int Arch Allergy Immunol 2004; 133:255–260.

76. Suh YJ, Yoon SH, Sampson AP, et al. Related articles, links specific immunoglobulin E for staphylococcal enterotoxins in nasal polyps from patients with aspirin-intolerant asthma. Clin Exp Allergy 2004; 34(8):1270–1275.

77. Jankowski R. Eosinophils in the pathophysiology of nasal polyposis. Acta Otolaryngol 1996; 116:160–163.

78. Nasser SM, Pfister R, Christie PE, et al. Inflammatory cell populations in bronchial biopsies from aspirin-sensitive asthmatic subjects. Am J Respir Crit Care Med 1996; 153(1):90–96.

79. Kowalski ML, Lewandowska A, Wozniak J, Makowska J, Jankowski A, DuBuske L. Inhibition of nasal polyp mast cell and eosinophil activation by desloratadine. Allergy 2005; 60:80–85.

80. Sousa AR, Lams BE, Pfister R, Christie PE, Schmitz M, Lee TH. Expression of interleukin-5 and granulocyte-macrophage colony-stimulating factor in aspirin-sensitive and non-aspirin-sensitive asthmatic airways. Am J Respir Crit Care Med 1997; 156(5): 1384–1389.

81. Hamilos DL, Leung DY, Huston DP, Kamil A, Word R, Hamind Q. GM-CSF, IL-5 and RANTES immunoreactivity and mRNA expression in chronic hyperplastic sinusitis with nasal polyposis. Clin Exp Allergy 1998; 28:1145–1152.

82. Varga EM, Jacobson ER, Masuyama K, et al. Inflammatory cell populations and cytokine mRNA expression in the nasal mucosa in aspirin-sensitive rhinitis. Eur Respir J 1999; 14:610–615.
83. Pods R, Ross D, van Hulst S, Rudack C, Maune S. RANTES, eotaxin and eotaxin-2 expression and production in patients with aspirin triad. Allergy 2003; 58(11): 1165–1170.
84. Bachert C, Gevaert P, van Cauwenberge P. Nasal polyposis – a new concept on the formation of polyps. ACI Int 1999; 11:130–135.
85. Kowalski ML, Grzegorczyk J, Pawliczak R, Kornatowski T, Wagrowska-Danilewicz M, Danilewicz M. Decreased apoptosis and distinct profile of infiltrating cells in the nasal polyps of patients with aspirin hypersensitivity. Allergy 2002; 57:493–500.
86. Kowalski ML, Lewandowska-Polak A, Wozniak J, et al. Association of stem cell factor expression in nasal polyp epithelial cells with aspirin sensitivity and asthma. Allergy 2005; 60:631–637.
87. Otsuka H, Kusumi T, Kanai S, Koyama M, Kuno Y, Takizawa R. Stem cell factor mRNA expression and production in human nasal epithelial cells: contribution to the accumulation of mast cells in the nasal epithelium of allergy. J Allergy Clin Immunol 1998; 102:757–764.
88. Hamilos DL, Leung DYM, Wood R, et al. Evidence for distinct cytokine expression in allergic versus nonallergic chronic sinusitis. J Allergy Clin Immunol 1995; 96:537–544.
89. Bachert C, Wagenmann M, Hauser U, Rudack C. IL-5 synthesis is upregulated in human nasal polyp tissue. J Allergy Clin Immunol 1997; 99:837–842.
90. Conlon K, Osborne J, Morimoto C, Ortaldo J, Young H. Comparison of lymphokine secretion and mRNA expression in the CD45RA+ and CD45RO+ subsets of human peripheral blood CD4+ and CD8+ lymphocytes. Eur J Immunol 1995; 25:644–648.
91. Picado C, Bioque G, Roca-Ferrer J, et al. Related nuclear factor-kappaB activity is down-regulated in nasal polyps from aspirin-sensitive asthmatics. Allergy 2003; 58(2):122–126.
92. Pujols L, Mullol J, Alobid I, Roca-Ferrer J, Xaubet A, Picado C. Related articles, links dynamics of COX-2 in nasal mucosa and nasal polyps from aspirin-tolerant and aspirin-intolerant patients with asthma. J Allergy Clin Immunol 2004; 114(4):814–819.
93. Smith CM, Hawksworth RJ, Thien FC, Christie PE, Lee TH. Urinary leukotriene E4 in bronchial asthma. Eur Respir J 1992; 5(6):693–699.
94. Kumlin M, Dahlen B, Bjorck T, Zetterstrom O, Granstrom E, Dahlen SE. Urinary excretion of leukotriene E4 and 11-dehydro-thromboxane B2 in response to bronchial provocations with allergen, aspirin, leukotriene D4, and histamine in asthmatics. Am Rev Respir Dis 1992; 146(1):96–103.
95. Sladek K, Dworski R, Soja J, et al. Eicosanoids in bronchoalveolar lavage fluid of aspirin-intolerant patients with asthma after aspirin challenge. Am J Respir Crit Care Med 1994; 149(4 Pt 1):940–946.
96. Szczeklik A, Sladek K, Dworski R, et al. Bronchial aspirin challenge causes specific eicosanoid response in aspirin-sensitive asthmatics. Am J Respir Crit Care Med 1996; 154(6 Pt 1):1608–1614.
97. Cowburn AS, Sladek K, Soja J, et al. Overexpression of leukotriene C4 synthase in bronchial biopsies from patients with aspirin-intolerant asthma. J Clin Invest 1998; 101(4):834–846.
98. Cai Y, Bjermer L, Halstensen TS. Related articles, links bronchial mast cells are the dominating LTC4S-expressing cells in aspirin-tolerant asthma. Am J Respir Cell Mol Biol 2003; 29(6):683–693 [Epub 2003 Jun 19].
99. Yamashita T, Tsuji H, Maeda N, Tomoda K, Kumazawa T. Etiology of nasal polyps associated with aspirin-sensitive asthma. Rhinol Suppl 1989; 8:15–24.
100. Jung TT, Juhn SK, Hwang D, Stewart R. Prostaglandins, leukotrienes, and other arachidonic acid metabolites in nasal polyps and nasal mucosa. Laryngoscope 1987; 97:184–189.
101. Perez-Novo CA, Watelet JB, Claeys C, Van Cauwenberge P, Bachert C. Prostaglandin, leukotriene, and lipoxin balance in chronic rhinosinusitis with and without nasal polyposis. J Allergy Clin Immunol 2005; 115(6):1189–1196.

102. Higashi N, Taniguchi M, Mita H, et al. Clinical features of asthmatic patients with increased urinary leukotriene E4 excretion (hyperleukotrienuria): involvement of chronic hyperplastic rhinosinusitis with nasal polyposis. J Allergy Clin Immunol 2004; 113(2):277–283.
103. Corrigan C, Mallett K, Ying S, et al. Expression of the cysteinyl leukotriene receptors cysLT(1) and cysLT(2) in aspirin-sensitive and aspirin-tolerant chronic rhinosinusitis. J Allergy Clin Immunol 2005; 115(2):316–322.
104. Arm JP, O'Hickey SP, Spur BW, Lee TH. Airway responsiveness to histamine and leukotriene E4 in subjects with aspirin-induced asthma. Am Rev Respir Dis 1989; 140(1):148–153. Cai Y, Bjermer L, Halstensen TS. Related articles, links bronchial mast cells are the dominating LTC4S-expressing cells in aspirin-tolerant asthma. Am J Respir Cell Mol Biol 2003; 29(6):683–693.
105. Dahlen SE, Niżankowska E, Dahlen B. The Swedish-Polish treatment study with the 5-lipoxygenase inhibitor Zileuton in aspirin-intolerant asthmatics. Am J Respir Crit Care Med 1995; 151:A376–A370.
106. Ragab S, Parikh A, Darby YC, Scadding GK. An open audit of montelukast, a leukotriene receptor antagonist, in nasal polyposis associated with asthma. Clin Exp Allergy 2001; 31:1385–1391.
107. Chiang N, Arita M, Serhan CN. Related articles, links anti-inflammatory circuitry: lipoxin, aspirin-triggered lipoxins and their receptor ALX. Prostaglandins Leukot Essent Fatty Acids 2005; 73(3–4):163–177.
108. Sanak M, Levy BD, Clish CB, et al. Aspirin-tolerant asthmatics generate more lipoxins than aspirin-intolerant asthmatics. Eur Respir J 2000; 16:44–49.
109. Sanak M, Szczeklik A. Related articles, links leukotriene C4 synthase polymorphism and aspirin-induced asthma. J Allergy Clin Immunol 2001; 107(3):561–562.
110. Choi JH, Park HS, Oh HB, et al. Related articles, links leukotriene-related gene polymorphisms in ASA-intolerant asthma: an association with a haplotype of 5-lipoxygenase. Hum Genet 2004; 114(4):337–344.
111. Kim SH, Choi JH, Park HS, et al. Association of thromboxane A2 receptor gene polymorphism with the phenotype of acetyl salicylic acid-intolerant asthma. Clin Exp Allergy 2005; 35(5):585–590.
112. Jinnai N, Sakagami T, Sekigawa T, et al. Related articles, links polymorphisms in the prostaglandin E2 receptor subtype 2 gene confer susceptibility to aspirin-intolerant asthma: a candidate gene approach. Hum Mol Genet 2004; 13(24):3203–3217.
113. Sanak M, Simon HU, Szczeklik A. Related articles, links leukotriene C4 synthase promoter polymorphism and risk of aspirin-induced asthma. Lancet 1997; 350(9091): 1599–1600.
114. Kedda MA, Shi J, Duffy D, et al. Characterization of two polymorphisms in the leukotriene C4 synthase gene in an Australian population of subjects with mild, moderate, and severe asthma. J Allergy Clin Immunol 2004; 113(5):889–895.
115. Asano K, Shiomi T, Hasegawa N, et al. Leukotriene C4 synthase gene A(−444)C polymorphism and clinical response to a CYS-LT(1) antagonist, pranlukast, in Japanese patients with moderate asthma. Pharmacogenetics 2002; 12(7):565–570.
116. Choi JH, Lee KW, Oh HB, et al. Related articles, links HLA association in aspirin-intolerant asthma: DPB1∗0301 as a strong marker in a Korean population. J Allergy Clin Immunol 2004; 113(3):562–564.
117. Park HS, Kim SH, Sampson AP, Lee KW, Park CS. The HLA-DPB1∗0301 marker might predict the requirement for leukotriene receptor antagonist in patients with aspirin-intolerant asthma. J Allergy Clin Immunol 2004; 114(3):688–689.
118. Melillo G, Balzano G, Bianco S, et al. Oral and inhalation provocation tests for the diagnosis of aspirin-induced asthma. Allergy 2001; 56:899–911.
119. Stevenson DD. Approach to the patient with a history of adverse reactions to aspirin or NSAIDs: diagnosis and treatment [Review]. Allergy Asthma Proc 2000; 21(1):25–31.
120. Cormican LJ, Farooque S, Altmann DR, Lee TH. Improvements in an oral aspirin challenge protocol for the diagnosis of aspirin hypersensitivity. Clin Exp Allergy 2005; 35(6):717–722.

121. Stevenson DD, Simon RA, Mathison DA, Christiansen SC. Montelukast is only partially effective in inhibiting aspirin responses in aspirin-sensitive asthmatics. Ann Allergy Asthma Immunol 2000; 85(6 Pt 1):477–482.
122. Bianco SR, Robuschi M, Petrini G. Aspirin induced tolerance in aspirin asthma detected by a new challenge test. IRCS J Med Sci 1977; 5:129–136.
123. G Melillo et al. Dosimeter inhalation test with lysine acetylsalicylate for the detection of aspirin-induced asthma. Ann Allergy 1993; 71:61–65.
124. Dahlen B, Zettestrom D. Comparison of bronchial and peroral provocations with aspirin in aspirin-sensitive asthmatics. Eur Resp J 1990; 3:527–534.
125. Nizankowska E, Bestyska-Krypel A, Cmiel A, Szczeklik A. Oral and bronchial provocation tests with aspirin for diagnosis of aspirin-induced asthma. Eur Respir J 2000; 15:863–869.
126. Makowska J, Kowalski ML, Grzegorczyk J, et al. Mobilization of hemopoietic precursors in aspirin sensitive asthmatics following bronchial provocation with aspirin. In press.
127. Jang AS. Severe reaction to lysine aspirin. Allergy 2000; 55(6):1092–1093.
128. Lee DK, Haggart K, Lipworth BJ. Reproducibility of response to nasal lysine-aspirin challenge in patients with aspirin-induced asthma. Ann Allergy Asthma Immunol 2004; 93(2):185–188.
129. Milewski M, Mastalerz L, Nizankowska E, Szczeklik A. Nasal provocation test with lysine-aspirin for diagnosis of aspirin-sensitive asthma. J Allergy Clin Immunol 1998; 101(5):581–586.
130. Alonso-Llamazares A, Martinez-Cocera C, Dominguez-Ortega J, Robledo-Echarren T, Cimarra-Alvarez M, Mesa del Castillo M. Nasal provocation test (NPT) with aspirin: a sensitive and safe method to diagnose aspirin-induced asthma (AIA). Allergy 2002; 57(7):632–635.
131. Casadevall J, Ventura PJ, Mullol J, Picado C. Intranasal challenge with aspirin in the diagnosis of aspirin intolerant asthma: evaluation of nasal response by acoustic rhinometry. Thorax 2000; 55(11):921–924.
132. Okuda Y, Hattori H, Takashima T, et al. Basophil histamine release by platelet-activating factor in aspirin-sensitive subjects with asthma. J Allergy Clin Immunol 1990; 86(4 Pt 1):548–553.
133. Lebel B, Messaad D, Kvedariene V, Rongier M, Bousquet J, Demoly P. Related articles, links cysteinyl-leukotriene release test (CAST) in the diagnosis of immediate drug reactions. Allergy 2001; 56(7):688–692.
134. Demoly P, Lebel B, Messaad D, et al. Related articles, links predictive capacity of histamine release for the diagnosis of drug allergy. Allergy 1999; 54(5):500–506.
135. Czech W, Schopf E, Kapp A. Release of sulfidoleukotrienes in vitro: its relevance in the diagnosis of pseudoallergy to acetylsalicylic acid. Inflamm Res 1995; 44(7):291–295.
136. Mewes T, Riechelmann H, Klimek L. Increased in vitro cysteinyl leukotriene release from blood leukocytes in patients with asthma, nasal polyps, and aspirin intolerance. Allergy 1996; 51(7):506–510.
137. Celik G, Bavbek S, Misirligil Z, Melli M. Related articles, links release of cysteinyl leukotrienes with aspirin stimulation and the effect of prostaglandin E(2) on this release from peripheral blood leucocytes in aspirin-induced asthmatic patients. Clin Exp Allergy 2001; 31(10):1615–1622.
138. Abrahamsen O, Haas H, Schreiber J, Schlaak M. Differential mediator release from basophils of allergic and non-allergic asthmatic patients after stimulation with anti-IgE and C5a. Clin Exp Allergy 2001; 31(3):368–378.
139. May A, Weber A, Gall H, Kaufmann R, Zollner TM. Related articles, links means of increasing sensitivity of an in vitro diagnostic test for aspirin intolerance. Clin Exp Allergy 1999; 29(10):1402–1411.
140. Sanz ML, Gamboa P, de Weck AL. Related Articles, Links A new combined test with flowcytometric basophil activation and determination of sulfidoleukotrienes is useful for in vitro diagnosis of hypersensitivity to aspirin and other nonsteroidal anti-inflammatory drugs. Int Arch Allergy Immunol 2005; 136(1):58–72.

141. Pierzchalska M, Mastalerz L, Sanak M, Zazula M, Szczeklik A. A moderate and unspecific release of cysteinyl leukotrienes by aspirin from peripheral blood leucocytes precludes its value for aspirin sensitivity testing in asthma. J Clin Exp Allergy 2000; 30:1785–1791.

142. Gamboa P, Sanz ML, Caballero MR, et al. The flow-cytometric determination of basophil activation induced by aspirin and other non-steroidal anti-inflammatory drugs (NSAIDs) is useful for in vitro diagnosis of the NSAID hypersensitivity syndrome. Clin Exp Allergy 2004; 34(9):1448–1457.

143. Settipane RA, Stevenson DD. Cross sensitivity with acetaminophen in aspirin-sensitive subjects with asthma. J Allergy Clin Immunol 1989; 84(1):26–33.

144. Bavbek S, Celik G, Ozer F, Mungan D, Misirligil Z. Safety of selective COX-2 inhibitors in aspirin/nonsteroidal anti-inflammatory drug-intolerant patients: comparison of nimesulide, meloxicam, and rofecoxib. J Asthma 2004; 41(1):67–75.

145. Quaratino D, Romano A, Di Fonso M, et al. Tolerability of meloxicam in patients with histories of adverse reactions to nonsteroidal anti-inflammatory drugs. Ann Allergy Asthma Immunol 2000; 84(6):613–617.

146. Kosnik M, Music E, Matjaz F, Suskovic S. Relative safety of meloxicam in NSAID-intolerant patients. Allergy 1998; 53(12):1231–1233.

147. Dahlen B, Szczeklik A, Murray JJ. Celecoxib in patients with asthma and aspirin intolerance. The Celecoxib in Aspirin-Intolerant Asthma Study Group. N Engl J Med 2001; 344(2):142.

148. Szczeklik A, Nizankowska E, Bochenek G, Nagraba K, Mejza F, Swierczynska M. Safety of a specific COX-2 inhibitor in aspirin-induced asthma. Clin Exp Allergy 2001; 31(2):219–225.

149. Woessner KM, Simon RA, Stevenson DD. Safety of high-dose rofecoxib in patients with aspirin-exacerbated respiratory disease. Ann Allergy Asthma Immunol 2004; 93(4):339–344.

150. Nussmeier NA, Whelton AA, Brown MT, et al. Complications of the COX-2 inhibitors parecoxib and valdecoxib after cardiac surgery. N Engl J Med 2005; 352(11): 1081–1091.

151. Johnsen SP, Larsson H, Tarone RE, et al. Risk of hospitalization for myocardial infarction among users of rofecoxib, celecoxib, and other NSAIDs: a population-based case-control study. Arch Intern Med 2005; 165(9):978–984.

152. Kowalski ML, Makowska J. Use of non steroidal anti-inflammatory drugs in patients with aspirin-hypersensitivity: safety of cyclooxygenase-2 inhibitors treatments. Resp Med. In press.

153. Fokkens W, Lund V, Bachert C, et al. EAACI position paper on rhinosinusitis and nasal polyps executive summary. Allergy 2005; 60(5):583–601.

154. McFadden EA, Woodson BT, Fink JN, Toohill RJ. Surgical treatment of aspirin triad sinusitis. Am J Rhinol 1997; 11(4):263–270.

155. Amar YG, Frenkiel S, Sobol SE. Related articles, links outcome analysis of endoscopic sinus surgery for chronic sinusitis in patients having Samter's triad. J Otolaryngol 2000; 29(1):7–12.

156. Batra PS, Kern RC, Tripathi A, et al. Outcome analysis of endoscopic sinus surgery in patients with nasal polyps and asthma. Laryngoscope 2003; 113(10):1703–1706.

157. Nakamura H, Kawasaki M, Higuchi Y, Takahashi S. Effects of sinus surgery on asthma in aspirin triad patients. Acta Otolaryngol 1999; 119(5):592–598.

158. Dahlen SE, Malmstrom K, Nizankowska E, et al. Improvement of aspirin-intolerant asthma by montelukast, a leukotriene antagonist: a randomized, double-blind, placebo-controlled trial. Am J Respir Crit Care Med 2002; 165(1):9–14.

159. Dahlen B, Nizankowska E, Szczeklik A, et al. Benefits from adding the 5-lipoxygenase inhibitor zileuton to conventional therapy in aspirin-intolerant asthmatics. Am J Respir Crit Care Med 1998; 157(4 Pt 1):1187–1194.

160. Mastalerz L, Nizankowska E, Sanak M, et al. Related articles, links clinical and genetic features underlying the response of patients with bronchial asthma to treatment with a leukotriene receptor antagonist. Eur J Clin Invest 2002; 32(12):949–955.

161. Pleskow WW, Stevenson DD, Mathison DA, Simon RA, Schatz M, Zeiger RS. Aspirin desensitization in aspirin-sensitive asthmatic patients: clinical manifestations and characterization of the refractory period. J Allergy Clin Immunol 1982; 69(1 Pt 1):11–19.

162. Szmidt M, Grzelewska-Rzymowska I, Kowalski ML, Rozniecki J. Tolerance to acetylsalicylic acid (ASA) induced in ASA-sensitive asthmatics does not depend on initial adverse reaction. Allergy 1987; 42(3):182–185.

163. Kowalski ML, Grzelewska-Rzymowska I, Rozniecki J, Szmidt M. Aspirin tolerance induced in aspirin-sensitive asthmatics. Allergy 1984; 39(3):171–178.

164. Berges-Gimeno MP, Simon RA, Stevenson DD. Early effects of aspirin desensitization treatment in asthmatic patients with aspirin-exacerbated respiratory disease. Ann Allergy Asthma Immunol 2003; 90(3):338–341.

165. Stevenson DD, Pleskow WW, Simon RA, et al. Aspirin-sensitive rhinosinusitis asthma: a double-blind crossover study of treatment with aspirin. J Allergy Clin Immunol 1984; 73(4):500–507.

166. Stevenson DD. Aspirin desensitization in patients with AERD [Review]. Clin Rev Allergy Immunol 2003; 24(2):159–168.

167. Sweet JA, Stevenson DD, Simon RA, Marhison DA. Long term effects of aspirin desensitization treatment for aspirin sensitive rhinosinusitis asthma. J Allergy Clin Immunol 1990; 86:59–65.

168. Berges-Gimeno MP, Simon RA, Stevenson DD. Related articles, links long-term treatment with aspirin desensitization in asthmatic patients with aspirin-exacerbated respiratory disease. J Allergy Clin Immunol 2003; 111(1):180–186.

169. Stevenson DD, Hankammer MA, Mathison DA. Long term ASA desensitization-treatment of aspirin sensitive asthmatic patients: clinical outcome studies. J Allergy Clin Immunol 1996; 98:751–758.

170. Gosepath J, Schafer D, Mann WJ. Aspirin sensitivity: long term follow-up after up to 3 years of adaptive desensitization using a maintenance dose of 100 mg of aspirin a day. Laryngorhinootologie 2002; 81(10):732–738.

171. Kowalski ML, Grzelewska-Rzymowska I, Szmidt M, Rozniecki J. Clinical efficacy of aspirin in "desensitized" aspirin-sensitive asthmatics. Eur J Respir Dis 1986; 69(4): 219–225.

172. Kowalski ML. Management of aspirin-sensitive rhinosinusitis-asthma syndrome: what role for aspirin desensitization? Allergy Proc 1992; 13(4):175–184.

173. Gollapudi RR, Teirstein PS, Stevenson DD, Simon RA. Related articles, links aspirin sensitivity: implications for patients with coronary artery disease. JAMA 2004; 292(24): 3017–3023.

174. Patriarca G, Bollioni P, Nucera E, et al. Intranasal treatment with lysine actylsalicylate in patients with nasal polyposis. Ann Allergy 1991; 67:588–591.

175. Scadding GK, Hassab M, Darby YC, et al. Intranasal lysine aspirin in recurrent nasal polyposis. Clin Otolaryngol Allied Sci 1995; 20(6):561–563.

176. Parikh AA, Scadding GK. Intranasal lysine-aspirin in aspirin-sensitive nasal polyposis: a controlled trial. Laryngoscope 2005; 115(8):1385–1390.

10 Viral and Bacterial Rhinitis

William J. Doyle
Department of Otolaryngology, University of Pittsburgh School of Medicine, and Department of Pediatric Otolaryngology, Children's Hospital of Pittsburgh, Pittsburgh, Pennsylvania, U.S.A.

Deborah A. Gentile
Department of Pediatric, Division of Allergy, Asthma, and Immunology, Allegheny General Hospital, Pittsburgh, Pennsylvania, U.S.A.

David P. Skoner
Department of Pediatrics, Drexel University College of Medicine, Philadelphia, Pennsylvania, and Division of Allergy, Asthma, and Immunology, Allegheny General Hospital, Pittsburgh, Pennsylvania, U.S.A.

"God heals and the doctor takes the fee"   B. Franklin, Poor Richard's Almanic

NOSOLOGY OF RHINITIS

"Hence the saying: If you know the enemy and know yourself, you need not fear the result of a hundred battles." Sun Tzu, *The Art of War*

Rhinitis, inflammation of the nasal mucosa, is a pathological condition[a] that is often associated with a constellation of symptoms (if identifiable only by self-assessment) and signs (if also identifiable by observer assessment) that we term the rhinitis symptom-sign complex (rSSC). In discussing rhinitis, it is important to identify the referenced disease condition as either that embodied by the Old French derivation, *desaise*[b] corresponding to the rSSC or the broader, more contemporary usage as pathology[c]. This distinction creates a nested definition, wherein the rSSC is a (presumably) sufficient but not sole marker of disease. Nonetheless, in the usual clinical setting, rhinitis diagnosis by an rSSC is common because patients present on that basis.

---

[a] Rhinitis (noun): Inflammation of the mucous membrane of the nose; also any of various conditions characterized by such inflammation. *Source*: Merriam-Webster's Medical Dictionary , 2002 Merriam-Webster, Inc.

[b] Disease (noun): from O.Fr. *desaise*, from *des*- "without, away" + *aise* "ease" ("discomfort"). Sense of "sickness, illness" first recorded 1393; the word was still used in its literal sense in the early 17c. *Source*: Online Etymology Dictionary. http://www.etymonline.com

[c] Disease (noun): A pathological condition of a body part, an organ, or a system resulting from various causes, such as infection, genetic defect, or environmental stress, and characterized by an identifiable group of signs or symptoms. *Source*: The American Heritage[R] Stedman's Medical Dictionary. Copyright© 2002, 2001, 1995 by Houghton Mifflin Company. Published by Houghton Mifflin Company.

Included in this definition of rhinitis is the regional area delimited by the "nasal mucosa." However, like a Mobius surface[d], the mucosa covering the nasal airway is continuous with that for the mucosa lining the paranasal sinuses, the nasopharynx, the Eustachian tubes, and the middle ears, among others, which makes boundary definition somewhat arbitrary. Boundaries can be assigned based on regional differences in subepithelial vascular anatomy and physiology wherein the mucosa lining the nasal airway and contained structures (e.g., turbinates and septum) is anatomically more complex than that of its extensions (e.g., the paranasal sinuses and middle ear) (1–5) and is capable of rapidly responding to environmental (e.g., cold air) and autonomic (e.g., nasal cycle) stimuli by fold changes in blood flow, relative thickness, and secretory capability (6–15). Incorporation of this regional distinction allows rhinitis to be defined as an inflammation of the mucosa covering the nasal airway and contained structures that may (*desaise*), but need not (disease), be accompanied by an rSSC.

Clinically, rhinitis diagnosed by the presence of an rSSC localizes pathology but does not guide treatment. There, it is well established that the components of the rSSC do not discriminate among the different causal etiologies [e.g., nasal allergy, cold air, and viral upper respiratory tract infection (vURI)] (16–19). For example, the etymology of the phrase "common cold" which is now recognized to be the rSSC of virus infection[e] derives from the similarity of that presentation to the rSSC associated with cold air exposures[f] (12,20,21). For this reason, it is common practice to precede the term "rhinitis" with an etiological modifier thereby supplementing the diagnostic information (e.g., allergic rhinitis, viral rhinitis, idiopathic rhinitis, vasomotor=neurogenic? rhinitis) (22). Other modifiers can be attached, which indicate seasonality (e.g., perennial) or the duration of the diagnosed condition (e.g., acute, recurrent, persistent, and chronic). However, the usefulness of some of these descriptors is compromised by informational redundancy (e.g., acute, viral rhinitis, or recurrent, seasonal allergic rhinitis); by default assignment to ambiguous categories reflecting mechanistic ignorance (e.g., idiopathic rhinitis); and by overreliance on the rSSC for defining presentations (Fig. 1).

The topic of this chapter is viral and bacterial rhinitis. From the above, we focus on the discussion on inflammation of the mucosa bounding the nasal airway caused by viral or bacterial infection of that mucosa. Consequently, we first provide a brief description of the relevant mucosal defense mechanisms since their activation is believed by many to be causally responsible for the rSSC (9,23–29).

---

[d] Mobius surface, named after the astronomer and mathematician August Ferdinand Möbius (1790–1868), is a nonorientable, boundariless surface typically illustrated in one dimension by a "Mobius strip."

[e] Common Cold (noun): an acute contagious disease of the upper respiratory tract that is marked by inflammation of the mucous membranes of the nose, throat, eyes, and Eustachian tubes with a watery then purulent discharge and is caused by any of several viruses. *Source*: Merriam-Webster's Medical Dictionary[c], 2002 Merriam-Webster, Inc.

[f] Cold (noun): from O.E. *cald* (Anglian), *ceald* (W. Saxon), from P.Gmc. *kaldaz*, possibly pp. adj. of *kal-/kol-*, from PIE base *gel-/gol-* "cold." Sense in *common cold* first recorded 1537 from symptoms resembling those of exposure to cold. *Source*: The American Heritage[B] Dictionary of Idioms by Christine Ammer. Copyright[c] 1997 by The Christine Ammer 1992 Trust. Published by Houghton Mifflin Company.

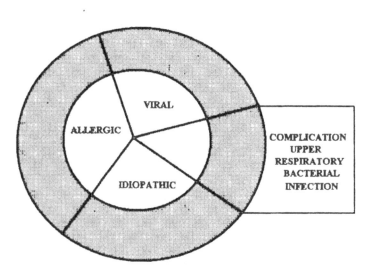

FIGURE 1 Partitioning by etiology of all nasal symptoms/sign complexes sufficient to be identified as rhinitis (note the absence of a segment defined by "bacterial").

NASAL MUCOSAL DEFENSE MECHANISMS

> *"... ensure that your whole host may withstand the brunt of the enemy's attack and remain unshaken—this is effected by maneuvers direct and indirect ..."*
>
> Sun Tzu, The Art of War

The nasal airway represents a portal of entry for environmental irritants, pollutants, allergens, bacteria, and viruses to the host's internal environment (17,30,31). Providentially, the nose is equipped with a series of successive barriers to prevent these inhalants from entering the nose (e.g., filtration by nares hairs, directed airflow to impact first upon and deposit materials on keratinized surfaces) and/or from coming into physical contact with the nasal mucosal epithelium (e.g., presence of a superficial mucous layer) (32,33). The mucous layer overlying the epithelial cells contains host-produced chemicals that: (i) physically bind and entrap inhaled particles, chemicals, and microorganisms; (ii) limit the free availability of nutrients required for bacterial metabolism (e.g., iron scavaging by lactoferrin); and (iii) exhibit nonspecific (e.g., defensins and lysozyme) and specific [e.g., secretory immunoglobulin A (sIgA)] antimicrobial properties (34–40). Like the river of Heraclitus[8], the mucous barrier is temporally dynamic yet functionally stable as the existing layer is propelled by ciliary beat to the nasopharynx for expectoration or swallowing, and replacement mucus is continuously produced by epithelial cells and glands (9,41–43). Alternatively, forcible prograde nasal expulsion of particle-laden mucus accompanies the "sneeze reflex," a rapid forced expiration through the nose initiated when certain irritants or other chemicals contact epithelial cells (32,44).

If these physical/temporal barriers are breached and an infectious agent makes physical contact with the cells of the nasal epithelium, a phylogenetically old, yet

---

[8] Heraclitus: Greek Philosopher (540 BCE–480 BCE) concerned with the dynamics of stasis and who is quoted as saying "Upon those who step into the same rivers different and ever different waters flow down."

functionally sophisticated "innate" immune response is activated to prevent colonization (for bacteria, molds, etc.) or infection (for all pathogens) and to limit and localize infection (45). There, germline-encoded, conserved pattern recognition molecules (PRRs) expressed on epithelial cells (and on other surveillance cells likely to encounter foreign proteins and chemicals) bind to conserved pathogen-associated molecular patterns (PAMPs) of bacteria, viruses and presumably other pathogens (46–50). This binding causes the cells to upregulate the synthesis and release of defensive proteins (e.g., ICAM as a decoy for rhinovirus attachment) and nonspecific antimicrobials (e.g., lysozyme, lactoferrin), to alter the function of transcellular ion pumps that indirectly control mucociliary transport, and to initiate the signaling pathways of the classic inflammatory cascade. These and other cell-specific changes facilitate the recruitment, localization, and activation of phagocytes that engulf and kill the invader to neutralize the threat (51).

While usually considered to be relatively nonspecific, there are a wide variety of host PRRs that can be secreted, expressed on the cell surface or resident in intracellular compartments, and a PAMP conserved within a certain class of pathogens (e.g., gram-positive organisms) can engage multiple PRRs (52). The specific location and number of PRRs bound by a PAMP yield a degree of host response specificity, for example, discrimination between intracellular and extracellular pathogens. Epithelial cells also continuously "sample" their internal environments and present the processed sample complexes on their surfaces to surveillance cells for threat evaluation. Complexes indicative of intracellular infection can bind to receptors on natural killer cells and activate synthesis cascades that cause death in the infected cell (53–56). Cellular lysis by this process is accompanied by the generation of "death" signals that upregulate the degree of immune surveillance, increase the synthesis of defense chemicals by adjacent epithelial cells, and initiate and reinforce the pathways for inflammation (57,58).

Engagement of the innate immune system also functions to activate and shape the adaptive immune response whose effector function to novel stimuli is typically delayed by four to seven days (54,59). There, the vascular and cellular effects of the inflammatory cascade allow antigen-presenting cells (e.g., macrophages and dendritic cells) greater access to the site of infection for environmental sampling by engulfment (59). This is followed by their subsequent migration to lymphoid centers (e.g., the adenoids) with surface presentation of sample complexes to resident T-lymphocytes (35,56,60). The nature of the presentation complex selects the type of adaptive response to be elicited (antibody or cytotoxic T-cell mediated) and the effector cell populations (B- or T-lymphocytes) to be expanded. Unlike the more general PRRs of the innate immune system, those of the adaptive immune system are tailored to a specific PAMP of the invader by clonal expansion of those lymphocyte populations that express molecular complexes with high binding affinities to the target PAMP.

The candidates for clonal expansion consist of millions of relatively small pools of lymphocytes, each derived from a single prelymphocyte that had undergone random, somatic gene rearrangements to yield a unique antigen receptor for environmental presentation. The expanded population of effector lymphocytes either migrates to the site of infection and directly kills infected cells (if T-cell mediated) or produces antibodies (if B-cell mediated) that are introduced into the circulation and then bind and neutralize toxins, bacterial attachment molecules, and viruses or mark the pathogen for host killing by other means (e.g., cytolysis secondary to complement fixation).

To appropriately coordinate the initiation, maintenance, and downregulation of these responses, a plethora of neuronal and biochemical signals is generated by each of the involved cell types (61–64). The interactions of these signals are highly complex with significant cross talk and feedback modulation (65,66). Of primary importance to illness expression and the risk for complications is the phase delay between signals responsible for tracking threat evaluation and those that initiate, maintain, and/or downregulate the appropriate responses. For example, premature downregulation of the defense responses predisposes to disseminating infection while delayed downregulation leads to complications attributable to persistent inflammation.

VIRAL RHINITIS

"In war, then, let your great object be victory, not lengthy campaigns."
                                              Sun Tzu, The Art of War

Epidemiology

By definition, viral rhinitis is an inflammation of the mucosa bounding the nasal airway caused by viral infection of that mucosa whose presentation may or may not include an rSSC. The incidence of viral rhinitis as estimated by counting the number of presentations of an acute, temporally limited rSSC is approximately two to four episodes per year in adults and four to ten episodes per year in children (67). By viral culture of recovered nasal secretions and/or nasal lavage fluids, these rSSC presentations were shown to be attributable to infection with any of a large number of viruses (e.g., more than 100 types for rhinovirus alone), the majority of which can be assigned to type variants of rhinovirus, influenza virus, respiratory syncytial virus, adenovirus, coxsackie virus, and parainfluenza virus (68). While the usual duration of the infection is not well defined for most viruses, the maximum duration of viral shedding for rhinovirus infection is approximately 20 days with a modal value of approximately five days (27,69). Thus, these infections of the nasal mucosa are acute and self-limited with no known example cases of chronic "carriage" in humans. Indeed, in clinical practice, the limited duration of an acute rSSC is the hallmark discriminating feature for a diagnosis of viral rhinitis (70).

For these reasons, viral rhinitis is not directly associated with mortal consequences and the magnitude and period of morbidity is limited. Despite this, the total yearly dollar expenditures by the U.S. population for palliative "treatment" of these infections are enormous and, more recently, large additional "hidden" costs associated with work absenteeism and decreased productivity were enumerated (71–73). Epidemiological and experimental studies show conclusively that virus infection of the nasal mucosa predisposes to secondary bacterial/viral infections of the mucosa lining the paranasal sinuses, the middle ears, and the lungs (74–82). These secondary presentations predominate in the very young, the elderly, and the immune-compromised patient, and the diagnosed conditions of sinusitis, otitis media, and pneumonia are associated with significant and prolonged periods of morbidity, with loss of function (e.g., hearing acuity), and, for pneumonia, with excess mortality (71). Also, there is a large body of work supporting a link between viral rhinitis and exacerbations of asthma (81,83–85). When considered to be complications of viral rhinitis, the diagnosis and treatment of these illnesses drive the total dollar costs to the U.S. population for viral rhinitis to the tens of billions of dollars.

Illness Susceptibility

Susceptibility to viral rhinitis and the magnitude and duration of the rSSC are variable in the population. An individual's risk for infection and illness depends both on past exposure history for similar viruses and on the ability of the innate and adaptive immune systems to upregulate, coordinate, and appropriately downregulate the requisite responses. The effect of past exposures depends on "recall immunity" wherein viruses previously presented to the adaptive immune system establish circulating levels of specific antibodies that bind virus to prevent and/or limit infection and long-lived "memory" T-cells that recognize a characteristic PAMP of the virus and quickly upregulate adaptive immunity to abort the infection. In studies on humans, high serum levels of virus-specific IgG antibodies or high nasal levels of virus-specific sIgA antibodies were shown to protect from detectable reinfection with an antigenically identical virus and to lessen the rSSC in those who become infected (78,86–90). Limited protection may also be afforded by previous exposure(s) to antigenetically related viruses (e.g., rhinoviruses within either of the two main classes for receptor binding) (91). Data from our laboratories for human volunteers with elevated serum homotypic antibody titers support antibody-mediated protection from infection but a cell-mediated immune limitation on virus shedding (87,89,90).

The other risk-limiting factor for infection and illness is usually referred to as "immunocompetence," a broad category that encompasses all moderating influences on the threat-appropriate host defense response. Such influences include not only the predictable effects of age (immune immaturity in infants and immune senescence in the elderly), socioeconomic status (immune fatigue?), and nutritional adequacy (92), but also genetic factors such as the haplotype for the human leukocyte antigens (codes for components of the antigen presentation complex) and other genotypes that influence the production of signaling molecules (e.g., cytokines) (93,94), psychosocial characteristics (e.g., perceived stress level, degree of social supports, and personality markers) (95–97), and the type of adaptive immune conditioning imposed by exposures to infectious agents during infancy (98). While much of the earlier work on these factors was done in animals, a body of literature is developing on the role they play in moderating viral rhinitis and its complications in humans. For example, in adult volunteers experimentally exposed to influenza, rhinovirus, or respiratory syncytial virus, we reported that chronic stress, less diverse social networks, and low levels of positive emotional style all predicted an increased probability of developing illness in infected persons (95–97). Analyses done to test hypothesized mediational pathways for the observed psychosocial–somatic interaction ruled out a number of candidates, though many exerted independent effects (e.g., cortisol, epinephrine and norepinephrine, cigarettes/day, alcoholic drinks/day, and zinc and vitamin C intake), but supported linkage mediation by interleukin (IL)-6 (99).

Transmission

Virus infection of nasal epithelial cells is associated with internalization of the viral genome, which hijacks the cell's replication/transcription/translation machinery for replication of the viral genomic sequence and synthesis of viral proteins. The proteins and genome are assembled as virons and then released (shed) to the extracellular environment during host cell lyses (e.g., influenza) or by other mechanisms (e.g., exocytosis). This process geometrically increases the number of infectious virons available for secondary infection of adjacent cells and for transmission to the host's external environment by sneezing, coughing (aerosolized particle dispersion), or other means.

Interpersonal spread of these viruses[h] is usually by contact transfer of the infectious virons between an infected person and a potentially susceptible individual. This can occur by aerosolized spray-recipient transfers, by aerosolized spray-object-recipient transfers, by nasal–hand-recipient transfers, by nasal–hand-object-recipient transfers, or by other routes (100). A required act in this process is the within recipient transfer of virons from keratinized epithelial surfaces (e.g., hand) or other contact surfaces to the nasal mucosa (101). Experimental observations suggest that this frequently occurs during hand-nasal or hand-ocular contacts, a route that explains the documented prophylactic efficacy of frequent hand washing (102,103).

Contagious spread of viral rhinitis within a population is facilitated by the reluctance or inability of persons with an rSSC to absent themselves from social intercourse[i] and by the decoupling of infection (with viral shedding) from the temporal and/or magnitude expression of the rSSC (104,105). In the former situation, contact avoidance may not be feasible (e.g., required parental involvement with young infants), while in the latter, viral shedding precedes and/or continues after the rSSC (69,70) and/or the rSSC is of such limited magnitude that the typical alert signals for contact avoidance are masked (104,105). These factors underlie current theories to explain the patterned seasonality for viral rhinitis where prevalence is much higher in the winter months as compared to the summer months (106,107). There, it is argued that colder temperatures favor restricted individual activities, more confined social spaces, and more extensive and intimate interpersonal contacts (107).

INFECTION AND THE rSSC

Studies in adult volunteers experimentally exposed to rhinovirus, influenza virus, and respiratory syncytial virus show that despite evidence of viral replication by shedding, an accompanying rSSC is observed in only about 50% of the subjects (104). When present, rSSC expression is phase delayed relative to infectious exposure by about two days for rhinovirus, by three days for influenza virus, and by as long as seven days for RSV, though the typical "time to resolution" of the rSSC is approximately four to ten days for all of these viruses (23). With the exceptions of nonrequisite but diagnostic (for influenza?) signs/symptoms of fever

---

[h] Interpersonal transfer of the "common cold" was discussed more than 200 years ago by Benjamin Franklin (1706–1790), American printer, publisher, philosopher, scientist, inventor, and diplomat who pointed out that colds are "caught" from other people, not from exposure to a cold environment.

[i] "The Masque of the Red Death," a short story written by Edgar Allan Poe in 1842 that presages the potentially devastating consequences of a temporal disjunction between "infection" and "illness signaling." Set during a time of ravaging pestilence—the Red Death—a wealthy prince, Prospero, isolates himself and his favorites within a fortress to protect them from contact with the ill of the countryside. "The scarlet stains upon the body and especially upon the face of the victim were the pest ban, which shut him out from the aid and from the sympathy of his fellow-men. And the whole seizure, progress and termination of the disease, were the incidents of half an hour." After six months of revelry, Prospero realizes to his horror that one of his favorites "carried" the Red Death and "...now was acknowledged the presence of the Red Death. He had come like a thief in the night. And one by one dropped the revellers in the blood-bedewed halls of their revel, and died each in the despairing posture of his fall." *Source*: http://bau2.uibk.ac.at/sg/poe/works/reddeath.html

and chills, and the nonrequisite/nondiagnostic symptoms of muscle and joint "aches," the components of the rSSC for these viruses are similar and include sneezing, nasal blockage (congestion), runny nose (rhinorrhea), sore throat, and cough. Typically, patients make a self-diagnosis of a "common cold" if their rSSC is of short duration and without fever, chills, and body aches or a "flu" if the rSSC is of longer duration and/or those symptoms/signs are included.

The rSSC components directly relate to the underlying mucosal changes effected by the inflammatory cascade of the innate and adaptive immune responses (41,108). These include nasal epithelial sensitization for low threshold activation of the "sneeze reflex"; nasopharyngeal sensitization to upregulate expectoration by coughing; intercellular tight juncture remodeling with upregulated epithelial mucin production to allow subepithelial fluids to wash the surface of the mucosa-environment boundary while maintaining a functional mucous barrier; and altered regulation of the subepithelial vasculature to promote venous pooling that in turn drives mucosal swelling and an accompanying decrease in nasal airway cross section.

A temporal decoupling of nasal infection and the rSSC was demonstrated for viral rhinitis in experimental studies where virus shedding is observed both before and after the rSSC (69). However, the possibility of decoupling by suppression of rSSC magnitude remains an open question. While viral shedding in the absence of an rSSC is well established, documentation that the nasal mucosa is the source of the shed viruses (i.e., pathology) has not been confirmed (109). Experimental work with rhinovirus shows that cells in the adenoid tissue may be the first to be infected after virus deposition on the nasal mucosa by ocular and nasal routes which is then followed by secondary anterior spread of infection to the nasal mucosa (110,111). Because detection of shedding in asymptomatic persons is usually done by assay of nasal wash fluids and/or expelled secretions (that have come into contact with the adenoid tissues), it is possible that viral recovery does not necessarily reflect infection of the nasal mucosa and consequently is neither a sole nor sufficient marker of viral rhinitis as defined by the adopted nosology.

This possibility is reinforced by the above discussed relationship between the rSSC and pathological changes in the mucosa attributable to the consequences of virus infection. There, we can question if viral rhinitis in the absence of an rSSC is a true disease entity, or, if such presentations are better described as viral adenititis (111). We suggest that until these issues are resolved, the more inclusive term, vURI, be used to describe all cases where virus is recovered from nasal secretions/washings and that "viral rhinitis" be reserved for those infections with either an expressed rSSC or documented nasal mucosal pathology.

SIGNALING PATHWAYS FOR RESPONSE REGULATION

As can be appreciated from the above overview, the signal-response pathways that control the host response to virus infection of the nasal mucosa are quite complex and, for this reason, poorly understood. While not representative of the degree of physiological integration, the involved pathways can be grouped into those associated with viral detection, upregulation of defense responses, threat monitoring and inflammatory downregulation, into those that involve primarily biochemical event sequences (e.g., the cytokine network), and those that include a neural component (e.g., neurogenic inflammation). For discussion, we make a distinction between "signals" that inform the global system with respect to nodal status and "effectors" that translate the nodal value to a recognizable component of the rSSC (Fig. 2).

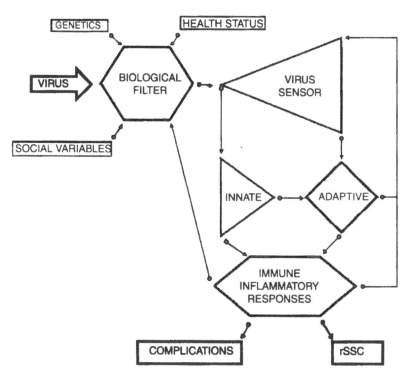

FIGURE 2 Hypothetical network pathway for the generation of the rSSC and development of complications after exposure to a virus capable of infecting the nasal mucosa.

Because of similarities in the rSSC across etiologies, early work on pathway signaling in viral rhinitis focused on the known chemical effectors of the allergic rSSC. In those studies, a chemical was considered to be a candidate effector if its concentration in nasal secretions varied systematically over the course of natural or experimental viral rhinitis and if direct application of the chemical to the nasal mucosa provoked a physiological response consistent with the expected rSSC (112,113). Previously, we argued that the first of these criteria is too strict given the possibility for significant dilution of highly potent, low concentration chemicals with serum transudates and the few compartments sampled for effector chemicals (e.g., typically limited to mucosal surface). Therefore, we modified the first criteria to include those host-derived chemicals whose expected physiological expressions (based on nasal exposure studies) are modified by treatment of viral rhinitis with effector-specific antagonists (23).

In that regard, components of the rSSC can be elicited by nasal mucosal challenge with histamine, bradykinin, platelet activating factor, and members of the prostaglandin (Pg) and leukotriene families (114). There is also evidence that some of these host-derived chemicals activate neurogenic inflammation as well as other neural reflex pathways (e.g., histamine and sneezing) (6). While the responses provoked by these effectors exhibit a high degree of overlap (e.g., secretion production and nasal congestion), the elements of the rSSC show some degree of effector specificity as, for example, sneezing with histamine, sinus pain with bradykinin, cough with PgD2, and nasal decongestion with PgF2-ά (114).

Assays of nasal wash fluids recovered from persons with viral rhinitis for these potential effector chemicals documented consistent patterning only for bradykinin production, but assay of other compartments (e.g., urine for histamine metabolites) and modulation of appropriate rSSC components by specific viral rhinitis "treatments" support an effector role for histamine and certain members of the prostaglandin and leukotriene families, as well as a contribution of neural circuit activation (e.g., parasympathetic induction of mucous secretion and decreased histamine-provoked effects after capsaicin pretreatment) (23,112,113).

More recently, the focus of studies exploring pathway mediation has shifted to the cytokines and chemokines, a family of host-derived chemicals that orchestrate and coordinate the immune/inflammatory responses (23,63–65). Because these chemicals are involved in cell–cell communication, they represent signals in our classification. So, their activity cannot be easily assessed by direct application to the nasal mucosa because they have a short half-life, are highly potent at low molar concentrations and, with few exceptions (e.g., INF which upregulates mucosal defense and elicits select components of the rSSC when topically applied), the elicited response is context dependent (e.g., requires a specific system state for downstream effects). Nonetheless, there is a large literature documenting: (i) the elaboration of biologically active cytokines and other intercellular signaling chemicals including IL-1β, tumor necrosis factor (TNF)-α, IL-6, IL-8, and NO by epithelial cells, leukocytes and other cell populations after virus infection or exposure to cytokine stimuli (115), (ii) patterned expression of these chemicals in nasal secretions recovered from humans with viral rhinitis (28,98,116–118), and (iii) modulation of the local expression for some of these chemicals (e.g., IL-6, but not IL-8) by antiviral treatments and by psychosocial factors that affect the rSSC (23,118).

In perhaps the most inclusive study of these signaling chemicals in viral rhinitis, Hayden et al. measured the nasal lavage and blood levels of IL-1β, IL-2, IL-6, IL-8, INF-α, TGF-β, and TNF-α in 19 volunteers over the course of an experimental influenza infection (28). They reported that nasal IL-6 and INF-α peaked early (day two) and correlated directly with viral titers, temperature, mucous production, and symptom scores; TNF-α peaked later when viral titer was dropping (day 4), and IL-8 peaked late (days 4–6) and correlated only with lower respiratory symptoms. No infection-related changes in nasal lavage IL-1β, IL-2, or TGF-β levels were observed. In a comparative study of rhinovirus, influenza A virus, and respiratory syncytial virus infection, we reported a similar sequential pattern for IL-1, IL-6, IL-8 and IL-10, with IL-1 and IL-6 tracking the rSSC of all viruses despite the large differences among viruses in the postexposure times to maximum rSSC (23).

Relating these and other observations to the outlined, simple functional description of pathway signaling, a parsimonious, but hypothetical, interpretation of these data is that INF-α signals viral detection, IL-1 and IL-6 signal an upregulation of the inflammatory response, TNF-α signals an upregulation of antiviral activity, IL-8 signals inflammatory downregulation and IL-10 signals mucosal healing processes (Fig. 3). Future research is needed to test the validity of this broad outline and, if valid, to characterize the branched pathways activated by each of these primary chemical signals that culminate in a coordinated antiviral response.

Treatment

The rSSC is the entity referenced by the general population in their demand for a "cure for the common cold" because viral rhinitis in the absence of an rSSC is not self-assessable. Existing common cold and flu "treatments" include the folk

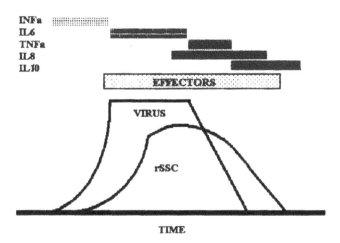

FIGURE 3 Suggested temporal relationships between viral load, cytokine signals, intermediate effectors, and the magnitude of the rhinitis symptom sign complex for a hypothetical viral rhinitis episode.

admonitions to "feed a cold, starve a fever," "eat your chicken soup" and "stay warm and drink plenty of fluids," herbal and nutritional supplements (e.g., echinacea, zinc, vitamin C, and selenium), as well as single component (e.g., antihistamine) and multi-ingredient (e.g., antihistamine, decongestant, anti-inflammatory, and antiviral) pharmaceutical formulations that target effector chemicals (22,102,119). However, with the exception of the multi-ingredient formulations (that include an antiviral), demonstrable efficacy with respect to the global rSSC is lacking, but, for some treatments, modulation of select rSSC components was observed (26). This treatment limitation is expected given the large number of effector chemicals, the relatively few effector-specific responses, and the redundancy of effectors for a given response (see above).

Interestingly, treatment studies with an effective antiviral (i.e., documented decrease in viral shedding) consistently report an earlier resolution of the rSSC by about one day for both influenza and rhinovirus infection when compared to placebo treatment (87,120,121). Again, this is expected because the maximum impact of even highly effective treatments is expected to be low given the typically short interval between self-assessment of rSSC presence (a signal indicating need for treatment) and the self-resolution of that complex (105). This maximum efficacy is expected to be even less in "real world" applications given that the initiation of some of these treatments will be delayed by the need for physician approval and pharmacist release of the "prescribed" treatment.

Accepting the process of interpersonal virus transmission described above, treating or curing the rSSC without concomitantly decreasing viral replication may be detrimental to the general population and to the individual. For example, such treatments mask the markers of infectious status that usually limit an infected individual's willingness to participate in social intercourse and that identify the infected individual as a contact "risk." If widely adopted, such "cures" can be expected to increase the prevalence of the infection and to drive increases in the more serious complications of the subclinical epidemic. Also, it is expected that highly effective rSSC treatments will need to target upstream events (e.g., cytokine) that are biological signals for downstream activation of effector pathways. Because of our poor understanding regarding the specifics of this signaling network, such interventions are unwise and may lead to concomitant downregulation of host defense allowing for dissemination of virus and/or synergistic bacterial pathogens to adjacent anatomical compartments (e.g., lungs, sinuses, and middle ear) (105).

A number of investigators have expressed optimism that viral rhinitis can be prevented by vaccination and/or antiviral prophylaxis (122). However, the large number of rhinovirus serotypes, the yearly changes in circulating influenza subtype within a population, and the poor immune memory response to respiratory syncytial virus infection as well as the significant risks associated with antiviral vaccination dampen our enthusiasm for that option. Prophylactic antiviral treatment (e.g., capsid-binding agents and infusion of monoclonal antibodies) over a viral season may endanger the health of treated patients (as experience with long-term use of these potent chemicals is limited) and may represent a societal hazard by selecting for resistant virus strains and, perhaps of greater concern, virus strains with altered infectious and/or trophic properties. Application of these strategies should remain limited to those "at risk" for serious complications of vURIs (the young, elderly, and immunocompromised).

Perhaps the best treatment option is to recognize the population as the infected organism and to educate its members regarding their individual obligations to actively participate in preventing infectious dissemination. While contrary to contemporary lifestyles, routine adoption of simple hygienic practices (e.g., frequent hand washing), absenting oneself and especially one's children from social interactions during a concurrent rSSC, and palliative treatment for discomforts can be expected to promote rapid resolution of an infection in that organism.

BACTERIAL RHINITIS

> *"The general, unable to control his irritation, will launch his men to the assault like swarming ants..."*
>
> Sun Tzu, *The Art of War*

With, perhaps the exception of obligate intracellular bacteria (e.g., Chlamydia), there is little direct evidence supporting bacterial colonization or infection of the normal nasal mucosa (123–126). There, the requisite bacteria-epithelial cell attachment for "infection" is made difficult by the temporal–physical barrier of the overlying mucus and its potent antibacterial properties (secondary bacterial infection of a pathological nasal mucosa, rhinitis caused by toxin exposure, etc., is excluded from our definition of bacterial rhinitis by reference to primacy of etiology). Nasal culture of bacterial pathogens typical of the nasopharyngeal environment can be explained by contamination from adjacent compartments (nasopharynx and sinuses) during sample collection, and pathogen identification by polymerase chain reaction (PCR) amplification of nasal mucosal biopsies does not fulfill Koch's postulate[j] for disease causation (127–131). The latter is especially true when the specific biological compartment sampled for PCR amplification is

---

[j]Koch's postulate, named after the German physician, Robert Koch (1843–1910), Nobel Laureate and discoverer of the cause of tuberculosis holds two premises: 1) that an organism which is said to cause a disease must be found in every case of that disease, 2) that the organism must be isolated in the laboratory, injected into a healthy animal, cause illness and then be re-isolated from that animal.

unknown (e.g., epithelium, submucosa, and intracellular environment) since phagocytes containing engulfed pathogens are free to migrate throughout the contiguous mucosa of the upper respiratory tract and detection of bacteria within a phagocyte (as is possible with PCR) does not evidence engulfment at that site (60,132). Adopting our defined nosology, bacterial rhinitis caused by typical upper respiratory pathogens, if it exists, is a rare entity with presentations limited to the severely immune compromised patient (127,130).

Bacterial rhinitis is better described as rhinitis secondary to acute bacterial infection of the mucosa lining adjacent compartments (18,133,134). The most well-developed mechanistic description supporting this nosology is sinusitis complicated by rhinitis. There, pathogens colonizing the nasospharynx are freed from local sequestration by a precipitating event, most typically, a viral upper respiratory infection. By one of several possible mechanisms, the bacterial pathogens gain access to the paranasal sinuses where they establish infectious colonization, i.e., bacterial sinusitis. This initiates the typical immune/inflammatory responses including the production and release of proinflammatory effector chemicals and activation of neural reflex circuits (36,41). The provoked inflammation does not localize to the sinus mucosa but extends to the contiguous mucosa of the nasal airway by neurogenic inflammation (135). Moreover, the major route for clearance of the produced inflammatory chemicals and detritus (e.g., pus) is by way of the sinus osteum to the nasal mucosa and then to the pharynx where they are expectorated or swallowed (5,32). Direct mucosal contact with these chemicals reinforces the rSSC and also provokes symptoms and signs referable to the nasopharynx/ pharynx (sore throat and cough), an entity classified as bacterial sinusitis complicated by pharyngitis.

Bacterial sinusitis complicated by rhinitis usually resolves spontaneously with host killing of the pathogen and downregulation of the inflammatory component of host defense. Published studies suggest that antimicrobial therapy is effective in promoting a more rapid eradication of the usual bacterial pathogens (*Streptococcus pneumoniae*, *Haemophilis influenzae*, and *Bramanella catarhalis*, among others) and may cause an earlier resolution of the rSSC (80,131,136). However, questions remain regarding the appropriate choice of an antimicrobial; the timing for initiation of therapy; and the potential for anaerobes and bacterial biofilms to establish long-term infections indistinguishable in presentation from other causes of persistent rhinitis (128,137–141).

SUMMARY

" .... *Amid the turmoil and tumult of battle, there may be seeming disorder and yet no real disorder at all; amid confusion and chaos, your array may be without head or tail, yet it will be proof against defeat.*"

Sun Tzu, The Art of War

In contradistinction to the poetically inspired disjunction between the name and quality of a rose recited by Juliet in the famous quote from Shakespeare's play[k],

---

[k] Juliet: *"Tis but thy name that is my enemy; thou art thyself though, not a Montague. What's Montague? It is nor hand, nor foot, nor arm, nor face, nor any other part belonging to a man. O! Be some other name: What's in a name? That which we call a rose by any other name would smell as sweet; so Romeo would, were he not Romeo call'd."* W. Shakespeare, Romeo and Juliet

disease labels used in the medical sciences need to have exact meaning to ensure that they communicate an accurate diagnosis and a valid treatment approach. Above, we presented a consistent nosology for rhinitis consequent to infection. There, we argued that the term "rhinitis" should be used to describe the condition of nasal mucosal pathology and that the rSSC be used to describe the appreciated expression of that pathology. In discussing viral and bacterial rhinitis, we conclude that former is consistent with a strict application of our nosology where the accompanying rSSC is usually referred to as cold or flu, but that the latter is not. Lacking direct evidence for bacterial infection of the nasal mucosa, bacterial rhinitis is better referred to as an acute bacterial infection of an adjacent compartment complicated by rhinitis (e.g., sinusitis complicated by rhinitis) or as "toxic rhinitis" complicated by bacterial infection. Interestingly, bacterial infection of the adjacent compartments is a frequent complication of viral rhinitis making "bacterial" rhinitis a complication of a complication of viral rhinitis.

The antiviral and antibacterial host-defense mechanisms available to the nasal mucosa are multilayered and formidable. For this reason, nasal mucosal infection with extracellular bacterial pathogens is rarely established and infection with a broad range of upper respiratory viruses is self-limited with short duration morbidity and no mortality. However, in select subpopulations, those infections predispose to more serious complications associated with secondary bacterial, and perhaps viral, infection of the sinuses, middle ears, and lungs. The morbidity and mortality of these complications remains a concern, and strategies to decrease their frequency need to be formulated and tested in clinical trials.

Because the viruses causing rhinitis are spread by interpersonal contact, the most appropriate and least expensive prophylactic measures are good hygiene and contact avoidance. Prophylactic efficacy for vaccination and passive immunoglobulin therapy was demonstrated for influenza and RSV infections, respectively. However, these approaches hold little promise for other viruses and are associated with some risks, making them less acceptable for populations "at low risk" for the more serious complications of viral rhinitis. Existing pharmacological treatments for viral rhinitis target the effector chemicals of the rSSC and therefore are largely palliative, whereas antiviral treatment has limited theoretical and realized efficacy, and no treatment has been shown to decrease the risk of complications. Indeed, given the small treatment window available (time between rSSC onset and typical resolution) and the poor understanding of the immune/inflammatory pathways of host defense, it is doubtful that the general population's demand for a cure will be satisfied in the near future, but then, viral rhinitis by any other name is still just a cold.

REFERENCES

1. Cauna N. Electron microscopy of the nasal vascular bed and its nerve supply. Ann Otol Rhinol Laryngol 1970; 79(3):443–450.
2. Grevers G. Electron-microscopic observations on the muscular coat of swell bodies in human nasal mucosa. Laryngoscope 1994; 104(10):1285–1289.
3. Grevers G, Herrmann U. Cavernous tissue of the nasal mucosa. Laryngol Rhinol Otol (Stuttg) 1987; 66(3):152–156.
4. Ritter FN. The vasculature of the nose. Ann Otol Rhinol Laryngol 1970; 79(3):468–474.
5. Rohr AS, Spector SL. Paranasal sinus anatomy and pathophysiology. Clin Rev Allergy 1984; 2(4):387–395.
6. Baraniuk JN. Neural control of human nasal secretion. Pulm Pharmacol 1991; 4(1): 20–31.

7. Davies AM, Eccles R. Reciprocal changes in nasal resistance to airflow caused by pressure applied to the axilla. Acta Otolaryngol 1985; 99(1–2):154–159.
8. Eccles R. The central rhythm of the nasal cycle. Acta Otolaryngol 1978; 86(5–6):464–468.
9. Eccles R. Plasma exudation in rhinitis. Clin Exp Allergy 1992; 22(3):319–320.
10. Falck B, et al. The effect of physical work on the mucosal blood flow and gas exchange in the human maxillary sinus. Rhinology 1989; 27(4):241–250.
11. Hasegawa M. Nasal cycle and postural variations in nasal resistance. Ann Otol Rhinol Laryngol 1982; 91(1 Pt 1):112–114.
12. Le Merre C, et al. Effects of cold dry air nasal stimulation on airway mucosal blood flow in humans. Arch Physiol Biochem 2003; 111(4):327–329.
13. Olsson P, Bende M. Influence of environmental temperature on human nasal mucosa. Ann Otol Rhinol Laryngol 1985; 94(2 Pt 1):153–155.
14. Olsson P, Bende M. Sympathetic neurogenic control of blood flow in human nasal mucosa. Acta Otolaryngol 1986; 102(5–6):482–487.
15. Toppozada HH, Talaat MA. The normal human maxillary sinus mucosa. An electron microscopic study. Acta Otolaryngol 1980; 89(3–4):204–213.
16. Connell JT. Nasal disease: mechanisms and classification. Ann Allergy 1983; 50(4):227–235.
17. Geurkink N. Nasal anatomy, physiology, and function. J Allergy Clin Immunol 1983; 72(2):123–128.
18. Hueston WJ, et al. Criteria used by clinicians to differentiate sinusitis from viral upper respiratory tract infection. J Fam Pract 1998; 46(6):487–492.
19. Corey JP, Houser SM, Ng BA. Nasal congestion: a review of its etiology, evaluation, and treatment. Ear Nose Throat J 2000; 79(9):690–693, 696, 698 passim.
20. Proctor DF, Andersen I, Lundqvist GR. Human nasal mucosal function at controlled temperatures. Respir Physiol 1977; 30(1–2):109–124.
21. White MD, Cabanac M. Nasal mucosal vasodilatation in response to passive hyperthermia in humans. Eur J Appl Physiol Occup Physiol 1995; 70(3):207–212.
22. Dykewicz MS. 7. Rhinitis and sinusitis. J Allergy Clin Immunol 2003; 111(2 Suppl):S520–S529.
23. Doyle WJ, Skoner DP, Gentile D. Nasal cytokines as mediators of illness during the common cold. Curr Allergy Asthma Rep 2005; 5(3):173–181.
24. Turner RB, Hendley JO, Gwaltney JM Jr. Shedding of infected ciliated epithelial cells in rhinovirus colds. J Infect Dis 1982; 145(6):849–853.
25. Gwaltney JM Jr. Combined antiviral and antimediator treatment of rhinovirus colds. J Infect Dis 1992; 166(4):776–782.
26. Gwaltney JM. Viral respiratory infection therapy: historical perspectives and current trials. Am J Med 2002; 112(Suppl 6A):S33–S41.
27. Gwaltney JM. Clinical significance and pathogenesis of viral respiratory infections. Am J Med 2002; 112(Suppl 6A):S13–S18.
28. Hayden FG, et al. Local and systemic cytokine responses during experimental human influenza A virus infection. Relation to symptom formation and host defense. J Clin Invest 1998; 101(3):643–649.
29. Winther B, et al. Viral-induced rhinitis. Am J Rhinol 1998; 12(1):17–20.
30. Widdicombe G. The physiology of the nose. Clin Chest Med 1986; 7(2):159–170.
31. Proctor DF, Swift DL. The nose—a defence against the atmospheric environment. Inhaled Part 1970; 1:59–70.
32. Proctor DF. The upper airways. I. Nasal physiology and defense of the lungs. Am Rev Respir Dis 1977; 115(1):97–129.
33. Proctor DF. The upper airways. II. The larynx and trachea. Am Rev Respir Dis 1977; 115(2):315–342.
34. Naumann HH. On the defense mechanisms of the respiratory mucosa towards infection. Acta Otolaryngol 1980; 89(3–4):165–176.
35. Bernstein JM. Mucosal immunology of the upper respiratory tract. Respiration 1992; 59(Suppl 3):3–13.
36. Kaliner MA. Human nasal host defense and sinusitis. J Allergy Clin Immunol 1992; 90(3 Pt 2):424–430.

37. Cole AM, Dewan P, Ganz T. Innate antimicrobial activity of nasal secretions. Infect Immun 1999; 67(7):3267–3275.
38. Cole AM, et al. Cationic polypeptides are required for antibacterial activity of human airway fluid. J Immunol 2002; 169(12):6985–6991.
39. Chen PH, Fang SY. Expression of human beta-defensin 2 in human nasal mucosa. Eur Arch Otorhinolaryngol 2004; 261(5):238–241.
40. Kirkeby L, et al. Immunoglobulins in nasal secretions of healthy humans: structural integrity of secretory immunoglobulin A1 (IgA1) and occurrence of neutralizing antibodies to IgA1 proteases of nasal bacteria. Clin Diagn Lab Immunol 2000; 7(1):31–39.
41. Widdicombe JG. Nasal pathophysiology. Respir Med 1990; 84(Suppl A):3–9; discussion 9–10.
42. Proctor DF, Adams GK III. Physiology and pharmacology of nasal function and mucus secretion. Pharmacol Ther (B) 1976; 2(3):493–509.
43. Persson CG, et al. Extravasation, lamina propria flooding and lumenal entry of bulk plasma exudate in mucosal defence, inflammation and repair. Pulm Pharmacol 1996; 9(3):129–139.
44. Thurauf N, et al. Nociceptive and reflexive responses recorded from the human nasal mucosa. Brain Res 1993; 629(2):293–299.
45. Tosi MF. Innate immune responses to infection. J Allergy Clin Immunol 2005; 116(2):241–249; quiz 250.
46. Triantafilou M, Triantafilou K. The dynamics of LPS recognition: complex orchestration of multiple receptors. J Endotoxin Res 2005; 11(1):5–11.
47. Worthley DL, Bardy PG, Mullighan CG. Mannose-binding lectin: biology and clinical implications. Intern Med J 2005; 35(9):548–555.
48. Zanetti M. The role of cathelicidins in the innate host defenses of mammals. Curr Issues Mol Biol 2005; 7(2):179–196.
49. Wang CS, Dong Z. Expression of toll-like receptor mRNA in epithelial cell of nasal mucosa. Zhonghua Er Bi Yan Hou Ke Za Zhi 2003; 38(4):243–246.
50. Soderblom T, et al. Bacterial protein toxins and inflammation. Scand J Infect Dis 2003; 35(9):628–631.
51. Gordon SB, Read RC. Macrophage defences against respiratory tract infections. Br Med Bull 2002; 61:45–61.
52. Xu D, Komai-Koma M, Liew FY. Expression and function of Toll-like receptor on T cells. Cell Immunol 2005; 233(2):85–89.
53. Walzer T, et al. Natural killer cell-dendritic cell crosstalk in the initiation of immune responses. Expert Opin Biol Ther 2005; 5(Suppl 1):S49–S59.
54. Wan H, Dupasquier M. Dendritic Cells in vivo and in vitro. Cell Mol Immunol 2005; 2(1):28–35.
55. Van Kaer L, Joyce S. Innate immunity: NKT cells in the spotlight. Curr Biol 2005; 15(11):R429–R431.
56. Brandtzaeg P. Immunocompetent cells of the upper airway: functions in normal and diseased mucosa. Eur Arch Otorhinolaryngol 1995; 252(Suppl 1):S8–S21.
57. Proud D, Sanders SP, Wiehler S. Human rhinovirus infection induces airway epithelial cell production of human beta-defensin 2 both in vitro and in vivo. J Immunol 2004; 172(7):4637–4645.
58. Biron CA, Brossay L. NK cells and NKT cells in innate defense against viral infections. Curr Opin Immunol 2001; 13(4):458–464.
59. Vliagoftis H, Befus AD. Rapidly changing perspectives about mast cells at mucosal surfaces. Immunol Rev 2005; 206:190–203.
60. Bachert C, Moller P. The tonsils as MALT (mucosa-associated lymphoid tissue) of the nasal mucosa. Laryngorhinootologie 1990; 69(10):515–520.
61. Freihorst J, Ogra PL. Mucosal immunity and viral infections. Ann Med 2001; 33(3):172–177.
62. Alfano M, Poli G. Role of cytokines and chemokines in the regulation of innate immunity and HIV infection. Mol Immunol 2005; 42(2):161–182.
63. Banyer JL, et al. Cytokines in innate and adaptive immunity. Rev Immunogenet 2000; 2(3):359–373.

64. Biron CA. Role of early cytokines, including alpha and beta interferons (IFN-alpha/beta), in innate and adaptive immune responses to viral infections. Semin Immunol 1998; 10(5):383–390.
65. Salazar-Mather TP, Hokeness KL. Calling in the troops: regulation of inflammatory cell trafficking through innate cytokine/chemokine networks. Viral Immunol 2003; 16(3):291–306.
66. Yoshimura A. Negative regulation of cytokine signaling. Clin Rev Allergy Immunol 2005; 28(3):205–220.
67. Gwaltney JM Jr. Epidemiology of the common cold. Ann N Y Acad Sci 1980; 353:54–60.
68. Heikkinen T, Jarvinen A. The common cold. Lancet 2003; 361(9351):51–59.
69. Harris, JM II, Gwaltney JM Jr. Incubation periods of experimental rhinovirus infection and illness. Clin Infect Dis 1996; 23(6):1287–1290.
70. Gwaltney JM Jr., Hendley JO, Patrie JT. Symptom severity patterns in experimental common colds and their usefulness in timing onset of illness in natural colds. Clin Infect Dis 2003; 36(6):714–723.
71. Monto AS, Fendrick AM, Sarnes MW. Respiratory illness caused by picornavirus infection: a review of clinical outcomes. Clin Ther 2001; 23(10):1615–1627.
72. Bertino JS. Cost burden of viral respiratory infections: issues for formulary decision makers. Am J Med 2002; 112(Suppl 6A):S42–S49.
73. Bramley TJ, Lerner D, Sames M. Productivity losses related to the common cold. J Occup Environ Med 2002; 44(9):822–829.
74. Gwaltney JM Jr., et al. Computed tomographic study of the common cold. N Engl J Med 1994; 330(1):25–30.
75. Alho OP, arttunen R, Karttunen TJ. Nasal mucosa in natural colds: effects of allergic rhinitis and susceptibility to recurrent sinusitis. Clin Exp Immunol 2004; 137(2):366–372.
76. Buchman CA, et al. Otologic manifestations of experimental rhinovirus infection. Laryngoscope 1994; 104(10):1295–1299.
77. Henderson FW. Pulmonary infections with respiratory syncytial virus and the parainfluenza viruses. Semin Respir Infect 1987; 2(2):112–121.
78. Hendley JO, Edmondson WP Jr., Gwaltney JM Jr. Relation between naturally acquired immunity and infectivity of two rhinoviruses in volunteers. J Infect Dis 1972; 125(3):243–248.
79. Kristo A, et al. Paranasal sinus findings in children during respiratory infection evaluated with magnetic resonance imaging. Pediatrics 2003; 111(5 Pt 1):e586–e589.
80. Anon JB. Acute bacterial rhinosinusitis in pediatric medicine: current issues in diagnosis and management. Paediatr Drugs 2003; 5(Suppl 1):25–33.
81. Tan WC, et al. Epidemiology of respiratory viruses in patients hospitalized with near-fatal asthma, acute exacerbations of asthma, or chronic obstructive pulmonary disease. Am J Med 2003; 115(4):272–277.
82. Moody SA, Alper CM, Doyle WJ. Daily tympanometry in children during the cold season: association of otitis media with upper respiratory tract infections. Int J Pediatr Otorhinolaryngol 1998; 45(2):143–150.
83. Lemanske RF Jr., et al. Rhinovirus upper respiratory infection increases airway hyperreactivity and late asthmatic reactions. J Clin Invest 1989; 83(1):1–10.
84. Mygind N, et al. The common cold and asthma. Allergy 1999; 54(Suppl 57):146–159.
85. Tarlo SM, et al. The role of symptomatic colds in asthma exacerbations: Influence of outdoor allergens and air pollutants. J Allergy Clin Immunol 2001; 108(1):52–58.
86. Renegar KB, Small PA Jr. Passive transfer of local immunity to influenza virus infection by IgA antibody. J Immunol 1991; 146(6):1972–1978.
87. Doyle WJ, et al. Effect of rimantadine treatment on clinical manifestations and otologic complications in adults experimentally infected with influenza A (H1N1) virus. J Infect Dis 1998; 177(5):1260–1265.
88. Reynolds HY. Host defense impairments that may lead to respiratory infections. Clin Chest Med 1987; 8(3):339–358.
89. Alper CM, et al. Prechallenge antibodies moderate disease expression in adults experimentally exposed to rhinovirus strain hanks. Clin Infect Dis 1998; 27(1):119–128.

90. Alper CM, et al. Prechallenge antibodies: moderators of infection rate, signs, and symptoms in adults experimentally challenged with rhinovirus type 39. Laryngoscope 1996; 106(10):1298–1305.
91. Gern JE, et al. Rhinovirus-specific T cells recognize both shared and serotype-restricted viral epitopes. J Infect Dis 1997; 175(5):1108–1114.
92. Cohen S. Keynote Presentation at the Eight International Congress of Behavioral Medicine: the Pittsburgh common cold studies: psychosocial predictors of susceptibility to respiratory infectious illness. Int J Behav Med 2005; 12(3):123–131.
93. Gentile DA, et al. Cytokine gene polymorphisms moderate illness severity in infants with respiratory syncytial virus infection. Hum Immunol 2003; 64(3):338–344.
94. Gentile DA, et al. Cytokine gene polymorphisms moderate responses to respiratory syncytial virus in adults. Hum Immunol 2003; 64(1):93–98.
95. Cohen S, et al. State and trait negative affect as predictors of objective and subjective symptoms of respiratory viral infections. J Pers Soc Psychol 1995; 68(1):159–169.
96. Cohen S, et al. Social ties and susceptibility to the common cold. Jama 1997; 277(24):1940–1944.
97. Cohen S, et al. Types of stressors that increase susceptibility to the common cold in healthy adults. Health Psychol 1998; 17(3):214–223.
98. Gentile DA, Skoner DP. Effect of respiratory syncytial virus infection during early infancy on the ontogeny of cytokine immune responses. Allergy Asthma Proc 2002; 23(6):399–405.
99. Cohen S, Doyle WJ, Skoner DP. Psychological stress, cytokine production, and severity of upper respiratory illness. Psychosom Med 1999; 61(2):175–180.
100. Gwaltney JM, Hendley JO. Rhinovirus transmission: one if by air, two if by hand. Trans Am Clin Climatol Assoc 1977; 89:194–200.
101. Hendley JO, Wenzel RP, Gwaltney JM Jr. Transmission of rhinovirus colds by self-inoculation. N Engl J Med 1973; 288(26):1361–1364.
102. Turner RB. New considerations in the treatment and prevention of rhinovirus infections. Pediatr Ann 2005; 34(1):53–57.
103. Turner RB, Hendley JO. Virucidal hand treatments for prevention of rhinovirus infection. J Antimicrob Chemother 2005; 56(5):805–807.
104. Doyle WJ, et al. Illness and otological changes during upper respiratory virus infection. Laryngoscope 1999; 109(2 Pt 1):324–328.
105. Doyle WJ, Alper CM. Prevention of otitis media caused by viral upper respiratory tract infection: vaccines, antivirals, and other approaches. Curr Allergy Asthma Rep 2003; 3(4):326–334.
106. Arruda E, et al. Frequency and natural history of rhinovirus infections in adults during autumn. J Clin Microbiol 1997; 35(11):2864–2868.
107. Eccles R. An explanation for the seasonality of acute upper respiratory tract viral infections. Acta Otolaryngol 2002; 122(2):183–191.
108. Bende M, et al. Changes in human nasal mucosa during experimental coronavirus common colds. Acta Otolaryngol 1989; 107(3–4):262–269.
109. Arruda E, et al. Localization of human rhinovirus replication in the upper respiratory tract by in situ hybridization. J Infect Dis 1995; 171(5):1329–1333.
110. Turner RB, et al. Sites of virus recovery and antigen detection in epithelial cells during experimental rhinovirus infection. Acta Otolaryngol Suppl 1984; 413:9–14.
111. Rihkanen H, et al. Rhinovirus in adenoid tissue. Int J Pediatr Otorhinolaryngol 2004; 68(7):903–908.
112. Naclerio RM, et al. Is histamine responsible for the symptoms of rhinovirus colds? A look at the inflammatory mediators following infection. Pediatr Infect Dis J 1988; 7(3):218–222.
113. Naclerio RM, et al. Kinins are generated during experimental rhinovirus colds. J Infect Dis 1988; 157(1):133–142.
114. Doyle WJ, Boehm S, Skoner DP. Physiologic responses to intranasal dose-response challenges with histamine, methacholine, bradykinin, and prostaglandin in adult volunteers with and without nasal allergy. J Allergy Clin Immunol 1990; 86(6 Pt 1):924–935.
115. Das S, et al. Cytokine amplification by respiratory syncytial virus infection in human nasal epithelial cells. Laryngoscope 2005; 115(5):764–768.

116. Kaiser L, et al. Symptom pathogenesis during acute influenza: interleukin-6 and other cytokine responses. J Med Virol 2001; 64(3):262–268.
117. Gentile D, et al. Increased interleukin-6 levels in nasal lavage samples following experimental influenza A virus infection. Clin Diagn Lab Immunol 1998; 5(5):604–608.
118. Skoner DP, et al. Evidence for cytokine mediation of disease expression in adults experimentally infected with influenza A virus. J Infect Dis 1999; 180(1):10–14.
119. Turner RB, et al. An evaluation of Echinacea angustifolia in experimental rhinovirus infections. N Engl J Med 2005; 353(4):341–348.
120. Hedrick JA, et al. Zanamivir for treatment of symptomatic influenza A and B infection in children five to twelve years of age: a randomized controlled trial. Pediatr Infect Dis J 2000; 19(5):410–417.
121. Fendrick AM. Viral respiratory infections due to rhinoviruses: current knowledge, new developments. Am J Ther 2003; 10(3):193–202.
122. Kibble A. 18th International Conference on Antiviral Research. Respiratory viruses. IDrugs 2005; 8(6):465–466.
123. Boot JM, et al. Congenital syphilis. Int J STD AIDS 1992; 3(3):161–167.
124. Iskandar NM, Naguib MB. Chlamydia trachomatis: an underestimated cause for rhinitis in neonates. Int J Pediatr Otorhinolaryngol 1998; 42(3):233–237.
125. Shinkwin CA, Gibbin KP. Neonatal upper airway obstruction caused by chlamydial rhinitis. J Laryngol Otol 1995; 109(1):58–60.
126. Toppozada H, Talaat M, Elwany S. The human respiratory nasal mucosa in nasal syphilis. An ultra-microscopic study. Acta Otolaryngol 1985; 99(3–4):272–279.
127. Cole AM, et al. Determinants of Staphylococcus aureus nasal carriage. Clin Diagn Lab Immunol 2001; 8(6):1064–1069.
128. Morinaka S, Ichimiya M, Nakamura H. Detection of Helicobacter pylori in nasal and maxillary sinus specimens from patients with chronic sinusitis. Laryngoscope 2003; 113(9):1557–1563.
129. Efremova SA, et al. Microflora of the nasal cavity and its sensitivity to antibiotics in patients with chronic rhinitis treated by cryotherapy. Antibiotiki 1977; 22(4):324–327.
130. Holbrook KA, et al. Staphylococcus aureus nasal colonization in HIV-seropositive and HIV-seronegative drug users. J Acquir Immune Defic Syndr Hum Retrovirol 1997; 16(4):301–306.
131. Hickner JM, et al. Principles of appropriate antibiotic use for acute rhinosinusitis in adults: background. Ann Emerg Med 2001; 37(6):703–710.
132. Braunstahl GJ. The unified immune system: respiratory tract-nasobronchial interaction mechanisms in allergic airway disease. J Allergy Clin Immunol 2005; 115(1):142–148.
133. Fox RW, Lockey RF. The impact of rhinosinusitis on asthma. Curr Allergy Asthma Rep 2003; 3(6):513–518.
134. Keech DR, Ramadan H, Mathers P. Analysis of aerobic bacterial strains found in chronic rhinosinusitis using the polymerase chain reaction. Otolaryngol Head Neck Surg 2000; 123(4):363–367.
135. Baraniuk JN. Neurogenic mechanisms in rhinosinusitis. Curr Allergy Asthma Rep 2001; 1(3):252–261.
136. Poole MD, et al. Antimicrobial guidelines for the treatment of acute bacterial rhinosinusitis in immunocompetent children. Int J Pediatr Otorhinolaryngol 2002; 63(1):1–13.
137. Sanclement JA, et al. Bacterial biofilms in surgical specimens of patients with chronic rhinosinusitis. Laryngoscope 2005; 115(4):578–582.
138. Scheid DC, Hamm RM. Acute bacterial rhinosinusitis in adults: Part II. Treatment. Am Fam Physician 2004; 70(9):1697–1704.
139. Scheid DC, Hamm RM. Acute bacterial rhinosinusitis in adults: Part I. Evaluation. Am Fam Physician 2004; 70(9):1685–1692.
140. Kennedy DW. Pathogenesis of chronic rhinosinusitis. Ann Otol Rhinol Laryngol Suppl 2004; 193:6–9.
141. Kalcioglu MT, et al. Bacteriology of chronic maxillary sinusitis and normal maxillary sinuses: using culture and multiplex polymerase chain reaction. Am J Rhinol 2003; 17(3):143–147.

11 Nonallergic Rhinitis in Children

William E. Berger
Department of Pediatrics, Division of Allergy and Immunology, University of California, Irvine, California, U.S.A.

J. Ellen Schonfeld
Allergy and Asthma Associates of Southern California, Mission Viejo, California, U.S.A.

INTRODUCTION

It is not unusual in an allergy practice to see a child with persistent rhinitis symptoms, negative skin tests, and a variable response to therapy. Because pure nonallergic rhinitis is a common condition affecting approximately 20% of all patients with rhinitis (1), it would be reasonable to assume that there would be a vast body of publications in the medical literature to help the clinician assess and treat this condition appropriately in all affected age groups. Surprisingly, however, information available concerning pediatric patients with this medical condition has been extremely sparse in comparison to the considerable literature published regarding adult patients with nonallergic rhinitis. As a result, the approach to the diagnosis and treatment of children with nonallergic rhinitis is a relatively limited endeavor for the practitioner, and nonallergic rhinitis is a medical condition that has not been dealt with adequately in previously published reviews of rhinitis.

Data suggests that non-immunoglobulin (Ig) E-mediated (perennial nonallergic) rhinitis is more prevalent in individuals over 20 years of age, but there is no definitive database that provides reliable information regarding the true incidence of pediatric nonallergic rhinitis patients in clinical practice. The age of onset still remains vague, and no reliable epidemiologic data on this condition in children have been firmly established. In addition, as with age distribution, the gender distribution of nonallergic rhinitis in children is not well established, while several studies in adult populations have suggested a higher incidence among females (1–3). With this in mind, our approach to this topic is based on the limited amount of available information. Hopefully, this review will encourage other investigators to contribute to the present body of knowledge and eventually establish definitive practice parameters for the diagnosis and treatment of nonallergic rhinitis in children.

CHRONIC NONALLERGIC RHINITIS IN CHILDREN

Pathophysiology

Under normal physiologic conditions, children react with an inflammatory response when exposed to infectious or irritant substances. This response is characterized by obstruction and rhinorrhea. This vasomotor reaction results from a series of complex, neuroendocrine pathways interacting at the level of the nasal mucosa—part of an exquisite defense system designed to enhance retention of offending agents so that non-IgE antibody responses can be initiated. When the presentation of these symptoms cannot be associated with a known trigger, the term "nonallergic rhinitis" is used (4).

Nonallergic rhinitis has been defined as an inflammation of the mucosal surface of the nose, not associated with an IgE-mediated mechanism, generally characterized by nasal congestion, postnasal drip, and rhinorrhea. Less frequently, pruritis and sneezing are also present. In this disorder, symptoms tend to be perennial and are often associated with changes in temperature, weather, humidity, and strong odors (1). Researchers have classified nonallergic rhinitis disorders in several different ways, including grouping them by cytological features [e.g., nonallergic rhinitis with eosinophilia syndrome (NARES)], frequency of occurrence, and causality (e.g., inflammatory and metabolic) (4,5).

Due to the fact that very little is known about the actual pathogenesis of perennial nonallergic rhinitis, it is frequently described as a nonspecific nasal hyperreactivity (1). Some researchers believe overactive parasympathetic nerve discharge could lead to vasodilatation of submucosal venous sinusoids, resulting in congestion and excess seromucous production (6).

In a study by Berger et al., the tissue of 39 adults with symptoms of perennial rhinitis, most with negative skin tests, and classified as medical treatment failures, underwent a turbinate reduction. Normal subjects having elective rhinoplasty served as controls. Nasal turbinate samples were examined for any relevant histological differences between allergic and nonallergic subjects. Both groups demonstrated inflammatory changes consisting of the presence of macrophages, polymorphonuclear leukocytes, and plasma cells, with lymphocyte proliferation predominating. Both allergic and nonallergic patients with turbinate hypertrophy demonstrated a greater number of mast cells in the lamina propria when compared to normal controls. Although not a surprising finding in patients with allergic rhinitis, the significance of mast cells in the lamina propria of nonallergic patients is not well understood. Possibly, mast cells in nonallergic patients may play a role in the homeostatic regulation of the nasal mucosa by the release of histamine, helping to regulate vascular tone and mucosal permeability (7).

The presence of nasal eosinophils is not pathognomonic for either allergic or nonallergic rhinitis. In one clinical trial by Mullarkey et al., 42% of patients identified as having allergic rhinitis based on positive skin tests and markedly elevated levels of IgE, demonstrated elevated levels of nasal eosinophils. This same study, however, uncovered a substantial number of patients expressing symptoms similar to perennial nonallergic rhinitis, yet also showing elevated levels of eosinophils (NARES). Therefore, nasal eosinophil levels were not found to be useful for differentiating between allergic and nonallergic rhinitis (8).

Evaluation

When considering causality of chronic rhinitis in the nonallergic child, a thorough history and a physical examination as well as pertinent diagnostic tests should be conducted.

The clinician should begin with a discussion of the patient's overall health and well-being, level of physical and emotional development, and general demeanor. The history should include a review of the quality of sleep, presence/absence of snoring, existence of daytime somnolence, and level of school performance.

If the patient is an infant, the discussion needs to include a review of the birth history. Trauma to the nasal passages can occur during the birthing process, giving rise to chronic nasal congestion. The history should also include a review of any pregnancy complications, such as chlamydia infections, which can present as chronic rhinitis. Other considerations should include a history of craniosynostosis or cleft palate repair, because both conditions can contribute to a mechanical etiology of nasal congestion (4).

In the adolescent, inquiring about the onset of puberty is important because hormonal changes can cause nasal congestion (5). If the adolescent is sexually active, sexually transmitted diseases should be discussed because syphilis can present with chronic rhinitis (9).

In all patients, any recent sinus surgery or head trauma should be reviewed, the latter being associated with cerebrospinal fluid leakage, presenting as clear rhinorrhea. The discharge can be easily identified as cerebrospinal fluid by dipstick; the presence of glucose would confirm the diagnosis (4).

Inquiring about the chronicity of rhinitis is paramount. Intermittent nasal congestion is most closely associated with self-limiting infections such as a rhinovirus. Chronic nasal congestion is representative of more complex disorders such as adenoid hypertrophy or immotile cilia syndrome.

Information regarding the onset of symptoms can be important. The existence of a foreign body tends to present with sudden onset of symptoms and continuation with little variation (4), while most other conditions are associated with exacerbations and remissions of nasal symptoms.

Exploring all possible etiologic factors is crucial. Inquiry regarding exposure to potential triggers commonly associated with nasal hyperreactivity, such as odors, drafts, cold air, temperature changes, fatigue, stress, and spicy foods will help the clinician confirm the diagnosis. Discussing the patient's physical environment, including exposure to severe air pollution and secondhand cigarette smoke, will also provide valuable information.

Review of past medication usage and the degree of relief provided may also aid in the diagnosis. Response to specific therapies will vary based on the underlying disease mechanism (8). Rhinitis medicamentosa or rebound nasal blockage from overuse of topical decongestants (e.g., oxymetazoline) will be easily identified by asking about over-the-counter nasal spray usage. It is important to also inquire about compliance with prescribed medications, because patients will often stop taking their medication if they feel better, resulting in the eventual return of symptoms and the perception that the medication is ineffective.

Physical Exam

Examination of each nasal passage includes noting the color and consistency of any discharge, the amount of mucosal edema, the presence or absence of turbinate hypertrophy, and the degree of patency. Visualization of the oropharynx may provide additional information regarding the degree of throat irritation and the severity of postnasal drip. Also, examination of the middle ear should include observation of the color, contour, and mobility of the tympanic membrane. The presence and character of any fluid behind the eardrum should be noted.

Differential Diagnosis

The most common trigger of rhinitis in infants and children is the common cold, very often caused by rhinovirus or adenovirus. However, rhinitis can also represent a typical prodromal symptom of other common viral illnesses such as measles or erythema infectiosum (4). Various conditions may also present with chronic rhinitis in the nonallergic pediatric patient. These include irritant rhinitis from environmental pollutants, obstruction from foreign bodies in the nose, thyroid disorders, adenoid hypertrophy, rhinosinusitis, nasal polyps, immotile cilia syndrome, midline granulomas, immunodeficiency diseases, cystic fibrosis, and reflux disorders.

Pollutants and Environmental Irritants

The role of pollutants and environmental irritants in nasal inflammation has primarily been studied in atopic patients. Researchers have found that ozone and endotoxins have a significant effect on nonallergic nasal airways. In a study by Graham, a 0.4 ppm exposure of ozone induced a neutrophilic inflammation in nonallergic patients (10), which could manifest as chronic rhinitis. In nonatopic subjects, Togias found that endotoxins induce neutrophilic inflammation in nasal passages and lower airways, which could contribute to chronic inflammatory symptoms such as nasal obstruction and rhinorrhea (11).

Foreign Bodies in the Nose

Foreign bodies in the nose can initiate an inflammatory response that will result in nasal congestion and rhinorrhea. Typically, the discharge will be unilateral and malodorous. If the substance is organic, such as a pea, discharge will occur soon after the object is lodged in the nose. An inorganic substance, such as a bead, tends to form rhinoliths (4).

Thyroid Disorders

Thyroid disorders are associated with nasal symptoms because diminished thyroxine levels lead to altered adrenergic receptor function, inhibiting normal vasoconstrictor mechanisms. This condition results in chronic nasal congestion (12).

In congenital hypothyroidism, nasal congestion is part of a spectrum of respiratory manifestations including noisy respirations and · apneic episodes. Fortunately, due to newborn screening, this disorder is usually detected early in life. Thyroiditis is also associated with chronic nasal symptoms. This disorder occasionally occurs during the first three years of life but is more common after the age of six. Thyroiditis is often autoimmune in nature (13).

Adenoid Hypertrophy

Adenoid hypertrophy is the most common cause of anatomic nasal obstruction in infants and children and can present with marked nasal congestion (14). The obstruction creates stasis of mucus and a chronic cycle of inflammation. In children with adenoidal disease, symptoms include those of nonallergic rhinitis but may also be characterized by the presence of cough, halitosis, and irritability. These children also mount intermittent fevers, require frequent courses of antibiotics, and clinically are often heavy snorers or daytime mouth breathers (14). In addition, adenoid hypertrophy is a significant risk factor for developing chronic sinus disease (15).

Rhinosinusitis

It is estimated that children have six to eight viral upper respiratory infections per year and, as a result, 5% to 13% will develop an acute bacterial sinusitis (15). The upper respiratory infection causes mucosal injury, swelling, and obstruction. Ciliary activity is reduced while concomitant hypersecretion increases. Severe nasal congestion and rhinorrhea are almost universally present.

Studies that have looked at the prevalence of acute sinus disease in the pediatric population have shown that the main risk factor in the nonallergic patient is a recent viral syndrome or adenoid disease. Chronic sinusitis is characterized by episodes that last more than three months and are associated with persistent, severe nasal congestion, intermittent rhinorrhea, cough, headache, postnasal drip, and halitosis (9). Inferior turbinate hypertrophy is often observed in these patients (15). Chronic sinus disease has a strong association with several other disorders including nasal polyps, immotile cilia syndrome, and cystic fibrosis (16).

Nasal Polyps
Nasal polyps are moist glistening herniations of respiratory mucosa (16). They are found in the nasal chamber but can also protrude from the maxillary sinus. The space-occupying nature of these structures can contribute to chronic rhinitis (4). The presence of nasal polyps and chronic sinus disease can be associated with cystic fibrosis. The work-up of any child with nasal polyps under 12 years of age should include a sweat chloride test to rule out cystic fibrosis (17). Polyps are often present in ciliary disorders such as immotile cilia syndrome or Kartagener's syndrome (4).

Immotile Cilia Syndrome (Ciliary Dyskinesia)
Immotile cilia syndrome (ciliary dyskinesia) should be suspected when a child presents with chronic obstructive rhinitis and concomitant chronic bronchitis, sinusitis, otitis media, and nasal polyposis (4). Recently characterized as a genetic disorder (18), it is known to alter mucociliary clearance mechanisms critical to the normal function of the upper and lower airways. The degree of severity is highly variable and children may begin having respiratory symptoms in the neonatal period. Typically, signs and symptoms consistent with chronic rhinitis appear around six months of age. These children have persistent disease of the ear and lower airways as well. The nasal congestion observed in these patients has been described as showing little seasonal variation. Frequently, the clinical course includes the development of nasal polyps and some patients may develop bronchiectasis. The prevalence of this genetic disorder is estimated to be 1:16,000 (18).

Midline Granulomas
Midline granulomas are relatively uncommon idiopathic diseases that can affect the nasal passages and sinuses. They share similar clinical and morphological characteristics with other vasculitis disorders such as Churg–Strauss syndrome (4). Patients can present with nasal symptoms including rhinorrhea and nasal obstruction, but will also demonstrate crusting of the mucosa and frequent epistaxis. These lesions can be destructive and are difficult to treat. Cultures as well as biopsies may be necessary to distinguish them from other serious conditions such as fungal sinusitis (4).

Immunodeficiency Disease
Immunodeficiency disease, through genetic expression or spontaneously, can alter the body's immune function. The different disorders are usually described as humoral, cellular, or combined. The deficiencies that result are expressed as altered lymphocyte function, dysfunctional phagocytes, or disorders of the complement

system. Humoral immunodeficiencies are the most common and are usually associated with recurrent infections of the upper and lower respiratory tract. Although viral infections are handled normally, sinusitis and pneumonias can be recurrent, refractory to treatment, and severe. The site of infection, the type of organism, and the age at onset of infections dictate the type of disorder and will often determine the clinical course (17).

Immunoglobulin-A Deficiency

IgA deficiency is a common B-cell deficit with an incidence of 1:700 in the pediatric population. The hallmark of this disorder is chronic upper and lower respiratory tract infections. These infections can be characterized by chronic nasal inflammation, rhinorrhea, and obstruction (17). Although most individuals will be asymptomatic, those with symptoms require aggressive treatment for respiratory tract infections. There is a high association between IgA deficiency and the development of atopic or autoimmune disorders (19). Many individuals produce anti-IgA antibodies and should not routinely receive blood products without appropriate pretreatment of the material being used. Patients should be counseled about the importance of informing all health-care providers of their condition so that the potential for a transfusion reaction can be minimized.

The prognosis is excellent if the patient is followed closely, infections are promptly treated, and the patient is closely monitored for the development of any autoimmune disorder.

Cystic Fibrosis

Cystic fibrosis is a relatively common genetic disorder with variable degrees of expression. Its frequency is approximately 1:2300 in the general population. Multiple genetic defects alter the function of exocrine glands, leading to the variable organ system involvement observed. Patients with cystic fibrosis produce highly viscous mucus in their airways, which contributes to obstruction of mucus membrane surfaces including the nasal and sinus cavities (20). These individuals frequently suffer from chronic sinus disease, which may initially present as chronic rhinitis (18).

Reflux Disease

Reflux disease refers to the backflow of stomach contents into the esophagus. Reflux can be physiologic (infants may reflux 50 to 60 times per day) or pathologic. When reflux becomes pathologic, inflammatory changes are initiated by a complex interplay of neurophysiological mechanisms. The relationship between gastroesophageal reflux (GER) and respiratory tract disorders such as chronic cough and asthma has been well established in both adults and children (21,22).

Koufman has described an association between extraesophageal events and upper airway pathology (23). In the past, patients who did not experience typical heartburn symptoms but only presented with upper airway inflammation were diagnosed with "atypical reflux." Most clinicians felt that the inflammation observed in the upper airway structures was a function of vagally mediated pathways, rather than a direct result of the refluxate. With evidence mounting that extraesophageal reflux is a distinct entity, otolaryngologists are now defining this type of condition as "laryngopharyngeal reflux" (LPR) (24).

LPR differs in mechanism and presentation from traditional reflux. Whereas traditional GER is usually associated with lower esophageal sphincter dysfunction,

LPR is thought to be associated with upper esophageal sphincter dysfunction. Many patients with LPR do not present in ways that are consistent with traditional GER. As an example, many LPR patients reflux more when upright in contrast to the established supine pattern in GER. Although LPR is seldom associated with reports of heartburn, which is nearly universal in traditional GER, throat symptoms predominate, including hoarseness, globus pharyngeus, excessive throat clearing, and chronic cough. Patients with LPR can also experience significant tissue damage even with moderate reflux disease. Compared to the esophagus, the laryngeal tissue is a hundred times more sensitive to activated pepsin (25). Because of this hypersensitivity, LPR requires aggressive and prolonged treatment.

Tasker investigated the role of reflux disease in children with otitis media with effusion. It was postulated that contents from the nasopharynx could reach the middle ear when the child was supine, and therefore contribute to chronic inflammation. To test this hypothesis, he reasoned that if refluxate reaches the middle ear, there should be a difference between the concentrations of gastric enzymes in the effusions as compared to plasma levels. Fifty-four children aged two to eight years, undergoing myringotomy for the treatment of otitis media with effusion, had the fluid from their middle ear analyzed. The concentrations of pepsin and pepsinogen were 1000 times higher than the serum levels while the albumin level was equal to serum levels (26). These findings suggest that reflux disorders do contribute to chronic middle ear disease. If refluxate is present in the middle ear fluid, it seems logical that it could also pool in the nasopharynx. The presence of refluxate could contribute to chronic rhinitis through the same inflammatory pathways.

Barbero described 22 children between 15 months and 5 years, who were being followed for persistent nasal obstruction and chronic nasal discharge of unknown etiology. All patients had a long-standing history of upper airway symptoms. These symptoms included inflammation of the nasal mucosa, as well as cobblestoning of the posterior pharynx. All the children underwent pH monitoring to rule out reflux as a cause of their persistent symptoms. Sixteen of the 22 patients were found to have significant reflux. When the reflux was treated, these patients demonstrated a marked reduction in their rhinitis symptoms, further supporting the relationship between reflux and chronic rhinitis (27).

Contencin and Narcy performed 24-hour pH monitoring on a group of 31 infants and children suffering from chronic, recurrent rhinitis of unknown origin. Patients with reflux but without nasal symptoms served as controls. Upon analysis, the rhinitis group demonstrated only slightly decreased pH levels over the control group. There was, however, a statistically significant increase in the number of reflux events in the rhinitis group when compared to controls (28). Nasal congestion in a patient known to have GER may be a manifestation of LPR in the same patient. Although it is less common for an individual to have concomitant GER and LPR, this, in fact, has been reported (24,25).

In a meta-analysis by Weaver, 152 articles were reviewed to look for evidence in the literature that would support an association between reflux disorders and extraesophageal pathologies (sinusitis, otitis media, and laryngeal malignancy). The results of his evaluation demonstrated a strongly positive causal association between GER and sinusitis (29).

When determining the etiology of chronic nasal symptoms in nonatopic children, it appears that sufficient evidence exists in the literature to encourage the clinician to consider reflux disorders in the differential diagnosis of chronic nonallergic rhinitis.

DIAGNOSIS AND TREATMENT OF NONALLERGIC RHINITIS

Diagnosis

Nonallergic rhinitis is generally a disease of exclusion. Allergic etiologic factors must be ruled out before a diagnosis of nonallergic rhinitis can be considered. A detailed history and physical examination, as well as appropriate tests such as skin tests and nasal cytology are often required to make the definitive diagnosis.

A study by Mullarkey demonstrated that although the presence of eosinophils in nasal smears did not differentiate allergic rhinitis from nonallergic rhinitis, there was a strong correlation between the presence of eosinophils and a positive response to treatment with nasal steroids (30).

A blood test to examine total eosinophil counts and IgE levels may act as an additional screening tool for children who have persistent symptoms (31). Intranasal challenges and nasal lavage techniques (e.g., histamine and allergen) are more difficult in pediatric patients but have yielded important information in adult populations and should be considered (32).

Rhinomanometry provides an objective method for quantifying nasal obstruction. Utilization of this tool could assist the clinician in the initial diagnosis, as well as in assessing clinical response to treatment over time. The variables measured by rhinomanometry are airflow and nasal resistance. Measurements are taken during quiet breathing through the nose with the mouth closed. Nasal passages are tested independently with the alternate nostril occluded using a tight-fitting plug. Normal reference values have been calculated to allow for the physiological differences between nostrils (33).

In the past, pediatric reference values were not available, making interpretation of rhinomanometry results difficult. Data from adults cannot be used because the maturation process creates dynamic changes in the size of the airways reflected by changes in airflow and nasal resistance.

Zapletal and Chalupova performed rhinomanometry on 192 children and adolescents without respiratory or nasal disease. They found that increased nasal inspiratory flow and decreased nasal resistance were a function of growth, and that the most reliable predictor of nasal values was body height. Hopefully, their predicted values will allow rhinomanometry to become a useful measurement tool in the pediatric population (33).

Treatment

Treatment of pediatric nonallergic rhinitis is based on an accurate diagnosis and determination of all etiologic factors. The choice of pharmacotherapy will often closely follow the treatment guidelines established for adults. The second-generation topical nasal antihistamine, azelastine, and corticosteroids have received Food and Drug Administration (FDA) approval for treatment of chronic nonallergic rhinitis (3).

Azelastine is the first intranasal antihistamine medication approved for use in the United States. It has shown to be effective in treating the rhinorrhea associated with nonallergic rhinitis, as well as relieving congestion. Suggested mechanisms for its anti-inflammatory activity include inhibition of mediator release and reduction of inflammatory cell infiltration and activation (34). A second new topical nasal antihistamine, olopatadine, is presently under development.

Oral nonsedating antihistamines are not FDA approved for nonallergic rhinitis and are often found to be ineffective in relieving the nasal congestion in these patients. Data support the use of topical nasal antihistamines such as azelastine in children over the age of six with nonallergic rhinitis (3,35,36).

The nasal steroids approved by the FDA for use in nonallergic rhinitis include the aqueous preparations of budesonide, beclomethasone, and fluticasone propionate (1). The anti-inflammatory properties of these compounds have been clearly established in allergic rhinitis (37) but strong evidence suggests they may also be effective in treating the chronic inflammation associated with nonallergic rhinitis (1,7,30). Umland et al. have found that fluticasone propionate, budesonide, and beclomethasone are able to modulate interleukin (IL)4 and (IL)5 activity (38).

Oral decongestants prescribed in conjunction with intranasal corticosteroids can be helpful in treating the nasal congestion sometimes associated with chronic rhinitis (1,6). For those patients who experience more rhinorrhea, the use of anticholinergic medications can be helpful. Research targeting nonallergic rhinitis strongly suggests their applicability in these patients. Grossman et al. found decreased rhinorrhea with reduction of concomitant medications and improved quality of life in patients who used these medications (37). Ipratropium bromide nasal spray is an anticholinergic agent approved for ages six and older and has demonstrated a decrease in methacholine-induced nasal secretion in nonallergic patients. One recent study found that two-thirds of a pediatric population, 6 to 18 years of age, found substantial relief of their rhinorrhea after treatment with ipratropium bromide nasal spray (3,39).

CONCLUSION

Attempts to explain the different types of nonallergic rhinitis in adults have focused on the specific cytologic features of the different disorders (e.g., NARES). Additional research into neurophysiological events may be helpful. Recent work with capsaicin has shown that local neural defects such as altered nociceptor function might play a role in this disorder. As knowledge increases regarding the mechanisms of nonallergic rhinitis, we may be able to better define pediatric nonallergic rhinitis as a specific entity (1,40).

At present, pediatric nonallergic rhinitis is not well described in the medical literature. Information on the possible mechanisms and appropriate management is obtained mainly from adult studies. The Agency for Healthcare Research and Quality (41) recently reported that in the past 20 years only 13 nonallergic rhinitis trials have been completed, enrolling a total of 450 patients. Of these, no specific studies of pediatric populations were conducted.

A recent survey study among treating physicians found that among patients with rhinitis symptoms, 43% were diagnosed allergic, 23% were found to be nonallergic, and 34% were classified as mixed (1). Although the exact percentage might differ slightly in the pediatric population, it would be reasonable to assume that the same ratio also occurs in children. Clearly, additional studies are needed to examine the phenomenon of nonallergic rhinitis, especially in children. Considering the large number of pediatric patients with rhinitis, it appears that pediatric nonallergic rhinitis is a significant, yet ill-defined disease entity in children and certainly requires a better understanding of its etiology, appropriate diagnostic testing, and optimal treatment.

ACKNOWLEDGMENT

The authors wish to acknowledge the editorial assistance of Wendy Davidson-Southall in the writing of this manuscript.

REFERENCES

1. Settipane RA, Lieberman P. Update on nonallergic rhinitis. Ann Allergy Asthma Immunol 2001; 86:494–508.
2. Dykewicz M, Fineman S. Executive summary of joint task force practice parameters on diagnosis and management of rhinitis. Ann Allergy Asthma Immunol 1998; 81:463.
3. Lieberman P. Treatment update: nonallergic rhinitis. Allergy Asthma Proc 2001; 22: 199–202.
4. Belenky W, Madgy DO. Nasal obstruction and rhinorrhea. In: Bluestone C, Stool S, Kenna M, eds. Pediatric Otolaryngology. Philadelphia: WB Saunders, 1996:765–779.
5. Scadding GK. Non-allergic rhinitis: diagnosis and management. Curr Opin Allergy Clin Immunol 2001; 1:15–20.
6. Economides A, Kaliner MA. Vasomotor rhinitis: making the diagnosis and determining therapy. J Respir Dis 1999; 20(7):463–467.
7. Berger G, Goldberg A, Ophir D. The inferior turbinate mast cell population of patients with perennial allergic rhinitis and non-allergic rhinitis. Am J Rhinol 1997; 11:63–66.
8. Mullarkey MF, Hill JS, Webb RW. Allergic and nonallergic rhinitis: their characterization with attention to the meaning of nasal eosinophilia. J Allergy Clin Immunol 1980; 65(2):122–126.
9. Alobid I, Guilemany JM, Mullol J. Nasal manifestations of systemic illness. Curr Allergy Asthma Rep 2004; 4:208–216.
10. Graham DE. Biomarkers of inflammation in ozone-exposed humans: comparison of the nasal and bronchoalveolar lavage. Am Rev Resp Dis 1990; 142:152–156.
11. Togias A. Unique mechanistic features of allergic rhinitis. J Allergy Clin Immunol 2000; 105:S599–S604.
12. Oppenheimer JH. Tissue and cellular effects of thyroid hormones and their mechanism of action. In: Barow G, Oppenheimer JH, Volpe R, eds. Thyroid Function and Disease. Philadelphia: WB Saunders, 1989:90–123.
13. LaFranchi S. Disorders of the thyroid gland. In: Behrman RE, Kliegman RM, Jenson HB, eds. Nelson's Textbook of Pediatrics. 17th ed. Philadelphia: WB Saunders, 2004: 1870–1883.
14. Vandenberg SJ, Heathy DG. Efficacy of adenoidectomy in relieving symptoms of chronic sinusitis in children. Arch Otolaryngol Head Neck Surg 1997; 123:675–678.
15. Wald E, Bordley WC, Darrow D, et al. Clinical practice guideline: management of sinusitis. Pediatrics 2001; 108:798–808.
16. Magit AE. Tumors of the nose, paranasal sinuses, face and orbit. In: Bluestone C, Stool S, Kenna M, eds. Pediatric Otolaryngology. Philadelphia: WB Saunders, 1996:893–904.
17. Ballow M, O'Neil KM. Approach to the patient with recurrent infections. In: Middleton E, Reed C, Ellis E, Adkinson NF, Younginer J, Busse W, eds. Allergy Principles and Practice. 4th ed. St. Louis: Mosby, 1993:1027–1058.
18. Sturgess J, Turner JA. The immotile cilia syndrome. In: Cherick V, Kendig E, eds. Kendig's Disorders of the Respiratory Tract in Children. 5th ed. Philadelphia: WB Saunders, 1990:692–730.
19. Bonilla F. Antibody deficiency. In: Yeung D, Sampson H, Geha R, Szefler S, eds. Pediatric Allergy: Principles and Practice. St. Louis: Mosby, 2003:88–98.
20. McKlusky I. Cystic fibrosis. In: Cherick V, Kendig E, eds. Kendig's Disorders of the Respiratory Tract in Children. 5th ed. Philadelphia: WB Saunders, 1990:692–730.
21. Stein MR. Possible mechanisms of influence of esophageal acid on airway hyperresponsiveness. Am J Med 2003; 115(3A):555–595.
22. Harding S. The role of gastroesophageal reflux in chronic cough and asthma. Chest 1997; 111:1389–1402.

23. Koufman JA. Laryngopharyngeal reflux 2002: a new paradigm of airway disease. Ear Nose Throat J 2002; 1(2):2–5.
24. Bach K, McGuirt W, Postma G. Pediatric laryngopharyngeal reflux. Ear Nose Throat J 2002; 81(2):7–9.
25. Koufman JA. Laryngopharyngeal reflux is different from classic gastroesophageal reflux disease. Ear Nose Throat J 2002; 81(2):7–9.
26. Tasker A. Reflux of gastric juice and glue ear in children research (letter). Lancet 2002; 359:493.
27. Barbero GJ. GER and upper airway disease. Otolaryngol Clin North Am 1996; 29(1): 31–38.
28. Contencin P, Narcy P. Nasopharyngeal pH monitoring in infants and children with chronic rhinopharyngitis. Int J Pediatr Otorhinolaryngol 1991; 22:249–256.
29. Weaver EM. Association between GER and sinusitis, otitis media, and laryngeal malignancy: a systematic review of the evidence. Am J Med 2003; 115(3A):815–895.
30. Mullarkey MF. Eosinophilia non-allergic rhinitis. J. Allergy Clin Immunol 1988; 82(5):941–949.
31. Hsu PY, Lin YT, Chiang BL. Serum eosinophil cationic protein level and disease activity in childhood rhinitis. Asian Pac J Allergy Immunol 2004; 22(1):19–24.
32. Togias AG, Philip G. Nonallergic rhinitis. Pathophysiology and models for study. Eur Arch Otorhinolaryngol 1995; 252(1):S27–S32.
33. Zapletal A, Chalupova J. Nasal airflow and resistance measured by active anterior rhinomanometry in healthy children and adolescents. Pediatr Pulmonol 2002; 33:174–180.
34. Banov CH, Lieberman P. Efficacy of azelastine nasal spray in the treatment of vasomotor (perennial nonallergic) rhinitis. Ann Allergy Asthma Immunol 2001; 86:28–35.
35. Masieri S, Cavaliere F, Filiaci F. Nasal obstruction improvement induced by topical furosemide in subjects affected by perennial nonallergic rhinitis. Am J Rhinol 1997; 11(6):443–448.
36. Dockhorn R, Aaronson D, Bronsky E. Ipratropium bromide nasal spray 0.03% and beclomethasone nasal spray alone and in combination for the treatment of rhinorrhea in perennial rhinitis. Ann Allergy Asthma Immunol 1999; 82(4):349–356.
37. Grossman J, Banov C, Boggs P, et al. Use of ipratropium nasal spray in chronic treatment of nonallergic perennial rhinitis, alone and in combination with other perennial rhinitis medications. J Allergy Clin Immunol 1995; 95(5 Pt 2):1123.
38. Umland SP, Nahrebne DK, et al. The inhibitory effects of topically active glucocorticoids on IL-4 IL-5 and interferon-γ production by cultured primary CD4 T cells. J Allergy Clin Immunol 1997; 100(4):511–519.
39. Meltzer EO, Orgel AH, Biondi R, et al. Ipratropium nasal spray in children with perennial rhinitis. Ann Allergy Asthma Immunol 1997; 78:485–493.
40. Sanico A, Togias A. Noninfectious, nonallergic rhinitis (NINAR): considerations of possible mechanisms. Am J Rhinol 1998; 12(1):65–72.
41. Agency for Healthcare Research and Quality. Management of allergic and nonallergic rhinitis: summary AHRQ evidence report summary. http://www.ncbi,nlm.nih.gov/books/bv.fcgirid=hstat1chapter87435 (accessed July 2005).
42. Berger WE. Allergic rhinitis in children. Curr Allergy Asthma Rep 2001; 1:498–505.

12 | Rhinitis in the Elderly

A. Asli Sahin-Yilmaz and Jacquelynne P. Corey

Department of Surgery, Section of Otolaryngology—Head and Neck Surgery, University of Chicago, Chicago, Illinois, U.S.A.

INTRODUCTION

The U.S. population has a higher life expectancy than ever before. According to the National Center for Health Statistics, life expectancy at birth was 47.3 years in 1900, and by 2002, it had increased to 77.3 years (1). The U.S. residents over the age of 65 numbered 35 million in the year 2000 and that number is expected to reach 86 million by the year 2050. Persons over 65 will comprise about 20% of the U.S. population (2). A significant number of these people may experience rhinologic problems related to their age that could damage their quality of life.

During the past decades, geriatric medicine has experienced dramatic growth; however, little attention has been given to rhinologic diseases of the elderly (3,4). A search of English language articles on rhinologic diseases in the healthy aging group revealed a limited number of results (4–7). It is extremely important to increase the number of research and clinical studies in this field in order to enhance our basic knowledge of the aging nose, and meet the needs and demands of the older population with rhinologic problems.

In this article, the structural and physiological changes of the aging nose and the approach to common rhinological diseases of the elderly will be reviewed.

AGING AND NASAL ANATOMY

Nasal Structures

The aging nose undergoes changes in all of its structural components including the skin, muscles, cartilages, and bones. The skin quality changes and the dermis becomes thinner with diminished skin elasticity (8). Frequently, the alae and nasal tip take a fuller appearing character and this is possibly the outcome of increases in the density of sebaceous glands, which, may lead to the development of rhinophyma in male patients (9). Rhinophyma, which is the end stage of advanced rosacea, has a deep impact on patients' self-esteem and quality of life (10).

The fibroelastic attachments between the upper and lower cartilages of the nose fragment ossificate with aging. Because of maxillary alveolar hypoplasia, the columella shortens and the result is a droopy tip appearance (9,11). Edelstein found significant increases in the nasolabial angle and decreases in the height of the nose with age. The lower nasal width showed a trend toward widening in subjects who were 50 to over 80 years of age, but these changes were not statistically significant (4).

Nasal Mucosa

Information about the effect of aging on the changes of the nasal ciliated epithelium is very limited. Toppozada has studied postmenopausal subjects and showed that, although the nasal mucosa remains normal, the number of goblet cells decreases, resilient structures atrophy, and the basement membrane gets thicker with aging (12). Getchell et al. studied human respiratory and olfactory mucosa and noted an age-related decrement in the intensity and extent of immunoreactivity within the nasal cells (13). Edelstein found no significant age-related changes in gross and electron microscopic examination of the histopathology of the mucosa of either the septum or the turbinates (4).

Histologic analysis of the olfactory area in the elderly population reveals an increase in the number of patches of respiratory epithelium. This may represent a loss of primary olfactory receptor neurons (14). Robinson et al. showed age-induced changes in gene expression in the olfactory mucosa; this favored apoptosis of the olfactory neurons in older animals (15).

AGING AND NASAL PHYSIOLOGY

Airflow

Few studies have addressed the impact of age on nasal airflow. Edelstein evaluated elderly subjects with rhinomanometry and determined a significant correlation between aging and increasing nasal resistance both before and after the administration of a decongestant agent (4). In a more recent study, Kalmovich et al. measured the minimal cross-sectional areas and endonasal volumes of healthy elderly subjects by acoustic rhinometry and showed that there was an increase in minimal cross-sectional areas and endonasal volumes with age (16). It is unclear why there is a difference between the two studies—it may be due to differences in measurement techniques, or it may be that although the volume and area are increased, the mucosa functions less well and has increased resistance to airflow despite its larger size. The aging mucosa has less estrogen and is therefore less soft and less elastic and perhaps this leads to increased resistance.

The results of studies on the effect of aging on nasal mucociliary clearance (NMCC) and nasal ciliary beat frequency (NCBF) are controversial. In two studies, no particular trend in regard to NCBF and advancing age were observed (4,17). However, Edelstein reported that the standard deviation of the intrasubject NCBF varied significantly with age, which he suggested that may be an explanation of why the elderly often complain of fluctuating nasal symptoms (4). On the other hand, in a more recent study, Ho et al. showed that aging was associated with a decrease in NCBF and increase in NMCC time, which negatively reflects the efficiency of NMCC (18).

Olfactory Function

It is well known that the sense of smell diminishes with age. The prevalence of chronic olfactory problems from the National Health Interview Survey was estimated at 1.42% (2.7 million adults in US). In the age groups of 55 to 64 years, 65 to 74 years, and 75 years or older, the prevalence rates were 1.99%, 2.65%, and 4.60%, respectively (19). In a study by Murphy et al. the mean prevalence of disturbance of olfaction on a population of residents between 53 and 97 years of age was 24.5%. The prevalence increased with age and 62.5% of 80 to 97 year old subjects had olfactory impairment (20). In another study by Landis et al., gender and age were found to be the most important determinants of olfactory function, with women outperforming men and olfaction decreasing dramatically with age (21).

The sense of smell is composed of multiple sensations and predominantly mediated by two independent neural systems, the olfactory and somatosensory (trigeminal) system (22). Trigeminal afferents mediate sensations of touch, pressure, temperature, and nociception. It is suggested that older subjects not only show reduced olfactory sensitivities, but they also exhibit reduced trigeminal sensitivity of the intranasal system, which responds to the irritation of the nasal cavity and protects the respiratory tract from inhalation of potentially harmful irritants (22,23).

Data on the changes of the trigeminal system with aging are sparse. Hummel et al. have found that patients with olfactory dysfunction have lower trigeminal sensitivity compared with normosmic controls, independent of the cause of the olfactory loss. It was suggested that this observed decrease in trigeminal sensitivity could have been based on an interaction between the olfactory and intranasal trigeminal system. They further suggested that in normosmic subjects, there is an age-related decrease in trigeminal sensitivity (24). According to Frasnelli and Hummel, based on electrophysiological measures, age-related loss of intranasal trigeminal sensitivity seems to take place in the periphery of the intranasal trigeminal system (22,23).

Older individuals are susceptible to olfactory dysfunction, but it is imperative to remember that these symptoms may also be a signal of important underlying medical conditions. It is usually difficult to make a distinction between olfactory changes that result from losses due to the normal aging process and disease states, and medication effects that occur more commonly in the elderly. The causes of clinically observed olfactory impairment include local nasal inflammatory diseases (allergic rhinitis, rhinosinusitis, and nasal polyposis), prior viral upper respiratory tract infections, neurodegenerative diseases, nutritional deficiencies, endocrine diseases, surgical interventions, head trauma, environmental pollutants, and smoking (25). In a cross-sectional study of 2491 residents aged 53 to 97, stroke, epilepsy, current smoking, and nasal congestion at examination or having had an upper respiratory infection in the past week were associated with increased prevalence of olfactory impairment (20).

Accurate detection and characterization of olfactory deficits are of vital importance because defects in olfactory function have been described in the early phase of a number of neurodegenerative diseases including Alzheimer's disease, Parkinson's disease, and mild cognitive impairment (26–28). Olfactory dysfunction in Alzheimer's is thought to result from damage to the olfactory bulb and the medial temporal lobe (26,27). Olfactory dysfunction in Parkinson's disease is independent of the disease severity and duration and can be seen in 70% to 90% of nondemented patients with Parkinson's disease (29,30). Many researchers support the hypothesis that olfactory dysfunction is an early event in Parkinson's disease and may precede the development of motor dysfunction (29,30).

All of the above-mentioned alterations of the nasal anatomy and physiology due directly to the normal aging process result in symptoms of postnasal dripping, nasal drainage, sneezing, olfactory loss, and gustatory rhinitis (4). Edelstein investigated some other common nasal symptoms including nasal obstruction, headache, sinus pain, itching, and epistaxis, but none of these symptoms demonstrated a significant relationship to aging. Important etiologies of nasal problems in elderly patients will be evaluated under different headings.

NONALLERGIC RHINITIS IN THE ELDERLY

Vasomotor rhinitis, atrophic rhinitis, and gustatory rhinitis are common types of nonallergic rhinitis types that occur in older patients (31).

Vasomotor Rhinitis

Vasomotor rhinitis is the most common form of nonallergic rhinitis (32). Nasal mucosal reactivity is a balance of the sympathetic and parasympathetic systems and it controls vascularity and glandular expression (31). Autonomic dysfunction was shown to be significant in patients with vasomotor rhinitis (33). Neuropeptides, nitric oxide, ozone, cigarette smoke, and other environmental factors, and gastroesophageal reflux have been associated with vasomotor rhinitis (32–34).

Primary Atrophic Rhinitis

Primary atrophic rhinitis was commonly associated with infection from a bacterium called *Klebsiella ozaenae* prior to antibiotics. Today it is more commonly seen as a result of aggressive surgery, trauma, granulomatous diseases, and radiation therapy and is also associated with aging (31).

Gustatory Rhinitis

Gustatory rhinitis is a profuse watery rhinorrhea that may be exacerbated by eating. It is believed to arise from α-adrenergic activity stimulated by the regular use of antihypertensives.

ALLERGIC RHINITIS IN THE ELDERLY

It is suggested that the immune system undergoes characteristic changes with aging and most T-cell functions are depressed (35). Some investigators advocate that the incidence of onset of allergic symptoms and their severity decreases with age and there are significantly fewer cases of atopy among elderly subjects (60 years or older) compared with younger ones (36,37) Similarly, Jackola et al. observed a decline in serum total Immunoglobulin E (IgE) and atopic incidence in subjects older than 60 years. However, they failed to observe apparent age-related declines in parameters associated with specific mechanisms of atopy and suggested that in atopy prone families atopic humoral response is robust (38). Lately, Mediaty and Neuber measured specific and total IgE levels of 559 individuals with atopic dermatitis, asthma or allergic rhinitis, and insect allergies, and discovered that total and specific IgE production is reduced in the elderly with the exception of old patients with either high serum IgE or atopic dermatitis, indicating that atopic mechanisms with high serum IgE are vigorous and that atopic tendency among these patients remains into advanced age (37). In a cohort study by Burrows et al., the prevalence of positive skin testing was 36.6% among the elderly (39). Huss et al. found 74.7% positive test results to at least one allergen in 75 patients with asthma over the age of 65. It was found that 53.2% of these subjects were skin test positive to at least one indoor allergen (40). Unfortunately, there are no data available in the literature regarding the prevalence or course of allergic rhinitis in the elderly.

CHRONIC RHINOSINUSITIS IN THE ELDERLY

Rhinosinusitis is the sixth most common chronic condition of elderly persons, occurring more frequently than cataracts, diabetes, and general visual impairment (41). Settipane and Chafee reviewed their records of about 4900 patients with asthma and rhinitis and found that the frequency of nasal polyps increased with age (42).

RHINITIS DUE TO MEDICATIONS

Elderly adults have many health-care needs and therefore they require concurrent medications. According to a recent study by Roth and Ivey, the mean number of prescription medications used per patient is 9.6 (43). There is a myriad list of medications that may interfere with nasal functions in the elderly. The mechanism by which drugs affect the nasal functions is different and for some it is unidentified.

Rhinitis in the elderly due to "antihypertensives" is thought to be caused by α-adrenergic activity of the drugs. Antihypertensives, including methyldopa, hydralazine, clonidine, doxazosin, labetalol, reserpine, amiloride, guanabenz, terazosin, and guanethidine, and antihypertensives with diuretic effect cause nasal congestion, stuffiness, and dryness (44).

"Beta Blockers" bind to β-adrenoceptors to block the response to stimulation from sympathetic neurons and circulating catecholamines and have been reported to cause mild and transient nasal congestion (44).

Several "psychotropic agents" including thioridazine, amitriptyline, and perphenazine cause nasal symptoms and congestion most probably related to autonomic effects (31,44).

Aspirin-sensitive patients may experience rhinitis on taking this medication. Because of its antiplatelet action, aspirin may prolong epistaxis in the elderly.

A dry mucosal surface may be related to symptoms of congestion. The combined effect of many of the preceding disorders is drying of the mucosal surface. Many elderly patients present with no discernible etiology but with a visibly dry mucosa.

MANAGEMENT OF RHINITIS IN THE ELDERLY

Treatment of rhinological disorders of the aged can be aided by accurate diagnosis to decide on the correct treatment. Unfortunately, many disorders fall into the idiopathic category.

Clinical evaluation of elderly patients with rhinologic problems should start with a complete medical history. Patients should be questioned regarding the onset and duration of problems, whether they had been gradual, and other associations. A past medical, social, and family history should be included. A complete head and neck exam with particular attention to the nasal cavity including anterior rhinoscopy and nasal endoscopy should be performed. If there is no apparent etiology for olfactory dysfunction, neurodegenerative diseases must be ruled out with a cranial nerve exam, a neurologic exam, and a minimental test. Accurate differentiation of olfactory dysfunction due to Alzheimer's disease versus normal aging is possible using high magnetic field functional magnetic resonance imaging techniques (45).

Various types of inflammatory and noninflammatory rhinitis become prevalent in the elderly. Should the history and physical exam raise a suspicion of allergic rhinitis, in vivo or in vitro tests may be needed.

SYMPTOMATIC TREATMENT

Humidification
The main goal of treatment in the majority of older patients is to moisten the nasal mucosa. Nasal lavage with isotonic sodium chloride is usually the preferred method to reduce the nasal dryness and facilitate the clearing of thick mucus and crusts. Several randomized, controlled studies on saline nasal irrigation suggest that it is a safe, effective, well-tolerated method to use in inflammatory diseases of the nose.

Currently, many nasal irrigation methods are available. Wormald et al. compared the efficacy of three methods of nasal irrigation, which included metered nasal spray, nebulization, and nasal douching, and suggested that the nasal cavity is well irrigated by all three techniques (46). The nasal douche method is more effective in distributing irrigation solution to the maxillary sinus and frontal recess. Similarly, Passali et al. have shown that atomized nasal douches are efficacious in the normalization of nasal resistance and have a greater diffusion onto the nasal mucosa (47). Mucus thinning agents like guaifenesin and Alkolol (a nonprescription irrigating solution) may give relief to the elderly with dry nasal mucosa. Pure sesame oil has also been shown to decrease the complaints of people with nasal crusts (48).

Topical and Systemic Decongestants
Although they can improve congestion, topical and systemic decongestants should be avoided in the elderly because they may aggravate nasal dryness. They also may have systemic side effects such as confusion, difficulty in urination, irritability, and aggravation of glaucoma.

Antihistamines
First-generation antihistamines should not be used in the elderly due to risks of adverse effects and interactions with other medications. However, second-generation antihistamines such as loratadine, cetirizine, fexofenadine, desloratadine, and levocetirizine provide effective selective H1 blockade without anticholinergic or α-adrenoceptor antagonist activity. Use of the newer antihistamines is safe and effective in the elderly with allergic rhinitis (49,50).

Intranasal Ipratropium
Anticholinergic medications may provide relief in elderly patients with vasomotor or gustatory rhinitis. Ipratropium bromide, as a topical anticholinergic, acts locally and is effective in controlling rhinorrhea, and contributes to control of congestion, postnasal dripping, and sneezing (31,51). Ipratropium has few local side effects. Epistaxis and nasal dryness may occur but usually decrease in incidence with prolonged use (51).

Intranasal Steroids

Short-term studies both in children and in adults demonstrated no significant effect of intranasal steroids on bone mineral metabolism. Similarly, studies evaluating the effect of intranasal steroids on intraocular pressure and cataract formation have demonstrated that these side effects are similar to those in nonusers (52). Topical intranasal steroids are generally well tolerated by the elderly. The most commonly encountered side effects are epistaxis, dryness, and burning.

Intranasal steroids may be a treatment of choice in olfactory dysfunction due to infections of the upper respiratory tract or apparent sinonasal disease. Unfortunately, the response to either local or oral steroids is limited (53). Recent studies on the molecular biology of olfaction on mice have shown that the antibiotic minocycline may inhibit olfactory sensory neuron apoptosis, and may be efficacious in the management of peripheral olfactory loss (54).

Leukotriene Inhibitors

Montelukast has been approved in the United States for use in the treatment of nasal congestion due to allergic rhinitis. Although there is no study on the long-term therapeutic experience with montelukast use in the elderly, this drug is generally safe and well tolerated. Zafirlukast is another leukotriene inhibitor Zileuton (zyflow) is a 5-lipokygenase inhibitor that blocks leukotriene C4 and B4 synthesis.

Hormonal Replacement

Caruso et al. have shown that nasal respiratory epithelium has receptors for ovarian hormones, and that estrogen plays an important role in trophism (55). In another study, they also demonstrated that eight months of treatment with either oral or patch hormone therapy in postmenopausal women had a positive effect on olfactory thresholds of odors (56). Nappi et al. treated a group of postmenopausal women with nasal stuffiness by intranasal hormone therapy, and another group by intradermal hormonal therapy for six months and observed that both regimens improved nasal symptomatology and nasal mucosal appearance and reduced NMCC time. Intranasal application was more successful in improving nasal function compared to the transdermal route (57).

ALLERGIC RHINITIS TREATMENT

Treatment of allergies has three different components: environmental control, pharmacological therapy, and immunotherapy.

Huss et al. selected a sample of 80 elderly subjects with asthma and found high levels of house dust mites, cockroach evidence, cat dander and dog dander in samples collected in the homes. They suggested that the high allergen levels found in the home of older adults with asthma were related to living in homes with carpeting, older furnishings, high indoor relative humidities, and nonencased mattresses (40). Interventions to decrease the exposure to allergens may be done in order to accomplish environmental control for the elderly.

Pharmacological therapy includes humidification, antihistamines, intranasal steroids, ipratropium bromide, and leukotriene inhibitors, which have been mentioned above.

The efficacy of immunotherapy in the elderly has not really been studied. Asero assessed the efficacy of injection immunotherapy in patients older than 54 years who are monosensitized to birch and ragweed, and considered specific immunotherapy an effective therapeutic option in otherwise healthy elderly patients (58). More studies on immunotherapy of allergic rhinitis in the elderly are needed to develop strategies for successful management of these patients.

SURGICAL TREATMENT

Surgical reconstruction of the aging nose is aimed at reconstituting support for the nasal upper lateral cartilage and elevating the drooping nasal tip. Removal of turbinate mucosa should be avoided especially when excessive dryness is already a factor.

Busaba et al. assessed the clinical outcomes of septoplasty with or without inferior turbinate reduction in patients with nasal septal deviation 65 years or older and suggested that these surgical procedures are beneficial in this population (59).

Endoscopic sinus surgery (ESS) in the treatment of chronic sinusitis refractory to medical management in older persons has been established in a few studies. It has been shown that ESS is a relatively safe procedure in the elderly (5,6). However when considering revision ESS, surgeons and patients need to be aware of higher risk of complications in this population (6). Candidates for surgery should be assessed by their overall general health, rather than strictly by age alone.

ROSACEA TREATMENT

The effective treatment of rosacea starts with avoidance of triggers, including sun exposure, stress, and alcohol consumption. Topical metronidazole, oral tetracycline, or minocycline therapy have been shown to be effective. Both topical and oral retinoid therapy and topical vitamin C therapy are alternate treatment methods. Patients in the late stage of disease, with rhinophyma, should be treated with surgical methods using cryosurgery and laser therapy (10).

SUMMARY

Very little has been published regarding rhinitis in the elderly. Changes in the nose due to aging include structural, hormonal, mucosal, olfactory, and neural effects. The effects of polypharmacy may contribute to causing congestion and dryness. Physicians should look for treatable causes of rhinitis such as allergic rhinitis or rhinosinusitis, and rule out neurodegenerative disorders if applicable. Treatments that may provide symptomatic relief include humidification and antiallergy therapies. Surgery for structural and skin conditions of the external nose may also provide relief in some cases. As the U.S. population ages and remains in overall better health, we may learn more about the effects of aging on rhinitis.

REFERENCES

1. National Center for Health Statistics. Health, United States, 2004, Table 12. http://www.cdc.gov/nchs/data/dvs/nvsr53_06t12.pdf. Accessed November 5, 2005.
2. Administration on Aging. Statistics on the aging population. http://www.aoa.gov/prof/Statistics/future_growth/PopAge2050.xls. Accessed November 5, 2005.

3. Besdine R, Boult C, Brangman S, et al. American geriatrics society task force on the future of geriatric medicine. Caring for older Americans: the future of geriatric medicine. J Am Geriatr Soc 2005; 53:245–256.
4. Edelstein DR. Aging of the normal nose in adults. Laryngoscope 1996; 106:1–25.
5. Colclasure JC, Gross CW, Kountakis SE. Endoscopic sinus surgery in patients older than sixty. Otolaryngol Head Neck Surg 2004; 13:946–949.
6. Ramadan HH, VanMetre R. Endoscopic sinus surgery in geriatric population. Am J Rhinol 2004; 18:125–127.
7. Bassichis BA, Marple BF. Dry mouth and nose in the older patient. What every PCP should know. Geriatrics 2002; 57:22–24.
8. Vacher C, Accioli J, Lezy JP. Surgical anatomy of the nose in the elderly: value of conservative rhinoplasty by transoral route. Surg Radiol Anat 2002; 24:140–146.
9. Rohrich RJ, Hollier LH Jr., Janis JE, Kim J. Rhinoplasty with advancing age. Plast Reconstr Surg 2004; 114:1936–1944.
10. Cohen AF, Tiemstra JD. Diagnosis and treatment of rosacea. J Am Board Fam Pract 2002; 15:214–217.
11. Patterson CN. The aging nose: characteristics and correction. Otolaryngol Clin North Am 1980; 13:275–288.
12. Toppozada H. The human nasal mucosa in the menopause (a histochemical and electron microscopic study) [abstr]. J Laryngol Otol 1988; 102:314–318.
13. Getchell ML, Chen Y, Ding X, Sparks DL, Getchell TV. Immunohistochemical localization of a cytochrome P-450 isozyme in human nasal mucosa: age-related trends. Ann Otol Rhinol Laryngol 1993; 102:368–374.
14. Paik SI, Lehman MN, Seiden AM, Duncan HJ, Smith DV. Human olfactory biopsy. The influence of age and receptor distribution. Arch Otolaryngol Head Neck Surg 1992; 118:731–738.
15. Robinson AM, Conley DB, Shinners MJ, Kern RC. Apoptosis in the aging olfactory epithelium. Laryngoscope 2002; 112:1431–1435.
16. Kalmovich LM, Elad D, Zaretsky U, et al. Endonasal geometry changes in elderly people: acoustic rhinometry measurements. J Gerontol A Biol Sci Med Sci 2005; 60:396–398.
17. Agius AM, Smallman LA, Pahor AL. Age, smoking and nasal ciliary beat frequency. Clin Otolaryngol Allied Sci 1998; 23:227–230.
18. Ho JC, Chan KN, Hu WH, et al. The effect of aging on nasal mucociliary clearance, beat frequency, and ultrastructure of respiratory cilia. Am J Respir Crit Care Med 2001; 163:983–988.
19. Hofmann HJ, Ishii EK, Macturk RH. Age related changes in the prevalence of smell and taste problems among the US adult population: results of the 1994 disability supplement to the National Health Interview Survey. Ann N Y Acad Sci 1998; 855:716–722.
20. Murphy C, Schubert CR, Cruickshanks KJ, Klein BE, Klein R, Nondahl DM. Prevalence of olfactory impairment in older adults. JAMA 2002; 288:2307–2312.
21. Landis BN, Konnerth CG, Hummel T. A study on the frequency of olfactory dysfunction. Laryngoscope 2004; 114:1764–1769.
22. Hummel T, Livermore A. Intranasal chemosensory function of the trigeminal nerve and aspects of its relation to olfaction. Int Arch Occup Environ Health 2002; 75:305–313.
23. Frasnelli J, Hummel T. Age-related decline of intranasal trigeminal sensitivity: is it a peripheral event? Brain Res 2003; 987:201–206.
24. Hummel T, Futschik T, Frasnelli J, Huttenbrink KB. Effects of olfactory function, age, and gender on trigeminally mediated sensations: a study based on the lateralization of chemosensory stimuli. Toxicol Lett 2003; 140–141:273–280.
25. Seiberling KA, Conley DB. Aging and olfactory and taste function. Otolaryngol Clin North Am 2004; 37:1209–1228.
26. Peters JM, Hummel T, Kratzsch T, Lotsch J, Skarke C, Frolich L. Olfactory function in mild cognitive impairment and Alzheimer's disease: an investigation using psychophysical and electrophysiological techniques. Am J Psychiatry 2003; 160:1995–2002.
27. Kovacs T, Cairns NJ, Lantos PL. Olfactory centres in Alzheimer's disease: olfactory bulb is involved in early Braak's stages. Neuroreport 2001; 12:285–288.

28. Eibenstein A, Fioretti AB, Simaskou MN, et al. Olfactory screening test in mild cognitive impairment. Neurol Sci 2005; 26:156–160.
29. Double KL, Rowe DB, Hayes M, et al. Identifying the pattern of olfactory deficits in Parkinson disease using the brief smell identification test. Arch Neurol 2003; 60:545–549.
30. Tissingh G, Berendse HW, Bergmans P, et al. Loss of olfaction in de novo and treated Parkinson's disease: possible implications for early diagnosis [abstr]. Mov Disord 2001; 6:41–46.
31. Joe S, Benson A. Nonallergic rhinitis. In: Cummings CW, ed. Otolaryngology Head and Neck Surgery. Philadelphia: Elsevier Mosby, 2005:990–1000.
32. Lal D, Corey JP. Vasomotor rhinitis update. Curr Opin Otolaryngol Head Neck Surg 2004; 2:243–247.
33. Loehrl TA, Smith TL, Darling RJ, et al. Autonomic dysfunction, vasomotor rhinitis, and extraesophageal manifestations of gastroesophageal reflux. Otolaryngol Head Neck Surg 2002; 126:382–387.
34. Giannessi F, Ursino F, Fattori B, et al. Immunohistochemical localization of 3-nitrotyrosine in the nasal respiratory mucosa of patients with vasomotor rhinitis. Acta Otolaryngol 2005; 125:65–71.
35. Pawelec G, Barnett Y, Forsey R, et al. T cells and aging. Front Biosci 2002; 1:1056–1183.
36. Hanneuse Y, Delespesse G, Hudson D, de Halleux F, Jacques JM. Influence of ageing on IgE-mediated reactions in allergic patients [abstr]. Clin Allergy 1978; 8:165–174.
37. Mediaty A, Neuber K. Total and specific serum IgE decreases with age in patients with allergic rhinitis, asthma and insect allergy but not in patients with atopic dermatitis. Immun Ageing 2005; 31:9.
38. Jackola DR, Pierson-Mullany LK, Daniels LR, et al. Robustness into advanced age of atopy-specific mechanisms in atopy-prone families. J Gerontol A Biol Sci Med Sci 2003; 58:99–107.
39. Burrows B, Barbee RA, Cline MG, Knudson RJ, Lebowitz MD. Characteristics of asthma among elderly adults in a sample of the general population. Chest 1991; 100:935–942.
40. Huss K, Naumann PL, Mason PJ, et al. Asthma severity, atopic status, allergen exposure and quality of life in elderly persons. Ann Allergy Asthma Immunol 2001; 86:524–530.
41. Calkins E, Davis PJ, Ford AB. The Practice of Geriatrics. Philadelphia: W.B. Saunders, 1986.
42. Settipane GA, Chafee FH. Nasal polyps in asthma and rhinitis. A review of 6,037 patients [abstr]. J Allergy Clin Immunol 1977; 59:17–21.
43. Roth MT, Ivey JL. Self-reported medication use in community-residing older adults: a pilot study. Am J Geriatr Pharmacother 2005; 3:196–204.
44. Bateman ND, Woolford TJ. The rhinological side-effects of systemic drugs. Clin Otolaryngol Allied Sci 2003; 28:381–385.
45. Wang J, Eslinger PJ, Smith MB, Yang QX. Functional magnetic resonance imaging study of human olfaction and normal aging. J Gerontol A Biol Sci Med Sci 2005; 60:510–514.
46. Wormald PJ, Cain T, Oates L, Hawke L, Wong I. A comparative study of three methods of nasal irrigation. Laryngoscope 2004; 114:2224–2227.
47. Passali D, Damiani V, Passali FM, Passali GC, Bellussi L. Atomized nasal douche vs nasal lavage in acute viral rhinitis. Arch Otolaryngol Head Neck Surg 2005; 31:788–790.
48. Johnsen J, Bratt BM, Michel-Barron O, Glennow C, Petruson B. Pure sesame oil vs isotonic sodium chloride solution as treatment for dry nasal mucosa. Arch Otolaryngol Head Neck Surg 2001; 127:1353–1356.
49. Kaliner MA. H1-antihistamines in the elderly. Clin Allergy Immunol 2002; 17:465–481.
50. Hansen J, Klimek L, Hormann K. Pharmacological management of allergic rhinitis in the elderly: safety issues with oral antihistamines. Drugs Aging 2005; 22:289–296.
51. Kaiser HB, Findlay SR, Georgitis JW, et al. Long-term treatment of perennial allergic rhinitis with ipratropium bromide nasal spray 0.06%. J Allergy Clin Immunol 1995; 95:1128–1132.
52. Benninger MS, Ahmad N, Marple BF. The safety of intranasal steroids. Otolaryngol Head Neck Surg 2003; 129:739–750.
53. Heilmann S, Huettenbrink KB, Hummel T. Local and systemic administration of corticosteroids in the treatment of olfactory loss. Am J Rhinol 2004; 18:29–33.

54. Kern RC, Conley DB, Haines GK III, Robinson AM. Treatment of olfactory dysfunction. II: Studies with minocycline. Laryngoscope 2004; 114:2200–2204.
55. Caruso S, Roccasalva L, Di Fazio E, et al. Cytologic aspects of the nasal respiratory epithelium in postmenopausal women treated with hormone therapy. Fertil Steril 2003; 79:543–549.
56. Caruso S, Grillo C, Agnello C, Di Mari L, Farina M, Serra A. Olfactometric and rhinomanometric outcomes in post-menopausal women treated with hormone therapy: a prospective study. Hum Reprod 2004; 19:2959–2964.
57. Nappi C, Di Spiezio Sardo A, Guerra G, et al. Comparison of intranasal and transdermal estradiol on nasal mucosa in postmenopausal women. Menopause 2004; 11:447–455.
58. Asero R. Efficacy of injection immunotherapy with ragweed and birch pollen in elderly patients. Int Arch Allergy Immunol 2004; 135:332–335.
59. Busaba NY, Hossain M. Clinical outcomes of septoplasty and inferior turbinate reduction in the geriatric veterans' population. Am J Rhinol 2004; 18:343–347.

13 Rhinitis of Granulomatous and Vasculitic Diseases

Isam Alobid and Joaquim Mullol

Department of Otolaryngology, Rhinology Unit, University of Barcelona, and Institut d'Investigacions Biomèdiques August Pi i Sunyer (IDIBAPS), Barcelona, Catalonia, Spain

Maria Cinta Cid

Department of Internal Medicine, Vasculitis Research Unit, Hospital Clínic, University of Barcelona, and Institut d'Investigacions Biomèdiques August Pi i Sunyer (IDIBAPS), Barcelona, Catalonia, Spain

INTRODUCTION

There are a variety of systemic diseases including vasculitic, granulomatous, and autoimmune diseases that, among other body parts, also affect the lower and upper airways, including nasal mucosa and paranasal sinuses. The nasal symptoms and signs of these diseases are usually not specific and may mimic an allergic or nonallergic rhinitis, or even a chronic rhinosinusitis. When appropriate tests such as allergic skin-prick tests or blood tests give negative results, a systemic disease involving the nasal or paranasal layers should be suspected. In the present chapter, the authors have tried to provide a short but useful overview of the main vasculitic, granulomatous, and autoimmune systemic disorders to be included in the differential diagnosis of nonallergic rhinitis and chronic rhinosinusitis.

VASCULITIC DISEASES

The systemic vasculitides encompass a heterogeneous group of disorders with a common histopathologic substrate: inflammation of blood vessels. The inflammatory process may involve vessels of any magnitude, although different entities tend to preferentially target vessels of a particular size, and this feature has been considered in several classification/definition systems (Table 1) (1). The inflammatory process leads, in some instances, to the generation of extravascular inflammatory masses and, frequently, to the occlusion of involved vessels with the ensuing ischemia and necrosis of supplied tissues.

Among the systemic vasculitides, Wegener's granulomatosis (WG) and Churg-Strauss syndrome (CSS) typically involve the nasal cavity and paranasal sinuses. Less frequently, other necrotizing vasculitides such as microscopic polyangiitis, polyarteritis nodosa (PAN), and mixed cryoglobulinemia may generate lesions in the ear, nose, and throat (ENT) area.

Wegener's Granulomatosis

WG is an infrequent disease with an annual incidence of 6 to 58 per million, according to epidemiologic studies conducted in Europe (2). WG can arise in a wide range of ages from childhood to old age. Men and women are equally affected.

TABLE 1 The Chapel-Hill Nomenclature of the Systemic Vasculitides

Large-vessel vasculitis	
Giant-cell (temporal) arteritis	Granulomatous arteritis of the aorta and its major branches, with a predilection for the extracranial branches of the carotid artery. It often involves the temporal artery. Usually occurs in patients older than 50 yr and is associated with polymyalgia rheumatica
Takayasu's arteritis	Granulomatous inflammation of the aorta and its major branches. Usually occurs in patients younger than 50 yr
Medium-sized vessel vasculitis	
Polyarteritis nodosa	Necrotizing inflammation of medium-sized or small arteries without glomerulonephritis or vasculitis in arterioles, capillaries, or venules
Kawasaki disease	Arteritis involving large, medium sized, and small arteries, and associated with mucocutaneous lymph node syndrome. Coronary arteries are often involved. Aorta and veins may be involved. Usually occurs in children
Small-vessel vasculitis	
Wegener's granulomatosis	Granulomatous inflammation involving the respiratory tract, and necrotizing vasculitis affecting small-to-medium-sized vessels (i.e., capillaries, venules, arterioles, and arteries). Necrotizing glomerulonephritis is common
Churg-Strauss Syndrome	Eosinophil-rich and granulomatous inflammation involving the respiratory tract, and necrotizing vasculitis affecting small-to-medium-sized vessels, and associated with asthma and eosinophilia
Microscopic polyangiitis	Necrotizing vasculitis, with few or no immune deposits, affecting small vessels (i.e., capillaries, venules, or arterioles). Necrotizing vasculitis involving small- and medium-sized arteries may be present. Necrotizing glomerulonephritis is very common
Henoch-Shönlein purpura	Vasculitis, with IgA-dominant immune deposits, affecting small vessels (i.e., capillaries, venules, or arterioles); typically involves skin, gut, and glomeruli, and is associated with arthralgias or arthritis
Mixed cryoglobulinemic vasculitis	Vasculitis with cryoglobulin immune deposits affecting small vessels and associated with cryoglobulins in serum. Skin and glomeruli are often involved
Cutaneous leukocytoclastic vasculitis	Isolated cutaneous leukocytoclastic vasculitis without systemic vasculitis or glomerulonephritis

Source: From Ref. 1.

WG is characterized by granulomatous involvement of the upper and lower respiratory airways. Microscopic examination typically discloses necrosis, mixed inflammatory infiltrates that frequently undergo granulomatous differentiation with multinucleated giant-cells, and inflammation of blood vessels. Vasculitis may involve capillary vessels, small- and medium-sized arteries and veins, and may affect a variety of organs, leading to a protean array of disease manifestations.

Rhinosinusal manifestations are the presenting symptoms of WG in about 73% of patients and develop at some point during the course of the disease in 90% or more (3–5). Infiltration of the nasal mucosa by granulomatous, necrotizing inflammation causes nasal obstruction, crusting, and bloody nasal discharge. Ulcers may also develop, and the progression of inflammatory lesions may lead to necrosis of the nasal septum and to saddle nose deformity (Fig. 1). Nasal mucosa disruption may lead to anosmia. Cacosmia due to tissue necrosis aggravated by secondary infection may also be present. Paranasal sinuses are frequently involved, and recurrent episodes of sinusitis with bloody/purulent nasal discharge frequently precede the appearance of other disease manifestations (Fig. 2). Lesions may be destructive, leading to the development of fistulae, and disrupted sinus architecture facilitates bacterial and fungal colonization and infection, which is also favored by immunosuppressive therapy. Distinction between active disease and secondary infection may be challenging during the course of the disease. Chronic nasal carriage of *Staphylococcus aureus* is associated with higher relapse rates in these patients (6). Additional ENT manifestations include recurrent serous otitis and mastoiditis. Hearing loss may appear and can be conductive, caused by recurrent serous, granulomatous or infectious otitis, or sensorineural, the latter presumably due to vasculitis.

Subglottic stenosis by granulomatous tissue or its resulting scars is a typical complication of WG (Fig. 3A). This complication is more frequent in children and adolescents and may critically impair the airflow, requiring transient or permanent tracheostomy (7).

The lower respiratory tract is involved in 85% of patients. Pulmonary nodules, cavities, and atelectasia secondary to bronchial stenosis are the most typical manifestations (Fig. 3B). Diffuse alveolar hemorrhage is a life-threatening complication.

Eye involvement is frequent (50%) and may include a variety of lesions including episcleritis, granulomatous conjunctivitis, scleritis, keratitis, uveitis, and nasolacrimal duct obstruction. Granulomatous masses in the orbits may cause proptosis and impairment in ocular motion, leading to diplopia. Patients may lose

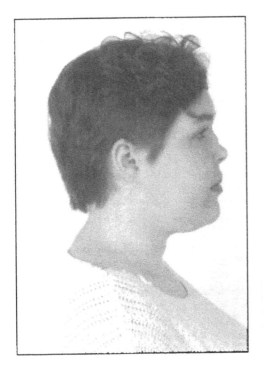

FIGURE 1 Saddle nose deformity in a patient with Wegener's granulomatosis. Cushing's features (round face and obesity) due to corticosteroid treatment can also be appreciated. *Source:* Courtesy of Dr. Gary S. Hoffman, Cleveland Clinic, Cleveland, Ohio, U.S.A.

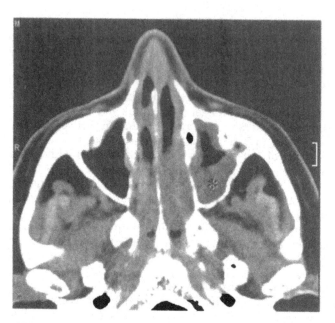

FIGURE 2 Computed tomography scan disclosing inflammatory tissue occupying both nasal cavities and the left maxillary sinus in a patient with Wegener's granulomatosis.

vision due to ulcerative keratitis or scleritis, orbit pseudotumor, or vasculitis, leading to optic nerve or retinal ischemia.

Systemic vasculitis may involve any organ. The kidney is involved in 75% of cases, and pauci-immune–necrotizing glomerulonephritis is the underlying lesion. However, identical lesions can be found in other vasculitides such as microscopic polyangiitis and renal-limited vasculitis. Granulomatous lesions can be found in some biopsies, and this finding supports the diagnosis of WG. Early manifestations may consist only of urinary sediment abnormalities (microhematuria with red cell casts) and mild proteinuria. However, impairment of renal function is common and rapidly progressive renal failure may occur. Skin and peripheral nerve involvement are not infrequent, and systemic symptoms such as fever, arthritis, or weight loss may be observed in 30% to 50% of patients.

The diagnosis and management of WG requires a multidisciplinary approach. WG can be diagnosed when typical lesions (necrosis, granuloma, and vasculitis) are demonstrated in the upper or lower respiratory airways. Mycobacterial or fungal infection must be ruled out with specific stainings, cultures, or molecular techniques. Although biopsies from ENT lesions are easier to obtain than open lung biopsies, the diagnostic yield is lower. In a survey from 126 biopsies taken from the ENT area, mostly nose and paranasal sinuses, Devaney et al. found typical lesions in only 16% of WG patients; in 23%, granuloma and vasculitis were found. Twenty-three percent showed only necrosis and the remaining, nonspecific inflammatory changes (Fig. 4) (8). Antineutrophil cytoplasmic antibodies (ANCA) are typically detected in sera from patients with WG and are thought to contribute to the development of vessel inflammation and injury. ANCA can be detected by indirect immunofluorescence and, in WG, almost invariably display a cytoplasmic

(A)

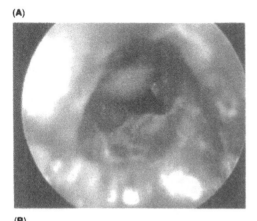

(B)

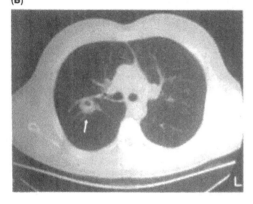

FIGURE 3   Involvement of other organs by Wegener's granulomatosis. (A) Subglottic stenosis by granulomatous tissue in a patient with Wegener's grannulomatosis. (B) Computed tomography scan showing a pulmonary cavity (arrow) in a patient with Wegener's granulomatosis. Source: Courtesy of Dr. Gary S. Hoffman, Cleveland Clinic, Cleveland, Ohio, U.S.A.

pattern on ethanol-fixed neutrophils and recognize proteinase 3 (PR3). In an appropriate clinical context, ANCA-PR3 detection strongly suggests the diagnosis of WG.

Several disorders must be considered in the differential diagnosis of WG. Destructive ENT lesions can be found in other processes such as nasal lymphoma of T/natural killer (TNK) phenotype, relapsing polychondritis (RPC) and granulomatous infections. Lung infections and angiocentric lymphoma may mimic WG pulmonary lesions.

WG is a chronic, relapsing, and potentially a life-threatening disease. Treatment relies, at present, on corticosteroids and immunosuppressive agents, which have proved to be lifesaving and efficient in inducing disease remission, but not in curing the disease. Patients cumulate disease and treatment-derived morbidity over the years (3). Cyclophosphamide must be given to patients with severe generalized disease, but must be switched to a safer immunosuppressive agent (azathioprine, mycophenolate, or methotrexate) when remission is obtained (9). These agents can be tried as a first option in patients without kidney involvement (10). Biologic therapies are under investigation. In spite of the expectations raised by experimental data and open-label studies, blocking TNF-α with etanercept has failed to add additional efficacy to the standard therapy in a large multicenter, randomized, placebo-controlled, double-blind study performed in patients with

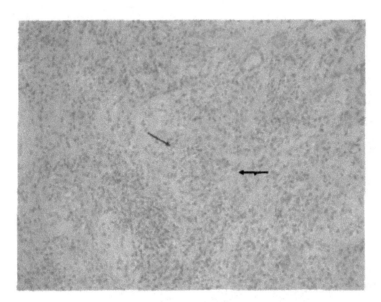

FIGURE 4 Nasal mucosa biopsy from a patient with Wegener's granulomatosis. Vasculitis (*arrows*) with chronic inflammation in the surrounding tissue can be appreciated. Granulomas could not be demonstrated in this specimen.

WG (11). Preliminary results have suggested the potential efficacy of B-cell depletion, and clinical trials are ongoing to assess this point.

Churg-Strauss Syndrome

CSS is a rare condition that may complicate the outcome of patients with asthma. Annual incidence of CSS in the general population is six cases per million and 64 per million among patients with asthma. CSS most frequently appears in patients between 30 and 50 years, but may affect people within a wide spectrum of ages (5,12,13).

CSS frequently progress through three stages, which may appear gradually over the years, may develop in a subacute or, in some cases, abrupt presentation. The first stage is characterized by asthma and increased blood eosinophil counts. In this stage, ENT abnormalities are common and include allergic rhinitis, nasal polyps, and recurrent sinusitis (Fig. 5A). Eustachian tube dysfunction and secondary middle ear infection may also occur. Anosmia is very frequent. This stage may last from months to years before CSS fully develops. At this point, the diagnosis of CSS syndrome must be considered, and patients must be carefully evaluated and followed, but a definite diagnosis of CSS cannot be established if no additional features are present because many patients never progress to subsequent stages. The following stage is characterized by tissue eosinophilia. Infiltration by eosinophils may involve the nasal and sinusal mucosa (Fig. 5A), lungs (Fig. 5B), skin, the gastrointestinal tract, and the heart. At this stage, CSS may be difficult to distinguish from other hypereosinophilic conditions such as primary hypereosinophilic syndrome, fleeting lung infiltrates due to parasitic diseases, eosinophilic gastroenteritis, and chronic eosinophilic pneumonia. The existence of asthma and ENT

(A)

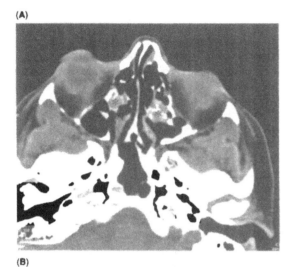

(B)

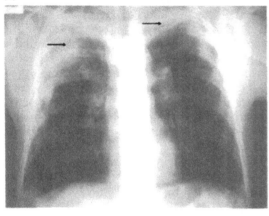

FIGURE 5 Patient with Churg-Strauss syndrome: **(A)** incipient ethmoidal sinusitis, and **(B)** pulmonary infiltrates with predominant apical involvement of both lungs.

symptoms is an important clue for the diagnosis. Fully developed disease includes manifestations related to systemic necrotizing vasculitis, which may involve a variety of territories leading to a wide array of clinical manifestations. Involvement of peripheral nerves manifesting as mononeuritis multiplex is frequent. Skin, gastrointestinal, heart, and kidney involvement are also common.

From the histopathologic point of view, vasculitis in CSS may involve small- and medium-sized vessels and may be indistinguishable from other systemic necrotizing vasculitis. The presence of accompanying extravascular eosinophilic granulomas is highly suggestive of CSS. The diagnosis of CSS requires both clinical and histopathologic features. Diagnostic criteria are not fully established (14). According to the American College of Rheumatism classification criteria, a patient with vasculitis can be classified as having CSS, if four of the following are present: asthma, eosinophilia >10%, peripheral neuropathy, pulmonary infiltrates, paranasal sinus abnormality, or extravascular eosinophil infiltration on biopsy findings (15). ANCA with a perinuclear pattern (pANCA) can be detected in about 40% to 70% of patients and usually have specificity for myeloperoxidase.

Patients with CSS require treatment with corticosteroids. Several factors indicating poor prognosis have been identified and include cardiac, gastrointestinal tract, central nervous system (CNS) involvement, and proteinuria >1 g/24 hr (16). If at least two of these are present, immunosuppressive agents are warranted. Pulse IV cyclophosphamide is usually used for these patients. Relapses are common when corticosteroids are tapered and frequently involve the ENT area. Rhinitis, nasal stuffiness due to congestion or polyps, sinusitis, and Eustachian tube dysfunction with secondary otitis are common forms of smouldering activity in these patients. About one-third of patients require sustained oral steroids to control asthma and rhinosinusal manifestations. Severe clinical manifestations related to vascular involvement are fortunately less common during relapses. CSS patients may eventually benefit from investigational products tested in the field of vasculitis or asthma. The rarity of this disease makes the performance of clinical trials difficult.

Microscopic Polyangeiitis

Microscopic polyangeiitis (MPA) is a systemic necrotizing vasculitis involving small vessels. Blood vessel inflammation may target a variety of organs, but kidneys are the most characteristically involved. Renal lesions consist of necrotizing crescentic glomerulonephritis. Vasculitis in the interstitial vessels can be also found. Alveolar capillaritis is a typical pulmonary lesion and may lead to diffuse alveolar hemorrhage, which is a severe complication. Vessels supplying additional territories such as skin, perineural vessels, or the gastrointestinal tract can be also involved (5). Glomerulonephritis and alveolar capillaritis are indistinguishable from those found in WG. The most distinctive feature differentiating both entities is the granulomatous involvement of the respiratory tract, characteristic of WG, and absent in MPA. MPA may involve the ENT area. Rhinitis and nasal crusting can be seen in MPA, but are usually much less prominent than in WG. Histopathologic examinations disclose chronic inflammation or vasculitis but not granulomatous lesions. ANCA can be detected in about 70% of patients with MPA. ANCA positivity assessed by indirect immunofluorescence on ethanol-fixed neutrophils discloses a perinuclear distribution (pANCA) in MPA and usually recognizes myeloperoxidase.

Patients with MPA must be treated with corticosteroids and immunosuppressive agents. When kidney or lung involvement patients are present, they must receive cyclophosphamide, either in a daily oral or monthly IV pulse regime, depending on the severity. For less severe cases or for maintenance of remission, less-aggressive immunosuppressive agents such as methotrexate or azathioprine can be used (9,10,17).

Polyarteritis Nodosa

Classical PAN is a systemic necrotizing vasculitis involving medium-sized arteries. ENT involvement is rare in this disease. Some cases, reported in the literature, with nasal ulcers or septum necrosis, may correspond to other necrotizing vasculitis because they were published prior to the recognition of MPA as a separate entity or prior to the availability of ANCA testing (18).

Cryoglobulinemic Vasculitis

Cryoglobulinemia is defined by the presence of circulating immunoglobulins (Igs) able to reversibly precipitate at cold temperatures. Cryoglobulinemias may be classified into three types. In Type I, cryoglobulins are monoclonal and usually are generated by late B-cell differentiation stage malignancies such as multiple myeloma or Waldeström macroglobulinemia. Type II or mixed cryoglobulinemias have a monoclonal component forming complexes with polyclonal Igs. The monoclonal component is usually an IgM with anti-IgG activity, leading to the formation of immune complexes with rheumatoid factor activity. Type III cryoglobulins are complexes formed by polyclonal Igs. Type II and Type III cryoglobulins can be found in association with chronic infections and lymphoproliferative or autoimmune diseases. The most common cause of Type II cryoglobulinemia is hepatitis C virus (HCV) infection. Circulating Type II cryoglobulins can be found in about 30% of patients infected by HCV, but a minority of these patients develop cryoglobulinemic vasculitis (19,20).

Cryoglobulinemia can produce tissue injury through two main mechanisms: vascular occlusion by cryoprecipitates or inflammatory vessel damage (vasculitis) triggered by immune complexes. Vascular occlusion due to cryoprecipitates usually occurs in Type I monoclonal cryoglobulinemias in which the concentration of circulating cryoglobulins is high. Small vessels appear occluded by hyaline thrombi, and the resulting necrotic lesions appear in distal body regions, where temperature is lower, such as fingertips, ears, or nose. Vascular inflammation (vasculitis) mainly develops in the context of mixed cryoglobulins, which typically form immune complexes and is a much more frequent mechanism of vessel injury. Vasculitis frequently involves small vessels (capillaries and postcapillary venules) in the skin, leading to palpable purpura that can be seen at some point in 90% of patients. When arterioles or small arteries are involved in the deep dermis, necrotic skin ulcers may appear (Fig. 6). Kidney involvement (membranoproliferative glomerulonephritis) and peripheral neuropathy presenting as mononeuritis multiplex or symmetrical polyneuropathy are common.

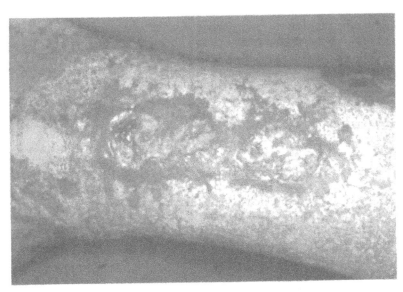

FIGURE 6 Cutaneous necrotic ulcers in a patient with hepatitis C virus–associated cryoglobulinemic vasculitis.

A variety of nonspecific nasal manifestations may be present: nasal obstruction, epistaxis, postnasal discharge, whistling, and crusting. Cases of nasal septal perforation secondary to cryoglobulinemic vasculitis have been reported (21). Because HCV-associated cryoglobulinemia is the most frequent, some of the nasal manifestations found in patients with cryoglobulinemia such as crusting may be related to Sjögren's syndrome (SS), a recognized extrahepatic complication of HCV infection.

Treatment of patients with cryoglobulinemia is complex and is frequently unsatisfactory. The main efforts must be addressed to treat the underlying condition. HCV infection is by far the most common cause of cryoglobulinemic vasculitis. Combination therapy with interferon alpha and ribavirin leads to a decrease in viral burden and improvement of clinical symptoms in a substantial proportion of patients, but relapses are frequent and side effects are remarkable. Current efforts are addressed to more efficiently reduce the viral load and delete B-cell clonalities. The management of patients with prominent manifestations derived from vascular inflammation/occlusion is difficult and, regardless of the underlying disease, requires the administration of corticosteroids and, in the most severe cases, immunosuppressive agents or plasmapheresis to remove circulating cryoglobulins. There are no clinical trials definitely supporting particular treatment regimens.

GRANULOMATOUS DISEASES

Granulomatosus Diseases of Unknown Etiology

Sarcoidosis

Sarcoidosis is a chronic multisystemic disorder of unknown etiology, which commonly affects young- and middle-aged adults, characterized histologically by noncaseating epithelioid granulomas involving various organs or tissues, with symptoms dependent on the site and degree of involvement. Sarcoidosis occurs commonly in mediastinal and peripheral lymph nodes, lungs, liver, eyes, and skin and less often in the spleen, bones, joints, skeletal muscle, heart, and CNS. The incidence of sarcoidosis greatly varies with race and country. Prevalence as high as 50 per 100,000 people has been reported, and females are affected more often than males (22). African-American women are at particular risk. Approximately 50% of patients are asymptomatic at diagnosis. Symptoms depend on the site of involvement and may be absent, slight, or severe. Fever, weight loss, and arthralgias may occur initially. Sinonasal involvement occurs with an incidence of 1%, but is not a typical presenting symptom of sarcoidosis. Nonspecific symptoms such as nasal obstruction, postnasal drip, crusting, congestion, epistaxis, chronic sinusitis, and headache are the typical initial complaints. The most consistent finding in the nose and sinuses is an erythematous, edematous, friable, hypertrophied mucosa. Subcutaneous granulomatous infiltration may also occur in the form of yellowish nodules predominantly in the septum and inferior turbinate. Epiphora or anosmia may also occur due to an occupation of lachrymal or olfactory cleft, respectively. Nasal polyposis, rhinophyma, and septal perforations can also exist in sarcoidosis. Aggressive noncaseating granulomas can cause hard and/or soft palate erosions creating an oral nasal fistula, as well as provoke a saddle nose deformity (23,24).

Chest X-ray findings of bilateral hilar and right paratracheal adenopathy occur in 90% of patients. Bronchoalveolar lavage shows lymphocytosis in most patients with active disease and the CD4/CD8 ratio on bronchoalveolar lavage is elevated. The Kveim reaction, a granulomatous reaction appearing four weeks after intradermal injection of sarcoid spleen or lymph node extracts, is positive in 50% to 60% of patients. Lung biopsy and histologic examination are essential for the diagnosis. When superficial or palpable lesions (e.g., in skin, lymph nodes, or conjunctiva) are present, biopsy is positive for sarcoidosis in more than 85% of such specimens. Leukopenia is frequently present, and serum uric acid elevation is common. In the earlier stages of sarcoidosis, there is no treatment. However, systemic steroids are needed as the disease progresses. Other treatments are the administration of chloroquine, immunosupressing agents, and lung transplantation. Although immunosuppressive drugs are often more effective in refractory cases, relapse is frequent after their cessation.

Idiopathic Midline Granuloma

In 1982, Tsokos et al. (25) identified a group of patients with idiopathic midline granuloma (IMG) who had distinctive clinicopathologic features that were aggregated under the term "idiopathic midline destructive disease." This was characterized as a locally destructive lesion limited to the upper respiratory tract and with no systemic involvement. In the current proposed World Health Organization classification of lymphoid malignancies, these tumors are classified as nasal-type extranodal NK/T-cell lymphoma (26). IMG presents over a wide range of ages, peaking in the sixth decade, with males predominating. The initial symptoms are usually those of a nonspecific rhinitis or sinusitis (with nasal obstruction and nasal discharge). Epistaxis and facial swelling may enter into the clinical spectrum as well. With disease progression, ulcerations spread, destroying the soft tissues, cartilage, and bone. Subsequently, facial pain and facial deformities develop (27). On physical examination, the most typical finding is the presence of a nasal septal perforation. The lesions are gray or yellow with a friable granular surface and arise on the nasal septum or midline palate. Large amounts of necrotic tissues are often present in the affected structures. Paranasal sinus computed tomography and magnetic resonance imaging are indicated to evaluate bone changes and to determine the extent of soft tissue, orbital, and intracranial involvement. After assessing the extent of the disease via radiographic imaging studies, the next step should be to exclude more common etiologies. Each disease has its own treatment based on histopathologic diagnosis such as immunosuppressive therapy and radiotherapy.

Pyogenic Granuloma

Pyogenic granuloma (PG) is a scarlet, brown, or blue–black vascular nodule composed of proliferating capillaries in an edematous stroma (28). It was originally thought to be a botryomycotic infection, but now is thought to be a response to minor trauma (produced by nasogastric tube, nasal packing, or nose-boring) with secondary invasion by microorganisms. There is no sex or age predilection. Nasal obstruction, purulent secretion, and bleeding are the most common symptoms (29). The PG tends to be friable, bleeds easily, and does not blanch on pressure. Treatment consists of removal by excision or curettage and electrodesiccation, but the lesions may recur.

Infectious Granulomas

Tuberculosis

Mycobacterium tuberculosis is the organism that is the causative agent for tuberculosis (TB). There are other "atypical" mycobacteria such as *Mycobacterium kansasii* that may produce a similar clinical and pathologic appearance of disease. Case rates vary by country, age, race, sex, and socioeconomic status. In 2001, the Centers for Disease Control and Prevention reported approximately 16,000 cases of TB in the United States, a significant decrease from the 28,000 cases reported in 1981 (30). Most countries located in the eastern part of Europe, Portugal, and Spain, reported 20 cases per 100,000 people. The incidence of TB has increased alarmingly among persons infected with HIV. Primary TB may become active at any age, producing clinical TB in any organ, most often the apical area of the lung but also the kidney, long bones, vertebrae, lymph nodes, and other sites. Classic symptoms are often absent, particularly in patients who are immunocompromised or elderly. Up to 20% of patients with active TB may be asymptomatic. Classic features associated with active TB are productive cough, hemoptysis, fever, night sweats, anorexia, and weight loss. Nasal manifestations in TB-affected patients are similar to common catarrh with rhinorrhea and nasal obstruction. The nasopharynx is the nasal site most commonly involved. Nasal endoscopy may reveal an adenoid hypertrophy normally associated to rhinorrhea and nasal obstruction with no characteristic features. Nasopharyngeal TB is mainly a primary infection often accompanied by cervical adenopathies. Nasal polyps can be observed predominantly growing from the inferior turbinate. TB should also be included in the differential diagnosis of septal perforation. The laboratory diagnosis of TB is based on acid-fast smear, culture, and tuberculin skin test. Recently, polymerase chain reaction as a diagnostic and confirmatory test has been introduced (31). Chest radiography consistent with TB indicates active disease in the symptomatic patient even in the absence of a diagnostic sputum smear result. The treatment is based on a multidrug anti-TB regime.

Leprosy

Leprosy is a chronic granulomatous disease, caused by *Mycobacterium leprae*, which affects principally the skin and peripheral nervous system in the hands and feet, and mucous membranes of the nose, throat, and eyes. Approximately 6000 patients with leprosy live in the United States; 95% of these patients acquired their disease in developing countries. In the United States, 200 to 300 cases are reported each year. In adults, the lepromatous type of leprosy is more common in men than women, with a male-to-female ratio of 2:1. In children, the tuberculoid form predominates, and no sex preference exists (32). The nasal mucosa and cartilage are affected in lepromatous patients; untreated patients often complain of chronic nasal congestion and, at times, epistaxis. Although uncommon, nasal cartilage perforation and collapse may result if leprosy goes untreated. Lepromatous leprosy is characterized by a chronic stuffy nose due to invasion of the mucous membranes, and the presence of nodules and lesions all over the body and face (33). Diagnosis of leprosy is most commonly based on the clinical signs and symptoms. Skin scraping examination for acid-fast bacteria (typical appearance of *M. leprae*) is definitive. A Lepromin skin test can be used to distinguish lepromatous from tuberculoid leprosy but is not used for diagnosis. Medications used to eliminate the microorganism and to reduce symptoms include dapsone, rifampin, clofazimine, and ethionamide.

Syphilis

Syphilis is a contagious systemic disease caused by the spirochete *Treponema pallidum*, characterized by sequential clinical stages and by years of latency.

The prominent histologic features of the human response to the presence of *T. pallidum* are vascular changes with associated endarteritis and periarteritis. From 1990–2000, there was a 90% reduction in the number of reported cases of primary; secondary syphilis falling to 2.1 per 100,000, which is the lowest rate ever reported in the United States (34). The initial lesion of primary syphilis develops at the site of transmission; secondary syphilis develops about 4 to 10 weeks after the appearance of the primary lesion and has a wide range of presentations. The most common systemic manifestations include malaise, fever, myalgias, and arthralgias with a generalized body rash and lymphadenopathy. In the primary syphilis, the nose is not the typical location, although there exist reported cases with a nasal vestibule chancre. Secondary syphilis presents as an acute rhinitis with a great nasal discharge irritating the narines. Tertiary syphilis shows gummata of the nose, septum perforation and deformation, and saddle nose deformity, while nasopharynx is rarely involved. Nasal discharge is the main manifestation of congenital syphilis, occurring two weeks before the rash. Septum perforation and deformation can also occur (35). Diagnosis of syphilis is most commonly based on the clinical signs and symptoms, physical examination, lesion-based test (darkfield microscopy and fluorescent antibody staining), and nontreponemal [rapid plasma reagin (RPR) and Venereal Disease Research Laboratory (VDRL)] or treponemal [Fluorescent Treponemal Antibody Absorption (FTA-ABS), IgG, and Western Blot] serologic tests. Microorganism detection is useless for the diagnosis. The antibiotic of choice is penicillin-G. Doxycycline is an alternative in patients with penicillin allergy (36).

Invasive Fungal Sinusitis

Invasive fungal sinusitis (IFS) predominantly affects those with diabetes mellitus and immunodeficient (primary or acquired), oncologic, and elderly patients who present a high rate of mortality (50% to 80%). The *Mucor* family and *Aspergillus fumigatus* are the fungi most commonly associated with an aggressive behavior capable of inducing bone destruction. IFS includes the acute fulminant type, which has a high mortality rate if not recognized early and treated aggressively, and the chronic and granulomatous types (37). Acute IFS results from a rapid spread of fungi through vascular invasion into the orbit and CNS. Typically, patients with acute IFS are severely ill with fever, cough, nasal discharge, headache, and mental status changes. Chronic IFS is a slowly progressive fungal infection, a low-grade invasive process, and usually occurs in patients with diabetes. Orbital apex syndrome usually is associated with this condition. Granulomatous IFS has been reported in immunocompetent individuals who are almost exclusively from North Africa. Generally, proptosis is associated with granulomatous IFS. Early diagnosis for IFS is critical for survival. Histopathological evidence of hyphal forms within sinus mucosa, submucosa, blood vessels, or bone confirms the diagnosis. The treatment consists of a surgical aggressive debridement plus prolonged intravenous antifungal (amphotericin B) medication (38).

Rhinoscleroma

Rhinoscleroma (RS) is a chronic granulomatous condition of the nose and other structures of the upper respiratory tract. RS is a result of infection by the bacterium *Klebsiella rhinoscleromatis*. RS is contracted by means of the direct inhalation of droplets of contaminated material. The disease probably begins in areas of epithelial transition such as the vestibule of the nose, the subglottic area of the larynx, or the area between the nasopharynx and oropharynx (39). RS tends to affect females somewhat more often than it does males and typically appears in patients aged 10 to 30 years. Patients may present with nasal obstruction, rhinorrhea, epistaxis, nasal deformity, and anosmia. The diagnosis of RS requires a bacterial identification and positive result with culturing in MacConkey agar (positive in 50% to 60% of patients). The biopsy findings include large vacuolated Mikulicz cells (large macrophage with clear cytoplasm that contains the bacilli) and transformed plasma cells with Russell bodies. Treatment should include long-term antimicrobial therapy (ciprofloxacin) and surgical intervention in patients with symptoms of obstruction (40). The course of RS is usually chronic, and relapses can occur.

Rhinosporidiosis

Rhinosporidiosis is a chronic granulomatous infection of the mucous membranes, which usually manifests as vascular friable polyps that arise from the nasal mucosa. Infection usually results from a local traumatic inoculation with the *Rhinosporidium seeberi* (41). Rhinosporidiosis can cause prolonged painless disease with limited morbidity. Men (between 15 and 40 years) are affected more commonly than women, with a male-to-female ratio of 4:1. Nose and nasopharynx were the commonest (85%) sites involved followed by ocular tissue (9%) (42). Eye involvement initially is asymptomatic. Increased tearing may be reported as the disease progresses. Photophobia, redness, and secondary infection may occur. Nasal manifestations may present with unilateral nasal obstruction, epistaxis, sneezing, rhinorrhea, or postnasal discharge. Diagnosis is made by identifying the typical structures of *R. seeberi* directly on microscopic examination of macerated tissue or histology of prepared biopsy sections. The treatment of choice is wide surgical excision to avoid recurrences.

AUTOIMMUNE DISEASES

Systemic Lupus Erythematosus

A multisystem, autoimmune inflammatory condition characterized by a fluctuating, chronic course that can affect virtually any body system. The cause of SLE remains elusive. Predisposing factors include genetic factors (certain types of human leukocyte antigens and null complement alleles), environmental factors including sun exposure, some drugs such as sulfa antibiotics, and hormonal factors. The incidence of SLE is 5.6 per 100,000 people, with an estimated prevalence of 130 per 100,000 (43). SLE is more common in blacks and is obviously more common in women than in men (ratio: 10:1). It varies from mild to severe and may be lethal (CNS and renal forms). The most common symptoms include extreme fatigue, painful or swollen joints (arthritis), unexplained fever, skin rashes, and kidney problems. The skin of the nose and nasal vestibule can be involved in the skin rashes. Shallow ulcers of the nasal mucosa and chronic bacterial sinusitis have been reported with increasing frequency (44). Nasal perforations are uncommon.

The diagnosis of SLE requires a thorough history, a physical examination, and laboratory tests, including a complete blood cell count, chemistry panel, and urinalysis. Serologic tests such as antinuclear antibodies, anti-Rh$_o$, anti-La, anti-ribonuclease protein, anti-Sm, anti-dsDNA, and antiphospholipid antibodies are helpful to confirm the diagnosis. There is no cure for SLE, but corticosteroid therapy or medications to suppress the immune system may be prescribed to control the various symptoms of this severe disease. The more severe the disease, the greater the risk of iatrogenic drug-induced complications, which further increase morbidity and mortality. The prognosis for patients with SLE has greatly improved over the last few decades, and this improvement reflects the general advancements in health care (i.e., dialysis, antibiotics, antihypertensives, and newer immunosuppressives with more favorable efficacy to toxicity ratio), but also the specialized care available for patients with SLE.

Sjögren's Syndrome

SS is an autoimmune disorder of unknown cause characterized by lymphocytic infiltration of salivary and lachrymal glands leading to xerostomia and keratoconjunctivitis sicca, and systemic production of autoantibodies (45). An association between SS and the HLA class II markers DR3 and DQ2 has been found (46). SS affects 1% to 3% of general population and predominates in women. SS may affect only the eyes or mouth (primary SS, sicca complex, and sicca syndrome), or generalized collagen vascular disease (secondary SS) may be present. Arthritis occurs in about 33% of patients. The most common nasal symptoms are epistaxis, crusting, hyposmia/anosmia, and hypogeusia. Nasal mucosa atrophy may be found in approximately 50% of patients at nasal endoscopy. Chronic sinusitis and nasal perforations are less common (47).

Once SS is suspected, the physician should request a variety of blood tests including antinuclear antibody, rheumatoid factor, erythrocyte sedimentation rate, and Igs. Other tests may also be of help: Schirmer test measures tear production, parotid gland flow, sialography, and lip biopsy used to confirm lymphocytic infiltration of the minor salivary glands. Treatment is based on the symptoms. Dry eyes are treated with artificial tears, a tear stimulant, or eye lubricant. Dry mouth may be helped by frequent small drinks of water, or chewing gum to stimulate saliva production. Arthritis symptoms are treated with corticosteroids and immunosuppressive drugs (48). Prognosis in SS is often related to the associated connective tissue disorder, although the disease is chronic and death may also occasionally result from pulmonary infection and, rarely, from renal failure or lymphoma.

Scleroderma

Scleroderma (systemic sclerosis) is a chronic disorder characterized by degenerative changes and scarring in the skin, joints, and internal organs and by blood vessel abnormalities (49). The cause of scleroderma is not known. The disorder is four times more common in women than in men. The peak onset occurs in patients aged 30 to 40 years. Scleroderma can damage large areas of skin or only the fingers (sclerodactyly). One form of scleroderma, called limited scleroderma, tends to stay restricted to the skin of the hands. In another form, called diffuse scleroderma, the disorder progresses; the skin becomes more widely taut, shiny, and darker than usual. The nasal mucosa of patients with scleroderma show initial goblet cell hyperplasia, loss of cilia and microvilli, exfoliation of the superficial epithelial layers, increased glandular activity in cases with squamous metaplasia, and fibrous tissue deposition in the lamina propria (50,51). Laboratory tests alone cannot identify scleroderma because test results, like the symptoms, vary greatly. The course of scleroderma varies and is unpredictable, sometimes being fatal. Nonsteroidal anti-inflammatory drugs (NSAIDs) or immunosuppressive therapy help relieve severe muscle and joint pain. Digital sympathectomy may be used for patients with severe Raynaud's phenomenon. Physical therapy and exercise can help to maintain muscle strength.

Antiphospholipid Syndrome

Antiphospholipid syndrome (APS) is an autoimmune disorder of unknown cause characterized by a combination of clinical features that consist of thrombotic- or pregnancy-related events and autoimmune antiphospholipid antibodies (52). In the 1998 International Consensus Preliminary Criteria, APS is defined by the concomitant presence of these clinical features and laboratory tests, including solid immunoassay and lupus anticoagulant. Actual frequency in the general population is unknown. The most frequent clinical manifestation is renal dysfunction due to the presence of renal thrombotic microangiopathy. Pulmonary manifestations range from multiple pulmonary emboli to the fatal acute respiratory distress syndrome. Nasal examination occasionally demonstrates a silent nasal septum perforation (53). The hallmark result from laboratory tests, which defines APS, is the presence of antiphospholipid (aPL) antibodies or abnormalities in phospholipid-dependent tests of coagulation. It is now accepted that unfractionated or low-molecular-weight heparin in combination with low-dose aspirin represents the current standard treatment for pregnant women with antiphospholipid antibodies, and high-dose Ig is considered as a salvage therapy for refractory APS.

Relapsing Polychondritis

RPC is characterized by episodes of painful, destructive inflammation of the cartilage and other connective tissues in many organs (54). By 1997, 600 cases of RPC had been reported worldwide. It may occur at any age with no gender distribution difference. At least three of the following criteria are needed for the diagnosis of RPC of the pinna, nose, larynx, or trachea: ocular alterations, sensorineural hearing loss, and seronegative arthritis. The etiology of this rare disease is unknown; however, the pathogenesis most likely is autoimmune. The evidence for an autoimmune etiology includes pathology findings of infiltrating T-cells, the presence of antigen–antibody complexes in affected cartilage, and cellular and humoral responses against collagen Type II and other collagen antigens. Nasal chondritis occurs in 48% to 72% of patients with RP. Typically, the onset of nasal chondritis is acute, painful, and accompanied by a feeling of fullness over the nasal bridge. Mild epistaxis may be present. No specific diagnostic laboratory findings exist in patients with RPC. A biopsy of the affected cartilage may show characteristic abnormalities. Mild RPC can be treated with aspirin or other NSAIDs. In more severe cases, daily doses of prednisone are given. Sometimes very severe cases are treated with immunosuppressives. These drugs treat the symptoms but have not been shown to alter the ultimate course of the disorder (55). Recently, Trentham and Le found a survival rate of 94% at five years (56).

CONCLUSIONS

A variety of granulomatous and vascular diseases are associated with nasal manifestations. Primary care physicians as well as ENT specialists and allergologists should keep in mind these differential diagnoses when treating nasal or paranasal sinus pathology.

ACKNOWLEDGMENTS

Dr. Isam Alobid is the recipient of the 2004 Award on Clinical Research by the European Rhinologic Society. Dr. M.C. Cid is supported by Ministerio de Educación y Ciencia (SAF 02/3307 and 05/6250). Dr. Joaquim Mullol's research is supported in part by Ministerio de Sanidad y Consumo–Instituto Carlos III (FIS 99-3121), Generalitat de Catalunya (2001SGR0384), and SEPAR—Red RESPIRA (C03/11).

REFERENCES

1. Jennette JC, Falk RJ, Andrassy K, et al. Nomenclature of systemic vasculitis. Proposal of an International Consensus Conference. Arthritis Rheum 1994; 37:187–192.
2. Watts R, Lane S, Scott DG. What is known about the epidemiology of systemic vasculitis? Best Pract Res Clin Rheumatol 2005; 19:191–207.
3. Hoffman GS, Kerr GS, Leavitt R, et al. Wegener's granulomatosis: an analysis of 158 patients. Ann Intern Med 1992; 116:488–498.
4. Metaxaris G, Prokopakis EP, Karatzanis AD, et al. Otolaryngologic manifestations of small vessel vasculitis. Auris Nasus Larynx 2002; 29(4):353–356.
5. Seo P, Stone JH. The anti-neutrophil cytoplasmic antibody-associated vasculitides. Am J Med 2004; 117:39–50.
6. Stegeman CA, Tervaert JW, Sluiter WJ, Manson WL, de Jong PE, Kallenberg CG. Association of chronic nasal carriage of Staphylococcus aureus and higher relapse rates in Wegener's granulomatosis. Ann Intern Med 1994; 120:12–17.
7. Langford CA, Sneller MC, Hallahan CW, et al. Clinical features and therapeutic management of subglottic stenosis in patients with Wegener's granulomatosis. Arthritis Rheum 1996; 39:1754–1760.
8. Devaney KO, Travis WD, Hoffman GS, Leavitt RY, Lebovics RS, Fauci AS. Interpretation of head and neck biopsies in Wegener's granulomatosis. A pathologic study of 126 biopsies in 70 patients. Am J Surg Pathol 1990; 14:555–564.
9. Jayne D, Rasmussen N, Anfrassy K, et al. European vasculitis study Group. A randomized trial of maintenance therapy for vasculitis associated with anti-neutrophil cytoplasmic antibodies. N Engl J Med 2003; 349:36–44.
10. De Groot K, Rasmussen N, Bacon PA, et al. Randomized trial of cyclophosphamide versus methotrexate for induction of remission in early systemic anti-neutrophil cytoplasmic antibody-associated vasculitis. Arthritis Rheum 2005; 52:2461–2469.
11. Wegener's granulomatosis etanercept trial (WGET) research group. Etanercept plus standard therapy for Wegener's granulomatosis. N Engl J Med 2005; 352:351–360.
12. Gross WL. Churg-Strauss Syndrome: update on recent developments. Curr Opin Rheumatol 2002; 14:11–14.
13. Noth I, Strek ME, Leff AR. Churg-Strauss syndrome. Lancet 2003; 361:587–594.
14. Keogh KA, Specks U. Churg-Strauss syndrome: clinical presentation, antineutrophil cytoplasmic antibodies, and leukotriene receptor antagonists. Am J Med 2003; 115:284–290.
15. Masi AT, Hunder GG, Lie JT, et al. The American College of Rheumatology 1990 criteria for the classification of Churg-Strauss syndrome (allergic granulomatosis and angiitis). Arthritis Rheum 1990; 33:1094–1100.
16. Guillevin L, Lhote F, Gayraud M, et al. Prognostic factors in polyarteritis nodosa and Churg-Strauss syndrome. A prospective study in 342 patients. Medicine (Baltimore) 1996; 75:17–28.
17. Jayne D. How to induce remission in primary systemic vasculitis. Best Pract Res Clin Rheumatol 2005; 19:293–305.

18. Oristrell SJ, Bosch JA, Valdes OM, Knobel FH. Polyarteritis nodosa and perforation of the nasal septum. Med Clin (Barc) 1985; 84:673–674.
19. Ferri C, Zignego AL, Pileri SA. Cryoglobulins. J Clin Pathol 2002; 55:4–13.
20. Sansonno D, Damacco F. Hepatitis C virus, cryoglobulinemia, and vasculitis: immune complex relations. Lancet Infect Dis 2005; 5:227–236.
21. Smith I, Smith M, Mathias D, Wallis J. Cryoglobulinaemia and septal perforation: a rare but logical cause. J Laryngol Otol 1996; 110:668–669.
22. James DG. Sarcoidosis and other granulomatous disorders. In: James DG, ed. Epidemiology. New York: Marcel Dekker, 1994:729–743.
23. Long CM, Smith TL, Loehrl TA, Komorowski RA, Toohill RJ. Sinonasal disease in patients with sarcoidosis. Am J Rhinol 2001; 15:211–215.
24. Rottoli P, Bargagli E, Chidichimo C, et al. Sarcoidosis with upper respiratory tract involvement. Respir Med 2005; 100(2):253–257.
25. Tsokos M, Fauci AS, Costa J. Idiopathic midline destructive disease (IMDD): a subgroup of patients with the "midline granuloma" syndrome. Am J Clin Pathol 1982; 77:162–168.
26. Chan JKC, Jaffe ES, Ralfkiaer E. Extranodal NK/T-cell lymphoma, nasal type. In: Jaffe ES, Harris NL, Stein H, Vardiman JW, eds. World Health Organization Classification of Tumours. Pathology and Genetics of Tumours of Haematopoietic and Lymphoid Tissues. Lyon: IARC Press, 2001:204–207.
27. Rodrigo JP, Suarez C, Rinaldo A, et al. Idiopathic midline destructive disease: fact or fiction. Oral Oncol 2005; 41:340–348.
28. Mooney MA, Janniger CK. Pyogenic granuloma. Cutis 1995; 55:133–136.
29. Neves-Pinto RM, Carvalho A, Araujo E, Alberto C, Basilio-De-Oliveira, De Carvalho GA. Nasal septum giant pyogenic granuloma after a long lasting nasal intubation: case report. Rhinology 2005; 43:66–69.
30. Centers of disease control. Core curriculum on tuberculosis. Available at: www.cdc.gov/nchstp/tb/pubs/corecurr/default.htm. Accessed 1/13/03.
31. Hup AK, Haitjema T, de Kuijper G. Primary nasal tuberculosis. Rhinology 2001; 39:47–48.
32. Lockwood DNJ, Bryceson ADM: Leprosy. In: Champion RH, et al., eds. Rook/Wilkinson/Ebling Textbook of Dermatology. 6th ed. Vol. 2. Malden (MASS): Blackwell Science, 1998:1215–1235.
33. Davis BD. Bacterial and mycotic infections: leprosy. In: Davis BD, et al., eds. Microbiology. 3rd ed. New York: Harper & Row Publishers, 1980.
34. Groseclose SL, Brathwaite WS, Hall PA, et al. Summary of notifiable diseases, United States, 2002. Morb Mortal Wkly Rep 2004; 51:1–84.
35. Pletcher SD, Cheung SW. Syphilis and otolaryngology. Otolaryngol Clin North Am 2003; 36:595–605.
36. Boot JM, Oranje AP, de Groot R, et al. Congenital syphilis. Int J STD AIDS 1992; 3:161–167.
37. deShazo RD, O'Brien M, Chapin K, Soto-Aguilar M, Gardner L, Swain R. A new classification and diagnostic criteria for invasive fungal sinusitis. Arch Otolaryngol Head Neck Surg 1997; 123:1181–1188.
38. Alobid I, Bernal M, Calvo C, et al. Successful treatment of rhinocerebral mucormycosis by combination of endoscopic sinus surgery and amphotericin B. Am J Rhinology 2001; 15:327–331.
39. Thompson LD. Rhinoscleroma. Ear Nose Throat J 2002; 81:506.
40. Ammar ME, Rosen A. Rhinoscleroma mimicking nasal polyposis. Ann Otol Rhinol Laryngol 2001; 110:290–292.
41. Arseculeratne SN. Rhinosporidiosis: what is the cause? Curr Opin Infect Dis 2005; 18:113–118.
42. Makannavar JH, Chavan SS. Rhinosporidiosis—a clinicopathological study of 34 cases. Indian J Pathol Microbiol 2001; 44:17–21.
43. Uramoto KM, Michet CJ Jr., Thumboo J, et al. Trends in the incidence and mortality of systemic lupus erythematosus, 1950–1992. Arthritis Rheum 1999; 42:46–50.
44. Robson AK, Burge SM, Millard PR. Nasal mucosal involvement in lupus erythematosus. Clin Otolaryngol 1992; 17:341–343.

45. Talal N. Sjögren's syndrome: historical overview and clinical spectrum of disease. Rheum Dis Clin North Am 1992; 18:507–515.
46. Gottenberg JE, Busson M, Loiseau P, et al. In primary Sjogren's syndrome, HLA class II is associated exclusively with autoantibody production and spreading of the auto-immune response. Arthritis Rheum 2003; 48:2240–2245.
47. Mahoney EJ, Spiegel JH. Sjogren's disease. Otolaryngol Clin North Am 2003; 36:733–745.
48. Rasmussen N, Brofeldt S, Manthorpe R. Smell and nasal findings in patients with primary Sjogren's syndrome. Scand J Rheumatol Suppl 1986; 61:142–145.
49. Mitchell H, Bolster MB, LeRoy EC. Scleroderma and related conditions. Med Clin North Am 1997; 81:129–149.
50. Elwany S, Talaat M, Kamel N, Stephanos W. Further observations on nasal mucosal changes in scleroderma. A histochemical and electron microscopic study. J Laryngol Otol 1984; 98:879–886.
51. Willkens RF, Roth GJ, Novak A, Walike JW. Perforation of nasal septum in rheumatic diseases. Arthritis Rheum 1976; 19:119–121.
52. Nishiguchi T, Kobayashi T. Antiphospholipid syndrome: characteristics and obstetrical management. Curr Drug Targets 2005; 6:593–605.
53. Callot V, Sirieix ME, Cohen P, et al. Recurrent leg ulcers, intra-alveolar hemorrhage, perforation of the nasal septum: primary antiphospholipid syndrome? Ann Med Int 1995; 146:366–369.
54. Zeuner M, Straub RH, Rauh G, Albert ED, Scholmerich J, Lang B. Relapsing polychondritis: clinical and immunogenetic analysis of 62 patients. J Rheumatol 1997; 24:96–101.
55. Michet CJ Jr., McKenna CH, Luthra HS, O'Fallon WM. Relapsing polychondritis. Survival and predictive role of early disease manifestations. Ann Intern Med 1986; 104:74–78.
56. Trentham DE, Le CH. Relapsing polychondritis. Ann Intern Med 1998; 129:114–122.

14 Nonallergic Occupational Rhinitis

Johan Hellgren
Department of Otolaryngology, Head and Neck Surgery, Capio Lundby Hospital, University of Gothenburg, Göteborg, Sweden

Kjell Torén
Department of Occupational and Environmental Medicine, Sahlgrenska University Hospital, Göteborg, Sweden

INTRODUCTION

The nasal mucosa is the first line of defense that protects the lower airways from potentially harmful effects from the inhaled air, such as chemicals and particles. The activation of defensive nasal reflexes can cause nasal blockage, secretion, itching, and sneezing. Up to 40% of the population experience symptoms of this kind every day as an effect of the changes in the air surrounding us (1,2). The occupational environment constitutes a special challenge to the nasal defense, with exposures to dusts and chemicals in a prolonged and repetitive way. This can result in the development of occupational rhinitis.

The term "occupational rhinitis" has been in use since the beginning of the last century and refers specifically to rhinitis caused by exposure to irritants and sensitizers in the occupational environment (3,4). Occupational rhinitis can be of either allergic or nonallergic origin, but in this chapter we shall be focusing on nonallergic occupational rhinitis. The mechanism behind most occupational rhinitis is still unknown and several occupational exposures are known to cause symptoms through both allergic and nonallergic pathways. Because of this, and to clarify the role of nonallergic occupational rhinitis in the overall assessment of occupational rhinitis, allergic occupational rhinitis will be included to some extent in this chapter.

DEFINITION AND CLASSIFICATION OF NONALLERGIC OCCUPATIONAL RHINITIS

The symptoms of occupational rhinitis are identical to those of other forms of non-infectious rhinitis, e.g., nasal congestion, rhinorrhea, sneezing, and itching (2). In occupational rhinitis, there may be additional symptoms, such as an impaired sense of smell, nosebleeds, crust formation, and a reduced mucociliary transport rate (5). From a clinical point of view, nonallergic occupational rhinitis is occupational rhinitis without an immunoglobulin (Ig)E-mediated sensitivity to the exposed substance, as demonstrated by a negative radioallergosorbent test (RAST) or skin-prick test. The picture is, however, more complicated, because skin-prick test positivity to common aeroallergens has been found in 15% of asymptomatic individuals (6). This means that exposed subjects with nonallergic occupational rhinitis can be skin-prick test positive against specific exposures in the occupational environment without having an allergy.

The pathophysiology behind nonallergic rhinitis is thoroughly addressed elsewhere in this book, but the hypothesis behind nonallergic rhinitis includes a non–IgE-mediated inflammatory response with increased permeability of the nasal epithelium and an imbalance in the autonomous regulation of nasal patency, abnormal sensory nerve fibers, and C-fiber stimulation (7). Morphological changes in nasal mucosa, such as the loss of cilia, hyperplasia, and metaplasia, have also been associated with occupational exposure to airborne irritants and the development of nonallergic occupational rhinitis (3).

To identify patients with nonallergic occupational rhinitis, it is important to have a precise definition of the disease, because large population-based, epidemiological studies show that up to 20% of the population in the Western World have nonallergic rhinitis (8,9). Bachert has suggested a classification of nonallergic rhinitis into (i) idiopathic rhinitis or vasomotor rhinitis, (ii) irritative toxic or "occupational rhinitis," (iii) hormonal rhinitis, (iv) drug-induced rhinitis, and (v) other forms such as nonallergic rhinitis with eosinophilia syndrome. He has specified occupational rhinitis as rhinitis caused by airborne particles or gases in the workplace, such as chemicals, glues, solvents, and cigarette smoke, causing the stimulation of or damage to epithelial cells in the nasal mucosa via nonimmunologic mechanisms (10).

Baraniuk and Kaliner have suggested the further classification of occupational rhinitis into annoyance, immunological, irritational, and corrosive rhinitis (11). "Annoyance reaction" refers to a negative psychological state, at times with other transient physical symptoms related to the perception of offensive air quality, particularly offensive odors. "Immunological reaction" denotes allergic occupational rhinitis, such as allergy to laboratory animals, and is often characterized by rhinoconjunctivitis. "Irritational" occupational rhinitis denotes a neurogenic inflammation with a stinging or burning sensation in the eyes, nose, and throat and is caused by prolonged exposure to irritating chemicals. Neurogenic inflammation can be accompanied by reflex hypersecretion or nasal blockage, but is rapidly reversible and does not involve anatomic alterations on pathologic examination. Finally, "corrosive" occupational rhinitis denotes reversible or permanent damage to the respiratory or olfactory epithelium due to exposure to high concentrations of gases, vapors, smokes, or dusts. The entity "reactive upper-airways dysfunction syndrome (RUDS)" has been described after a single exposure to strong irritants such as chlorine and is modeled on the diagnosis of reactive airways dysfunction syndrome (12). Irritational and corrosive rhinitis are examples of nonallergic occupational rhinitis, where the effect depends mainly on the chemical properties of the substance and its ability to penetrate the nasal mucosa. In particular, a combination of high water solubility and chemical reactivity predispose such chemicals as chlorine, sulphur dioxide, ammonia, and formaldehyde toward producing upper airway irritative effects (4).

In contrast to allergic occupational rhinitis, where the sensitization involves repeated exposure and where symptoms are sometimes delayed in relation to the exposure, the nonallergic reaction can take place immediately after exposure and often improves as exposure is reduced. Nonallergic occupational rhinitis is often accompanied by nasal hyperreactivity, making the nasal mucosa sensitive to nonspecific irritation such as cold air exposure. Plavec et al. have demonstrated increased nasal hyperreactivity in workers exposed to several irritants such as fluorine, chlorine, phosphate dust, sulfur, ammonia, and urea compared with unexposed controls, without any relation to atopy (13).

EPIDEMIOLOGY OF OCCUPATIONAL RHINITIS

Occupational rhinitis is a common disease and the overall prevalence of occupational rhinitis has been estimated at 5% to 15% (4). In a population-based interview study from Singapore comprising 2868 adults, self-reported exposure to occupational irritants, without any further specification, was associated with a doubled risk of rhinitis (14). Population-based studies evaluating occupational rhinitis are, however, scarce and most data relating to occupational rhinitis are therefore derived from workplace studies.

To further evaluate the epidemiological data relating to occupational rhinitis, it is important to be familiar with the different study designs that are used. The three most common types of study design, "population-based questionnaire studies, workplace-based cohort studies, and nasal challenge studies," are shown in Table 1.

The Population-Based Questionnaire Study

The population-based (or cross-sectional) study is preferred when surveying an occupational exposure as a potential risk factor for occupational rhinitis. A large random population can readily be addressed at a comparatively low cost. One major advantage of this study design is that individuals who are no longer under exposure (but previously have been) at the time of the study are included. The weakness of the population-based questionnaire study is that it relies on self-reported data and is therefore subject to recall bias, especially if a long time has passed since the exposure (15). This means that subjects who have developed rhinitis are probably more prone to report exposure than those who have not.

The Workplace-Based Cohort Study

The most common study design in the identification of occupational rhinitis is the workplace-based cohort study. A group of workers who are exposed to a potential airborne irritant are compared with a matched sample (age, gender, smoking habits, etc.) of unexposed workers. This study design offers an excellent opportunity for an accurate diagnosis and a good exposure assessment, making it possible to evaluate dose–response relationships between symptoms and exposure. The main disadvantage of this study design is that workers who have developed symptoms from an exposure may have left the workplace or they may have changed jobs and are thus not included in the risk evaluation. This phenomenon is called "the healthy worker effect" and may lead to the risk being underestimated.

TABLE 1 Different Study Designs to Assess Nonallergic Occupational Rhinitis

Type of study design	Advantages	Disadvantages
Population-based questionnaire study	Low cost Large population All exposed individuals	Uncertain exposure data Recall bias Lack of clinical diagnosis
Nasal challenge	Symptoms on exposure Dose response Differential diagnosis	Expensive Time consuming Few centers
Workplace-based cohort studies	Good exposure data Individual exposure assessment Clinical diagnosis	Selection bias (healthy worker bias) Expensive Time consuming

Nasal Challenge

Some of the most reliable data relating to allergic occupational rhinitis come from nasal challenge studies (16). The nasal challenge test includes an initial provocation by instilling normotonic NaCl into the nose as placebo in the detection of nasal hyperreactivity. The allergens or substances that are tested are either soaked into small cotton disks that are placed on the inferior turbinate, or else the test solution is dropped directly onto the inferior turbinate (if cotton is expected to give a reaction). The challenge substance can also be introduced as an aerosol in a challenge chamber. The effect of the nasal challenge is assessed with anterior rhinoscopy, scoring swelling of the mucous membrane, secretion, and sneezing. Objective assessments of the reaction can be made with anterior or posterior rhinomanometry, acoustic rhinometry, or nasal peak flow measurements. A significant change in the scores evaluated by rhinoscopy or a 50% increase in nasal resistance by rhinomanometry is usually regarded as a positive provocation test (16,17).

Exposures

As previously outlined, there is no clear-cut border between occupational rhinitis of nonallergic and allergic origin and several known airborne sensitizers and irritants therefore exhibit both allergic and nonallergic properties. There is a tendency, however, for low-molecular-weight compounds to act primarily through nonallergic mechanisms, whereas high-molecular-weight compounds show a higher degree of specific sensitization (Table 2) (18). Nasal and ocular symptoms that precede or coexist with asthma are a feature of IgE-modulated conditions and are more frequently linked to high-molecular-weight compounds (19). The degree of sensitization in relation to particle size for some common exposures causing occupational rhinitis is shown in Table 2.

A list of substances known to cause nonallergic occupational rhinitis, on the basis of data from workplace-based studies, is given in Table 3. For comparison, the "Finnish Register of Occupational Disease" has registered most new cases of allergic occupational rhinitis in Finland since 1964 on the basis of nasal challenge tests. In the Finnish material (1244 cases of occupational rhinitis), animal dander, flours, wood dust and textile dust, food, spices, storage mites, enzymes, natural rubber latex, and chemicals were the most common types of exposure associated with allergic occupational rhinitis (21).

TABLE 2 Extensive Survey of Workplace-Based Studies of Exposed Workers

	Type of exposure	Prevalence of occupational rhinitis in exposed workers (%)	Prevalence of specific sensitization (%)
Low-molecular-weight compounds	Diisocyanates	36–42	1
	Anhydrides	10–60	5–16
	Platinum salts	12	14
	Reactive dyes	20–30	8–30
High-molecular-weight compounds	Laboratory animal allergens	10–33	6–46
	Flour dust	18–29	10–38
	Latex	9–12	5–20
	Biological enzymes	7–87	22–52
	Fish proteins	5–22	24–38

Source: From Ref. 18.

TABLE 3 Substances Known to Cause Nonallergic Occupational Rhinitis

Gases	VOCs	Dusts	Combustion products	Various
Ozone	Formaldehyde	Phosphate dust	Tobacco smoke	Urea
Sulfur dioxide	Toluene	Coal dust	Wood smoke	Phosphate fertilizers
Chlorine	Xylene	Western red cedar dust	Polymer pyrolysis products	Pesticides
Oxides of nitrogen	Miscellaneous VOCs	Talc dust	–	Cleaning agents
Ammonia	–	–	–	Acid aerosols
Hydrogen chloride	–	–	–	Cold air
Hydrogen fluoride	–	–	–	Fragrance products
–	–	–	–	Anhydrides

Abbreviation: VOCs, volatile organic compounds.
Source: From Refs. 4,20.

Surveys

When looking for new hazards in the occupational environment, the workplace-based study is less suitable for surveys because of the costs and organization associated with it. In a population-based questionnaire study, on the other hand, a large random population can be addressed and several exposures can easily be assessed. The authors' group has evaluated the risk of rhinitis after occupational exposure to several substances in 2044 adults in an industrialized county in Sweden. The subjects were asked whether they had problems with nasal symptoms, such as nasal congestion, itching/sneezing, and secretion without having a cold, which we defined as "noninfectious rhinitis," and the year the symptoms began. The time each subject was under exposure until the start of nasal symptoms or until the end of follow-up (for those under exposure, who did not develop symptoms) was regarded as the time at risk. This group was compared with the rest of the population who were not exposed during the same follow-up period. The results showed a significant increase in the risk of developing rhinitis after exposure to fire smoke, paint hardeners, and rapid glues, and working as a cleaner (22). In the absence of a nasal examination, nasal challenge, or skin-prick test, it is of course not possible to determine whether this association is allergic or nonallergic and the relationship therefore has to be further evaluated in a clinical study.

DIAGNOSING NONALLERGIC OCCUPATIONAL RHINITIS

Several objective methods have been used in the study of nonallergic occupational rhinitis to detect signs of nasal inflammation. These methods analyze the nose from different aspects of its function, such as inspection of the nasal mucosa (rhinoscopy), nasal airflow (peak nasal expiratory and inspiratory flow and anterior and posterior rhinomanometry), intranasal geometry (acoustic rhinometry), mucociliary transport rate, and inflammatory markers in secretion. A detailed review of these methods goes beyond the scope of this chapter. The overall conclusion is that objective assessment of nasal patency and inflammatory reactions in the nasal mucosa are vital to the understanding of the nonallergic reaction in occupational rhinitis, but the correlations between the objective methods and nasal symptoms are contradictory (23).

The lack of a gold standard method to diagnose nonallergic occupational rhinitis, however, makes the medical history especially important. The temporal relationship between the onset of exposure and the onset of nasal symptoms should therefore be analyzed thoroughly in nonallergic occupational rhinitis. Symptoms that started before the onset of the occupational exposure are not indicative of occupational rhinitis. In the early stages of nonallergic occupational rhinitis, there is often deterioration in symptoms during the working week, with an improvement during weekends and holidays (5). As the disease progresses, these patterns may become less apparent. In a study of woodwork teachers, Ahman and Soderman showed how the nasal symptoms deteriorated and the peak nasal expiratory flow decreased during the working week, only to return to basal values after the weekend (24).

Objective exposure assessment is of great importance in occupational rhinitis (4). At some workplaces, occupational exposure may be very complex, requiring detailed assessments with an industrial hygiene consultant, whereas simple questioning may elicit the suspect agent in many work practices (25). For example, acrylates should be suspected as a potential exposure whenever the use of rapid glues is reported. In cases where exposure to a single high-level irritant has triggered new-onset rhinitis, RUDS, an exposure history should be clear cut. This requires an extended occupational history. Information about the pattern of exposure can be important for some agents. In dye-house operators, a dose-response relationship has been demonstrated (18).

Allergy

Associated symptoms from the bronchi, conjunctiva, and skin are common in allergic occupational rhinitis and should be the subject of inquiry (4). A positive skin-prick test and/or RAST may indicate allergic occupational rhinitis. Sensitization may take from weeks to 20 years to develop. In a prospective study of 125 trainee bakers, the number of skin-prick–positive individuals to α-amylase increased from 4 to 10 in 30 months (26). It is, however, important, to differentiate between sensitization in subjects without symptoms and sensitized individuals with rhinitis. "Standard panel" skin-prick tests can be used to exclude nonoccupational forms of rhinitis, such as allergy to cats or mites. The possibility that several forms of rhinitis coexist in the same patient must, however, be taken into consideration. In paper recycling workers with a high prevalence of nasal catarrh, 54.5% of the workers were skin-prick test positive to mites and molds, while only 15.8% were positive to paper extracts (13).

Nasal provocation tests can be conducted in the workplace or in the laboratory (17,18,27). The provocation should be made when the rhinitis symptoms are at a minimum and in the absence of anti-inflammatory medication to avoid confounding (4). It has been suggested that monitoring the effect with symptom evaluation, rhinoscopy, and rhinomanometry should be standard (17). In Finland, legislation demands nasal provocation as a routine for diagnosis and several authors advocate its use (18,21,27).

TREATMENT OF NONALLERGIC OCCUPATIONAL RHINITIS

The treatment of nonallergic rhinitis will be thoroughly examined elsewhere in this book and does not differ when the cause is occupational rhinitis. The value of preventive measures to reduce exposure to hazardous substances in the occupational environment cannot, however, be overemphasized. As previously mentioned, symptoms in nonallergic occupational rhinitis usually disappear when exposure ceases, but it should be remembered that nonallergic rhinitis often includes nasal hyperreactivity as well. This means that unspecific irritants such as tobacco smoke and cold air may still be a problem for these patients long after the occupational exposure is over and this may still require medical treatment.

CONCLUSION

Nonallergic occupational rhinitis is a common disease characterized by a non–IgE-mediated inflammation in the nasal mucosa after exposure to occupational airborne irritants, predominantly low-molecular-weight chemicals. The diagnosis is based primarily on a thorough exposure and symptom history, the exclusion of other forms of rhinitis such as allergy and, if possible, confirmation by objective exposure measurements and a positive nasal challenge test.

REFERENCES

1. Eccles R. Rhinitis as a mechanism of respiratory defense. Eur Arch Otorhinolaryngol 1995; 252(suppl 1):S2–S7.
2. International Rhinitis Management Working Group. International Consensus Report on the diagnosis and management of rhinitis. Allergy 1994; 49(19):1–34.
3. Welch AR, Birchall JP, Stafford FW. Occupational rhinitis—possible mechanisms of pathogenesis. J Laryngol Otol 1995; 109(2):104–107.
4. Puchner TC, Fink JN. Occupational rhinitis. Immunol Allergy Clin North Am 2000; 20(2):303–322.
5. Drake-Lee A, Ruckley R, Parker A. Occupational rhinitis: a poorly diagnosed condition. J Laryngol Otol 2002; 116:580–585.
6. Droste J, Kerhof M, de Monchy J, Schouten J, Rijcken B. Dutch ECRHS group, 1996. Association of skin test reactivity, specific IgE, total IgE, and eosinophils with nasal symptoms in a community-based population study. J Allergy Clin Immunol 1997; 97(4):922–932.
7. Garay R. Mechanisms of vasomotor rhinitis. Allergy 2004; 59(suppl 76):4–10.
8. Jessen M, Janzon L. Prevalence of non-allergic nasal complaints in an urban and a rural population in Sweden. Allergy 1989; 44(8):582–587.
9. Olsson P, Berglind N, Bellander T, Stjarne P. Prevalence of self-reported allergic and non-allergic rhinitis symptoms in Stockholm: relation to age, gender, olfactory sense and smoking. Acta Otolaryngol 2003; 123(1):75–80.
10. Bachert C. Persistent rhinitis—allergic or nonallergic? Allergy 2004; 59(suppl 76):11–15.
11. Baraniuk JN, Kaliner MA. Functional activity of upper-airway nerves. In: Busse W, Holgate S, eds. Asthma and Rhinitis. Cambridge, Massachusetts: Blackwell Scientific, 1995:652–667.
12. Meggs WJ. RADS and RUDS—the toxic induction of asthma and rhinitis. J Toxicol Clin Toxicol 1994; 32(5):487–501.
13. Plavec D, Somogyi-Zalud E, Godnic-Cvar J. Nonspecific nasal responsiveness in workers occupationally exposed to respiratory irritants. Am J Ind Med 1993; 24(5):525–552.
14. Ng TP, Tan WC. Epidemiology of allergic rhinitis and its associated risk factors in Singapore. Int J Epidemiol 1994; 23(3):553–558.
15. Fritschi L, Siemiatycki J, Richardson L. Self-assessed versus expert-assessed occupational exposures. Am J Epidemiol 1996; 144(5):521–527.
16. Litvyakova L, Baraniuk J. Nasal provocation testing: a review. Ann Allergy Asthma Immunol 2001; 86:355–365.

17. Hytonen M, Sala E. Nasal provocation test in the diagnostics of occupational allergic rhinitis. Rhinology 1996; 34(2):86–90.
18. Siracusa A, Desrosiers M, Marabini A. Epidemiology of occupational rhinitis: prevalence, aetiology, and determinants. Clin Exp Allergy 2000; 30(11):1519–1534.
19. Malo JL, Lemiere C, Desjardins A, Cartier A. Prevalence and intensity of rhinoconjunctivitis in subjects with occupational asthma. Eur Respir J 1997; 10(7):1513–1515.
20. Baraniuk JN, Meltzer EO, Spector SL. Is it allergic, infectious, or nonallergic/noninfectious? Getting the cause of chronic rhinitis. J Respir Dis 1996; 17(suppl):24–33.
21. Hytonen M, Kanerva L, Malmberg H, Martikainen R, Mutanen P, Toikkanen J. The risk of occupational rhinitis. Int Arch Occup Environ Health 1997; 69(6):487–490.
22. Hellgren J, Lillienberg L, Jarlstedt J, Karlsson G, Torén K. Population-based study of non-infectious rhinitis in relation to occupational exposure, age, sex, and smoking. Am J Ind Med 2002; 42(1):23–28.
23. Hellgren J, Karlsson G, Torén K. The dilemma of occupational rhinitis: management options (review article). Am J Respir Med 2003; 2:333–341.
24. Ahman M, Soderman E. Serial nasal peak expiratory flow measurements in woodwork teachers. Int Arch Occup Environ Health 1996; 68(3):177–182.
25. Teschke K, Kennedy SM, Olshan AF. Effect of different questionnaire formats on reporting of occupational exposures. Am J Ind Med 1994; 26(3):327–337.
26. De Zotti R, Bovenzi M. Prospective study of work related respiratory symptoms in trainee bakers. Occup Environ Med 2000; 57(1):58–61.
27. Slavin RG. Occupational and allergic rhinitis: impact on worker productivity and safety. Allergy Asthma Proc 1998; 19(5):277–284.

15 Environmental Nonallergic Rhinitis

Dennis Shusterman

Occupational and Environmental Medicine Program, University of Washington, Seattle, Washington, U.S.A.

INTRODUCTION

"Environmental nonallergic rhinitis" can be defined by the occurrence of nasal symptoms, with or without inflammation, triggered nonallergically by physical or chemical factors in the inspired atmosphere. ["Nonallergically," in turn, signifies a lack of immunoglobulin (Ig)E-mediated mast cell degranulation in the acute response.] The term "irritant rhinitis" can be treated as a subset of environmental nonallergic rhinitis, referring to rhinitis, triggered (or initiated) by chemical irritants. Nasal symptoms can be classified as "primary" (irritation > pruritus) as well as "secondary" or reflex (airflow obstruction, and rhinorrhea). Related symptoms and signs (headache, earache) may derive from pressure disequilibrium in the paranasal sinuses and middle ear. The subset of environmental nonallergic rhinitis occurring in specific occupational settings is dealt with in a separate chapter by Hellgren and Toren. In this chapter, we consider the upper airway health effects of: *ambient air pollutants* (including gases, vapors, and particulate matter) as well as *the indoor environment* [(including "problem buildings"/"sick building syndrome" and environmental tobacco smoke (ETS)]. Finally, we briefly consider potential reflex response mechanisms to upper airway irritants as well as evidence for population variability in irritant susceptibility.

The organization of this chapter is as follows: the Background section reviews types and sources of irritants in ambient and indoor air, relevant nasal anatomy and physiology, and study techniques applied to the upper airway. Studies of environmental nonallergic rhinitis are then reviewed in the following order: (i) controlled human exposure studies, (ii) observational studies of air quality and the upper airway, and (iii) intervention studies. Finally, consideration is given to alternative mechanisms involved in irritant-related upper airway reflexes. Because of space limitations, the mechanistic discussion will include "downstream" (reflex) events but not "upstream" events such as neural transduction of chemical irritant signals.

BACKGROUND

Potential Exposures in Ambient and Indoor Air
Individuals with idiopathic nonallergic rhinitis typically give a history of nonspecific reactivity to physical and/or chemical factors in the air. Included in the former are changes in temperature, humidity, and barometric pressure, and extremes of air movement. The latter category—chemical irritants—includes indoor and outdoor (ambient) air pollutants; these are briefly reviewed below.

Prior to discussing air pollution sources, a review of basic terminology is in order. Environmental scientists classify air pollutants as gases, aerosols ("particulates"), or mixed-phase pollutants. Gaseous air pollutants include compounds that are gases under normal atmospheric conditions ("true" gases), as well as compounds that are liquids under normal conditions but have significant vapor pressures ("vapors"). Among aerosols, there are dusts (finely divided solids), mists (suspended liquid particles), and condensation nuclei (e.g., acid aerosols and "fumes"—the latter being strictly defined as nascent oxides of metals or polymers subjected to combustion, pyrolysis, or other heating processes). Among the above terms, the one that is subject to the greatest abuse in everyday language is the word "fume" (e.g., "paint fumes" instead of "paint-derived vapors"). "Smokes," also derived from combustion processes, typically involve a dynamic mixture of gases and particulate matter.

Ambient air pollutants are traditionally classified in the United States as either "criteria air pollutants" or "air toxics." *Criteria air pollutants* include the oxides of nitrogen, sulfur dioxide (SO_2), ozone, and particulate matter, with carbon monoxide (CO) and lead also being regulated for reasons unrelated to the respiratory tract. In addition to federal ambient air quality standards for criteria air pollutants, individual states can maintain more stringent standards and/or promulgate standards for other pollutants (e.g., the hydrogen sulfide standard in the state of California). Standards for criteria air pollutants are defined in terms of average and/or peak community air concentrations as documented by air-monitoring networks. Criteria air pollutant standards in the United States are health based and, in contrast to occupational standards, must take into consideration vulnerable subpopulations. *Air toxics* include carcinogens, reproductive toxicants, and respiratory irritants and, when regulations exist, they are generally aimed at emission sources ("smokestack standards" or total facility emissions). In addition, reference exposure levels and emergency planning levels have been promulgated for many air toxics to deal with episodic releases in industrial or transportation accidents. Ambient air irritant compounds affecting the upper airway (and therefore pertinent to environmental nonallergic rhinitis) include both criteria air pollutants and air toxics.

Indoor air can be problematic with regard to its physical, chemical, or biological properties. Identified physical factors include extremes of temperature, humidity, or air movement (1–3). Chemical agents in indoor air can include combustion products (ETS, exhaust from malfunctioning combustion appliances, and reintrained vehicular exhaust) as well as volatile organic compounds (VOCs) (from building materials, interior furnishings, and building maintenance products such as cleaners and floor waxes). In addition, active microbial growth can produce microbial VOCs (MVOCs), some of which are specific with regard to source (i.e., "unique MVOCs") (4–6). Potent irritants can also be formed indoors from chemical reactions between ozone or nitrogen oxides and VOCs (especially terpenes) (7–9). Finally, indoor aeroallergens may infiltrate from ambient air (pollens and mold spores), be passively transferred from homes via wearing apparel (pet danders), or originate indoors from dust mites or from microbial growth. As these allergens can coexist with irritants, the distinction between allergic and nonallergic symptoms may be problematic in specific cases.

Anatomy and Innervation of the Upper Airway

Given the detailed treatment this subject has received elsewhere in this volume by Dr. Baroody, an abbreviated discussion of anatomy and physiology is offered here. The nasal cavity is invested with a highly vascular lining which, in combination with the extended surface area conveyed by the turbinates, facilitates the transfer of heat and moisture to inspired air. The complex anatomy of the turbinates also optimizes filtration of particles by the process of impaction (Fig. 1) (11,12). The presence of a ciliated epithelium further provides for transport and elimination of these particles, either to the anterior nares or to the nasopharynx (where they are either expectorated or swallowed).

Beyond this "air conditioning" and filtering function, the large surface area of the upper airway provides for the clearance of gaseous/vapor phase pollutants ("scrubbing") with surprising efficiency. For example, a single breath of chlorine (Cl_2) gas at up to three parts per million (ppm) concentration will be absorbed in the upper airway with greater than 95% efficiency, compared to approximately 50% efficiency for ozone (13,14). This scrubbing function is, in turn, dependent upon the water solubility and chemical reactivity of the pollutant in question, such that increasing solubility provides for early activation of mucous membrane irritant sensors, alerting individuals to avoid prolonged exposure (Fig. 2). The ability of an air pollutant to produce immediate upper airway/mucous membrane irritation, along with its olfactory potency, is an important component of its "warning properties" (15).

Noteworthily, many of the air pollutants that are encountered in indoor environments are both highly water soluble and chemically reactive. Principal among these are aldehydes (from building materials and cigarette smoke or produced by indoor chemical reactions). Further, common cleaning products used in indoor settings, including ammonia, sodium hypochlorite (bleach), and phenolic disinfectants, share these physicochemical properties and also produce initial warning sensations in the upper airway. Thus, the observed predominance of upper versus lower airway symptoms in problem buildings is understandable given both the anatomy of the upper airway and the nature of the pollutants present (16).

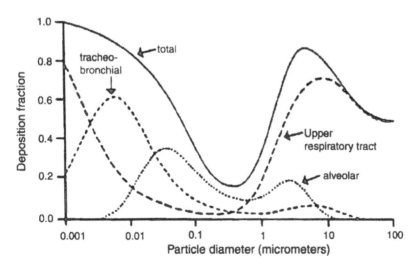

FIGURE 1 Regional deposition of particles within the respiratory tact, by particle diameter. *Source:* From Ref. 10.

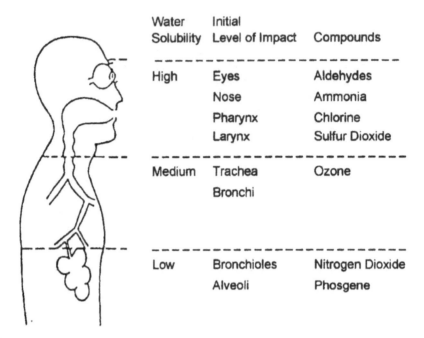

Water Solubility	Initial Level of Impact	Compounds
High	Eyes	Aldehydes
	Nose	Ammonia
	Pharynx	Chlorine
	Larynx	Sulfur Dioxide
Medium	Trachea	Ozone
	Bronchi	
Low	Bronchioles	Nitrogen Dioxide
	Alveoli	Phosgene

FIGURE 2 Initial site of impact of gaseous air pollutants within the respiratory tract. Among chemically reactive compounds, the major determinant of target site is water solubility, with highly water-soluble agents depositing in the upper respiratory tract. *Source:* Adapted from Ref. 15.

The neural apparatus stimulated by these pollutants includes two main structures: the olfactory nerve (cranial nerve I—providing for the sense of smell) and the trigeminal (cranial nerve V—providing for the sense of irritation in the eyes, nose, oral cavity, and nasopharynx). In addition, the glossopharyngeal and vagal nerves (Cr. N.'s IX and X) convey the sense of irritation for the hypopharynx and larynx. Just as our appreciation of foods involves a combination of the senses of taste and smell, our appreciation of many inhaled compounds involves aspects of olfaction and trigeminal stimulation (17,18). The latter carries sensations ranging from "freshness" or "cooling" (in response to menthol) to "burning" or "stinging" (as elicited by ammonia or Cl_2) (19).

Study Methods for Upper Airway End Points
Before reviewing the findings of selected experimental and observational studies, a summary of specialized upper airway study techniques is in order.

Measures of Nasal Patency
Nasal "congestion" ("stuffiness" or "blockage") is a prime symptom in rhinitis— along with pruritus and rhinorrhea. Although subjective nasal congestion and objective nasal patency should have a strong inverse relationship, the observed relationship between these two variables has been quite weak empirically (20,21). Notwithstanding their limitations, however, measures of nasal patency have an important role in evaluating nasal function, as outlined below (22).

An important methodologic issue that spans the various techniques for measuring nasal patency is the lack of predictive norms for nasal—as contrasted to pulmonary—function tests. In the lower respiratory tract, such parameters as forced expiratory volume in one second, forced vital capacity, and various lung volumes can be meaningfully compared with published norms based upon the age, sex, ethnicity, and height of the subject (or patient) being tested. Such is not the case in the upper respiratory tract, with such parameters as nasal airway resistance (NAR) or nasal inspiratory peak flow (PIFn) varying by as much as threefold between demographically similar subjects (23). This fact introduces an element of statistical variance that must be addressed in potential study designs.

The simplest measure of nasal patency is PIFn, which involves the use of a nasal peak flow meter (24). The flow meter is attached to a facemask; the subject exhales maximally (to residual volume or RV), places the mask over the nose, and then inspires with maximal effort, with the mouth closed, to total lung capacity (TLC). The meter reading is noted, the pointing device reset, and the procedure repeated. Typically, a total of three measurements are made (with the highest flow rate being recorded), and the procedure is repeated at various time intervals, with or without symptom correlations.

Rhinomanometry involves the simultaneous measurement of transnasal pressure (P) and flow (V), yielding a direct index of NAR: $NAR = P/V$. Rhinomanometry is divided into anterior and posterior rhinomanometry. Anterior rhinomanometry involves the separate measurement of NAR in each of the two heminasal cavities, whereas posterior rhinomanometry yields a global measure of upper airway resistance. Anterior rhinomanometry is generally preferred by otolaryngologists who are concerned with unilateral/asymmetric nasal pathologies. Posterior rhinomanometry, on the other hand, gives a direct measure of global nasal patency, without intervening calculations. However, subject cooperation can be a factor in posterior rhinomanometry, with a small minority of potential subjects being unable to produce meaningful tracings (25).

Acoustic rhinometry (AR) is a technique in which sharply demarcated pulses of sound ("clicks") are directed along a tube ("sound tube") into each nostril individually. The apparatus then records the reflected sound energy with a microphone in such a way that a map is generated of "cross-sectional area" of each heminasal cavity as a function of distance from the termination of the nosepiece of the sound tube. Integrating area over distance then yields *nasal volume* (26). Although there is a general expectation that nasal volume and NAR will relate in an inverse manner, the complexities of the anatomy of the nasal cavity militate against there being a universal relationship between these two variables across individuals.

Measures of Nasal Inflammation

Inflammation is a variable feature of nonallergic rhinitis, and, in fact, in its absence, the condition is more properly termed *"nonallergic rhinopathy."* One can document inflammation in the nose in a variety of manners. Biopsies can be obtained, yielding anatomically intact tissue (histologic specimens). Alternatively, the superficial mucosa can yield cytologic specimens by scraping, wiping, or brushing (27,28). Histologic or cytologic specimens can then be examined microscopically using conventional or immunochemical stains to document cell populations (including their state of activation). Cells so obtained can also be lysed, cellular RNA extracted, and assays of gene expression carried out (29).

Less invasively, exfoliated cells, biochemical mediators, and inflammatory markers can be retrieved from the nasal lumen by washing ("lavage") using a variety of techniques (30). Lavage specimens, in turn, can be separated into fractions for cytologic and biochemical analysis (31,32). With standardization of both sampling (lavage) and dilution (specimen handling), quantitative indices of cellular and biochemical responses can be validated for use in both cross-sectional and longitudinal study designs. A variant of this technique involves the collection of unaugmented nasal secretions using a nasal sponge, with microelution and analysis of the collected fluid (33). Finally, gaseous markers of airway inflammation [i.e., nitric oxide (NO) and exhaled breath condensates] can be obtained from the airway, with specific sampling techniques governing whether the gas so sampled is predominantly of upper or lower airway origin (34–36).

Measures of Nasal Mucociliary Clearance

The nasal cavity, posterior to the tip of the inferior turbinate, is invested with a ciliated respiratory epithelium whose function is to transport large particles that are filtered (by the process of "impaction") from the inspired airstream. Various techniques have been devised to assess mucociliary function. Radiographic visualization of the transit of radio-opaque microspheres placed on the inferior turbinate, as well as scintigraphic visualization of Tc 99m aerosol clearance, involves exposure of subjects to ionizing radiation (37). A simpler technique involves the placement of a grain of saccharine on the anterior tip of the inferior turbinate, with notation of the time between instillation of the substance and the appearance of a sweet taste in the mouth of the subject ("saccharine transit time"). While inhibition of mucocilary clearance is a hallmark of primary ciliary dyskinesia (an inherited condition), attempts to document *systematic* mucociliary alterations after exposures to air pollutants have met with variable success (see below).

CONTROLLED HUMAN EXPOSURE STUDIES

A number of studies have examined subjective and/or objective nasal responses to environmental incitants in controlled human exposure protocols (Table 1). Although many of these studies have compared the response of allergic rhinitics with that of normal controls, only one was identified, which utilized a subgroup with a diagnosis of "nonallergic rhinitis" (see below). Nevertheless, non-IgE-mediated responses to physical or chemical incitants are, by definition, "nonallergic" in nature regardless of the subpopulations studies, and hence are relevant to the scope of this chapter.

Barometric Pressure/Altitude

Barry et al. simulated ascent to over 8000 m in a hyperbaric chamber having controlled temperature and humidity, and measured peak inspiratory flow both nasally (PIFn) and orally (PIFo) at the equivalent of 0, 5000, and 8000 m. As expected (given decreasing air density at altitude), both PIFn and PIFo increased. However, the increase in PIFn was less than that in PIFo, interpreted as showing a relative airflow limitation in the nose related to altered barometric pressure (40).

Environmental Tobacco Smoke

Bascom et al. exposed 21 adult subjects to sidestream tobacco smoke (STS) for 15 minutes, and rated symptoms pre- and postexposure. The intensity of exposure

TABLE 1 Controlled Human Exposure Studies of Nonallergic Stimuli in the Upper Airway

Pollutant	Nasal patency	Nasal lavage	Mucociliary clearance	References
Acetic acid	↑NAR[a]			38
Ammonia	↑NAR			39
Barometric pressure	↓ PIFn vs. PIFo			40
Carbonless copy paper	↑NAR[b]			41
Chlorine gas	↑NAR[a]			42–46
Environmental tobacco smoke	↑NAR[b]	nc histamine albumin, kinins, nc PMNs	↓ clearance[b]	47–49
Ozone	nc NAR	↑PMNs, ↑ PMNs, ↑ PMNs, IL-8		50–52
Sulfur dioxide	↑NAR, nc NAR		↓ clearance	53,54
Volatile organic compounds	↓ NV	↑PMNs, cytokines, ↑ nc cytokines, ↑ cytokines	nc clearance, ↓ clearance, nc clearance	55,56, 57–59

Note: ↑, increased; ↓, decreased.
[a]Allergic rhinitic subjects only.
[b]Historically sensitive subjects only.
Abbreviations: NV, nasal volume; NAR, nasal airway resistance; nc, no change; PIFn, nasal peak inspiratory flow; PIFo, oral peak inspiratory flow.

corresponded to a CO concentration of 45 ppm (equivalent to a smoky bar). The subjects were subdivided into 10 historically sensitive to ETS (ETS-S) and 11 historically nonsensitive ETS (ETS-NS). (Noteworthily, the majority of the ETS-S subjects were atopic, whereas the majority of the ETS-NS were not.) ETS-S subjects reported significantly more (combined nose–throat) irritation than ETS-NS subjects. In addition, the ETS-S group showed significant increases in NAR by posterior rhinomanometry when compared with the ETS-NS group. The investigators then repeated the exposure with nasal lavage, rather than rhinomanometry, as the outcome of interest. Neither subgroup showed evidence of a true "allergic" (IgE-mediated) or vascular reaction, as evidenced by the lack of elevation of histamine, kinins, tosyl-L-arginine methyl ester (TAME)-esterase, and albumin in nasal lavage fluid postexposure (47).

The same laboratory examined the endpoint of mucociliary clearance after STS exposure. 99mTc-sulfur colloid was aerosolized into the nose after STS and air exposures, and clearance by scintillation detector was compared between the two exposure conditions. One-half of the subjects showed increased clearance, a quarter showed no change, and a quarter showed decreased clearance after STS exposure. The group with decreased clearance all gave a history of ETS-related rhinitis symptoms. The mechanism(s) underlying this heterogeneous response were not immediately apparent to the authors (48).

Nowak et al. performed nasal lavage on 10 mild asthmatics before and after exposure to STS at 22 ppm CO, analyzing for histamine, albumin, eosinophil cationic protein (ECP), myeloperoxidase (MPO), hyaluronic acid, and tryptase. Bronchoscopy was also performed the morning after exposure. Despite an increase in respiratory symptoms postexposure, no systematic changes were observed in spirometry, nasal lavage, or bronchoalveolar lavage fluid (49).

Junker et al. studied 24 subjects exposed to a constant source of STS with variable dilution rates, depending upon the experimental condition. They found a dose response for self-rated odor intensity, eye irritation, and annoyance as a function of airborne particle, polycyclic aromatic hydrocarbons (PAH), and VOC concentrations. Subjective nasal irritation, on the other hand, related only to particle concentration. Neither breathing pattern nor eye blink rate varied significantly with STS exposure concentration (60). The mean threshold for STS odor detection among these subjects corresponded to a $PM_{2.25}$ concentration of 0.6 to 1.4 mg/m^3.

Volatile Organic Compounds

Kjaergaard et al. exposed 18 each "hayfever" and normal subjects to a mixture of 22 different VOCs at an aggregate concentration of 20 mg/m^3 (the so-called "Molhave cocktail") for four hours. Exposure to control conditions—"clean air"—occurred on a separate day. Hayfever subjects showed greater increases in combined subjective (eye-nose-throat) irritation over the course of the exposure than did nonallergic subjects. With regard to nasal volume by AR, however, rhinitics and nonrhinitics (NRs) showed equivalent decreases in nasal volume after VOC challenge (55).

Hudnell et al. compared the response of adult male volunteers exposed to the "Molhave cocktail" over a 2.75-hour period, and found increasing eye and throat irritation, headache, and drowsiness, whereas odor ratings decreased (adapted) during exposure (61). In the same laboratory, Koren et al. extended VOC exposures over four hours and performed nasal lavage before and after. Investigators found increases in polymorphonuclear leukocytes (PMNs) in nasal lavage fluid both immediately postexposure and 18 hours later (56).

Muttray et al. exposed 12 healthy subjects to 1,1,1-trichloroethane (TCA) at 20 and 200 ppm for four hours, assessing nasal mucociliary transport time (by saccharine instillation) and sampling nasal secretions (via sponges) 20 minutes postexposure. Various cytokines, including interleukin IL-1β, IL-6, and IL-8 were analyzed in nasal secretions, and ciliary beat frequency determined on sampled cells studied ex vivo. Although neither measure of mucociliary function was significantly altered postexposure, all three cytokines were elevated in concentration (57).

The same group studied 19 healthy volunteers exposed to 0 and 200 ppm methyl ethyl ketone, again analyzing secretions for cytokines and documenting mucociliary transport time (saccharine method). Mucociliary transport time was significantly elevated postexposure, but cytokines showed no significant changes (58). Also from this laboratory, Mann et al. studied the response of 12 healthy subjects to 20 and 200 ppm of methanol, examining cytokines, mucociliary clearance, and ciliary beat frequency of nasal epithelial cells. Both IL-1β and IL-8 concentrations were elevated postexposure, whereas IL-6 and PGE2 were unchanged; neither measure of mucociliary function was altered by the exposure (59).

Andersen et al. studied NAR and mucociliary clearance, along with psychometric end points, during six-hour exposures to 10, 40, or 100 ppm of toluene vapor. No significant exposure-related changes were noted in either physiologic parameter (62).

Ammonia

McLean et al. measured NAR among 33 seasonal allergic rhinitic (SAR) and NR subjects pre- and postexposure to ammonia (100 ppm × 5 seconds per nostril). Exposures were repeated at 15-minute intervals, with successively longer durations of exposure (10, 15, and 20 seconds) in separate subexperiments. Mean NAR increased after NH_3 exposures, and a dose response was evident for exposure duration; however, no difference was apparent between subgroups by rhinitis status (39).

Chlorine

Shusterman et al. compared the response of eight each, SAR and NR subjects, to a 15-minute exposure by nasal mask to Cl_2 at 0.5 ppm. The experiment was counterbalanced with respect to both subject gender and order-of-exposure (Cl_2 vs. control first), and SAR subjects were tested out-of-season. After Cl_2 provocation, SAR subjects only showed significant increases in self-rated nasal irritation, as well as a significant congestive response (approximately 20% increase in NAR after Cl_2 compared to control condition) (42). In a larger sample of subjects stratified by age, gender, and allergy status studied in the same laboratory, both allergic rhinitics and older subjects showed augmented congestion, but no gender-related differences in reactivity to Cl_2 were apparent (43).

The above Cl_2 exposure paradigm was applied by Shusterman et al. to identify underlying mechanism(s) of irritant-induced nasal airway obstruction. In their first pathophysiologic study, subjects were pretreated with either ipratropium bromide nasal spray or placebo on a double-blinded manner prior to Cl_2 or air exposure. Differential congestion by rhinitis status was still apparent, suggesting that cholinergic reflexes were not responsible for the observed response (44). In a separate experiment, nasal lavage fluid was analyzed for evidence of mast cell degranulation (tryptase) and neuropeptide release substance P, calcitonin gene-related peptide, vasoactive intestinal peptide, and neuropeptide (SP, CGRP, VIP, and NPY), but neither set of markers was systematically affected by exposure. Thus, no evidence was generated that either mast cell degranulation or neuropeptide release was responsible for Cl_2's effect on nasal patency (45,46).

Sulfur Dioxide

Tam et al. studied 22 allergic rhinitics exposed nasally to 4 ppm of SO_2 for 10 minutes, as well as 8 combined asthmatic/rhinitics exposed to 1 to 2 ppm SO_2 by mouthpiece. There were no significant exposure-related changes in either NAR or nasal symptoms (54). These results contrasted with an earlier study by Andersen et al., which had documented SO_2-induced nasal airflow obstruction as well as alterations in mucociliary clearance (53).

Ozone

Graham et al. exposed 20 subjects to filtered air and 19 subjects to 0.5 ppm O_3 for four hours on two successive days. Subjects had nasal lavage performed preexposure on both days, as well as immediately postexposure on day 1 and 22 hours postexposure on day 2. The O_3-exposed group only showed increased PMNs on all postexposure samples, including an elevated baseline prior to the second day's exposure (50).

Graham and Koren compared the upper and lower respiratory tract responses of 10 nonsmoking nonasthmatic subjects exposed to 0.4 ppm O_3 for two hours with exercise. Parallel increases in PMNs and albumin were apparent in both nasal lavage and bronchoalveolar lavage at 18 hours postexposure, in addition to an early rise in PMNs documented on nasal lavage (51).

McBride et al. exposed 10 atopic asthmatic subjects to 0, 0.12, and 0.24 ppm O_3 for 90 minutes during intermittent exercise. Nasal lavage and nasal work-of-breathing were obtained preexposure, immediately postexposure, and at 6- and

24-hours postexposure. At the higher exposure level (0.24 ppm), a significant increase in nasal lavage white blood corpuscles (WBC) count was observed at the earliest and latest postexposure sampling time, but not at six hours. In addition, a significant correlation was found between nasal lavage WBC count and IL-8 levels. However, no significant changes in either nasal work-of-breathing or pulmonary function were observed postexposure (52).

Acetic Acid
Shusterman et al. compared eight SARs and eight NR subjects exposed to either acetic acid vapor (15 ppm) or filtered air for 15 minutes. The allergic rhinitics obstructed significantly compared to NRs, with responses evident both immediately postexposure and 15 minutes postexposure (38).

Carbonless Copy Paper
Morgan and Camp studied 30 workers with self-reported skin and/or respiratory sensitivity to carbonless copy paper. Air was passed through shredded carbonless copy paper and bond paper and supplied to the breathing zone of subjects. Mean NAR by rhinomanometry increased by 34% after carbonless copy paper exposure versus 8% after bond paper exposure. Symptoms, however, did not correlate with the magnitude of NAR changes (41). No comparison was attempted between subjects with and without self-reported nasal reactivity to this agent.

Paper Dust
Theander and Bender studied 15 nonallergic rhinitics who reported nasal symptoms to newspapers, and compared them with six healthy controls. Subjects inhaled either vapors from printing ink or paper dust, and then registered nasal symptoms on visual analog scales, as well as having their NAR measured by anterior rhinomanometry. The nonallergic rhinitic subjects reported significantly greater symptoms after paper dust, but not ink vapor, exposure. However, neither group showed significant changes in NAR (63). It appears that there was no attempt to achieve "blinding" with these exposures.

OBSERVATIONAL STUDIES

Numerous observational (epidemiologic) studies have addressed the nasal effects of physical and/or chemical aspects of ambient or indoor air quality. In some studies, individual factors (age, gender, or rhinitis status) were considered as potential markers of differential susceptibility. Although many of these studies have focused on single aspects of the inspired atmosphere (e.g., meteorology, O_3 levels, and presence of wet and/or moldy indoor conditions), potential confounding is always a concern in epidemiologic investigations. The following is a selective sample of these studies (Table 2).

Ambient Air Quality
Braat et al. (64) performed a time-series analysis of nasal symptoms recorded on a daily basis over a seven-month period among 16 nonallergic rhinitics and 7 normals, correlating symptoms with daily measurements of temperature, humidity,

TABLE 2 Observational Studies of Air Quality and the Upper Airway

Exposure	End point	Observation	References
Meteorologic conditions	Nasal symptoms	Symptoms in nonallergic rhinitic subjects varied with minimum daytime temperature, relative humidity, and air pollutant levels	64
Ambient air pollutants	Nasal biopsy	Squamous metaplasia comparing Mexico City vs. rural residents	65
	Nasal biopsy	Short-term visitors to Mexico City developed nasal neutrophilia	66
	Nasal biopsy	Children from Mexico City vs. unpolluted area showed squamous metaplasia, ciliary disorientation, intraepithelial exudate	67
	Nasal symptoms and biopsy	Children from Mexico City vs. unpolluted area reported greater nasal symptoms and showed squamous metaplasia, neutrophilia, +p53 expression	68
	Nasal lavage	Austrian school children underwent serial nasal lavage during air pollution season. An increase in white blood corpuscles count and ECP concentration was apparent with increasing O_3 (early season only)	69
	Nasal brushings	Adults from Florence, Italy (high-O_3) vs. Sardinia (low-O_3) showed more DNA damage	70
Indoor air pollutants	Acoustic rhinometry; nasal lavage	Cross-sectional study of school personnel in which nasal patency, nasal ECP, and lysozyme levels varied by building characteristic	71
	Nasal symptoms and lavage	Increased nasal symptoms, cytokines (interleukin-6, TNF-α) and nitric oxide during occupancy of mold-damaged vs. control building	72

Abbreviation: ECP, eosinophilic cationic protein.

and air pollutant levels. After correcting for autocorrelation and introducing optimal lag times, symptoms were predicted by minimum daytime temperature, average daytime relative humidity (%), O_3 levels, and PM_{10} levels among the nonallergic rhinitics only. Comparisons were hampered by the small number of subjects, however.

In a series of related studies, Calderon-Garciduenas et al. have examined the upper airway impact of air pollutants (including O_3, particulate matter, and aldehydes) in Mexico City. One such study compared urban residents with residents of an unpolluted locale, revealing squamous metaplasia, loss of normal cilia, vascular congestion, and glandular atrophy on nasal biopsy of the urban residents (65). Another study examined visitors to the city, who came from more rural areas; such short-term visitors developed epithelial desquamation and neutrophilic inflammation that took more than two weeks to resolve after returning to their hometowns (66). More recent studies have identified ultrastructural abnormalities of both cellular maturation and ciliary morphology, as well as evidence of p53 tumor suppressor protein activation among Mexico City residents versus controls (67,68).

Kopp et al. (69) studied the effects of varying atmospheric O_3 levels on the upper airway by examining serial nasal lavage specimens collected over a seven-month period from *nonatopic* school children in Germany. The investigators found an initial increase in nasal leukocytes and ECP with the initial seasonal increase in O_3 levels, but an apparent adaptation effect with continued high O_3 exposures.

Pacini et al. (70) compared nasal mucosal cells taken by brushing from residents of Florence, Italy (a high O_3 area) versus rural residents of Sardinia. They found higher levels of DNA damage and more inflammatory changes among cytologic specimens from the Florence residents than from the rural Sardinians.

Indoor Air Quality

Studies of indoor air quality documenting, subjectively or objectively, nonallergic upper airway responses are quite numerous. What follow are a few relatively recent representative studies:

Walinder et al. (71) studied 234 primary school personnel (adults) from 12 randomly selected Swedish schools. Background health information was obtained by structured interview, and nasal symptoms ascertained using a self-administered questionnaire. Environmental measures included room temperature and levels of carbon dioxide, nitrogen dioxide, formaldehyde, and other VOCs, and dust. AR was performed in the school/work setting after at least one hour of building occupancy. Nasal lavage was performed, and fluid analyzed for ECP, lysozyme, MPO, and albumin. Symptomatically, there were significant relationships between ventilation type (mechanical vs. natural), as well as dust concentrations, with self-reported nasal obstruction. On AR, nasal cross-sectional area was smaller as a function of dust concentrations, formaldehyde levels, the presence of PVC flooring, and the use of mechanical (vs. natural) ventilation. On nasal lavage, lysozyme levels were higher with mechanical ventilation and wet mopping of floors. ECP levels were higher with decreased frequency of floor cleaning and with increasing levels of formaldehyde and nitrogen dioxide. The authors state that these findings are unchanged after controlling for "personal factors," but the actual covariates considered were not spelled out in this report.

In Finland, Hirvonen et al. (72) obtained symptom histories and performed nasal lavage on 32 school personnel, including both teachers and support staff, near the end of the spring term, at the end of summer vacation, and again at the end of the fall term. All subjects came from a single school with visible mold growth. Eight unexposed controls (from a public health institute) were also studied on multiple occasions. Symptoms of rhinitis and eye irritation were significantly more frequent in the exposed group, particularly during spring and fall terms. Similarly, nitrite levels in NL fluid (equivalent to nasal NO) were also seasonally elevated in the exposed workers only. IL-6 and tumor necrosis factor alpha were both significantly elevated at the end of the spring term in exposed staff, whereas only the former was elevated at the end of the fall term. There were no differences in differential cell counts, either between the exposed and control subjects or within the former group on a seasonal basis. The interpretation of these findings is hampered by the noncomparability of the exposed and control groups.

INTERVENTION STUDIES

Two studies were identified in which the effects of various interventions were evaluated on nonallergically mediated nasal symptoms or pathology. In one, atopic asthmatic children in Mexico City exposed to urban air pollution (see above) were given either antioxidant dietary supplements (vitamins C and E) or placebo, and concentrations of cytokines (IL-6 and IL-8) and antioxidants (glutathione and uric acid) in nasal lavage fluid were evaluated. The antioxidant-treated group showed significantly lower levels of IL-6 (and borderline lower levels of IL-8) during high-O_3 days compared to placebo-treated children (73).

The second interventional study involved office workers who reported mucous membrane irritation at work. Their offices were subjected to either comprehensive or superficial (sham) cleaning on a blinded basis, resulting in significant reductions in airborne dust levels in the former group. Both subjective irritation and objective airway patency (by AR) were recorded. The active intervention group reported a significant reduction in upper airway irritative symptoms postintervention, and some measures of nasal patency increased in that group as well (74).

SUMMARY AND CONCLUSIONS

The upper airway occupies a sentinel position with respect to the physical and chemical qualities of the inspired atmosphere. Responses of the upper airway can be acute or chronic, as well as primary (sensory) or secondary (physiologic). Olfaction and sensory irritation are cofactors in the perception of air quality. Secondary reflex responses to airborne irritants may include blockage (airflow obstruction), secretion (with or without associated inflammation), and alterations in mucociliary clearance. Of the above end points, obstruction has been documented in response to a variety of agents, including acetic acid vapor, ammonia, Cl_2, ETS, mixed VOCs, vapors from carbonless copy paper, and (variably) SO_2. Alterations in mucociliary clearance have been variably observed with SO_2 and ETS exposure. A neutrophilic inflammatory response has been documented after acute exposure to either ozone or VOCs, and metaplastic mucosal changes after prolonged exposures to photochemical mixed air pollutants.

Augmented reactivity to irritants is a phenotypic characteristic of both nonallergic and allergic rhinitis; however, understanding of underlying mechanisms remains elusive (75–78). Differential physiologic responsiveness to environmental irritant stimuli has been documented by allergic rhinitis status for acetic acid and Cl_2 (objectively) and for mixed VOCs (subjectively only). Differential responsiveness by nonallergic rhinitis status has, to our knowledge, been documented for paper dust only, although a somewhat wider array of pollutants (including ETS and carbonless copy paper) has been studied in groups differing by self-reported pollutant reactivity.

Interestingly, although the congestive response to allergens and irritants is similar, the underlying mechanisms appear to differ, with neither mast cell degranulation nor cholinergic parasympathetic reflexes appearing critical to the response (Fig. 3). Although neuropeptide release does not accompany Cl_2-induced nasal obstruction, in one model system (hypertonic saline challenge), substance P release accompanied augmented secretions (80,81). In yet another hypertonic model (dry mannitol powder challenge), arachidonic acid metabolites characteristic of epithelial cell activation accompanied nasal obstruction (82). The relevance of these model systems to environmentally realistic (airborne) irritants remains unclear at this time.

Overall, nonallergic rhinitis has received considerably less attention than has allergic rhinitis in the context of descriptive, pathophysiologic, and intervention studies. This statement applies equally in the context of environmental nonallergic

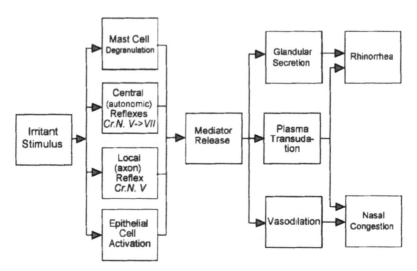

FIGURE 3 Potential mechanisms involved in the secondary (reflex) response to inhaled irritants. Evidence for involvement of alternative reflex mechanisms is reviewed in the text. Not illustrated are upstream processes involved in the initial mucosal impact of irritants (i.e., receptor- and nonreceptor-based irritant mechanisms), which are beyond the scope of this review. *Source*: Adapted from Ref. 79.

rhinitis. As is hopefully evident from the above discussion, many potential research questions in this area remain to be addressed.

REFERENCES

1. Hodgson MJ, Frohliger J, Permar E, et al. Symptoms and microenvironmental measures in nonproblem buildings. J Occup Med 1991; 33(4):527–533.
2. Nagda NL, Hodgson M. Low relative humidity and aircraft cabin air quality. Indoor Air 2001; 11(3):200–214.
3. Seppanen O, Fisk WJ. Association of ventilation system type with SBS symptoms in office workers. Indoor Air 2002; 12(2):98–112.
4. Gao P, Korley F, Martin J, Chen BT. Determination of unique microbial volatile organic compounds produced by five Aspergillus species commonly found in problem buildings. AIHA J (Fairfax, Va) 2002; 63(2):135–140.
5. Korpi A, Pasanen AL, Pasanen P. Volatile compounds originating from mixed microbial cultures on building materials under various humidity conditions. Appl Environ Microbiol 1998; 64(8):2914–2919.
6. Wilkins K, Larsen K, Simkus M. Volatile metabolites from mold growth on building materials and synthetic media. Chemosphere 2000; 41(3):437–446.
7. Clausen PA, Wilkins CK, Wolkoff P, Nielsen GD. Chemical and biological evaluation of a reaction mixture of R-(+)-limonene/ozone: formation of strong airway irritants. Environ Int 2001; 26(7–8):511–522.
8. Fan Z, Lioy P, Weschler C, Fiedler N, Kipen H, Zhang J. Ozone-initiated reactions with mixtures of volatile organic compounds under simulated indoor conditions. Environ Sci Technol 2003; 37(9):1811–1821.
9. Wolkoff P, Clausen PA, Wilkins CK, Nielsen GD. Formation of strong airway irritants in terpene/ozone mixtures. Indoor Air 2000; 10(2):82–91.
10. Snipes MB. Biokinetics of inhaled radionuclides. In: Raabe OG, ed. Internal Radiation Dosimetry. Madison, WI: Medical Physics Publishing, 1994:181–196.

11. Morawska L, Barron W, Hitchins J. Experimental deposition of environmental tobacco smoke submicrometer particulate matter in the human respiratory tract. Am Ind Hyg Assoc J 1999; 60(3):334–339.
12. Rasmussen TR, Andersen A, Pedersen OF. Particle deposition in the nose related to nasal cavity geometry. Rhinology 2000; 38(3):102–107.
13. Nodelman V, Ultman JS. Longitudinal distribution of chlorine absorption in human airways: comparison of nasal and oral quiet breathing. J Appl Physiol 1999; 86(6): 1984–1993.
14. Ultman JS, Ben-Jebria A, Hu SC. Noninvasive determination of respiratory ozone absorption: the bolus-response method. Res Rep Health Eff Inst 1994(69):1–27.
15. US Department of Health and Human Services. The Health Consequences of Involuntary Smoking: A Report of the Surgeon General. US DHHS, Public Health Service, Centers for Disease Control, 1986. Report No. (CDC) 87–8398.
16. Shusterman D. Toxicology of nasal irritants. Curr Allergy Asthma Rep 2003; 3(3):258–265.
17. Cain WS, Cometto-Muniz JE. Irritation and odor as indicators of indoor pollution. Occup Med 1995; 10(1):133–145.
18. Cometto-Muniz JE, Cain WS. Relative sensitivity of the ocular trigeminal, nasal trigeminal and olfactory systems to airborne chemicals. Chem Senses 1995; 20(2):191–198.
19. Laska M, Distel H, Hudson R. Trigeminal perception of odorant quality in congenitally anosmic subjects. Chem Senses 1997; 22(4):447–456.
20. Eccles R. Nasal airway resistance and nasal sensation of airflow. Rhinol Suppl 1992; 14:86–90.
21. Jones AS, Willatt DJ, Durham LM. Nasal airflow: resistance and sensation. J Laryngol Otol 1989; 103(10):909–911.
22. Nathan RA, Eccles R, Howarth PH, Steinsvag SK, Togias A. Objective monitoring of nasal patency and nasal physiology in rhinitis. J Allergy Clin Immunol 2005; 115(3 Pt 2):S442–S459.
23. Morris S, Jawad MS, Eccles R. Relationships between vital capacity, height and nasal airway resistance in asymptomatic volunteers. Rhinology 1992; 30(4):259–264.
24. Youlton LJF. The peak nasal inspiratory flow meter: a new instrument for the assessment of the response to immunotherapy in seasonal allergic rhinitis. Allergol Immunopathol 1980; 8(335).
25. Solomon WR. Nasal provocative testing. In: Spector SL, ed. Provocation Testing in Clinical Practice. New York: Marcel Dekker, 1995:647–692.
26. Hilberg O, Jackson AC, Swift DL, Pedersen OF. Acoustic rhinometry: evaluation of nasal cavity geometry by acoustic reflection. J Appl Physiol 1989; 66(1):295–303.
27. Meltzer EO, Jalowayski AA. Nasal cytology in clinical practice. Am J Rhinol 1988; 2(2):47–54.
28. Ronchetti R, Villa MP, Martella S, et al. Nasal cellularity in 183 unselected schoolchildren aged 9 to 11 years. Pediatrics 2002; 110(6):1137–1142.
29. Tarun AS, Bryant B, Zhai W, Solomon C, Shusterman D. Gene expression for carbonic anhydrase isoenzymes in human nasal mucosa. Chem Senses 2003; 28(7):621–629.
30. Klimek L, Rasp G. Norm values for eosinophil cationic protein in nasal secretions: influence of specimen collection. Clin Exp Allergy 1999; 29(3):367–374.
31. Peden DB. The use of nasal lavage for objective measurement of irritant-induced nasal inflammation. Regul Toxicol Pharmacol 1996; 24(1 Pt 2):S76–S78.
32. Wang DY, Yeoh KH. The significance and technical aspects of quantitative measurements of inflammatory mediators in allergic rhinitis. Asian Pac J Allergy Immunol 1999; 17(3):219–228.
33. Cain WS, Jalowayski AA, Kleinman M, et al. Sensory and associated reactions to mineral dusts: sodium borate, calcium oxide, and calcium sulfate. J Occup Environ Hyg 2004; 1(4):222–236.
34. Bartley J, Fergusson W, Moody A, Wells AU, Kolbe J. Normal adult values, diurnal variation, and repeatability of nasal nitric oxide measurement. Am J Rhinol 1999; 13(5): 401–405.
35. Djupesland PG, Chatkin JM, Qian W, et al. Aerodynamic influences on nasal nitric oxide output measurements. Acta Otolaryngol 1999; 119(4):479–485.

36. Olthoff A, Rohrbach S, Faber M, Gotz W, Laskawi R. Neuronal nitric oxide synthase immunoreactivity in the nasal mucosa of patients with idiopathic and allergic rhinitis. Otorhinolaryngol Relat Spec 2002; 64(3):180–185.
37. Di Giuda D, Galli J, Calcagni ML, et al. Rhinoscintigraphy: a simple radioisotope technique to study the mucociliary system. Clin Nucl Med 2000; 25(2):127–130.
38. Shusterman D, Tarun A, Murphy MA, Morris J. Seasonal allergic rhinitic and normal subjects respond differentially to nasal provocation with acetic acid vapor. Inhal Toxicol 2005; 17(3):147–152.
39. McLean JA, Mathews KP, Solomon WR, Brayton PR, Bayne NK. Effect of ammonia on nasal resistance in atopic and nonatopic subjects. Ann Otol Rhinol Laryngol 1979; 88(2 Pt 1):228–234.
40. Barry PW, Mason NP, Richalet JP. Nasal peak inspiratory flow at altitude. Eur Respir J 2002; 19(1):16–19.
41. Morgan MS, Camp JE. Upper respiratory irritation from controlled exposure to vapor from carbonless copy forms. J Occup Med 1986; 28(6):415–419.
42. Shusterman DJ, Murphy MA, Balmes JR. Subjects with seasonal allergic rhinitis and nonrhinitic subjects react differentially to nasal provocation with chlorine gas. J Allergy Clin Immunol 1998; 101(6 Pt 1):732–740.
43. Shusterman D, Murphy MA, Balmes J. Influence of age, gender, and allergy status on nasal reactivity to inhaled chlorine. Inhal Toxicol 2003; 15(12):1179–1189.
44. Shusterman D, Murphy MA, Walsh P, Balmes JR. Cholinergic blockade does not alter the nasal congestive response to irritant provocation. Rhinology 2002; 40(3):141–146.
45. Shusterman D, Balmes J, Avila PC, Murphy MA, Matovinovic E. Chlorine inhalation produces nasal congestion in allergic rhinitics without mast cell degranulation. Eur Respir J 2003; 21(4):652–657.
46. Shusterman D, Balmes J, Murphy MA, Tai CF, Baraniuk J. Chlorine inhalation produces nasal airflow limitation in allergic rhinitic subjects without evidence of neuropeptide release. Neuropeptides 2004; 38(6):351–358.
47. Bascom R, Kulle T, Kagey-Sobotka A, Proud D. Upper respiratory tract environmental tobacco smoke sensitivity. Am Rev Respir Dis 1991; 143(6):1304–1311.
48. Bascom R, Kesavanathan J, Fitzgerald TK, Cheng KH, Swift DL. Sidestream tobacco smoke exposure acutely alters human nasal mucociliary clearance. Environ Health Perspect 1995; 103(11):1026–1030.
49. Nowak D, Jorres R, Martinez-Muller L, et al. Effect of 3 hours of passive smoke exposure in the evening on inflammatory markers in bronchoalveolar and nasal lavage fluid in subjects with mild asthma. Int Arch Occup Environ Health 1997; 70(2):85–93.
50. Graham D, Henderson F, House D. Neutrophil influx measured in nasal lavages of humans exposed to ozone. Arch Environ Health 1988; 43(3):228–233.
51. Graham DE, Koren HS. Biomarkers of inflammation in ozone-exposed humans. Comparison of the nasal and bronchoalveolar lavage. Am Rev Respir Dis 1990; 142(1):152–156.
52. McBride DE, Koenig JQ, Luchtel DL, Williams PV, Henderson WR Jr. Inflammatory effects of ozone in the upper airways of subjects with asthma. Am J Respir Crit Care Med 1994; 149(5):1192–1197.
53. Andersen IB, Lundqvist GR, Jensen PL, Proctor DF. Human response to controlled levels of sulfur dioxide. Arch Environ Health 1974; 28(1):31–39.
54. Tam EK, Liu J, Bigby BG, Boushey HA. Sulfur dioxide does not acutely increase nasal symptoms or nasal resistance in subjects with rhinitis or in subjects with bronchial responsiveness to sulfur dioxide. Am Rev Respir Dis 1988; 138(6):1559–1564.
55. Kjaergaard S, Rasmussen TR, Molhave L, Pedersen OF. An experimental comparison of indoor air VOC effects on hayfever and healthy subjects. Proceedings of Healthy Buildings '95. Milan. 1995.
56. Koren HS, Graham DE, Devlin RB. Exposure of humans to a volatile organic mixture: III. Inflammatory response. Arch Environ Health 1992; 47(1):39–44.
57. Muttray A, Klimek L, Faas M, Schafer D, Mann W, Konietzko J. The exposure of healthy volunteers to 200 ppm 1,1,1-TCA increases the concentration of proinflammatory cytokines in nasal secretions. Int Arch Occup Environ Health 1999; 72(7):485–488.

58. Muttray A, Jung D, Klimek L, Kreiner C. Effects of an external exposure to 200 ppm methyl ethyl ketone on nasal mucosa in healthy volunteers. Int Arch Occup Environ Health 2002; 75(3):197–200.
59. Mann WJ, Muttray A, Schaefer D, Klimek L, Faas M, Konietzko J. Exposure to 200 ppm of methanol increases the concentrations of interleukin-1beta and interleukin-8 in nasal secretions of healthy volunteers. Ann Otol Rhinol Laryngol 2002; 111(7 Pt 1):633–638.
60. Junker MH, Danuser B, Monn C, Koller T. Acute sensory responses of nonsmokers at very low environmental tobacco smoke concentrations in controlled laboratory settings. Environ Health Perspect 2001; 109(10):1045–1052.
61. Hudnell HK, Otto DA, House DE, Molhave L. Exposure of humans to a volatile organic mixture: II. Sensory. Arch Environ Health 1992; 47(1):31–38.
62. Andersen I, Lundqvist GR, Molhave L, et al. Human response to controlled levels of toluene in six-hour exposures. Scand J Work Environ Health 1983; 9(5):405–418.
63. Theander C, Bende M. Nasal hyperreactivity to newspapers. Clin Exp Allergy 1989; 19(1):57–58.
64. Braat JP, Mulder PG, Duivenvoorden HJ, Gerth Van Wijk R, Rijntjes E, Fokkens WJ. Pollutional and meteorological factors are closely related to complaints of non-allergic, non-infectious perennial rhinitis patients: a time series model. Clin Exp Allergy 2002; 32(5):690–697.
65. Calderon-Garciduenas L, Osorno-Velazquez A, Bravo-Alvarez H, Delgado-Chavez R, Barrios-Marquez R. Histopathologic changes of the nasal mucosa in southwest Metropolitan Mexico City inhabitants. Am J Pathol 1992; 140(1):225–232.
66. Calderon-Garciduenas L, Rodriguez-Alcaraz A, Garcia R, et al. Human nasal mucosal changes after exposure to urban pollution. Environ Health Perspect 1994; 102(12):1074–1080.
67. Calderon-Garciduenas L, Valencia-Salazar G, Rodriguez-Alcaraz A, et al. Ultrastructural nasal pathology in children chronically and sequentially exposed to air pollutants. Am J Respir Cell Mol Biol 2001; 24(2):132–138.
68. Calderon-Garciduenas L, Rodriguez-Alcaraz A, Valencia-Salazar G, et al. Nasal biopsies of children exposed to air pollutants. Toxicol Pathol 2001; 29(5):558–564.
69. Kopp MV, Ulmer C, Ihorst G, et al. Upper airway inflammation in children exposed to ambient ozone and potential signs of adaptation. Eur Respir J 1999; 14(4):854–861.
70. Pacini S, Giovannelli L, Gulisano M, et al. Association between atmospheric ozone levels and damage to human nasal mucosa in Florence, Italy. Environ Mol Mutagen 2003; 42(3):127–135.
71. Walinder R, Norback D, Wieslander G, Smedje G, Erwall C, Venge P. Acoustic rhinometry in epidemiological studies—nasal reactions in Swedish schools. Rhinol Suppl 2000; 16:59–64.
72. Hirvonen MR, Ruotsalainen M, Roponen M, et al. Nitric oxide and proinflammatory cytokines in nasal lavage fluid associated with symptoms and exposure to moldy building microbes. Am J Respir Crit Care Med 1999; 160(6):1943–1946.
73. Sienra-Monge JJ, Ramirez-Aguilar M, Moreno-Macias H, et al. Antioxidant supplementation and nasal inflammatory responses among young asthmatics exposed to high levels of ozone. Clin Exp Immunol 2004; 138(2):317–322.
74. Skulberg KR, Skyberg K, Kruse K, et al. The effect of cleaning on dust and the health of office workers: an intervention study. Epidemiology 2004; 15(1):71–78.
75. Bascom R. Differential responsiveness to irritant mixtures. Possible mechanisms. Ann N Y Acad Sci 1992; 641:225–247.
76. Sanico A, Togias A. Noninfectious, nonallergic rhinitis (NINAR): considerations on possible mechanisms. Am J Rhinol 1998; 12(1):65–72.
77. Shusterman D. Individual factors in nasal chemesthesis. Chem Senses 2002; 27(6):551–564.
78. Tai CF, Baraniuk JN. Upper airway neurogenic mechanisms. Curr Opin Allergy Clin Immunol 2002; 2(1):11–19.
79. Shusterman D. Upper respiratory tract disorders. In: LaDou J, ed. Current Occupational and Environmental Medicine. 3rd. NY: McGraw-Hill, 2004:307–319.

80. Baraniuk JN, Ali M, Yuta A, Fang SY, Naranch K. Hypertonic saline nasal provocation stimulates nociceptive nerves, substance P release, and glandular mucous exocytosis in normal humans. Am J Respir Crit Care Med 1999; 160(2):655–662.

81. Baraniuk JN, Ali M, Naranch K. Hypertonic saline nasal provocation and acoustic rhinometry. Clin Exp Allergy 2002; 32(4):543–550.

82. Koskela H, Di Sciascio MB, Anderson SD, et al. Nasal hyperosmolar challenge with a dry powder of mannitol in patients with allergic rhinitis: Evidence for epithelial cell involvement. Clin Exp Allergy 2000; 30(11):1627–1636.

16 Cold Air–Induced Rhinitis

Alkis Togias

Department of Medicine, Divisions of Allergy and Clinical Immunology and Respiratory and Critical Care Medicine, Johns Hopkins University School of Medicine, Baltimore, Maryland, U.S.A.

Robert M. Naclerio

Department of Surgery, Section of Otolaryngology, Head and Neck Surgery, University of Chicago School of Medicine, Chicago, Illinois, U.S.A.

INTRODUCTION

Upon exposure to cold weather, many individuals develop nasal symptoms, primarily rhinorrhea and nasal congestion. A burning sensation inside the nose frequently precedes or accompanies these symptoms. This problem becomes accentuated in windy conditions. For example, rhinorrhea and nasal congestion are common during winter skiing and this condition has been termed "skier's nose" (1). Individuals who report cold air sensitivity may or may not be atopic and do not necessarily fall under the category of persistent or perennial rhinitis, because cold air exposure may be their only symptom trigger. Another clinical problem probably related to cold air rhinitis is the intolerance to nasal continuous positive airway pressure (CPAP) treatment, which many patients with sleep apnea develop (2). Although the air inhaled through the CPAP equipment is at room air temperature, nasal symptoms are most probably generated because of its relative low water content, as will be discussed below. This has led to the recommendation that the air delivered by CPAP equipment be warmed to body temperature and fully humidified. This approach has offered substantial amelioration of the problem (3).

Interest in cold air–induced rhinitis stems not only from the clinical problem per se, but also from the possibility that the mechanism through which nasal symptoms are induced may be the same as the mechanism of cold air–induced bronchospasm in patients with asthma (4). This reflects the structural and functional similarities between the nasal and the lower airway mucosa (5). Notably, one study has documented that individuals with asthma, compared to those with chronic rhinitis alone, develop stronger nasal responses when breathing cold air (6).

The prevalence of cold air–induced rhinitis is not clear, but in a 1980–1981 survey of 912 police officers in Paris, France, 5.4% reported this problem (7). A database of 206 individuals with objectively confirmed perennial allergic rhinitis and 150 with seasonal allergic rhinitis indicates that cold air is considered a stimulus for nasal symptoms by 55% and 28%, respectively (8).

One concept that will be discussed below is that the nasal reaction to cold air represents the high end of a spectrum of physiologic responses to a stimulus that perturbs the homeostasis of the nasal mucosa; this notion is supported by the fact that many individuals develop the problem when exposed to extreme conditions (skiers) while others report this sensitivity upon exposure to a stimulus of lower magnitude (higher temperature and less windy conditions).

THE AIR-CONDITIONING CAPACITY OF THE HUMAN NOSE

A major function of the nose is to warm and humidify air before it is presented to the lung for gas exchange (9). The air-conditioning capacity of the nasal passages is quite remarkable. For example, when inhaling air through the nose at subfreezing temperatures and at high flow (20 L/min), the average airstream temperature in the nasopharynx is 26°C, but it can be as high as 30°C (10,11). In the 1950s, Ingelstedt showed that, even when human subjects are exposed to a cold chamber (0 to −4°C), the relative humidity of inhaled air below the pharynx is around 99% (12). It remained unknown, however, what portion of air humidification takes place in the nasal cavities.

Recently, one of the authors (RMN) has developed a methodology to measure the ability of the nasal mucosa to warm and humidify air (11). This method involves the insertion in one nostril of a nasal catheter with a rounded tip so that the tip touches the posterior nasopharyngeal wall. The catheter is equipped with a temperature and a relative humidity sensor placed in small holes at 1 cm from its tip. Measurements of temperature and relative humidity of the air in the nasopharynx are conducted while air is being delivered to the opposite nostril under various flow rates (5, 10, and 20 L/min). The temperature of inhaled air at the entrance of the nostril is around 20°C, 10°C, and 0°C for each of the above flow rates, respectively. During the cold air exposure, study participants are instructed to breathe through their mouth; cold air enters through the nose and exits through the mouth; therefore, exhaled air does not enter the nasal cavity and does not provide water and heat back to the nasal mucosa. Measurements are made after seven minutes of breathing air at each of the above flow rates because this is the time required for the temperature in the probe to reach a steady state.

Using this methodology, it has been shown that the relative humidity of air in the nasopharynx is consistently around 100%, irrespective of the temperature and flow of inhaled air. However, the temperature of air at the nasopharynx varies significantly; therefore, and because the relative humidity remains constant, the water content of air varies as well. Subtraction of the water content of inhaled air from that in the nasopharynx yields a water gradient that can be used as a measure of the air-conditioning ability of the human nose. That ability does not correlate with baseline nasal airway resistance, nasal volume, nasopharyngeal mucosal temperature, or body temperature. Therefore, it probably reflects an intrinsic capacity of the nasal surface to warm inhaled air. Using a similar methodology, but without applying cold air, Keck et al. have shown that most of the air-conditioning takes place in the anterior segments of the nose (13).

When air is inspired through the nose, not only the warming but also the humidification process lead to mucosal surface cooling (14), because vaporization of water from the epithelial lining fluid into the airstream requires heat. With water leaving the epithelial lining fluid, transient increases in the osmolarity of this fluid should also be expected, but experimental confirmation for this is lacking. With increasing ventilation rates through the nose or when the ambient air is at much lower temperature than room air temperature (and, consequently, water content), the nasal heat and water losses are increased, and the cooling as well as the drying effects on the nasal mucosa are greater. This poses a stress on the mucosa and probably activates a number of compensatory mechanisms.

With unidirectional cold, dry air breathing at 5, 10, and 20 L/min, the approximate water loss is 20, 33, and 53 mg/min, respectively (11). Therefore, at a cold air breathing rate of 5 L/min, the entire surface liquid volume, which has been estimated around 150 μL [nasal surface = 150 cm^2, depth of mucus layer = 10 μm (15,16)], needs to be replaced every seven to eight minutes. With a bidirectional breathing pattern (inhalation and exhalation through the nose), heat and water losses are smaller because a substantial percentage, approximately 30%, of the heat and water supplied to the airstream at inspiration is passively returned to the mucosa at expiration, as long as expiration also takes place through the nose and at resting respiratory rates (12,17,18).

The anatomy of the nasal mucosa is of major importance in the ability of the nasal passages to condition air while retaining mucosal heat and water homeostasis and should be briefly reviewed. One of the characteristic mucosal structures is the dense, subepithelial capillary network. These capillaries have fenestrations that are polarized toward the luminal surface (19). Blood flow through this network provides heat and the fenestrae probably facilitate water transportation into the interstitium, the epithelial cells, and the epithelial lining fluid. Another important structural element of the nasal submucosa is the venous sinusoid system, which lies below the subepithelial capillary network. These blood vessels have the ability to rapidly pool large volumes of blood, because they are supplied by many arteriovenous anastomoses and because their draining veins (cushion veins) can contract and stop blood outflow (20). Blood pooling leads to engorgement of the nasal mucosa and this increases the airstream contact surface. According to a theoretical model proposed by Hanna and Scherer, mucosal temperature and volume of the nasal cavity are the most important factors determining the air-conditioning capacity of the human nose (21). However, the numerous glands of the nasal mucosa, approximately 45,000 per nasal cavity (22), release mucus and provide for the gel phase of the epithelial lining fluid. The water content of mucus is more than 90% (23). Stimulation of the glandular apparatus above its baseline activity can produce, within minutes, large quantities of mucus, tens of times the resting volume of the epithelial lining fluid.

Application of vasoconstrictors decreases the temperature of the nasal mucosa (24) and the temperature of inspired air at the oropharynx (14). We do not have information, however, whether vasoconstrictors reduce the water gradient across the nasal passages. Application of an alpha-adrenoreceptor antagonist, on the other hand, had no impact on the ability of the nose to provide water to the airstream, despite the fact that it led to an increase in nasal mucosal temperature (24). Increased mucosal temperature has been achieved also by immersing the feet in warm water; in that case, increased water transportation into the airstream was demonstrated without a change in nasal volume (25). Based on these observations, the theoretical model of Hanna and Scherer is only partially supported (21). It is quite possible that a factor that was only partially assessed in that model, the water transportation capacity across the nasal mucosa, may be of higher importance than mucosal temperature and nasal cavity volume.

There is no agreement on which structural element of the nasal mucosa mainly contributes to water transportation and air humidification. The abundance of seromucus submucosal glands, especially in the anterior portions of the nasal cavity, suggests that their secretions could provide most of the water needed for humidification. In support of this concept, it has been shown that subcutaneous injection of 1 mg atropine decreases the ability of the nose to humidify air (26). In other studies, however, application of homatropine or ipratropium bromide to the nasal surface did not impair its humidification function (27,28). Most recently, using the temperature and relative humidity monitoring system described above, Assanasen et al. showed that application of ipratropium bromide actually improved the ability of the nose to warm and humidify cold air, even at 20 L/min flow (29). This occurred despite the fact that the secretory response measured after the end of cold air exposure was decreased.

Cauna has contended that the role of humidification belongs to water from the fenestrated subepithelial capillaries, which continuously diffuses through the epithelium (30). However, Ingelstedt and Ivstam, who injected fluorescein intravenously in normal humans, were not subsequently able to detect it in their nasal secretions (31). Fluorescein is supposed to freely move across capillaries into the adjacent tissues and its absence in these experiments suggested that transudation does not occur. The possibility that fluorescein may not cross the nasal basement membrane and diffuse between epithelial cells was not examined. Osmotic drives generated by water loss during the inspiratory phase may move water from intraepithelial spaces into the airway lumen (32). At basal conditions, no osmotic drive for water to reach the lumen is generated by the apical surface of nasal epithelium, which predominantly absorbs sodium ions (33). However, hypertonicity of the periciliary fluid, which may occur as a result of water loss into the airstream, may lead to reduction of sodium absorption followed by induction of chloride secretion (33). Agents that induce cAMP also cause increased chloride secretion. These include α_2- and β-agonists and prostaglandins (PG) E_1, E_2, and F_{2a}. In addition, bradykinin, adenosine, eosinophil major basic protein, substance P, and mast cell mediators have shown similar effects (34,35). From this list, it becomes evident that sympathetic and neuropeptide-containing nerve activation as well as allergic or nonallergic inflammation can increase chloride secretion leading to osmotic water diffusion into the airway lumen. It is also worth noting that methacholine-induced human nasal secretions are hyperosmolar (approximately 340 mosm/kg H_2O) (36) and that, in vitro, acetylcholine induces a large secretory flow of both sodium and chloride (33) suggesting that cholinergic stimulation also results in the generation of an osmotic drive to provide water to the airway surface.

The above considerations are very important because they may explain some interesting in vivo observations: using the nasal air-conditioning monitoring system we described above, it was shown that individuals with seasonal allergic rhinitis, when tested out of the pollen season, while asymptomatic, had reduced ability to condition inhaled air, compared to healthy controls (11). However, 24 hours after a nasal allergen provocation, these individuals showed a 15% to 20% increase in the water gradient between the entrance of the nose and the nasopharynx (37). In addition, testing seasonal rhinitic subjects outside and during the pollen season (natural allergen exposure) resulted in the same effects (37). The allergen challenge–induced observation was subsequently confirmed by another group of investigators in subjects with perennial allergic rhinitis (38). The improvement in air-conditioning was not related to changes in nasal volume. In the opposite direction, a recent study demonstrated that treatment of the nose with topical glucocorticosteroids for two weeks decreases water transportation into the airstream, in nonsmoking subjects (39). Collectively, this work indicates that allergic inflammation increases nasal air-conditioning; this may be the result of increased blood flow through the mucosa, which provides increased amounts of water to the epithelium, but the possibility that inflammatory products may alter ionic transportation across the epithelium leading to better water availability should not be disregarded.

MECHANISMS OF NASAL REACTIONS TO COLD AIR

A fundamental question regarding the generation of nasal symptoms by cold air is whether the actual stimulus to the mucosa is related to heat loss, water loss, or to mechanical irritation from high airflow through the nose. Although mechanical irritation can induce nasal symptoms, it is unlikely that high flow of air per se can act as an irritant, unless the mucosa is highly inflamed. As will be discussed below, in an experimental model of cold air rhinitis in which air is inhaled at high flow rates through the nose, warm and moist air is used as a negative control and causes minimal, if any, nasal symptoms in the subjects who are sensitive to cold air. The second question is how the stimulus results in nasal symptoms and the third question regards the underlying cause of differential susceptibility to cold air.

The Nasal Cold Air Provocation Model

A model of cold, dry air nasal provocation was developed more than 20 years ago (40). The design calls for study participants to breathe air for 15 minutes, at subfreezing temperatures, through the nose and in a unidirectional manner (inhalation through the nose, exhalation through the mouth), at relatively high flow (26 L/min). These elements of the experimental protocol aim at maximizing the potency of the stimulus [e.g., exhalation through the nose would lead to 30% recovery of heat and water by the nasal mucosa (12,17,18)]. Prior to and after the cold air breathing period, nasal symptoms are recorded and nasal lavages are performed. Under various experimental protocols, analysis of the returned lavage fluids has included measurements of inflammatory mediators or biomarkers, cellular analyses and measurement of the osmolarity of the fluids. As a negative control, we have used nasal inhalation of warm and moist air (around 37°C, 100% relative humidity). Participants in these studies were divided into two categories: individuals with cold air rhinitis and individuals who deny any nasal symptoms upon exposure to cold, windy environments.

The nasal cold air–breathing model has provided us with information that has shed insights into the pathophysiology of cold air–induced rhinitis. The original observation was that the returned lavage fluids after cold air challenge contained increased levels of mast cell activation markers such as histamine and PGD_2 (40). We later found that mast cell tryptase was also elevated in nasal lavage fluids following cold air challenge (41). Mast cell activation markers were accompanied by biomarkers of glandular activation and plasma extravasation. All this activity was observed in the group of historically cold air–sensitive individuals, but not in the nonsensitive controls and correlated well with the development of nasal symptoms, even within the cold air–sensitive subjects. The reaction to cold air is specific in that it does not occur with warm, moist air breathing. Also, even if both inhalation and exhalation of air take place through the nose, reactions to cold air with qualitatively similar characteristics as those described above do occur in the same individuals (42).

An additional observation that was made with the use of this model was that cold air inhalation stimulates sensory nerves and generates a cholinergic secretory response. The sensorineural effect of cold air was first demonstrated with a model in which the challenge was performed only through one nostril; in that experimental setting, a secretory response was generated bilaterally. Furthermore, local anesthesia ipsilateral to the challenge reduced the contralateral response and a similar result was obtained when the contralateral nostril was pretreated with atropine (43). Even before this study, we had demonstrated that atropine could reduce rhinorrhea (but not nasal congestion) scores, as well as a biomarker of glandular activation after cold air challenge, without affecting plasma exudation (44).

Although it has been confirmed that the nasal reaction to cold air involves both mast cell activation and sensorineural stimulation, it has been difficult to demonstrate the clinical significance of the former pathway. In one study, we used a topical antihistamine that had been previously shown to block allergen-induced symptoms and mast cell activation in the human nose (45). This agent failed to inhibit the clinical response to cold air (46). In another study, the use of a topical glucocorticosteroid for seven days was not effective in reducing nasal symptoms after a cold air challenge, despite the fact that it reduced the level of H recovered in nasal lavage fluids (47). Nasal steroids are capable of inhibiting the acute allergic reaction in the human nose, and a reduction in the levels of mast cell numbers has been postulated as the mechanism for this action (48). On the basis of the above observations, it is reasonable to state that the clinical response to cold air challenge and, probably, the natural syndrome of cold air–induced rhinitis, are primarily mediated by neural mechanisms with a sensory element that is located in the nasal mucosa and an effector element that is mostly cholinergic. In support of this concept, objective measures of the nasal reaction (decreased nasal patency and secretion weight) to cold air have been successfully reduced with intranasal capsaicin treatment, which is meant to defunctionalize nociceptor c-fibers (49). Also, nasal atropine and ipratropium bromide have been effective in reducing rhinorrhea in skiers (1,50).

Mucosal Cooling or Drying?

The mechanism(s) through which inhalation of cold air leads to sensory nerve stimulation and mast cell activation in the nose is (are) not clear. Based on the fact that there is substantial mucosal heat and water loss during cold air breathing, the obvious candidate stimuli should be cooling and hyperosmolarity. Researchers in the field have been engaged in a two-decade-long and still ongoing debate between these two mechanisms in relation to the causes of exercise-induced asthma. This is because cold air hyperventilation not only potentiates exercise-induced bronchoconstriction, but can also induce bronchoconstriction in the absence of exercise (51–61). The reason behind this long debate is that it is quite difficult to separate the two stimuli, because as the mucosa heats the air in the nasal cavities (and, as a result, loses heat), water evaporates passively and humidifies the air (mucosal water loss). In addition, as previously mentioned, the evaporation process requires large amounts of heat and this further contributes to a cooling process. Most importantly, the temperature of the air determines the maximum amount of water that it can retain in vapor form; therefore, if the mucosa is capable of warming the air to a high degree, it will also be required to provide a large amount of water. Because delivery of heat and water to the airstream depends, to some extent, on different physiologic functions, the capacity of each of these functions should determine the overall air-conditioning ability. Based on the temperature and relative humidity measurements in the nasopharynx that we described above, it appears that the ability to warm the air is more of a limiting factor than the ability to humidify it (relative humidity remains around 100% over the entire range of recorded airstream temperatures). One could then argue that cooling is more likely to be the stimulus for the cold air reaction. However, what is most important from the standpoint of the clinical reaction to cold air is what happens at the nasal mucosal level.

With cold air breathing through the nose, there is good evidence that the temperature of the nasal mucosa can decrease substantially: Assanasen et al. have found that, whereas the temperature of the nasopharyngeal mucosa is 32°C at baseline, it can be reduced to approximately 23°C if cold air (−5°C) is inhaled in a unidirectional manner (inhalation through the nose and exhalation through the mouth) at a flow of 20 L/min, for eight minutes (29). This confirms that cooling of the nasal mucosa does take place with inhalation of cold air. What is unknown, however, is (i) whether a reduction in mucosal temperature of around 10°C is an adequate trigger for the generation of nasal symptoms, and (ii) whether individuals with cold air rhinitis experience a more substantial reduction in mucosal temperature when exposed to the cold air challenge. In other words, is increased cooling associated with a stronger symptomatic and biomarker response? Furthermore, one has to propose a mechanism through which cooling can trigger the two components of the nasal reaction to cold air: mast cell activation and sensory nerve stimulation. Mast cells, if anything, show reduced ability for activation when operating at lower temperatures: Studies have determined that optimal temperature is 37°C for lung and intestinal and 32°C for skin mast cells (62,63).

Cooling may not be able to activate mast cells, but it could activate nasal sensory nerves. Recently, cation channels that act as cold receptors have been identified and cloned (64–66). These include the transient receptor potential (TRP) melastatin 8 receptor and the TRP ankyrin-like 1 (TRPA1) receptor, the latter being regarded as a nociceptor and the former as a gentle cooling and menthol-sensing receptor (67). Additional cold-sensing receptors may exist. Although these receptors have been identified on rodent trigeminal sensory nerves and the TRPA1 receptor is strongly associated with the heat and capsaicin-sensing receptor TRP vanilloid 1 (TRPV1) (68), which is probably present in nasal mucosal sensory nerves (69), we do not know at this point whether these cold-sensing receptors are present in the sensory nerve endings of the human nose.

An increase in the osmolarity of the epithelial lining fluid has been demonstrated in the human nose at the end of a cold air breathing session (36,70). A most interesting observation that will be discussed below is that this change in osmolarity appears to occur only in cold air–sensitive subjects. The fact that increased osmolarity occurs despite the apparent unlimited ability of the nasal mucosa to provide water to inhaled air indicates that the mucosa does not provide water without an impact on its own homeostasis. Furthermore, hyperosmolarity is a known trigger for mast cell and sensory nerve activation in the human nose. Human lung mast cells release inflammatory mediators upon exposure to a hyperosmolar medium, in vitro (71,72) without the stimulus being toxic to the cells. Importantly, introduction of a hyperosmolar mannitol solution in the human nose results in histamine and PGD_2 release, indicating in vivo mast cell activation by a hypertonic stimulus (73,74). Yet, mast cell tryptase cannot be detected following hyperosmolar nasal challenge (41). Individuals with nasal sensitivity to cold air develop a stronger symptom and histamine release response to a hyperosmolar mannitol solution, when it is introduced in their nose, compared to cold air–nonsensitive subjects (75).

A hypertonic stimulus can induce nasal sensory nerve activation. In a study by Sanico et al. (76), 10-mm diameter filter paper discs carrying 50 μL of 5.13 M saline produced both an ipsilateral and a contralateral secretory response, when applied for one minute onto the nasal septal mucosa of one nostril. Unfortunately, that study did not compare subjects with cold air sensitivity to those without. In support of the concept of sensory nerve stimulation and generation of a central reflex, pretreatment of the ipsilateral to the challenge nostril with a topical anesthetic (lidocaine) substantially reduced the ipsilateral secretory response and almost completely abolished the contralateral response. Stimulation of sensory nerves by a hypertonic stimulus is probably mediated by capsaicin-sensitive, nociceptor nerves. In fact, it has been recently suggested that the osmotic stimulus acts on the nonselective cation channel TRPV1 (77), which is also the heat-sensing capsaicin receptor (78). This is not surprising, given that hypertonic challenge in the human nose causes a burning sensation that is qualitatively similar to that caused by capsaicin. Capsaicin-sensitive c-fibers do not only act as afferent nerves leading to the generation of central reflexes (such as the contralateral secretory response), but can also release inflammatory neuropeptides at their nerve endings where activation took place. This produces what has been conventionally termed "neurogenic inflammation" (79). Baraniuk et al. have clearly demonstrated substance P release in nasal secretions upon provocation with hyperosmolar saline (80), and neurogenic inflammation using the same stimulus in the trachea has been demonstrated in a rat model (81). Support for the concept of capsaicin-sensitive, c-fiber activation by hyperosmolar stimuli is offered by the finding that repetitive capsaicin application in the nasal mucosa leads to downregulation of the response to hypertonic saline (76). This defunctionalization action of capsaicin has been widely utilized in animal models to study the function of nociceptor c-fibers (82–84) and has even been used as a therapeutic tool in the management of nonallergic, noninflammatory rhinitis (85–92). The effect of capsaicin in the study of Sanico et al. was quite specific in that it did not influence the secretory response to a direct glandular stimulus, such as methacholine. As previously mentioned, the nasal cold air response in patients with nonallergic, noninfectious rhinitis is also suppressed by capsaicin treatment (49).

On the basis of the above information, one can conclude that, although both cooling and water loss/hypertonicity are, theoretically, good candidates as the primary stimulus for nasal reactions to cold air, water loss/hypertonicity has a stronger body of evidence in support of being the key stimulus. It is a good possibility, however, that the two stimuli work in concert. It is also possible that the relative importance of each stimulus is a function of individual susceptibility.

Does Cold Air–Induced Rhinitis Reflect a Specific Abnormality in Nasal Physiology?

Regardless what the stimulus is, the question should be why does cold air–induced rhinitis primarily affect a subgroup of humans and is not a universal phenomenon. The common conception that "everybody's nose runs in cold weather" does not appear to hold in surveys, as well as in experimental studies. The truth is that water condenses in the nose upon exhalation due to the rapid cooling of fully conditioned air that comes in contact with the cold environment and this is perceived as a "runny nose." As previously mentioned, only around 5% of individuals in a general population sample are bothered by rhinitis symptoms upon exposure to cold air (7,93). On the other hand, about 55% of individuals with perennial allergic rhinitis report cold air as a trigger of nasal symptoms (8). Furthermore, among individuals with perennial allergic rhinitis, those who also have asthma were shown, in one study, to have a stronger response to an experimental cold air challenge (6), compared to those with rhinitis alone, although this was not the case in another study (94); the intensity of the stimuli between the two studies, however, differed. Although the prevalence of cold air–induced rhinitis in individuals with other chronic nonallergic rhinitis symptoms is not known, the ability to differentiate nonallergic rhinitis patients from healthy controls on the basis of a cold air provocation (95) indicates that the problem is more prevalent in this population, as well. This apparent enrichment of nasal cold air sensitivity in individuals with allergic and nonallergic rhinitis and its possible further enrichment in those who also have asthma are very intriguing.

The first question that arises from the above observations is whether cold air–induced rhinitis reflects a nonspecific state of nasal hyperresponsiveness. In a study that we conducted several years ago, we found that individuals with nasal cold air sensitivity do not differ from those without in terms of their nasal responsiveness to histamine, a stimulus that is classically used to identify nasal hyperresponsiveness (75,96). Hyperresponsiveness to histamine is found in patients with allergic rhinitis (97) and can be induced with allergen provocation (98) or after seasonal natural allergen exposure (99). It is therefore, peculiar why, despite the apparent fact that compared to the general population, cold air sensitivity is reported more commonly among individuals with allergic rhinitis, no correlation between cold air sensitivity and histamine hyperresponsiveness exists. Part of the differentiation between cold air sensitivity and sensitivity to histamine may relate to differences in cellular targets. For example, H-1 receptors, which are responsible for histamine-induced sneezing and vascular permeability in the human nose (100), are not present, at least in the guinea pig, on the same sensory nerves as TRPV1, a receptor that may be important in the cold air reaction (69). On the other hand, stimuli that activate TRPV1, particularly capsaicin and possibly hypertonic stimuli, do generate augmented responses in individuals with allergic rhinitis (76,97,101). These observations suggest that, in the presence of allergic inflammation, there is upregulation of the nasal response to various forms of neural stimuli that do not necessarily act through the same pathways. It is conceivable, therefore, that, in these individuals, cold air rhinitis could at least partially fall under the general umbrella of nasal hyperresponsiveness. However, in many other individuals who do not have allergic airway disease, it does not appear that the answer to their susceptibility to cold air lies in the nonspecific hyperresponsiveness domain.

Other than developing significant nasal symptoms upon exposure to cold air, individuals with cold air rhinitis, compared to those without, are characterized by (i) increased responsiveness (measured through symptoms and mediator release in nasal fluids) to a hypertonic stimulus (75), (ii) increased tonicity of their nasal secretions at the end of a cold air provocation (70), and (iii) increased numbers of epithelial cells in nasal lavage fluids at the end of a cold air provocation (102). On the basis of these characteristics, one can propose the hypothesis that the primary abnormality underlying cold air rhinitis is a defect of the mucosa to compensate for the high water loss that occurs during exposure to the environmental stimulus (Fig. 1). Under such circumstance, water loss is not readily replenished, leading to a hypertonic environment. This scenario leads to two consequences: first, hypertonicity may stimulate mast cell mediator release as well as sensory nerve activation leading to the symptoms of cold air rhinitis, burning, rhinorrhea,

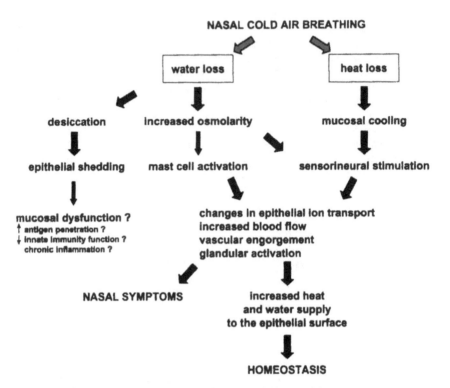

FIGURE 1 Schematic of a hypothesis on the pathophysiology of the nasal reaction to cold air.

and nasal congestion; second, hypertonicity may injure the nasal epithelium lead-ing to increased cell numbers in lavage fluids acutely after the end of cold air exposure. If this hypothesis is correct, one could further argue that both the secretory response and the congestion induced by the challenge represent mecha-nisms to restore mucosal homeostasis.

In relation to the above hypothesis, it is worth noting that the air-conditioning capacity of the nasal mucosa, as determined by the water gradient between the air-stream at the entrance of the nose and the nasopharynx, is decreased in allergic individuals, when their nose is not inflamed (i.e., in those with seasonal allergic rhi-nitis, when they are tested outside the pollen season) (11). This is not the case in the presence of induced or natural allergic inflammation (37,94), suggesting that inflam-mation plays a corrective role in this case. Most interestingly, however, the "defect" in air conditioning is also present in individuals with asthma (94), despite the fact that they tend to have chronic nasal inflammation. In other words, the magnitude of the underlying water transportation problem in patients with asthma may be such that it overwhelms the "corrective" function of inflammation. This observation may be important in view of the fact that the lower airways of asthmatics are also very sensitive to cold air exposure. As previously mentioned, in one study, the nasal reaction to cold air was found stronger in asthmatics with rhinitis than in subjects with rhinitis alone (6). It is, therefore, possible that in individuals who develop total airway disease (rhinitis and asthma), an air-conditioning defect of the respiratory mucosa may play a pathogenetic role. This hypothesis, which requires further testing, is even more interesting in view of the many reports of elite winter sport athletes developing asthma-like syndromes (103–105). There is no question that the long-term effects of cold air exposure on the human upper and lower respiratory tract should be studied more vigorously.

REFERENCES

1. Silvers WS. The skier's nose: a model of cold-induced rhinorrhea. Ann Allergy 1991; 67:32–36.
2. Nino-Murcia G, McCann C, Bliwise D, Guillemnault C, Dement W. Compliance and side effects in sleep apnea patients treated with nasal continuous positive airway pressure. West J Med 1989; 150:165–169.
3. Martins De, Araujo MT, Vieira SB, Vasquez EC, Fleury B. Heated humidification or face mask to prevent upper airway dryness during continuous positive airway pressure therapy. Chest 2000; 117:142–147.
4. Anderson S, Togias A. Dry air and hyperosmolar challenge in asthma and rhinitis. In: Busse WW, Holgate S, eds. Asthma and Rhinitis. Blackwell Scientific Publications Inc., 2000:1449–1468.
5. Baroody F, Canning B. Comparative anatomy of the nasal and tracheal/broncheal airways. In: Lenfant C, Corren J, Togias A, Bousquet J, eds. Upper and Lower Respiratory Disease. New York: Marcel Dekker, 2003:1–51.
6. Hanes L, Issa E, Proud D, Togias A. Stronger nasal responsiveness to cold air in individuals with rhinitis and asthma, compared with rhinitis alone. Clin Exp Allergy 2006; 36:26–31.
7. Kauffman F, Neukirch F, Anneis I, Korobaeff M, Dore A, Lellouch J. Relation of perceived nasal and bronchial hyperresponsiveness to FEV_1, basophil counts, and methacholine response. Thorax 1988; 43:456–461.
8. Diemer F, Sanico A, Horowitz E, Togias A. Non-allergenic inhalant triggers in seasonal and perennial allergic rhinitis. J Allergy Clin Immunol 1999; 103:S2.
9. Proctor D. The upper airways. I. Nasal physiology and defense of the lungs. Am Rev Respir Dis 1977; 115:97–130.
10. Jankowski R, Naclerio R, Andrews B, Thompson M, Knol M, Togias A. The ability of the nose to warm inhaled air is unrelated to its reactivity to cold dry air (CDA) [abstr]. J Allergy Clin Immunol 1993; 91:182.
11. Rouadi P, Baroody F, Abbott D, Naureckas E, Solway J, Naclerio R. A technique to measure the ability of the human nose to warm and humidify air. J Appl Physiol 1999; 87:400–406.
12. Ingelstedt S. Studies on the conditioning of air in the respiratory tract. Acta Otolaryngol 1956; 131:1–80.
13. Keck T, Leiacker R, Heinrich A, Kuhnemann S, Rettinger G. Humidity and temperature profile in the nasal cavity. Rhinology 2000; 38:167–171.
14. Cole P. Respiratory mucosal vascular responses, air conditioning and thermo regulation. J Laryngol Otol 1954; 68:613–622.
15. Baroody F, Naclerio R. A review of anatomy and physiology of the nose. A self instructional package from the committee on continuing education in otolaryngology. Alexandria, VA: American Academy of Otolaryngology-Head and Neck Surgery Foundation, Inc., 1990.
16. Dudley J, Cherry J. Scanning electron microscopic demonstration of goblet cell discharge and mucous layer on nasal ciliated respiratory epithelium. Otolaryngol Head Neck Surg 1980; 88:439–441.
17. Cole P. Modification of inspired air. In: Proctor DF, Andersen IB, eds. The Nose, Upper Airway Physiology and the Atmospheric Environment. Oxford: Elsevier Biomedical Press, 1982:351–376.
18. Cole P. Further observations on the conditioning of respiratory air. J Laryngol Otol 1953; 67:669–681.
19. Cauna N. Fine structure of the arteriovenous anastomosis and its nerve supply in the human nasal respiratory mucosa. Anat Rec 1970; 168:9–22.

20. Cauna N, Cauna D. The fine structure and innervation of the cushion veins of the human nasal respiratory mucosa. Anat Rec 1975; 181:1–16.

21. Hanna L, Scherer P. Regional control of local airway heat and water vapor losses. J Appl Physiol 1986; 61:624–632.

22. Tos M. Goblet cells and glands in the nose and paranasal sinuses. In: Proctor DF, Andersen IB, eds. The Nose. Upper Airway Physiology and the Atmospheric Environment. Amsterdam: Elsevier Biomedical Press B.V., 1982:99–144.

23. Kaliner M, Marom Z, Patow C, Shelhamer J. Human respiratory mucus. J Allergy Clin Immunol 1984; 73:318–323.

24. Pinto JM, Assanasen P, Baroody FM, Naureckas E, Naclerio RM. Alpha-adrenoreceptor blockade with phenoxybenzamine does not affect the ability of the nose to condition air. J Appl Physiol 2005; 99:128–133.

25. Abbott D, Baroody F, Naureckas E, Naclerio R. Elevation of nasal mucosal temperature increases the ability of the nose to warm and humidify air. Am J Rhinol 2001; 15:41–45.

26. Ingelstedt S, Ivstam B. Study in the humidifying capacity of the nose. Acta Otolaryngol 1951; 39:286–290.

27. Drettner B, Falck B, Simon H. Measurements of the air conditioning capacity of the nose during normal and pathological conditions and pharmacological influence. Acta Otolaryngol 1977; 84:266–277.

28. Kumlien J, Drettner B. The effect of ipratropium bromide (atrovent) on the air conditioning capacity of the nose. Clin Otolaryngol 1985; 10:165–168.

29. Assanasen P, Baroody F, Rouadi P, Naureckas E, Solway J, Naclerio R. Ipratropium bromide increases the ability of the nose to warm and humidify air. Am J Respir Crit Care Med 2000; 162:1031–1037.

30. Cauna N. Blood and nerve supply of the nasal lining. In: Proctor DF, Andersen IB, eds. The Nose. Oxford: Elsevier Biomedical Press, 1982:44–69.

31. Ingelstedt S, Ivstam B. The source of nasal secretion in infectious, allergic, and experimental conditions. Acta Otolaryngol 1949; 37:451–455.

32. Yankaskas J, Gatzy J, Boucher R. Effects of raised osmolarity on canine tracheal epithelial ion transport function. J Appl Physiol 1987; 62:2241–2245.

33. Knowles M, Clark C, Fischer N, et al. Nasal secretions: role of epithelial ion transport. In: Mygind N, Pipkorn U, eds. Allergic and Vasomotor Rhinitis: Pathophysiological Aspects. Copenhagen: Munksgaard, 1983:77–90.

34. Welsh M. Electrolyte transport by airway epithelia. Physiol Rev 1987; 67:1143–1184.

35. Boucher R, Chang E, Paradiso A, Strutts M, Knowles M, Earp H. Chloride secretory response of cystic fibrosis human airway epithelia. J Clin Invest 1989; 84:1424–1431.

36. Cruz A, Naclerio R, Lichtenstein L, Togias A. Further support for the role of hypertonicity on mast cell activation during nasal dry air reactions [abstr]. Clin Res 1990; 38:484A.

37. Assanasen P, Baroody F, Abbott D, Naureckas E, Solway J, Naclerio R. Natural and induced allergic responses increase the ability of the nose to warm and humidify air. J Allergy Clin Immunol 2000; 106:1045–1052.

38. Rozsasi A, Leicker R, Keck T. Nasal conditioning in perennial allergic rhinitis after nasal allergen challenge. Clin Exp Allergy 2004; 34:1099–1104.

39. Pinto J, Assanasen P, Baroody F, Naureckas E, Solway J, Naclerio R. Treatment of nasal inflammation decreases the ability of subjects with asthma to condition inspired air. Am J Respir Crit Care Med 2004; 170:863–869.

40. Togias A, Naclerio R, Proud D, et al. Nasal challenge with cold, dry air results in the production of inflammatory mediators: possible mast cell involvement. J Clin Invest 1985; 76:1375–1381.

41. Proud D, Bailey G, Naclerio R, et al. Tryptase and histamine as markers to evaluate mast cell activation during the responses to nasal challenge with allergen, cold, dry air, and hyperosmolar solutions. J Allergy Clin Immunol 1992; 89:1098–1110.

42. Naclerio R, Proud D, Kagey-Sobotka A, Lichtenstein L, Thompson M, Togias A. Cold, dry air-induced rhinitis: effect of inhalation and exhalation through the nose. J Appl Physiol 1995; 79:467–471.

43. Philip G, Jankowski R, Baroody F, Naclerio R, Togias A. Reflex activation of nasal secretion by unilateral inhalation of cold dry air. Am Rev Respir Dis 1993; 148: 1616–1622.
44. Cruz A, Togias A, Lichtenstein L, Kagey-Sobotka A, Proud D, Naclerio R. Local application of atropine attenuates the upper airway reaction to cold, dry air. Am Rev Respir Dis 1992; 146:340–346.
45. Togias A, Naclerio R, Warner J, et al. Demonstration of inhibition of mediator release from human mast cells by azatadine base. In vivo and in vitro evaluation. J Am Med Assoc 1986; 255:225–229.
46. Togias A, Proud D, Kagey-Sobotka A, Norman P, Lichtenstein L, Naclerio R. The effect of a topical tricyclic antihistamine on the response of the nasal mucosa to challenge with cold, dry air and histamine. J Allergy Clin Immunol 1987; 79:599–604.
47. Cruz A, Togias A, Lichtenstein L, Kagey-Sobotka A, Proud D, Naclerio R. Steroid-induced reduction of histamine release does not alter the clinical nasal response to cold, dry air. Am Rev Respir Dis 1991; 143:761–765.
48. Pipkorn U, Proud D, Lichtenstein L, Kagey-Sobotka A, Norman P, Naclerio R. Inhibition of mediator release in allergic rhinitis by pretreatment with topical glucocorticoids. N Engl J Med 1987; 316:1506–1510.
49. van Rijswijk J, Boeke E, Keizer J, Mulder P, Blom H, Fokkens W. Intransal capsaicin reduces nasal hyperreactivity in idiopathic rhinitis: a double-blind randomized application regimen study. Allergy 2003; 58:754–761.
50. Silvers W, Wiener M, Wood C, Paluch E. The skier's nose: a randomized, double blind placebo controlled study of ipratropium bromide (Atrovent MDI) administered intranasally for the prevention of cold-induced rhinorrhea [abstr]. J Allergy Clin Immunol 1988; 81:255.
51. Anderson S, Schoeffel R, Black J, Daviskas E. Airway cooling as the stimulus to exercise-induced asthma—a re-evaluation. Eur J Respir Dis 1985; 67:20–30.
52. Smith C, Anderson S. Hyperosmolarity as the stimulus to asthma induced by hyperventilation? J Allergy Clin Immunol 1986; 77:729–736.
53. Anderson S. Respiratory water loss as the mechanism of exercise-induced asthma. Folia Allergol Immunol Clin 1986; 33:271–277.
54. Smith C, Anderson S. An investigation of the hyperosmolar stimulus to exercise-induced asthma. Aust NZ J Med 1987; 17:A513.
55. Anderson S, Daviskas E, Smith C. Exercise-induced asthma: a difference in opinion regarding the stimulus. Allergy Proc 1989; 10:215–226.
56. Strauss R, McFadden E, Ingram R, Deal E, Jaeger J. Influence of heat and humidity in the airway obstruction induced by exercise in asthma. J Clin Invest 1978; 61:433–40.
57. Deal E, McFadden E, Ingram R, Strauss R, Jaeger J. Role of respiratory heat exchange in production of exercise-induced asthma. J Appl Physiol 1979; 46:467–475.
58. McFadden E, Pichurko B. Intraairway thermal profiles during exercise and hyperventilation in normal man. J Clin Invest 1985; 76:1007–1010.
59. McFadden E, Lenner K, Strohl K. Postexertional airway rewarming and thermally induced asthma. J Clin Invest 1986; 78:18–25.
60. Gilbert I, Pouke J, McFadden E. Intra-airway thermodynamics during exercise and hyperventilation in asthmatics. J Appl Physiol 1988; 64:2167–2174.
61. McFadden E. Hypothesis: exercise-induced asthma as a vascular phenomenon. Lancet 1990; 1:880–882.
62. Siraganian RP, Hazard KA. Mechanisms of mouse mast cell activation and inactivation for IgE-mediated histamine release. J Immunol 1979; 122:1719–1725.
63. Lawrence I, Warner J, Cohan V, Hubbard W, Kagey-Sobotka A, Lichtenstein L. Purification and characterization of human skin mast cells: evidence for human mast cell heterogeneity. J Immunol 1987; 139:3062–3069.
64. McKemy DD, Neuhausser WM, Julius D. Identification of a cold receptor reveals a general role for TRP channels in thermosensation. Nature 2002; 416:52–58.
65. Peier AM, Moqrich A, Hergarden AC, et al. A TRP channel that senses cold stimuli and menthol. Cell 2002; 108:705–715.

66. Story GM, Peier AM, Reeve AJ, et al. ANKTM1, a TRP-like channel expressed in nociceptive neurons, is activated by cold temperatures. Cell 2003; 112:819–829.
67. Reid G. ThermoTRP channels and cold sensing: what are they really up to? Pflugers Arch 2005; 451:250–263.
68. Kobayashi K, Fukuoka T, Obata K, et al. Distinct expression of TRPM8, TRPA1, and TRPV1 mRNAs in rat primary afferent neurons with a-delta/c-fibers and colocalization with trk receptors. J Comp Neurol 2005; 493:596–606.
69. Taylor-Clark T, Kollarik M, MacGlashan D, Undem B. Nasal sensory nerve populations responding to histamine and capsaicin. J Allergy Clin Immunol 2005; 116:1282–1288.
70. Togias A, Proud D, Kagey-Sobotka A, et al. The osmolality of nasal secretions increases when inflammatory mediators are released in response to inhalation of cold, dry air. Am Rev Respir Dis 1988; 137:625–629.
71. Eggleston P, Kagey-Sobotka A, Lichtenstein L. A comparison of the osmotic activation of basophils and human lung mast cells. Am Rev Respir Dis 1987; 135:1043–1048.
72. Eggleston P, Kagey-Sobotka A, Schleimer R, Lichtenstein L. Interaction between hyperosmolar and IgE-mediated histamine release from basophils and mast cells. Am Rev Respir Dis 1984; 130:86–92.
73. Silber G, Proud D, Warner J, et al. In vivo release of inflammatory mediators by hyperosmolar solutions. Am Rev Respir Dis 1988; 137:606–612.
74. Krayenbuhl M, Hudspith B, Scadding G, Brostoff J. Nasal response to allergen and hyperosmolar challenge. Clin Allergy 1988; 18:157–164.
75. Togias A, Lykens K, Kagey-Sobotka A, et al. Studies on the relationships between sensitivity to cold dry air, hyperosmolar solutions, and histamine in the adult nose. Am Rev Respir Dis 1990; 141:1428–1433.
76. Sanico AM, Philip G, Lai G, Togias A. Hyperosmolar saline induces reflex nasal secretions, evincing neural hyperresponsiveness in allergic rhinitis. J Appl Physiol 1999; 86:1202–1210.
77. Ahern GP, Brooks IM, Miyares RL, Wang XB. Extracellular cations sensitize and gate capsaicin receptor TRPV1 modulating pain signaling. J Neurosci 2005; 25:5109–5116.
78. Caterina M, Schumachert M, Tominaga M, Rosen T, Levine J, Julius D. The capsaicin receptor: a heat-activated ion channel in the pain pathway. Nature 1997; 389:816–824.
79. Pernow B. Role of tachykinins in neurogenic inflammation. J Immunol 1985; 135: 812–815.
80. Baraniuk J, Ali M, Yuta A, Fang S-Y, Naranch K. Hypertonic saline nasal provocation stimulates nociceptive nerves, substance P release, and glandular mucous exocytosis in normal humans. Am J Respir Crit Care Med 1999; 160:655–662.
81. Umeno E, McDonald D, Nadel J. Hypertonic saline increases vascular permeability in the rat trachea by producing neurogenic inflammation. J Clin Invest 1990; 85:1905–1908.
82. Jancso N, Jancso-Gabor A, Szolcsanyi J. Direct evidence for neurogenic inflammation and its prevention by denervation and by pretreatment with capsaicin. Br J Pharm Chemother 1967; 31:138–151.
83. Holzer P. Local effector functions of capsaicin-sensitive sensory nerve endings: involvement of tachykinins, calcitonin gene related peptide and other neuropeptides. Neuroscience 1988; 24:739–768.
84. Fuller R. The human pharmacology of capsaicin. Arch Int Pharmacodyn Ther 1990; 303:147–156.
85. Marabini S, Ciabatti G, Polli G, et al. Effect of topical nasal treatment with capsaicin in vasomotor rhinitis. Regul Pept 1988; 22:121.
86. Saria A, Wolf G. Beneficial effect of topically applied capsaicin in the treatment of hyperreactive rhinopathy. Regul Pept 1988; 22:167.
87. Wolf G, Saria A. Capsaicin in the Treatment of Hyperreflectory Rhinopathy (Vasomotor Rhinitis). VIII ISIAN, 1989.
88. Lacroix J, Buvelot J, Polla B, Lundberg J. Improvement of symptoms of non-allergic chronic rhinitis by local treatment with capsaicin. Clin Exp Allergy 1991; 21:595–700.
89. Marabini S, Ciabatti P, Polli G, Fusco B, Geppetti P. Beneficial effects of intranasal applications of capsaicin in patients with vasomotor rhinitis. Eur Arch Otorhinolaryngol 1991; 248:191–194.

90. Stjarne P, Lundblad L, Anggard A, Lundberg J. Local capsaicin treatment of the nasal mucosa reduces symptoms in patients with nonallergic nasal hyperreactivity. Am J Rhinol 1991; 5:145–151.

91. Blom H, Van Rijswijk J, Garrelds I, Mulder P, Timmermans T, Van Wijk R. Intranasal capsaicin is efficacious in non-allergic, non-infectious perennial rhinitis. A placebo-controlled study. Clin Exp Allergy 1997; 27:796–801.

92. Blom H, Severijnen A, Van Rijswijk J, Mulder P, Van Rijk R, Fokkens W. The long-term effects of capsaicin aqueous spray on the nasal mucosa. Clin Exp Allergy 1998; 28:1351–1358.

93. Annesi I, Neukirch F, Onoven-Friga E, et al. The relevance of hyperresponsiveness but not of atopy to FEV decline. Preliminary results in a working population. Bull Eur Physiopath Resp 1987; 23:397–400.

94. Assanasen P, Baroody F, Naureckas E, Solway J, Naclerio R. The nasal passage of subjects with asthma has a decreased ability to warm and humidify inspired air. Am J Resp Crit Care Med 2001; 164:1640–1646.

95. Braat J, Mulder P, Fokkens W, van Wijk R, Rijntjes E. Intranasal cold dry air is superior to histamine challenge in determining the presence and degree of nasal hyperreactivity in nonallergic noninfectious perennial rhinitis. Am J Respir Crit Care Med 1998; 157:1748–1755.

96. Togias A, Lichtenstein L, Norman P, et al. The relationship between atopy and the response to cold dry air (CDA) and histamine (H) challenge in perennial rhinitis (PR). J Allergy Clin Immunol 1988; 81:283.

97. Sanico AM, Koliatsos VE, Stanisz AM, Bienenstock J, Togias A. Neural hyperresponsiveness and nerve growth factor in allergic rhinitis. Int Arch Allergy Immunol 1999; 118:153–158.

98. Baroody F, Cruz A, Lichtenstein L, Kagey-Sobotka A, Proud D, Naclerio R. Intranasal beclomethasone inhibits antigen-induced nasal hyperresponsivess to histamine. J Allergy Clin Immunol 1992; 90:373–376.

99. Bedard P, Jobin M, Clement L, Mourad W, Hebert J. Evaluation of nonspecific nasal reactivity to histamine during and after natural ragweed pollen exposure. Am J Rhinol 1989; 3:211–215.

100. Togias A. H1-receptors: localization and role in airway physiology and in immune functions. J Allergy Clin Immunol 2003; 112:S60–S68.

101. Sanico A, Philip G, Proud D, Naclerio R, Togias A. Comparison of nasal mucosal responsiveness to neuronal stimulation in nonallergic and allergic rhinitis: effects of capsaicin nasal challenge. Clin Exp Allergy 1998; 28:92–100.

102. Cruz A, Naclerio R, Proud D, Togias A. Epithelial shedding is associated with nasal reactions to cold, dry air. J Allergy Clin Immunol. 2006; 117:1351–1358.

103. Davis MS, Schofield B, Freed AN. Repeated peripheral airway hyperpnea causes inflammation and remodeling in dogs. Med Sci Sports Exerc 2003; 35:608–616.

104. Heir T. Longitudinal variations in bronchial responsiveness in cross-country skiers and control subjects. Scand J Med Sci Sports 1994; 4:134–139.

105. Pabst R, Binns R. Lymphocytes migrate from the bronchoalveolar space to regional bronchial lymph nodes. Am J Respir Crit Care Med 1995; 151:495–499.

17 Pharmacological Provocation in Nonallergic Rhinitis

Roy Gerth van Wijk

Department of Internal Medicine, Section of Allergology, Erasmus Medical Center, Rotterdam, The Netherlands

THE CONCEPT OF NASAL HYPERREACTIVITY: RATIONALE BEHIND NASAL CHALLENGE TESTS WITH PHARMACOLOGICAL AGENTS

One of the first nasal challenge tests with a nonspecific agent was carried out by van Lier in 1960 (1). He challenged allergic subjects with veratrine, a mixture of plant alkaloids, in and outside the pollen season and observed a shift in dose–response curve, thereby concluding that patients with allergic rhinitis became more responsive to veratrine during the pollen season. This observation represents a phenomenon known as nasal hyperresponsiveness or nasal hyperreactivity. Hyperreactivity or hyperresponsiveness in the upper and lower airways refers to an increased sensitivity to nonspecific stimuli or irritants. In the case of hyperreactivity of the nasal mucosa, the most prominent symptoms of rhinitis patients are sneezes, rhinorrhea, and nasal blockage on exposure to low doses of stimuli, which do not induce symptoms in healthy subjects.

Nasal hyperreactivity can also be described as a clinical feature comprising occurrence of nasal symptoms on exposure to nonspecific stimuli such as dust particles, change of temperature, tobacco smoke, perfumes, and paint smells. The concept of nasal hyperreactivity either as a clinical characteristic of rhinitis or as hyperresponsiveness to pharmacological agents applied into the nose finds its counterpart? in lower airway hyperresponsiveness and bronchial asthma. Starting with clinical science in asthma, it is conceivable that many nasal challenge tests have been used to estimate nasal hyperreactivity.

Just as in studies in bronchial asthma, rhinitis patients and healthy subjects have undergone nasal challenge tests with agents such as histamine and methacholine. These and other substances will be discussed in the following sections.

PATHOPHYSIOLOGY

When we consider nasal hyperreactivity as an increased sensitivity to nonspecific stimuli or irritants, the question arises: what mechanisms are responsible for this phenomenon? Hyperreactivity of both upper and lower airways is a well-known feature of inflammatory disease (i.e., allergic rhinitis and bronchial asthma). Indeed, nasal responses to pharmacological agents have been studied mostly in allergic rhinitis compared to nonallergic rhinitis. It is known that allergen exposure or allergen challenge leads to increased nasal responsiveness to allergens but also to nonspecific agents.

In grass pollen–allergic patients during the pollen season, nasal sensitivity increased not only to allergen, but also to nonspecific stimuli such as histamine and methacholine (2). Also, in house dust mite allergy, a seasonal variation in nasal hyperreactivity in terms of nasal responsiveness to histamine can be observed (3). It appeared that during fall—the period of the highest exposure to house dust mites in The Netherlands—nasal reactivity to histamine was increased compared to the spring. Many investigators have shown that allergen provocation induced an increase in nasal sensitivity to nonspecific agents and stimuli such as histamine (4,5) and methacholine (6).

The increase of nasal sensitivity to histamine is very well correlated with increase in sensitivity to allergen (5), suggesting a common pathogenesis.

Several hypotheses have been advanced with respect to the mechanisms underlying hyperreactivity in allergic and nonallergic rhinitis. Having the sequence of events after stimulation of the nasal mucosa in mind, hyperresponsiveness could be located at several sites: (i) changes in epithelial barrier, (ii) altered neural sensitivity, (iii) changes at a central [central nervous system (CNS)] level, and (iv) changes at the endorgan level.

Increased Epithelial Permeability

Increased epithelial permeability would allow access for stimuli to sensory nerve endings, vessels, and nasal glands. In 1975, a better penetration of the mucosa was demonstrated in allergic rhinitis patients compared with healthy subjects, measured by application of topical albumin-^{125}I to the nasal mucosa (7). The concept of increased permeability has been challenged by Swedish investigators (8). Using a nasal pool device for concomitant provocation with histamine, they demonstrated a secretory hyperresponsiveness in both experimental and seasonal allergic rhinitis. However, neither nonspecific nor specific endorgan hyperresponsiveness could be explained by epithelial fragility or damage because nasal absorption permeability (measured with ^{51}Cr-labelled ethylene diaminetetra acetic acid and 1-deamino-8-D-arginine vasperssin) was decreased or unchanged in their studies of allergic and virus-induced rhinitis, respectively. They forwarded the

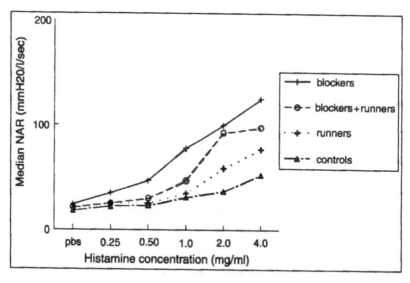

FIGURE 1 Histamine-induced nasal airway resistance in patients with nonallergic rhinitis. No statistically significant differences between subgroups. *Source:* Adapted from Ref. 50.

view of mucosal exudation of bulk plasma as a physiological airway tissue response with primarily a defense function. Plasma exudate entering the airway lumen immediately restores epithelial tight junctions, preventing luminal solutes from being reabsorbed.

Neural Hyperresponsiveness

Rapid allergen-induced changes in neural hyperresponsiveness involving sensory nerves have recently been demonstrated (9). It was shown that preceding allergen challenge in asymptomatic allergic subjects induced neural reflexes upon challenge with bradykinin persisting beyond the resolution of the acute allergic response. The data suggested that both afferent and efferent pathways were involved. These findings nicely fit with earlier experiments showing that bradykinin challenge led to contralateral secretory reflexes in subjects with symptomatic allergic rhinitis but not in subjects with seasonal allergic rhinitis who are asymptomatic and out of season (10). Others ascertained that the nasal response to hyperosmolar saline in allergic rhinitis was neural-mediated (11). Hyperosmolar saline-induced nasal secretions were significantly greater in the patients with rhinitis versus the healthy subjects. Sensory nerve desensitization with repeated application of capsaicin attenuated the hyperosmolar saline-induced secretions.

Changes at the Central or PNS Level

Changes at the central or peripheral nervous system (PNS) level have been proposed as a cause of hyperreactivity. Eccles and Lee (12) demonstrated in cats that stimulation of the hypothalamus leads to vasoconstriction in the nose, and they proposed that prolonged exposure to stress could result in loss of the hypothalamic control over sympathetic innervation. This condition would lead

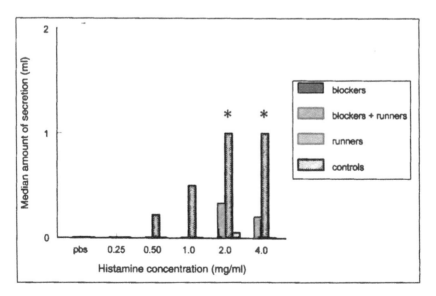

FIGURE 2 Histamine induced secretion in patients with nonallergic rhinitis. * represents a statistically significant difference compared to healthy controls ($p < 0.05$). Patients characterized by runny nose and sneezing (*runners*) react with increased secretory responsiveness to histamine. *Source:* Adapted from Ref. 50.

to a relative dominance of the parasympathetic system over the sympathetic pathways. Sanico proposed a hyper- or dysesthesia at the CNS or PNS level as a cause for nonallergic rhinitis. An increased nasal perceptual acuity would underlie the pathophysiology of nonallergic rhinitis. This would correspond with the observation that increased nasal irritant perceptual acuity for volatile organic compounds has been demonstrated in allergic rhinitis (13,14). Increased perception of irritants and environmental stimuli at the CNS level would lead to protective sneezing, rhinorrhea, and nasal congestion (15).

Changes in Endorgan Sensitivity at a Receptor Level

Changes in endorgan sensitivity at a receptor level could underlie nasal hyperreactivity. The presence of "histamine (H_1 and H_2) receptors" has been shown in the nasal mucosa (16). In patients with allergic rhinitis, the H_1 receptor mRNA is upregulated (17,18). In a recent study of seasonal allergic rhinitics, however, a difference in receptor gene expression versus normal controls could not be found, nor was it possible to correlate nasal reactivity to histamine with H_1 or H_2 receptor expression in superficial epithelial cells (19). In an animal model, it has been demonstrated that the number of H_1 receptors was correlated with hyperresponsiveness to antigen (20). Others (21) demonstrated that repeated allergen provocation in guinea pigs resulted in nasal hyperresponsiveness to histamine accompanied by an increased affinity of histamine for high-affinity agonist-binding sites in the hyperresponsive group. The authors suggested that this increased affinity might be induced by elevated G protein levels. From histamine H_3 receptors, it has been shown that the activation of these receptors inhibits sympathetic vasoconstrictor tone by inhibition of the release of noradrenaline from nerve terminals (22). Consistent with

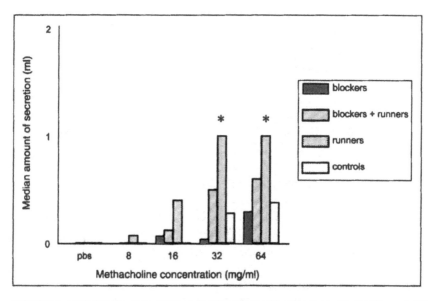

FIGURE 3 Methacholine-induced secretion in patients with nonallergic rhinitis. The asterisk represents a statistical significant difference compared to healthy controls ($p < 0.05$). Patients characterized by runny nose and sneezing (*runners*) react with increased secretory responsiveness to methacholine. *Source*: Adapted from Ref. 50.

this, a combination of histamine H_3 antagonists and histamine H_1 antagonists has been shown to display decongestant activity in a mast cell–dependent experimental feline model of nasal congestion (23). Although not known, it is conceivable that upregulation of H_3 receptors in nasal allergy might enhance the nasal response to both allergen and histamine.

An increased number of "muscarinic receptors" was found in patients with nasal allergy (24). As allergic patients are hyperresponsive to methacholine (24,25), it is possible that the increased number of muscarinic receptors plays a role in the exaggerated nasal discharge seen in allergic rhinitis patients. Also, increase of muscarinic receptors in nonallergic rhinitis patients might correspond with observations from challenge studies. In one study, the secretory response to capsaicin, which could be blocked by pretreatment with anticholinergic drugs, was found to be greater in nonallergic rhinitis patients, whereas the irritation of the nose was the same in both the healthy persons and in the patients with nonallergic rhinitis (26). These differences in effect were attributed to a change at the cholinoceptor site on the glandular cell and/or glandular hypertrophy, with an equal absorption of the test agents in healthy subjects and patients. In the past, research has been done on α- and β-receptor function in nasal vasculature. It was hypothesized that a decreased density of α_1-adrenergic receptors in the nasal mucosa might facilitate vasodilatation and swelling of the nasal mucosa in nasal allergy. Indeed, several groups revealed a decrease of α_1- and β-receptors in the nasal mucosa of allergic rhinitis patients compared with nonallergic patients with sinusitis (24,27). However, in contrast to these studies, Dutch researchers were unable to detect a decrease in α-adrenergic receptors in the nasal mucosa of allergic patients (28,29). They did demonstrate an increased sensitivity of muscarinic receptors and a decrease in number of β-adrenergic receptors in the nasal mucosa of allergic patients, but these shifts in sensitivity and number of cell receptors were small.

Nonimmunoglobulin E-Mediated Mast Cell Stimulation

Nonimmunoglobulin (Ig) E-mediated mast cell stimulation may be responsible for increased nasal responsiveness to certain stimuli. It is known that adenosine monophosphate (AMP) leads to mast cell degranulation. In particular, in allergic rhinitis nasal hyperresponsiveness to AMP has been shown (30). Another example of mast cell involvement regards nasal responsiveness to cold dry air (CDA). In several studies nasal challenge of the nose has been demonstrated in patients who experienced nasal symptoms after exposure to cold air. It was shown that in this subgroup of patients, nasal provocation with CDA will lead to mast cell activation and consequent mediator release (31–34). The assumption has been made that mast cells degranulate by an increased osmolality of the tissue due to evaporation. This is in agreement with the observation that CDA-induced mediator release is associated with an elevated osmolality in situ (35).

PHARMACOLOGICAL AGENTS

Provocation with Histamine

As previously mentioned, the nasal responses to histamine are mediated by three subtypes of histamine receptors (16,22). Histamine activates postjunctional H_1 receptors, which elicits an increase in vascular permeability, mucus production, and itch. H_2 receptors have been found in the nose, but their role has not been established yet. Prejunctional histamine H_3 receptors are abundantly expressed in the human nasal turbinate and mediate a significant sympathoinhibitory action of neurogenic vasoconstriction in human nasal mucosa (36). Attempts to discriminate patients with rhinitis from healthy subjects have been made particularly in patients with allergic rhinitis. In 1966 Grobler (37) could distinguish allergic patients from healthy subjects by topical application of histamine in the nose. In following studies, it appeared that it was not possible to distinguish asymptomatic patients from healthy subjects (38,39), which is opposite to the observation in bronchial asthma that patients free from symptoms may still be characterized by bronchial hyperresponsiveness. In contrast, symptomatic patients with allergic rhinitis appeared to be distinguished from controls (40–42). In a few studies nasal hyperresponsiveness to histamine could be demonstrated in patients with seasonal allergic rhinitis out of season (43,44). In several studies, considerable overlap between the healthy subjects and patients (45,46) have been found.

Fewer studies have been focused on nonallergic rhinitis. Clement et al. (47) found a statistically significant but small difference between nonallergic rhinitis patients and healthy subjects, using active and passive anterior rhinomanometry. One-sided measurements of the nasal airway resistance (NAR) and determination of a PD_{25} (the dose required to induce 25% increase in NAR) appeared to be superior in identifying nonallergic rhinitis patients to measurement of the total NAR and determination of a PD_{100} (48). Zambetti et al. (49) found hyperreactivity to histamine in 67.5% of patients with nonallergic rhinitis. We were able to discriminate between nonallergic patients with rhinitis and healthy subjects according to the history of patients. Patients characterized by sneezing and runny nose as could be distinguished in histamine challenge, whereas subjects with stuffy nose as the predominant symptom did not differ in nasal reactivity to histamine (50) (Figs. 1,2). Comparing different methods of nasal challenge with CDA appeared to be superior to histamine challenge in discriminating nonallergic rhinitis patients from healthy controls (51). Wuestenberg et al. (44) demonstrated clear-cut differences between healthy controls on the one hand and both allergic and nonallergic rhinitis patients on the other hand, using one-sided nasal challenge. By combining the results of symptom scores and rhinomanometry, a sensitivity of 100% and a specificity of 87% at a histamine concentration of 1 mg/mL for this procedure could be obtained.

Nasal responsiveness to histamine assessed with rhinostereometry has been used in a series of studies focused on the health impact of indoor environment. Nasal mucosal histamine reactivity among teachers working in a moisture-damaged school appeared to be increased compared to teachers working in a control school. Health complaints included general symptoms, irritation from eyes, nose, and throat, skin symptoms, and perceived "bad" air, dry air, and unpleasant smell (52,53). This nasal hyperreactivity persisted for years after remedial measures had been taken (54,55). Hyperresponsiveness to histamine appeared also to be present among tenants in a sick-building residential area (56). The observed hyperresponsiveness was not associated with the presence of allergic or nonallergic rhinitis. The increased responsiveness to histamine might be a sign of impending clinical disease.

Provocation with Methacholine

The first experiments with acetylcholine applied intranasally were performed by Grobler (37) who tested healthy subjects only. McLean et al. (38) and Borum (57) tested both healthy subjects and rhinitis patients with the stabler methacholine. It is well accepted that methacholine has an effect on muscarinic receptors only, therefore nasal challenge with methacholine may reveal endorgan glandular hyperresponsiveness. The results obtained from nasal challenge studies in both allergic and nonallergic rhinitis patients are inconsistent. Nasal allergy hyperresponsiveness to methacholine was shown by some (25,42,58) but not by others (11,38). Hyperresponsiveness to methacholine in patients with rhinitis of nonallergic origin was consistently shown in a series of studies (50,57,59,60) but not in all (58). In one study it was shown that methacholine hyperresponsiveness occured in nonallergic patients characterized by a history of watery rhinorrhea, whereas patients with predominantly nasal blockage were not captured with nasal methacholine challenge (50) (Fig. 3).

Other Agents and Stimuli

Nasal challenge with AMP, an agent known for its ability to release mediators from mast cells, has predominantly been used in patients with allergic rhinitis. Hyperresponsiveness to AMP has been shown in patients with nasal allergic rhinitis, but not in nonatopic subjects (30). AMP responsiveness could be attenuated by pretreatment with second-generation antihistamines such as desloratidine, fexofenadine, and levoceterizine (61). The involvement of inflammatory cells in nasal AMP responsiveness can be deduced from the observation that nasal steroids attenuate the response to AMP but not to histamine (62).

Other agents such as bradykinin and capsaicin, or stimuli as hypertonic saline have mostly been used in one-sided challenge tests to elucidate the neural pathways involved in nasal stimulation. These studies have been covered elsewhere.

One stimulus capable of clearly distinguishing between healthy subjects and well-characterized patients with severe nonallergic rhinitis is CDA. Nasal challenge with CDA proved to be more reproducible and better in discriminating than did histamine challenge (51). Moreover, it appeared that CDA hyperresponsiveness could be attenuated by repeated capsaicin desensitization (63).

COMMENTS ON PHARMACOLOGICAL PROVOCATION IN NAR

Surveying the literature in nonallergic rhinitis, the majority of studies point at an increased responsiveness to pharmacological and other stimuli. However, a few issues need to be addressed. First, the number of studies of allergic rhinitis exceeds the number of investigations of nonallergic rhinitis. This is not unexpected as there is much greater understanding of allergic rhinitis than of nonallergic rhinitis. However, concepts and findings may not be easily transferred from allergic to nonallergic rhinitis.

Secondly, in most studies, patients with nonallergic rhinitis are poorly defined or characterized. The definition is mainly based on the absence of other nasal disorders in the presence of symptoms. Less is known about the nature of symptoms, symptom severity, involvement of nasal inflammation, etc. In a Dutch series of investigations, patients with severe rhinitis, well defined in terms of symptom scores and a strict set of inclusion and exclusion criteria, were the subject of study. These patients appeared to be characterized by the absence of nasal inflammation (64,65) and resistance to nasal steroids (66). It is, however, not known whether these patients are representative of the total number of patients with nonallergic rhinitis. At least their characteristics diverge from the so-called nonallergic rhinitis with eosinophilia (NARES) syndrome marked by nasal eosinophilia and therapeutic responsiveness to nasal steroids. It is possible that patients from the latter group share other patterns of nasal hyperreactivity than, do patients from the former group, as in allergic rhinitis, involvement of inflammatory cells and mediators clearly augment the responses to nonspecific stimuli. The issue of careful characterization is valid, as methacholine responsiveness seems to be restricted to patients with predominantly runny nose (50).

Finally, all studies are characterized by a large variety of methods to assess nasal responsiveness to pharmacological agents. Histamine challenges have been monitored with rhinomanometry (41,42,44,47), acoustic rhinometry (43), and rhinostereometry (53,56), and by symptom scores (44,67). One-sided and two-sided challenges have been performed. This heterogeneity of methods and the heterogeneity in nonallergic rhinitis patients may explain the differences between a claimed sensitivity of 100% and specificity of 0% for histamine challenges in one study (51), in contrast to the sensitivity of 100% and a specificity of 87% found in another study (44).

So far, nasal challenge tests with nonspecific stimuli may give us insight into the pathophysiological backgrounds of nonallergic rhinitis. They can be used to monitor therapy, as has been done in treating patients with capsaicin and monitoring treatment with CDA challenges (63). We are, however, far away from being able to use them as an accepted diagnostic tool in the diagnosis and treatment of patients with nonallergic rhinitis.

REFERENCES

1. Lier LA. The influence of non-specific factors on the nasal mucous membranes in patients with rhinitis vasomotoria. Pract Otorhinolaryngol (Basel) 1960; 22:156–159.
2. Borum P, Gronborg H, Brofeldt S, Mygind N. Nasal reactivity in rhinitis. Eur J Respir Dis Suppl 1983; 128(Pt 1):65–71.
3. van Wijk RG, Dieges PH, van Toorenenbergen AW. Seasonal variability in nasal sensitivity to house dust mite extract. Rhinology 1987; 25:41–48.
4. Linder A, Venge P, Deuschl H. Eosinophil cationic protein and myeloperoxidase in nasal secretion as markers of inflammation in allergic rhinitis. Allergy 1987; 42:583–590.
5. Andersson M, Andersson P, Pipkorn U. Allergen-induced specific and non-specific nasal reactions. Reciprocal relationship and inhibition by topical glucocorticosteroids. Acta Otolaryngol 1989; 107:270–277.
6. Klementsson H, Andersson M, Pipkorn U. Allergen-induced increase in nonspecific nasal reactivity is blocked by antihistamines without a clear-cut relationship to eosinophil influx. J Allergy Clin Immunol 1990; 86:466–472.
7. Buckle FG, Cohen AB. Nasal mucosal hyperpermeability to macromolecules in atopic rhinitis and extrinsic asthma. J Allergy Clin Immunol 1975; 55:213–221.
8. Svensson C, Andersson M, Greiff L, Persson CG. Nasal mucosal endorgan hyperresponsiveness. Am J Rhinol 1998; 12:37–43.
9. Sheahan P, Walsh RM, Walsh MA, Costello RW. Induction of nasal hyper-responsiveness by allergen challenge in allergic rhinitis: the role of afferent and efferent nerves. Clin Exp Allergy 2005; 35:45–51.
10. Riccio MM, Proud D. Evidence that enhanced nasal reactivity to bradykinin in patients with symptomatic allergy is mediated by neural reflexes. J Allergy Clin Immunol 1996; 97:1252–1263.
11. Sanico AM, Philip G, Lai GK, Togias A. Hyperosmolar saline induces reflex nasal secretions, evincing neural hyperresponsiveness in allergic rhinitis. J Appl Physiol 1999; 86:1202–1210.

12. Eccles R, Lee RL. The influence of the hypothalamus on the sympathetic innervation of the nasal vasculature of the cat. Acta Otolaryngol 1981; 91:127–134.

13. Doerfler H, Hummel T, Klimek L, Kobal G. Intranasal trigeminal sensitivity in subjects with allergic rhinitis. Eur Arch Otorhinolaryngol 2006; 263(1):86–90.

14. Shusterman D, Murphy MA, Balmes J. Differences in nasal irritant sensitivity by age, gender, and allergic rhinitis status. Int Arch Occup Environ Health 2003; 76:577–583.

15. Sanico A, Togias A. Noninfectious, nonallergic rhinitis (NINAR): considerations on possible mechanisms. Am J Rhinol 1998; 12:65–72.

16. Uddman R, Moller S, Cardell LO, Edvinsson L. Expression of histamine H1 and H2 receptors in human nasal mucosa. Acta Otolaryngol 1999; 119:588–591.

17. Iriyoshi N, Takeuchi K, Yuta A, Ukai K, Sakakura Y. Increased expression of histamine H1 receptor mRNA in allergic rhinitis. Clin Exp Allergy 1996; 26:379–385.

18. Hamano N, Terada N, Maesako, et al. Expression of histamine receptors in nasal epithelial cells and endothelial cells—the effects of sex hormones. Int Arch Allergy Immunol 1998; 115:220–227.

19. Matovinovic E, Solberg O, Shusterman D. Epidermal growth factor receptor—but not histamine receptor—is upregulated in seasonal allergic rhinitis. Allergy 2003; 58: 472–475.

20. Ohkawa C, Ukai K, Miyahara Y, Takeuchi K, Sakakura Y. Histamine H1 receptor and reactivity of the nasal mucosa in sensitized guinea pigs. Auris Nasus Larynx 1999; 26:293–298.

21. Chiba Y, Saitoh N, Matsuo K, Misawa M. Elevated nasal mucosal G protein levels and histamine receptor affinity in a guinea pig model of nasal hyperresponsiveness. Int Arch Allergy Immunol 2002; 127:285–293.

22. Varty LM, Hey JA. Histamine H3 receptor activation inhibits neurogenic sympathetic vasoconstriction in porcine nasal mucosa. Eur J Pharmacol 2002; 452:339–345.

23. McLeod RL, Rizzo CA, West RE Jr., et al. Pharmacological characterization of the novel histamine H3-receptor antagonist N-(3,5-dichlorophenyl)-N'-[[4-(1H-imidazol-4-ylmethyl)phenyl]-methyl]-urea (SCH 79687). J Pharmacol Exp Ther 2003; 305: 1037–1044.

24. Konno A, Terada N, Okamoto Y. Changes of adrenergic and muscarinic cholinergic receptors in nasal mucosa in nasal allergy. ORL J Otorhinolaryngol Relat Spec 1987; 49:103–111.

25. Druce HM, Wright RH, Kossoff D, Kaliner MA. Cholinergic nasal hyperreactivity in atopic subjects. J Allergy Clin Immunol 1985; 76:445–452.

26. Stjarne P, Lundblad L, Lundberg JM, Anggard A. Capsaicin and nicotine-sensitive afferent neurones and nasal secretion in healthy human volunteers and in patients with vasomotor rhinitis. Br J Pharmacol 1989; 96:693–701.

27. Ishibe T, Yamashita T, Kumazawa T, Tanaka C. Adrenergic and cholinergic receptors in human nasal mucosa in cases of nasal allergy. Arch Otorhinolaryngol 1983; 238:167–173.

28. van Megen YJ, Klaassen AB, Rodrigues de Miranda JF, van Ginneken CA, Wentges BT. Alterations of adrenoceptors in the nasal mucosa of allergic patients in comparison with nonallergic individuals. J Allergy Clin Immunol 1991; 87:530–540.

29. van Megen YJ, Klaassen AB, Rodrigues de Miranda JF, van Ginneken CA, Wentges BT. Alterations of muscarinic acetylcholine receptors in the nasal mucosa of allergic patients in comparison with nonallergic individuals. J Allergy Clin Immunol 1991; 87:521–529.

30. Zeng D, Prosperini G, Russo C, et al. Heparin attenuates symptoms and mast cell degranulation induced by AMP nasal provocation. J Allergy Clin Immunol 2004; 114:316–320.

31. Togias AG, Naclerio RM, Proud D, et al. Nasal challenge with cold, dry air results in release of inflammatory mediators. Possible mast cell involvement. J Clin Invest 1985; 76:1375–1381.

32. Togias AG, Naclerio RM, Peters SP, et al. Local generation of sulfidopeptide leukotrienes upon nasal provocation with cold, dry air. Am Rev Respir Dis 1986; 133:1133–1137.

33. Togias A, Proud D, Kagey-Sobotka A, Norman P, Lichtenstein L, Naclerio R. The effect of a topical tricyclic antihistamine on the response of the nasal mucosa to challenge with cold, dry air and histamine. J Allergy Clin Immunol 1987; 79:599–604.

34. Iliopoulos O, Proud D, Norman PS, Lichtenstein LM, Kagey-Sobotka A, Naclerio RM. Nasal challenge with cold, dry air induces a late-phase reaction. Am Rev Respir Dis 1988; 138:400–405.
35. Togias AG, Proud D, Lichtenstein LM, et al. The osmolality of nasal secretions increases when inflammatory mediators are released in response to inhalation of cold, dry air. Am Rev Respir Dis 1988; 137:625–629.
36. Varty LM, Gustafson E, Laverty M, Hey JA. Activation of histamine H3 receptors in human nasal mucosa inhibits sympathetic vasoconstriction. Eur J Pharmacol 2004; 484:83–89.
37. Grobler NJ. Reactivity of the nasal mucosa. Thesis, Groningen, Drukkerij van Denderen, 1966.
38. McLean JA, Mathews KP, Solomon WR, Brayton PR, Ciarkowski AA. Effect of histamine and methacholine on nasal airway resistance in atopic and nonatopic subjects. Comparison with bronchial challenge and skin test responses. J Allergy Clin Immunol 1977; 59:165–170.
39. Guercio J, Saketkhoo K, Birch S, Fernandez R, Tachmes L, Sackner MA. Effect of nasal provocation with histamine, ragweed pollen and ragweed aerosol in normal and allergic rhinitis subjects. Am Rev Respir Dis 1979; 119(suppl):69.
40. Okuda M, Ohtsuka H, Sakaguchi K, Watase T. Nasal histamine sensitivity in allergic rhinitis. Ann Allergy 1983; 51:51–55.
41. Corrado OJ, Gould CA, Kassab JY, Davies RJ. Nasal response of rhinitic and non-rhinitic subjects to histamine and methacholine: a comparative study. Thorax 1986; 41:863–868.
42. Gerth Van Wijk R, Dieges PH. Comparison of nasal responsiveness to histamine, methacholine and phentolamine in allergic rhinitis patients and controls. Clin Allergy 1987; 17:563–570.
43. Hilberg O, Grymer LF, Pedersen OF. Nasal histamine challenge in nonallergic and allergic subjects evaluated by acoustic rhinometry. Allergy 1995; 50:166–173.
44. Wuestenberg EG, Hauswald B, Huettenbrink KB. Thresholds in nasal histamine challenge in patients with allergic rhinitis, patients with hyperreflectory rhinopathy, and healthy volunteers. Am J Rhinol 2004; 18:371–375.
45. Pipkorn U. Nasal provocation. Clin Rev Allergy 1988; 6:285–302.
46. Mygind N, Borum P, Secher C, Kirkegaard J. Nasal challenge. Eur J Respir Dis Suppl 1986; 143:31–34.
47. Clement PA, Stoop AP, Kaufman L. Histamine threshold and nasal hyperreactivity in non specific allergic rhinopathy. Rhinology 1985; 23:35–42.
48. Van de Heyning PH, Van Haesendonck J, Creten W, de Saegher D, Claes J. Histamine nasal provocation test. An evaluation of active anterior rhinomanometry and of threshold criteria of provocative dose. Allergy 1989; 44:482–486.
49. Zambetti G, Moresi M, Romeo R, Luce M, Filiaci F. Non-specific nasal provocation test with histamine Analysis of the dose-response curve. Rhinology 1999; 37:168–174.
50. Gerth van Wijk R, Dieges PH. Nasal hyper-responsiveness to histamine, methacholine and phentolamine in patients with perennial non-allergic rhinitis and in patients with infectious rhinitis. Clin Otolaryngol Allied Sci 1991; 16:133–137.
51. Braat JP, Mulder PG, Fokkens WJ, van Wijk RG, Rijntjes E. Intranasal cold dry air is superior to histamine challenge in determining the presence and degree of nasal hyperreactivity in nonallergic noninfectious perennial rhinitis. Am J Respir Crit Care Med 1998; 157:1748–1755.
52. Rudblad S, Andersson K, Stridh G, Bodin L, Juto JE. Slowly decreasing mucosal hyperreactivity years after working in a school with moisture problems. Indoor Air 2002; 12:138–144.
53. Rudblad S, Andersson K, Stridh G, Bodin L, Juto JE. Nasal hyperreactivity among teachers in a school with a long history of moisture problems. Am J Rhinol 2001; 15:135–141.
54. Rudblad S, Andersson K, Bodin L, Stridh G, Juto JE. Nasal mucosal histamine reactivity among teachers six years after working in a moisture-damaged school. Scand J Work Environ Health 2005; 31:52–58.

55. Rudblad S, Andersson K, Stridh G, Bodin L, Juto JE. Nasal histamine reactivity among adolescents in a remediated moisture-damaged school—a longitudinal study. Indoor Air 2004; 14:342–350.
56. Ohm M, Juto JE, Andersson K, Bodin L. Nasal histamine provocation of tenants in a sick-building residential area. Am J Rhinol 1997; 11:167–175.
57. Borum P. Nasal methacholine challenge. A test for the measurement of nasal reactivity. J Allergy Clin Immunol 1979; 63:253–257.
58. Asakura K, Enomoto K, Ara H, Azuma E, Kataura A. Nasal responsiveness to methacholine stimulation in allergic rhinitis patients. Arch Otorhinolaryngol 1984; 239: 273–278.
59. Filiaci F, Zambetti G. Aspecific nasal reactivity in allergic and non-allergic rhinopathy. Rhinology 1983; 21:329–334.
60. Marquez F, Sastre J, Hernandez G, et al. Nasal hyperreactivity to methacholine measured by acoustic rhinometry in asymptomatic allergic and perennial nonallergic rhinitis. Am J Rhinol 2000; 14:251–256.
61. Lee DK, Gardiner M, Haggart K, Fujihara S, Lipworth BJ. Comparative effects of desloratadine, fexofenadine, and levocetirizine on nasal adenosine monophosphate challenge in patients with perennial allergic rhinitis. Clin Exp Allergy 2004; 34:650–653.
62. Wilson AM, Sims EJ, Orr LC, Robb F, Lipworth BJ. An evaluation of short-term corticosteroid response in perennial allergic rhinitis using histamine and adenosine monophosphate nasal challenge. Br J Clin Pharmacol 2003; 55:354–359.
63. Van Rijswijk JB, Boeke EL, Keizer JM, Mulder PG, Blom HM, Fokkens WJ. Intranasal capsaicin reduces nasal hyperreactivity in idiopathic rhinitis: a double-blind randomized application regimen study. Allergy 2003; 58:754–761.
64. van Rijswijk JB, Blom HM, KleinJan A, Mulder PG, Rijntjes E, Fokkens WJ. Inflammatory cells seem not to be involved in idiopathic rhinitis. Rhinology 2003; 41:25–30.
65. Blom HM, Godthelp T, Fokkens WJ, et al. Mast cells, eosinophils and IgE-positive cells in the nasal mucosa of patients with vasomotor rhinitis. An immunohistochemical study. Eur Arch Otorhinolaryngol 1995; 252(suppl 1):S33–S39.
66. Blom HM, Godthelp T, Fokkens WJ, KleinJan A, Mulder PG, Rijntjes E. The effect of nasal steroid aqueous spray on nasal complaint scores and cellular infiltrates in the nasal mucosa of patients with nonallergic, noninfectious perennial rhinitis. J Allergy Clin Immunol 1997; 100:739–747.
67. de Graaf-in't Veld C, Garrelds IM, van Toorenenbergen AW, Gerth van Wijk R. Nasal responsiveness to allergen and histamine in patients with perennial rhinitis with and without a late phase response. Thorax 1997; 52:143–148.

Rhinitis Medicamentosa

Peter M. Graf

Karolinska University Hospital, Stockholm, Sweden

DEFINITION

Topical nasal decongestants have a long history of use. In the early 1900s, the substances were mainly derived from ephedrine. During the 1940s, nose-drop abuse was reported in a few studies and, in 1945 some authors found that rebound swelling developed after long-term use of topical vasoconstrictors (1). The substances used at that time had both α- and β-receptor activity as well as an indirect action because of the release of noradrenaline from the nerve terminals. In the 1960s, the modern vasoconstrictors, xylo- and oxymetazoline, were synthesized from the imidazole, naphazoline. They acted directly on the α-adrenoreceptors and were not thought to induce rebound swelling to the same extent as the earlier vasoconstrictors. Many studies of the effectiveness of modern vasoconstrictors were performed. Few studies, however, were made on the long-term effects of the drugs, and the results of these studies were contradictory.

Prolonged use of topical nasal decongestants may induce rebound swelling when the decongestive effect of the drug has disappeared. This phenomenon becomes more frequent the longer the vasoconstrictor is used. The nasal stuffiness is relieved by additional doses of the vasoconstrictor eventually in larger doses, indicating tolerance. The patient may then become uncertain as to whether congestion is still being caused by the nasal disease or by rebound congestion. In some cases, patients are unaware of the cause of nasal stuffiness, and the nose-drop overuse cannot be broken without professional help. The patient becomes increasingly dependent on the drug, and a vicious circle may be established with long-term daily overuse, i.e., rhinitis medicamentosa (RM). An abrupt cessation of topical decongestants in patients with RM induces marked nasal blockage because of rebound congestion. The pronounced nasal obstruction is hard to endure, and therefore patients usually start using the decongestants again after only a few days of withdrawal. Treatment of rhinitis medicamentosa is quite difficult; the condition is often referred to as "therapy-resistant rhinitis"; and should therefore be treated by rhinologists and not by general practitioners.

Thus, RM may be defined as "a condition characterized by symptoms of rhinitis caused by the same decongesting nose drops as the patients used to relieve the symptoms" (2). RM has also been defined as a condition of nasal hyperreactivity, mucosal swelling, and tolerance induced, or aggravated, by the overuse of topical vasoconstrictors with or without a preservative (3).

HISTORICAL BACKGROUND

The first topical vasoconstrictors were based on ephedrine with a brief decongestive effect. Even then Kully reported that prolonged use of these drugs could result in nasal stuffiness and tolerance, and the term "rhinitis medicamentosa" was coined in 1946 (1). With modern vasoconstrictors, such as oxy- and xylometazoline, the risk of developing RM was initially considered to be much less or even non-existent. Since 1981, it has been possible to purchase nose drops in single-dose pipettes containing oxymetazoline over-the-counter in Sweden, and, since 1989, there has been no need for a doctors' prescription for nasal sprays containing oxy- and xylometazoline. In contrast to nose drops in single-dose pipettes, all nasal decongestant sprays on the Swedish market then contained the preservative benzalkonium chloride (BKC) to prevent bacterial contamination. Since 1989 the sales of these drugs have increased tremendously. Because nasal sprays are preferred to single-dose pipettes, there was a switch after 1989 from the use of preservative-free to BKC preserved solutions. Since 1994, first oxymetazoline, and later also xylometazoline nasal sprays, became available without BKC in Sweden. These decongestants are now administered in a new type of spray bottle shown to prevent bacterial contamination.

INCIDENCE OF RM INDUCED BY OXY- AND XYLOMETAZOLINE

RM is more common in young middle-aged adults than in children and old people, but no difference between men and women has been reported. The incidence of RM in Sweden is unknown, but there is evidence indicating that the number of patients has increased in Sweden since 1989 when nasal decongestant sprays became available over-the-counter. Patients with some underlying chronic nasal obstruction, such as allergic- and vasomotor rhinitis, nasal polyposis, etc., run a greater risk of developing RM, but it has been reported that most patients start overusing the decongestants because of a common cold, sinusitis, or pregnancy rhinitis without previous nasal disease (4).

PATHOPHYSIOLOGY

The pathophysiology of the rebound swelling in RM is not known. However, several theories have been postulated, some of which are more plausible than others. It has been suggested that the rebound swelling occurs because of tissue hypoxia resulting in reacting hyperemia that is manifested as vasodilatation (5,6). It has been reported that oxymetazoline reduces nasal mucosal blood flow by about 50%. However this seems improbable because the resistance vessels regulating nasal mucosal blood flow are affected mainly by α2-adrenoreceptor agonists (7). Unlike the imidazoles, the α1-selective sympathomimetic amines cause decongestion without reducing mucosal blood flow (7). However, the sympathomimetic amines also induce rebound swelling after prolonged use (8). Complicating these explanations is the fact that the nasal vasculature consists of several compartments, which in turn may respond differently to different pharmacologic stimuli.

The rebound swelling has also been attributed to long-term use of α2-receptor agonists that may stimulate the negative feedback mechanism presynaptically, resulting in reduction of endogenous NA (9). The α-adrenergic tone would then persist only as long as the topical α2-receptor agonist is used. When the action of the drug disappears, rebound swelling follows. This may further be supported by evidence that, in the dog, the mucosal pretreatment with an α2-receptor agonist reduces the response to sympathetic nerve activation (10). However, vasoconstrictors without α2-receptor action also induce rebound swelling.

The rebound phenomenon has also been ascribed to alteration in the vaso-motor tone, which increased parasympathetic activity, vascular permeability, and edema formation. This hypothesis is in accordance with a study in guinea pigs that received naphazoline for four months (11). An increased activity of the cholinester-ase enzyme, which was interpreted as parasympathic hyperactivity, in the cholinergic nerves around the blood vessels was found. Marked vascular dilatation and edema were also present, indicating an increased vascular permeability. Simi-lar results have been reported by Talaat et al. (12), whereas no such histological changes were found in studies performed by others (13,14).

WHEN DOES RM OCCUR?

With modern vasoconstrictors, such as oxy- and xylometazoline, the risk of devel-oping RM was initially considered to be small or even nonexistent (15,16). This was further supported in a study by Petruson, indicating that xylometazolin contain-ing BKC could safely be used daily for six weeks in healthy subjects (13). In that study rhinomanometry was used to measure possible rebound mucosal swelling. However, Graf and Juto have shown that healthy subjects using oxymetazoline (0.5 mg/mL) nasal spray containing BKC three times daily for 30 days developed RM, evidenced both as rebound mucosal swelling and increased histamine sensi-tivity (17). The degree of increased histamine sensitivity was comparable to that seen in patients with idiopathic rhinitis, and it reflects the development of nasal hyperreactivity (18). In those studies, rhinostereometry and symptom scores of nasal stuffiness were used to assess rebound mucosal congestion. Åkerlund and Bende (2) found that patients with vasomotor rhinitis, but not healthy subjects, developed rebound swelling after three weeks of daily use of xylometazoline con-taining BKC. However, when investigating healthy subjects using oxymetazolin (0.5 mg/mL) nasal spray containing BKC three times daily for 10 days, no evidence of RM was found (19). Morris et al. (20) studied healthy subjects receiving oxyme-tazoline b.i.d. for seven days. These subjects did not develop rebound mucosal congestion after the end of treatment.

It has been suggested that patients with some chronic inflammation in the nasal mucosa are more susceptible to the development of RM than healthy subjects (2). Therefore, Graf et al. performed a study where patients with a chronic inflammation in the nasal mucosa, i.e., idiopathic rhinitis, used oxymetazoline with and without BKC for 10 days (19). Possible rebound congestion was measured both with rhinostereometry and acoustic rhinometry, and nasal stuffiness was subjec-tively estimated on visual analogue scales. We found no evidence of rebound congestion in either of the two groups with either of the two methods.

The incidence of RM has been increasing since 1989, when nasal sprays became available over-the-counter in Sweden. Long-term use of oxy- and xylome-tazoline nasal spray with or without BKC will probably induces RM in most or even all subjects/patients sooner or later. There is substantial evidence indicating that three- to four-week use of oxymetazoline 0.5 mg/mL three times daily should be avoided. Even oxymetazoline (0.5 mg/mL) containing BKC once daily at night for four weeks in healthy subjects induces RM (21). For long-term treatment with oxy- and xylometazoline, there is evidence indicating that RM develops faster and more pronounced if these solutions contain BKC (see below). However, there is no data suggesting that 10 days' use of oxymetazoline nasal spray with or without BKC, in healthy subjects or in patients with vasomotor rhinitis, induces RM.

Patients with common cold or allergic rhinitis have not been investigated regarding the development of RM, but it is unlikely that these patients would react differently and develop rebound mucosal swelling after 10 days' treatment with oxy- or xylometazoline with or without BKC.

There are no data indicating that there should be any difference between oxy- and xylometazoline regarding the development of RM; but in general, oxymetazoline has been more thoroughly investigated than xylometazoline regarding the development of RM.

TOLERANCE

In the literature on RM, the term tachyphylaxis has frequently been used instead of tolerance. By definition, tachyphylaxis is a rapid reduction in the effect of a drug after the administration of only a few doses. Tolerance, on the contrary, is a hyporeactivity acquired after longer exposure to the drug, which means that the decongestive effect fades after long-term use of the vasoconstrictor.

It has been shown that the decongestive effect of a single dose of oxymetazoline is significantly lower in patients with RM compared to healthy subjects (22). However, tolerance can also be expressed as a decreased duration of the decongestant after long-term use of the vasoconstrictor, which has been shown in healthy subjects (23) as well as patients with RM (22). Therefore, most patients with RM use the nasal sprays more often than two or three times daily, the dose recommended by the manufacturers. Thus in RM, tolerance is seen both as a reduction of the decongestive response and in the decongestive effect of a single dose of the vasoconstrictor.

BENZALKONIUM CHLORIDE

The preservative BKC is a quaternary ammonium compound which acts by damaging the cell wall of the microorganisms (24). It is used in nebulizer solutions for the lungs, in nasal sprays such as vasoconstrictors and corticosteroids, and in eye- and eardrops. In nasal solutions, BKC is ordinarily used in concentrations of 100 or 200 mg/L. The use of BKC has been questioned because of its reported bronchoconstrictive effects when inhaled by asthmatic patients (25). It has also been shown that exposure to 0.01% BKC for two minutes damages the corneal epithelium by cellular destruction (26), and BKC-induced contact allergy has been reported in patients with chronic external otitis (27). Moreover, 0.1% BKC applied to the serosal surface of the intestine of the rat for 30 minutes has been found to injure intramural nerve elements selectively, resulting in aganglionosis (28). In vitro studies in the nose have shown that BKC is toxic to the cilia (29). Deleterious effects on granulocyte chemotaxis and phagocytosis (30), and other important defence functions of the neutrophils in vitro (31) have also been reported.

BKC AND RM

Graf et al. have studied the effect of BKC on the development of RM (32). We studied healthy subjects receiving oxymetazoline nasal spray (0.5 mg/mL) three times daily with and without BKC (0.1 mg/mL) for 30 days. Rebound swelling was found in both groups, but it was significantly less marked in the group receiving oxymetazoline without BKC. These same two groups of subjects then had no nasal spray for three months and again were treated with the same nasal spray as before but this time for only 10 days (33). Only the group pretreated with oxymetazoline containing BKC for one to three months had earlier developed rebound mucosal swelling after 10 days. This was seen objectively using rhinostereometry and in the symptom scores. In the group receiving oxymetazoline without BKC, no rebound swelling was found; we concluded that BKC has long-lasting adverse effects on the nasal mucosa. Similarly, Graf and Hallén have reported that in patients with RM, one year after successful treatment (when these patients were without any nasal symptoms 7 days), use of oxymetazoline nasal spray containing BKC induced rebound swelling and nasal hyperreactivity (34). In another study of healthy subjects one group received oxymetazoline nasal spray without BKC; one group received BKC nasal spray alone; and the others were treated with placebo nasal spray for one month. The results showed that long-term use of BKC induces mucosal swelling, whereas oxymetazoline induces nasal hyperreactivity (35). Thus, both oxymetazoline and BKC per se are capable of inducing RM.

In conclusion, long-term use of BKC in oxymetazoline nasal spray accentuates the severity of RM and such a nasal spray has long-lasting adverse effects unlike oxymetazoline without BKC. Patients with RM induced by decongestants containing BKC, who have been able to stop using the decongestants, can easily reenter the vicious circle of RM again after only a few days use of the nasal decongestant sprays. This is of great clinical importance and is a common reason for "long-term" treatment failure. Patients successfully treated for RM may thus return months or years after treatment with a new episode of RM, if they use decongestants again even for a short period. All patients with RM must be informed about this risk when treatment is started.

DIAGNOSIS

RM is a common cause of nasal stuffiness. However, some patients are unaware of the connection between their nose drop overuse and their nasal stuffiness. There are also some patients who do not want to admit that they are "addicted" to nasal drops or sprays. Therefore, it is essential for the rhinologist to ask all patients with nasal stuffiness whether they use topical vasoconstrictors, how many doses daily, and for how long they have been using them. It is also important to ask patients with RM whether they have tried to stop using the decongestants, if they had professional help, etc.

Most patients who have a doctor's appointment have taken topical decongestants just before the appointment, resulting in decongestion of the nasal mucosa. When the nasal mucosa is decongested it almost looks "normal" and the diagnosis will easily be overlooked. If you know you are dealing with a patient with RM it is advisable to ask the patient not to take decongestants on the day of the first outpatient visit. Be sure to give these patients an appointment in the morning because these patients will have difficulty being without the decongestants until the afternoon. At the visit the nasal mucosa is severely swollen, and in severe cases the inferior turbinates are in direct contact with the nasal septum bilaterally. In fact, the actual severity of RM can be evaluated when inspected in the morning when the last dose of the decongestants was taken the evening before.

At the first visit, the nasal mucosa should be decongested and the nose must be endoscopically inspected. In severe cases, it is difficult to decongest the nasal mucosa sufficiently to be able to endoscopically investigate the nose. This may then be done at the next visit two weeks after treatment (see below).

In some cases, patients with RM have another nasal disease causing stuffiness. They may have nasal allergy, septal deviation, or an old nasal fracture causing nasal obstruction or nasal polyposis, and sometimes also malignancies. All these other diagnoses must be considered when patients are examined, and this is why these patients must be treated by rhinologists.

TREATMENT OF RM—THE "ACUTE PHASE"

The main aim of treatment is to convince the patient that the long-term use of vasoconstrictors is responsible for the nasal stuffiness and that overuse is harmful, regardless of the underlying nasal disease. Some patients have already unsuccessfully tried the therapy recommended by the physician, and in those cases it is particularly important not to compromise. It takes time and patience to explain the mechanisms of RM, but an explanation is essential for the treatment to be successful. The patient needs to fully understand the mechanism that causes the disorder, and the patient's cooperation should be assured before the actual treatment begins.

Management of RM requires withdrawal of the topical decongestant to allow the damaged nasal mucosa to recover, followed by treatment of the underlying nasal disease. In clinical practice, various methods to stop the overuse have been tried. Most authors discontinue the vasoconstrictors immediately and completely, whereas others recommend vasoconstrictor withdrawal from one nostril at a time. Nocturnal sedation has also been recommended during the withdrawal process, as nasal obstruction at night interferes with sleep. The most commonly used and most effective treatment is the application of intranasal steroids and/or systemic steroids. However, it has been suggested that no special treatment except vasoconstrictor withdrawal is needed in RM (36).

To the authors' knowledge, only one *controlled* study on treatment of RM has been performed (37). Graf et al. performed a parallel randomized, double-blind study to evaluate the treatment of RM. In two groups containing 10 patients with RM, each group stopped their overuse of nasal vasoconstrictor spray immediately and were treated with either fluticasone propionate nasal spray once daily 200 µg, or placebo nasal spray for 14 days. The nasal mucosal swelling was recorded with rhinostereometry, acoustic rhinometry, and a peak inspiratory flow meter. Nasal stuffiness was estimated on a visual analogue scale in the morning and in the evening of each day.

The study showed that the mucosal swelling was reduced after 7 and 14 days of treatment with fluticasone propionate as well as placebo, but the reduction was significantly greater after treatment with fluticasone propionate. The symptom scores for nasal stuffiness showed a marked reduction during the treatment period in both groups, but there was an earlier onset of symptom reduction after treatment with the topical steroid.

An abrupt cessation of topical decongestants in patients with RM induces marked nasal blockage because of rebound congestion. The pronounced nasal obstruction is hard to endure and therefore patients often start using the decongestants again after only a few days of withdrawal. This is another common reason why treatment of RM often fails. The first few days are crucial, and our results show that fluticasone propionate reduces nasal stuffiness significantly in as early as four days of treatment, unlike placebo, where symptom relief was not observed until seven days. In fact, a marked reduction in symptom scores occurred during the first three days of treatment with fluticasone propionate. This is in agreement with clinical practice, where the author's impression is that patients given topical corticosteroids, despite years of vasoconstrictor overuse, note a very fast reduction of the worst symptoms of nasal stuffiness, i.e., within three to seven days. It is of great importance for successful treatment and compliance to inform patients about this fast recovery.

The treatment study shows that vasoconstrictor withdrawal without treatment with active drug reduces nasal mucosal swelling and symptom scores after seven days of treatment and that no one used topical decongestants during the study period. Thus, the main aim of treatment was achieved even in the patients treated with a placebo nasal spray. However, this does not automatically mean that, in clinical practice, patients with RM will succeed in withdrawing the vasoconstrictors without any treatment except the instruction to discontinue the decongestant, which has been suggested (36). In the recent study, all patients naturally hoped that they had been given fluticasone propionate. They also received special attention and much more information about the disease than they would have been given on a regular visit to our outpatient department. Moreover, it has been suggested that placebo aqueous nasal spray per se may have a positive effect on RM.

An adequate treatment of patients with RM consists of a combination of vasoconstrictor withdrawal and a topical corticosteroid to alleviate the withdrawal process. It is the author's opinion that nocturnal sedation should not be used and that oral corticosteroids are usually not necessary. It is essential for successful treatment and compliance to give the patients adequate information about RM in general and especially about the rapid reduction in nasal stuffiness when given correct treatment. The study also shows that two-week treatment with a topical corticosteroid is sufficient. This is also the time for the second outpatient visit.

TREATMENT OF RM—THE "LONG-TERM" RESULT

Once the "acute phase" of treatment is achieved, the difficult long-term treatment result must be considered. As discussed earlier, patients successfully treated from RM will easily return days, months, or years after treatment with a new episode of RM if they use decongestants again even for a very short period. It is advisable to tell each patient after successful treatment (at the second outpatient visit) never to use topical decongestants again and also carefully explain the mechanisms behind such a statement. It is recommended to see these patients again after one to three months to see how the patient is doing.

Many patients make several attempts to stop using the vasoconstrictors, but like an alcoholic they reenter the nose drop overuse months or years after "acute phase" treatment. With each time of treatment failure, the patients get more and more convinced that they will never be able to once and for all stop using the decongestants. The best chance for successful long-term treatment is the first treatment attempt. This is why it is so important that the physician be an expert on RM for the treatment, and for information to be correct initially to be successful.

NASAL SURGERY AND RM

Some colleagues use nasal surgery such as turbinectomy, etc., to reduce nasal mucosal swelling, first making it easier for the patient to stop using the topical decongestants. It is my clinical experience, however, that nasal surgery does not cure RM. On the contrary, there may be a risk in performing nasal surgery on patients with RM. The patients will continue using the topical decongestants after surgery and there is a risk that the nasal mucosa will not heal properly after surgery and the situation will be worse than before surgery.

In general, patients with RM and some other nasal disorder that needs nasal surgery (septal deviation, nasal polyposis, etc.) should first receive adequate treatment for RM before surgery is performed. Nasal surgery may be performed three months after successful treatment of RM.

NEED FOR FURTHER STUDIES

It has been suggested that the severity of RM is directly proportional to the length of time the drug has been used, to the frequency of its use, and to the amount of drug administered. It is now also well established that RM depends on whether the nasal decongestant contains BKC, the period during which the decongestant has been used, and whether the nasal mucosa is healthy or pathologic.

It is possible that RM may be avoided if a lower dose of the vasoconstrictor is used. Thus, studies investigating the effect on the nasal mucosa of long-term use of oxymetazoline 0.25 and 0.1 mg/mL or xylometazoline 0.5 mg/mL for adults are important to perform. The goal must be to give the patient the least toxic decongestant. This is especially important for children.

CONCLUSION

Topical decongestants are helpful for symptomatic relief of nasal congestion during a common cold or sinusitis. However, RM is a serious complication after prolonged use of these drugs, and the condition is referred to as "therapy-resistant nasal blockage," because it is difficult to treat and the significant risk of recurrence after successful treatment. RM may in the end result in atrophic rhinitis, which is a serious condition. Adequate information must be given to the public and to doctors. Patients must be instructed that these drugs should only be used for symptomatic relief of nasal obstruction. Thus, in most cases the usage should be limited to only a few days when patients are bothered by nasal stuffiness during a common cold. Patients must be instructed that nasal decongestants do not have a curative effect on the common cold, sinusitis, or otitis media. Nasal stuffiness is most bothersome at night and in many cases it is sufficient to use it only before going to sleep. The lowest possible dose of the topical vasoconstrictor should be used.

It has been suggested that some patients are indeed more prone to develop RM. Thus, as a safety measure, there must be a warning in the product information of the risk of developing RM in some cases after only a few days.

Notwithstanding the above caution, there are no data indicating that 10-day use of oxymetazoline nasal spray with or without BKC, in healthy subjects or in patients having vasomotor rhinitis, induces RM. However, long-lasting adverse effects have been reported after the use of oxymetazoline nasal spray containing BKC, but not in oxymetazoline without BKC. In clinical practice, some patients get many episodes of common colds/sinusitis during one year, and we do not know whether RM develops if decongestants are used for two or more 10-day periods in succession. This has to be investigated further.

BKC has adverse effects on the nasal mucosa, and it should therefore be avoided as nasal decongestant sprays nowadays can safely be administered without BKC. This chapter refers to a number of well-performed studies showing adverse effects of BKC with and without oxymetazoline. Where possible, avoiding exposure of BKC is recommended.

REFERENCES

1. Lake C. Rhinitis medicamentosa. Mayo Clinic Proc 1946; 21:367–371.
2. Åkerlund A, Bende M. Sustained use of xylometazoline nose drops aggravates vasomotor rhinitis. Am J Rhinol 1991; 5(4):157–160.
3. Graf P. Overuse of oxy- and xylometazoline nasal sprays—changes in nasal mucosal swelling and histamine sensitivity in healthy subjects and in patients with rhinitis medicamentosa. Thesis, Karolinska Institute, 1994.
4. Walker J. Rhinitis medicamentosa. J Allergy 1952; 23:183–186.
5. Baldwin R. Rhinitis medicamentosa (an approach to treatment). J Med Assoc State Ala 1977; 47:33–35.
6. DeBernardis J, Winn M, Kerkman D, et al. A new nasal decongestant A-57219: a comparison with oxymetazoline. J Pharm Pharmacol 1987; 39:760–763.
7. Andersson K, Bende M. Adrenoreceptors in the control of human nasal mucosal blood flow. Ann Otol Rhinol Laryngol 1984; 93:179–182.
8. Osguthorpe D, Reed S. Neonatal respiratory distress from rhinitis medicamentosa. Laryngoscope 1987; 97:829–831.
9. Lacroix J. Adrenergic and nonadrenergic mechanisms in sympathetic vascular control of the nasal mucosa. Acta Physiol Scand Suppl 1989; 581:1–63.
10. Berridge T, Roach A. Characterization of alpha-adrenoreceptors in vasculature in the canine nasal mucosa. Br J Pharmacol 1986; 88:345–354.
11. Elwany S, Stephanos W. Rhinitis medicamentosa. An experimental histopathological and histochemical study. ORL 1983; 45:187–194.
12. Talaat M, Belal A, Aziz T, et al. Rhinitis medicamentosa; electron microscopic study. J Laryngol Otol 1981; 95:125–131.
13. Petruson B. Treatment with xylometazoline (Otrivin) nosedrops over a six-week period. Rhinology 1981; 19:167–172.
14. Rijntjes E. Nose-drop abuse; a functional and morphologic study. Thesis, University of Leiden, 1985.
15. Kuhn A. Evaluation of a new nasal decongestant. J Indiana State Med Assoc 1966; 59:1295–1296.
16. Mayer P. A prolonged acting topical nasal decongestant for various rhinitides. Illinois Med J 1966; 129:230–232.
17. Graf P, Juto J. Decongestion effect and rebound swelling of the nasal mucosa during four-week use of oxymetazoline. ORL 1994; 56:131–134.
18. Hallén H, Juto J. An objective method to record changes in nasal reactivity during treatment of non-allergic nasal hyperreactivity. ORL 1994; 56:92–95.
19. Graf P, Enerdal J, Hallén H. Ten days' use of oxymetazoline nasal spray with or without BKC in patients with vasomotor rhinitis. Arch Otolaryngol Head Neck Surg 1999; 125:1128–1132.
20. Morris S, Eccles R, Martez S, et al. An evaluation of nasal response following different treatment regimes of oxymetazoline with reference to rebound congestion. Am J Rhinol 1997; 11:109–115.
21. Graf P, Hallén H, Juto J. Four-week use of oxymetazoline nasal spray (Nezeril*) once daily at night induces rebound swelling and nasal hyperreactivity. Acta Otolaryngol (Stockh) 1995; 115:71–75.
22. Graf P, Hallén H, Juto J. The pathophysiology and treatment of rhinitis medicamentosa. Clin Otolaryngology 1995; 20:224–229.
23. Graf P, Juto J. Sustained use of xylometazoline nasal spray shortens the decongestive response and induces rebound swelling. Rhinology 1995; 33:14–17.

24. Richards R, Cavill R. Electron microscopic study of the effect of benzalkonium chloride and edete disodium on the cell envelope of *Pseudomonas aeruginosa*. J Pharm Sci 1976; 65:76–80.
25. Miszkiel K, Beasley R, Holgate S. The influence of ipratropiumbromide and sodium cromoglycate on benzalkonium chloride- induced bronchokonstriction in asthma. Br J Clin Pharmacol 1988; 26:295–301.
26. Tönjum A. Permeability of rabbit corneal epithelium to horseradish peroxidase after the influence of benzalkonium chloride. Acta Ophthal 1975; 53:335–347.
27. Fräki J, Kalimo K, Tuohimaa P, et al. Contact allergy to various components of topical preparations for treatment of external otitis. Acta Otolaryngol (Stockh) 1985; 100: 414–418.
28. Sato A, Yamamoto M, Imamura K, et al. Pathophysiology of aganglionic colon and anorectum: an experimental study on aganglionosis produced by a new method in the rat. J Ped Surg 1978; 13:399–405.
29. Batts A, Marriot C, Martin G, et al. The effect of some preservatives used in nasal preparations on mucociliary clearance. J Pharm Pharmacol 1989; 41:156–159.
30. Håkansson B, Forsgren A, Tegner H, et al. Inhibitory effects of nasal drop components on granulocyte chemotaxis. Pharmacol Toxicol 1989; 64:321–323.
31. Bjerknes R, Steinsvåg K. Inhibition of human neutrophil actin polymerization, phagocytosis and oxidative burst by components of decongestive nosedrops. Pharmacol Toxicol 1993; 73:41–45.
32. Graf P, Hallén H, Juto J. Benzalkonium chloride in a decongestant nasal spray aggravates rhinitis medicamentosa in healthy volunteers. Clin Exp Allergy 1995; 25:395–400.
33. Hallén H, Graf P. Benzalkonium chloride in nasal decongestive sprays has a long-lasting adverse effect on the nasal mucosa of healthy volunteers. Clin Exp Allergy 1995; 25:401–405.
34. Graf P, Hallén H. One week use of oxymetazoline nasal spray in patients with rhinitis medicamentosa one year after treatment. ORL 1997; 59:39–44.
35. Graf P, Hallén H. Effect on the nasal mucosa of long-term treatment with oxymetazoline, benzalkonium chloride and placebo nasal sprays. Laryngoscope 1996; 106:605–609.
36. Kumlien J. Rhinitis medicamentosa, a resurrected disease? Läkartidningen 1991; 88:4117.
37. Hallén H, Enerdal J, Graf P. Fluticasone propionate nasal spray is more effective and has a faster onset of action than placebo in treatment of rhinitis medicamentosa. Clin Exp Allergy 1997; 27:552–558.

19 Rhinitis in the Menstrual Cycle, Pregnancy, and Some Endocrine Disorders

Eva K. Ellegård

Department of Otolaryngology, Kungsbacka Hospital, Kungsbacka, Sweden

N. Göran Karlsson

Department of Otolaryngology, Sahlgrenska University Hospital, Göteborg, Sweden

Lars H. Ellegård

Department of Clinical Nutrition, Sahlgrenska University Hospital, Göteborg, Sweden

INTRODUCTION

The classification of rhinitis used in reviews and in consensus guidelines includes a subgroup of nonallergic rhinitis called "hormonal rhinitis" (1–3). Hypothyroidism and acromegaly are mentioned, but there are very few modern studies published on the subject, even though there is a clinical impression that such conditions do exist. Exclusively female causes of nasal symptoms of this "hormonal" type are the menstrual cycle and pregnancy. These two phenomena have been more studied in recent years. Nasal mucosal swelling can be caused by increased vascular pooling of blood due to a decrease in the alpha-adrenergic tonus to the venous sinusoids or by edema due to leakage of plasma from the vascular bed into the stroma. No hormone has been shown to activate any of these pathways in the nasal mucosa, although it could be a plausible mode of action.

MENSTRUAL CYCLE AND PREGNANCY: HISTORICAL BACKGROUND

In the late 19th century, several scientific papers reported observations connecting the female genitals with the nose. In 1881, Bresgen described a woman with ozena, which worsened during menstruation (4). In 1884, Mac Kenzie quoted the Ayurveda, Hippocrates, and Celsus, and quite a few 19th century writers, and presented multiple observations of his own on "the erection of the nasal turbinated structures" during menstruation and worsening of nasal symptoms during menstruation or sexual excitement (5). Expanding his theories, he included nasal congestion during pregnancy, in 1898 (6). In 1892, Endriss described epistaxis and worsening of nasal disease due to menstruation (7). The interest seems to have dropped at the turn of the century, and was not raised until 1943, when Mohun presented 20 cases of "vasomotor rhinitis" during pregnancy—appearing in the third to seventh month of gestation, persisting to term, all but one normalizing within 10 days postpartum. He concluded that there was a connection with estrogen, but also that "the acromegaly of pregnancy may in some way predispose the nasal structure to vasomotor rhinitis" (8). Estrogen was assumed to influence the nasal mucosa, and there were also case reports of successful nasal estrogen treatment of atrophic rhinitis (9,10). Holmes et al. stated in 1950: "the occurrence of hyperemia with swelling and hypersecretion in the nose as an accompaniment of menstruation does not require further confirmation." They emphasized the influence of psychological factors on the pathogenesis of those symptoms in menstruation as well as in pregnancy (11).

MENSTRUAL CYCLE

The theory of estrogen giving rise to nasal obstruction would imply a relative congestion during the preovulatory and luteal phases of the menstrual cycle, when the serum levels of estrogen are highest.

Toppozada et al. histochemical and electron microscopic study of the nasal mucosa in 10 females, during different phases of the menstrual cycle, did not reveal any cyclical changes (12). In a study on 41 normally menstruating women who registered subjective nasal congestion and nasal peak inspiratory flow (nPIF) for three to six months, significantly more congestion was found during the menstrual phase, when the estrogen levels are lowest (13). A similar study on 26 women who registered nPEF for two months did not show any cyclical changes. Neither did another part of that study comprising eight women, who registered acoustic rhinometry on two occasions during one menstrual cycle (14). Another study, using rhinostereometry and acoustic rhinometry on three occasions during one menstrual cycle in 10 women, failed to show any difference in nasal swelling in the different phases. However, an increased reaction to histamine at the time of ovulation was suggested (15). Rhinomanometry during three phases of one cycle in 60 women did not show any significant changes, but each woman had a higher airflow in the periovular phase (16). The latest published study on the subject measured nPIF, acoustic rhinometry, anterior rhinomanometry, mucociliary clearance time, and subjective scores on day 1 and in midcycle, during one menstrual cycle in 10 women. They found trends, not significant, for congestion at ovulation time (17).

In the evaluation of studies like these, which use methods with relatively large interindividual variation on few women, statistical methods comparing intraindividual data are more likely to find a difference, if there is one. The only study that used this way of evaluation was the study by Ellegård and Karlsson (13).

Variations of human growth hormone (hGH) secretion during the menstrual cycle have been suggested. A recent study on 43 women measured hGH in 10-minute intervals for 24 hours in either the follicular or the luteal phase showed that the hGH pulse frequency and the nocturnal hGH were higher in the follicular phase (18). However, a 24-hour study of integrated blood drawn in 30 minute intervals in 23 women studied both in the follicular and in the luteal phase, showed no difference (19), and another, less ambitious, study also failed to show any cyclic variation of daily morning hGH measured in nine women during one menstrual cycle (20). hGH has also been suggested as a possible cause of nasal congestion in acromegaly (see below).

Altogether, published studies do not show a clear picture of any cyclical pattern of the nasal mucosa in menstruating women.

PREGNANCY RHINITIS

Pregnancy rhinitis has only lately evolved as a defined condition worthy of being taken seriously, even though nasal congestion due to pregnancy has been known as a phenomenon for ages. It may seem to be a harmless condition compared with preeclampsia, the commonest cause of maternal and fetal morbidity and mortality (21). However, there is a possible connection between pregnancy rhinitis and preeclampsia, which makes the subject even more important to study.

Snoring is that possible connection. It is very common during pregnancy, and it may have negative effects such as maternal hypertension, preeclampsia, intrauterine growth retardation, and lower Apgar scores (22). It is well known that nasal congestion increases when the subject is in the supine position, especially in patients suffering from rhinitis (23), and that nasal congestion may result in snoring.

Air passing in through the nose is prepared to suit the lungs; it is filtered from particles, warmed, and humidified. Nasally inhaled air also transports nitric oxide (NO) from the sinonasal unit to the lungs, giving vasodilatation (24). Nasal congestion may force the subject into mouth breathing, which lacks these functions.

Quality-of-life scores can be worse in allergic rhinitis than in asthma, possibly influenced by problems such as daytime tiredness, thirst, poor concentration, and headache (25). The scores of pregnancy rhinitics have not yet been established.

Due to overuse of nasal decongestants, women with pregnancy rhinitis may develop an additional rhinitis medicamentosa, which persists after delivery (26).

Nasal congestion can result in mouth breathing, which gives a dry mouth with less saliva, which disturbs the dental protection system against caries. Long-standing nasal congestion can also induce sinusitis.

Knowledge of nasal congestion such as outlined above is probably confined to ear, nose, and throat–oriented physicians. Pregnant women are mainly in contact with their obstetricians, who may not be aware of the problems. A patient with a condition such as pregnancy rhinitis, within the purview of two specialties, is at risk of falling in between them. Information and further research may help to close this gap.

Definition

Many studies on the nasal congestion of pregnant women have been made without a proper definition. Some have presumed that it appears at the end of the first trimester and disappears after delivery (27,28). Others found that unspecified subjective nasal congestion was significantly increased during the third trimester compared with nonpregnant women (29).

To define pregnancy rhinitis, we followed 23 women, who daily, until one month after delivery, scored nasal congestion and registered nPEF (30). Their noses were more congested during than after pregnancy (excluding days with other signs of respiratory tract infection) (Fig. 1). We made the diagnosis in cases where we were convinced that there was a congestion caused by pregnancy. We then looked at the cases, and stated the criteria that would separate them from the rest of the women (Fig. 2). This resulted in our clinical definition: "nasal congestion present during the last six or more weeks of pregnancy without other signs of respiratory tract infection and with no known allergic cause, disappearing completely within two weeks after delivery." The diagnostic criteria for pregnancy rhinitis include the course after delivery, in order to make studies on etiology and epidemiology possible.

Nasal mucociliary transport speed was not affected in the group of pregnancy rhinitics. However, it was significantly decreased during pregnancy in the group of women without the condition (32). A similar (33) and a reverse (34) change have been reported.

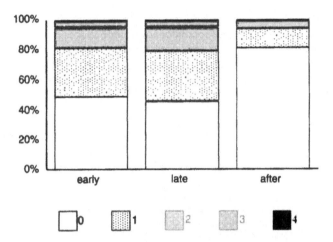

FIGURE 1 Subjective nasal congestion scores 0 to 4 of 23 women during two four-week periods; gestational weeks 15 to 18 (early), and the last month preceding delivery (late) were significantly higher than that observed the month after delivery (after), ($p = 0.001$, Wilcoxon signed rank test). Source: From Ref. 31.

Clinical Diagnosis

The diagnosis of pregnancy rhinitis is made when a pregnant woman presents with nasal congestion which is not due to any other condition. Watery or viscous clear nasal secretions are common additional symptoms. The swollen nasal mucosa responds to local decongestion, which facilitates complete inspection of the nasal cavities in order to sort out other conditions (Fig. 3). Measurements of nasal congestion are not needed for the clinical diagnosis.

Differential Diagnosis

Inspection of the nose is mandatory to rule out other causes of nasal obstruction. It is facilitated by decongestion and is best performed with an endoscope, but anterior rhinoscopy may be useful.

Rhinitis medicamentosa is both a differential diagnosis and a complication to pregnancy rhinitis. Nasal decongestants give good temporary relief, and patients generally do not spontaneously mention their long-standing use. The rebound congestion of induced rhinitis medicamentosa in healthy persons disappears within two days after the use of nasal decongestants has stopped (35). There is no study on pregnant women in this respect, but if congestion prevails after one week free of nasal decongestants, it could possibly not be attributed to the medication.

Sinusitis is also both a differential diagnosis and a complication. It is often a difficult diagnosis to make even in nonpregnant women, and the symptom of nasal congestion is not of any help. Purulent secretion in the middle meatus, a sensation of foul smell, and unilateral predominance of purulent secretion and of local pain have been proposed as strong diagnostic signs for sinusitis (36), but it may be more complicated—especially in the unselected primary care population (37). It may be even more difficult in pregnancy, as sinusitis then may give no other symptom than nasal congestion (38). Ultrasound examination of the sinuses can be a valuable tool in experienced hands, and in exceptional cases X ray may be needed. Antral puncture is the ultimate diagnostic method for sinus empyema.

Upper respiratory tract infection other than sinusitis is more obviously infective, is not confined to nasal congestion, and is not as long standing.

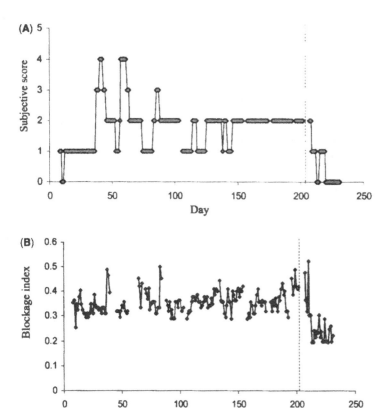

FIGURE 2 Daily subjective scores of nasal congestion (0 = no, 1 = slight, 2 = moderate, 3 = severe, and 4 = total congestion) (**A**) and objective "blockage index" (**B**). [(PEF-nPEF)/PEF] in a woman with pregnancy rhinitis show regression of nasal congestion after delivery. In her case, registrations started on study day 8 (gestational week 11 + 0). The vertical broken line indicates the day of delivery (gestational week 38 + 6). *Abbreviations:* PEF, peak expiratory flow; nPEF, nasal peak expiratory flow.

Airborne allergy is a common differential diagnosis, showing nasal congestion most often combined with excessive watery secretion and sneezing, which is not the case in pregnancy rhinitis. However, allergic rhinitis due to house dust mites frequently presents with nasal congestion as a single symptom. If it appears during pregnancy for the first time, it is difficult to differentiate from pregnancy rhinitis, and they may coexist. Allergy evaluation including in vitro tests for specific IgE or skin prick tests could be indicated.

Nasal granuloma gravidarum (pregnancy tumor, pregnancy granuloma, and telangiectatic polyp) is a benign rapidly growing tumor, histologically practically the same as pyogenic granuloma. In contrast to pregnancy rhinitis, it is almost always unilateral, and it may indeed grow to be seen from the outside. Besides nasal obstruction, it tends to cause recurrent nosebleed, and it easily bleeds to the touch. In case nosebleed or nasal obstruction is troublesome, excision under local anesthesia is indicated, but it may disappear spontaneously after delivery (39).

(A)

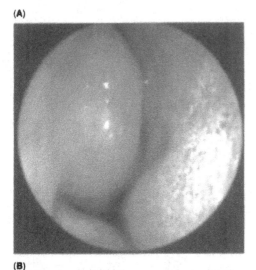

(B)

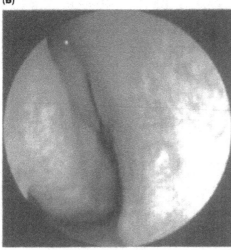

FIGURE 3 Endoscopic appearance of the right inferior turbinate in pregnancy rhinitis, before (A) and after (B) decongestion. *Source*: From Ref. 31.

Treatment

Information
Pregnant women who are prepared with the knowledge that pregnancy in itself can cause nasal congestion, and who are aware that this is a self-limited condition, are better prepared for this common complication of pregnancy. Information on pregnancy rhinitis should therefore be given to all pregnant women on their first visit to the antenatal care (40), either by the obstetrician or by the antenatal staff.

Physiological Measures
"Keep your head up when you have a stuffy nose"—most patients have heard this advice but they may need a reminder. The effective angle would be greater than

30° (23), or greater than 45° (41). The side position is desired, as it is in pregnancy both because of the vena cava syndrome and because it reduces the risk of snoring.

Mechanical devices of different designs can be used to dilate the nasal valve, which is the narrowest part of the airway. An external adhesive type dilator improved subjective nasal breathing in patients with "pregnancy-related nocturnal nasal congestion" (42). An internal type dilator significantly reduced snoring in men (43) and was as effective as a nasal decongestant in healthy subjects (44). As the negative effects of these devices are limited to local irritation of the skin by glue or pressure, they are well worth trying, especially when nasal congestion disturbs sleep. There is some suggestion that nasal valve muscular training (45) also proves to be an effective way to improve nasal breathing.

Physical exercise decongests the nasal mucosa (46) and the normal fatigue and well-being following exercise, including sexual activity, may have an additional positive effect on sleep problems caused by nasal congestion.

Nasal Saline
Nasal washings with saline solution (5 mL of salt in 0.5 L of water) are, in our clinical experience, often effective in reducing symptoms for women with pregnancy rhinitis, as they are in other sorts of rhinitis. The washings give temporary relief, as they reduce the amount of secretions and remove crusts, which block the nose. The patient can easily prepare the solution, and she leans forward when irrigating her nose. She can simply use her cupped hand or can use any of the different products available to make the procedure more comfortable.

Nasal Decongestants
Nasal decongestants have good temporary effect in pregnancy rhinitis. But as the condition does not resolve in a few days, like a common cold, women tend to use them for prolonged periods of time. This results in an additional rhinitis medicamentosa, which continues after delivery. Rebound swelling of the mucosa increases nasal congestion when the decongestive effect has disappeared. Therefore, patients gradually use larger doses of the vasoconstrictor more frequently (47). Patients get accustomed to the decongested state, and consider it normal, and they need to be informed of this misinterpretation (26). Even a dosage given only in the evenings, to healthy subjects, resulted in rhinitis medicamentosa (48). It is possible that a nose with rhinitis is more susceptible, and it has been suggested that nasal decongestants should not be used for more than five (49) or even three (50) days in a row during pregnancy. It is also possible that lower concentrations and unilateral, alternating administration may be used safely for longer periods of time.

Oral Decongestants
Vasoconstrictors administered orally, such as phenylpropanolamine and pseudo-ephedrine, are thought to reduce nasal congestion in various sorts of rhinitis (2). There are no data on whether they are efficient or not in pregnancy rhinitis. Recommendations for their use during pregnancy vary between countries. For example, in Sweden, phenylpropanolamine is the one classified to be safe, and pseudoephedrine is the one preferred in U.S. guidelines (2). A suspicion of an increased risk for the malformation gastroschisis could not be confirmed in a larger study on 206 cases compared with 798 controls (51). However, it is unwise to risk general

systemic adverse effects such as elevated blood pressure, palpitations, loss of appetite, tremor, and sleep disturbance.

Nasal Corticosteroids

Nasal corticosteroids are effective in allergic rhinitis (52,53), perennial, nonallergic rhinitis (54), rhinitis medicamentosa (55), and nasal polyps (56). Pregnant patients have not been included in any of these studies, and the documentation of treatment during pregnancy is limited.

Fluticasone propionate nasal spray did not show any positive effect on pregnancy rhinitis compared with placebo in 53 women treated for eight weeks in a randomized, double-blind study with parallel groups, evaluated by daily symptom scores and nPEF, as well as acoustic rhinometry. Furthermore, no side effects such as influence on maternal morning S-cortisol and overnight 12-hour U-cortisol, difference in ultrasound measures of fetal growth, or in pregnancy outcome could be detected (57).

Budesonide inhaled by women in early pregnancy for the treatment of asthma did not increase the rate of congenital malformations in their 2014 infants compared with the general population rate, according to figures from the Swedish Medical Birth Registry (58). Published data show that the currently available inhaled steroids used at clinically relevant doses do not impair intrauterine growth (59). Topical nasal therapy is probably just as safe in these respects.

Systemic Corticosteroids

Systemic corticosteroids have been used for various nasal conditions, but prolonged or repeated use should always be avoided because of side effects such as adrenal suppression. Mabry described his experiences of treating congested nasal mucosa in pregnancy. In his opinion, two weeks of oral corticosteroids may give temporary relief, allowing withdrawal of nasal decongestants, and intranasal submucosal injections of corticosteroids give effect within a few hours, which lasts for four to six weeks (27). No studies have been published on these treatments. The risk for side effects affecting both the fetus and the pregnant woman is obvious, including blindness after intranasal injections.

Antibiotics

Antibiotics are not indicated in pregnancy rhinitis. However, when sinusitis during pregnancy needs treatment with antibiotics, the dosage should be elevated. As renal clearance of betalactam antibiotics is increased, the dosage needs to be elevated by 50% (60). An extra dose per day is recommended, to increase the time over "minimum inhibitory concentration." Repeated antral irrigations are often useful, when the sinusitis has been long standing before diagnosis. This is facilitated by the use of a narrow catheter, left at the puncture site for a few days (e.g., SinoJect [R]).

Nasal Continuous Positive Airway Pressure

Nasal continuous positive airway pressure (CPAP) is not indicated in uncomplicated pregnancy rhinitis, but can be considered in cases of obstructive sleep apnea. As in nonpregnants, nasal CPAP has been used with excellent compliance for that diagnosis, and has proved to be effective in polysomnography studies. In the course of pregnancy, the CPAP pressure may need to be readjusted (61).

In a study of women with preeclampsia but without obstructive sleep apnea, nasal CPAP reduced nocturnal blood pressure significantly. The study was, however, not randomized (21).

Invasive Methods
Electrocautery, cryotherapy, laser, or radiofrequency treatment of the inferior turbinates can be used in pregnancy rhinitis (40), as can different types of surgical reduction. The effect may be temporary or permanent, and the frequency, degree, and lasting of side effects such as crusting, edema, and bleeding vary (62). Invasive methods should only be carefully considered in desperate cases, e.g., a woman with pregnancy rhinitis and obstructive sleep apnea, when CPAP is not tolerated, and other sorts of treatment of the nose have failed.

Etiology

Estrogen
The natural theory that estrogen causes nasal congestion is scientifically based mainly on the results of Toppozada et al. from biopsy studies on nasal mucosa in pregnancy (28), and from women taking contraceptive pills (63). However, serum levels of estradiol measured four times during pregnancy in 23 women were not more elevated in women with pregnancy rhinitis than in women without (64). Furthermore, only eight of the women had increasing congestion, and nine women, surprisingly, registered declining congestion in the course of pregnancy (30). A similar pattern was seen in a recent study, even though the mean results of different measurements indicated rising congestion during pregnancy (34). The parallel with asthma is obvious; about one-third of asthmatics improve during pregnancy, whereas one-third deteriorate (65). There was also a significant relationship between self-reported change in asthma course during pregnancy, and that of rhinitis in 568 patients (66). This agrees with the well-known concept of the "united airways," where upper and lower airway inflammatory events influence each other, as they are part of a systemic condition (67). Recent studies on postmenopausal women suggest that estrogen replacement therapy may indeed reduce subjective nasal congestion (68). The estrogen theory is not convincing.

Progesterone
Increased circulating blood volume, enhanced by a vasodilating effect of progesterone, was suggested to be responsible for pregnancy-induced nasal congestion (49), but serum levels of progesterone were similar in a group of women with pregnancy rhinitis, and a group without, which does not support this theory (64).

Prolactin
As prolactin production increases in the course of pregnancy, a role in the pathogenesis of pregnancy rhinitis is possible. This is contradicted by the absence of sinus pathology in prolactinoma patients (69). Furthermore, bromocriptine and quinagolide, which reduce prolactin, have nasal congestion as known side effects. On the other hand, this effect may be caused by the substances themselves.

Neuropeptides
Vasoactive intestinal polypeptide (VIP), associated with other sorts of rhinitis (70), has been proposed to be a mediator of vasodilatation in the nasal mucosa during

pregnancy, although a study on *serum* levels did not support the theory (71). After six months of hormone replacement therapy in postmenopausal women, there was an increased immunopositivity for VIP and substance P (SP), as well as for estradiol and estradiol receptor in nasal biopsies. Neuropeptide Y (NPY) was reduced. Thus, estrogen action in the nasal mucosa could be mediated by neuropeptides: an increase of gland secretion and vasodilatation by VIP and SP and a decrease of NPY-induced vasoconstriction. Nasal application induced stronger changes than did transdermal. Mucociliary transport time, and subjective nasal congestion decreased, but anterior rhinomanometry was unchanged (68).

Placental Growth Hormone

After the first trimester of pregnancy, the episodic bursts of hGH are replaced by a continuous secretion with rising values of a placental growth hormone (PGH) variant (72). In our study, serum levels of PGH were significantly higher in the pregnancy rhinitis group on all occasions throughout pregnancy (64). It is possible that PGH may stimulate mucosal growth in a similar way as is proposed for hGH in acromegaly, and thereby induce pregnancy rhinitis.

Incidence

Most incidence studies on nasal congestion due to pregnancy comprise small populations: 30% in 79 women (27), 18% in 66 women (73), and 21% in 160 women (42). Another study of 27 nonpregnant and 33 pregnant women failed to show any significantly increased frequency of nasal congestion during pregnancy. Undefined "prevalence of congestion" was compared using a visual analogue scale, once in each trimester. The resulting 33% (nonpregnant), 61%, 55%, and 55%, respectively, was not significantly different (74). The method is most certainly not appropriate for such a small number of women.

A larger study on 599 women registered subjective nasal congestion upon all visits to the midwife during and after pregnancy showed the incidence of pregnancy rhinitis to be 22%. Nasal congestion manifested itself in gestational weeks 7 through 36, i.e., from as early as it was possible to register, until as late as possible to obtain a six-week duration (Fig. 4). The incidence figure of pregnancy rhinitis may have been underestimated, as women with long-standing nasal problems before pregnancy were not included. But as their symptoms may have varied over time in the nonpregnant status, it was too difficult to evaluate what impact pregnancy may have had (75).

In an even larger study, 2264 pregnant women were asked whether they had had "daily nasal stuffiness during the last three weeks" on visits in gestational weeks 12, 20, 30, and 36. A positive answer to the question included all sorts of rhinitis, and sorted the woman into the "stuffiness" group. "Stuffiness" rate was 42% in week 36, and out of 1546 women who answered on all four occasions, 11% reported "stuffiness" every time (76).

Risk Factors

Smoking

In our questionnaire study, the incidence of pregnancy rhinitis was significantly higher in smokers than in nonsmokers (odds ratio 1.7, 95% confidence interval 1.1–2.5) (75). It is possible that the irritating effects of smoking add to other changes and thus induce nasal congestion.

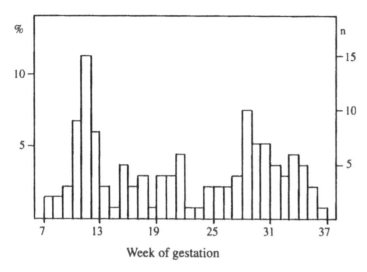

FIGURE 4 Pregnancy rhinitis appeared at any time during gestation in the 133 women. For details, see text. *Source:* From Ref. 75.

Allergy

Electron microscopic findings of nasal mucosa specimens from pregnant women with nasal symptoms, and from cases with allergic rhinitis were reported identical by Toppozada et al. (28). Mabry did not find any connection between reported constant or frequent nasal congestion during pregnancy, and previously documented allergic rhinitis (73).

Hay fever, asthma, and the month of conception were not associated with the diagnosis of pregnancy rhinitis in our questionnaire study (75). In vitro tests for 10 common airborne allergens were also performed on 165 of those women, 83 of whom had had pregnancy rhinitis. The sensitization rate was not raised in the group of women who had had pregnancy rhinitis compared with the group of women who had not, but sensitization to house dust mites was more frequent in the former group. It was impossible to differentiate their rhinitis from a subclinical allergic rhinitis with deterioration during pregnancy, but it was remarkable how they all recovered after delivery (77).

Serum levels of soluble intercellular adhesion molecule-1 (sICAM-1), elevated in perennial (78) and seasonal allergic rhinitis (79), can be used as a marker of allergic nasal disease. The mean serum values of sICAM-1 did not change significantly in the course of pregnancy in 23 women, and the group of women with pregnancy rhinitis had values similar to the group without (77).

Hyperreactivity

Identification of subjects with hyperreactive nasal mucosa, as measured by rhinostereometry, has been suggested at a cutoff limit of 0.4 mm congestion, five minutes after provocation with histamine 2 mg/mL in the same nostril (80). In this way, we compared 12 women who had had pregnancy rhinitis, with 13 who had not. The number of women exceeding that limit was not different between the two groups. Neither was there any difference between groups in reactions to increasing concentrations of histamine, as measured by rhinostereo-metry or acoustic rhinometry (77).

Possible Influence on the Fetus

It is well known that nasal congestion increases in the supine position, especially in patients suffering from rhinitis (23), and that nasal congestion increases the tend-ency to revert to mouth breathing and snoring. Regular snoring, which was reported by 9% of 73,231 women, was associated with hypertension independent of body mass index (81). Regular snoring during the previous week was reported by 23% of 502 women the day after delivery. There were more cases of hypertension, preeclampsia, and intrauterine growth retardation in the group of snorers, and the Apgar scores of their babies were lower (22). A possible factor in the pathogenesis of these pregnancy complications could be a reduction in inhaled NO. Inhaled NO, mainly produced in the maxillary sinuses, reduces pulmonary vascular resistance and increases pulmonary oxygenation (82). Mouth breathing in pregnancy rhinitis may possibly reduce this inhalation, and thereby affect the oxygen supply to the fetus by changes in maternal pulmonary vascular tone and/or oxygenation.

Furthermore, there is a risk that pregnancy rhinitis induces obstructive sleep apnea in women who are predisposed to that disease, but who normally can breathe through the nose. Hypertension in preeclampsia has primarily a rise in nocturnal blood pressure, a pattern previously experienced to be associated with snoring and obstructive sleep apnea (21).

In conclusion, pregnancy can induce nasal congestion. This is probably not mediated by estrogen or progesterone. A multifactorial etiology seems plausible.

HYPOTHYROIDISM

Common complaints such as long-standing nasal congestion, interminable colds, and excessive nasal discharge are not specific for patients with hypothyroidism, but seem to be a reminder for the physician to evaluate thyroid function. Increased amounts of connective tissue in the mucosa and hypertrophic mucus-secreting glands have been supposed to underlie the symptoms (83). Proetz, who studied 130 cases, noticed an increased tendency to nasal infection and allergy, with head-ache and nasal obstruction as prominent symptoms. In 66 of his cases, hypothyroidism was first suspected on the basis of nasal appearance alone, and the fact that usual nasal treatment failed was important (84).

Gupta et al. studied 66 patients with hypothyroidism. Nasal congestion, recurrent colds, and excessive discharge were common complaints (60%), and ede-matous nasal mucosa was a frequent finding (40%). Biopsies from the inferior turbinates in 16 cases showed abundant mucinous activity, proliferation of mucous glands, increased ground substance and submucous vascularity (85).

The impression from these studies is that hypothyroidism can induce nasal symptoms. The message so far would be to remind the physician to generously evaluate thyroid function in cases with unspecific nasal problems.

ACROMEGALY

In 1959, Beselin summarized earlier publications—"both the outside, and the inside of the nose grow in acromegaly"—and questioned whether nasal polyps, and turbi-nate hypertrophy also in nonacromegalics are caused by growth hormone (86).

A study by Skinner and Richards supports the theory that hGH may induce changes in the mucosa of the upper airways. In their study, acromegaly patients had an increased frequency of mucosal hypertrophy (submucosal edema) and polyps in the sinuses compared with patients with prolactinoma. No such pathology was found in the nasal mucosa, which, however, was examined after preoperative cocaine treatment (69).

hGH is an important regulator of insulin-like growth factor I (IGF-I), giving high circulating levels in acromegaly (87). Increased IGF-I-immunoreactivity has been demonstrated in different parts of nasal polyps from nonacromegalic patients. IGF-I could be a mediator important in the growth of nasal polyps, and the activity of IGF-I is inhibited by corticosteroids, which are effective in the treatment of nasal polyps (88).

Fatti et al. conclude that the high prevalence of obstructive sleep apnea syndrome in acromegalic patients (25% in female and 70% in male) is caused by congestion of the nasal mucosa, and nasal polyps, as well as by hypertrophy of the tongue and the pharyngeal soft tissue (89).

No significant nasal congestion was detected in 10 short bowel patients treated with low-dose hGH in a double-blind crossover trial with eight-week treatment periods (90). Maybe this was too short an exposure time, with too low a dose, to induce changes like the ones seen in manifest acromegaly.

These studies suggest an association with nasal congestion, but the causal relationship has not been established.

DIABETES

Diabetes mellitus does not per se induce a specific type of rhinitis, but is a risk factor for fungal rhinosinusitis, especially for chronic invasive rhinosinusitis and mucormycosis. Most invasive fungal rhinosinusitis begin in the nose, usually at the middle turbinate and can present with nasal congestion. The most common organisms are *Aspergillus* species and *Mucormycosis*. Treatment is optimized glycemic control, which may indeed be deteriorated by the infection, systemic antifungal therapy, and surgery (91).

SUMMARY

By clinical experience, rhinitis has been suggested as caused by some endocrine disorders, but the evidence for this is vague, and the few descriptions almost anecdotal. Rhinitis of the menstrual cycle has been more described, although a solid picture is still lacking. Pregnancy rhinitis is therefore so far the only clearly defined "hormonal rhinitis." However, the cause of pregnancy rhinitis is not simply estrogen or progesterone, but seems multifactorial, and may possibly be associated with the PGH. Treatment consists mainly of information, physiological measures, and nasal saline washings.

REFERENCES

1. Lund VJ. International consensus report on the diagnosis and management of rhinitis. Allergy 1994(suppl 19):5–34.
2. Dykewicz MS, Fineman S, Skoner DP, et al. Diagnosis and management of rhinitis: complete guidelines of the Joint Task Force on Practice Parameters in Allergy, Asthma and

Immunology. American Academy of Allergy, Asthma, and Immunology. Ann Allergy Asthma Immunol 1998; 81(5 Pt 2):478–518.

3. Settipane RA, Lieberman P. Update on nonallergic rhinitis. Ann Allergy Asthma Immunol 2001; 86(5):494–507.

4. Bresgen M. Der chronische Nasen- und Rachen- Katarrh. Wien: Urban & Schwarzenberg, 1881.

5. Mac Kenzie JN. Irritation of the sexual apparatus as an etiological factor in the production of nasal disease. Am J Med Sci 1884; 87:360–365.

6. Mac Kenzie JN. The physiological and pathological relations between the nose and the sexual apparatus of man. Alienist Neurol 1898; 19:219–239.

7. Endriss G. Die Bisherigen Beobachtungen von Physiologische und Pathologische Bezieungen der Obern Luftvage den Sexualorganismus. Würzburg, 1892.

8. Mohun M. Incidence of vasomotor rhinitis during pregnancy. Arch Otolaryngol 1943; 37:699–709.

9. Ruskin SL. Rationale of estrogen therapy of primary atrophic rhinitis (ozena). Arch Otolaryngol 1942; 36:632–649.

10. Bernheimer LB, Soskin S. Mechanism of effect of estrogen on nasal mucosa in atrophic rhinitis. Arch Otolaryngol 1940; 32:957–959.

11. Holmes TH, Goodell H, Wolf S, et al. The relation of nasal to sexual function. In: The Nose; An Experimental Study of Reactions Within the Nose in Human Subjects During Varying Life Experiences. Springfield, Ill.: Charles C Thomas, 1950:89–100.

12. Toppozada H, Michaels L, Toppozada M, et al. The human nasal mucosa in the menstrual cycle. J Laryngol Otol 1981; 95:1237–1247.

13. Ellegård E, Karlsson G. Nasal congestion during the menstrual cycle. Clin Otolaryngol 1994; 19(5):400–403.

14. Paulsson B, Gredmark T, Burian P, et al. Nasal mucosal congestion during the menstrual cycle. J Laryngol Otol 1997; 111(4): 337–339.

15. Haeggström A, Östberg B, Stjerna P, et al. Nasal mucosal swelling and reactivity during a menstrual cycle. ORL 2000; 62:39–42.

16. Grillo C, La Mantia I, Triolo C, et al. Rhinomanometric and olfactometric variations throughout the menstrual cycle. Ann Otol Rhinol Laryngol 2001; 110(8): 785–789.

17. Philpott CM, El-Alami M, Murty GE. The effect of the steroid sex hormones on the nasal airway during the normal menstrual cycle. Clin Otolaryngol Allied Sci 2004; 29(2): 138–142.

18. Kasa-Vubu JZ, Dimaraki EV, Young EA. The pattern of growth hormone secretion during the menstrual cycle in normal and depressed women. Clin Endocrinol (Oxf) 2005; 62(6):656–660.

19. Zadik Z, Chalew SA, McCarter RJ, et al. The influence of age on the 24-hour integrated concentration of growth hormone in normal individuals. J Clin Endocrinol Metab 1985; 60:513–516.

20. Stone BA, Marrs RP. Growth hormone in serum of women during the menstrual cycle and during controlled ovarian hyperstimulation. Fertil Steril 1991; 56:52–58.

21. Edwards N, Blyton DM, Kirjavainen T, et al. Nasal continuous positive airway pressure reduces sleep-induced blood pressure increments in preeclampsia. Am J Respir Crit Care Med 2000; 162(1):252–257.

22. Franklin KA, Holmgren PÅ, Jönsson F, et al. Snoring, pregnancy-induced hypertension, and growth retardation of the fetus. Chest 2000; 117:137–141.

23. Rundcrantz H. Postural variations of nasal patency. Acta Otolaryngol 1969; 68:435–443.

24. Silkoff PE, Robbins RA, Gaston B, et al. Endogenous nitric oxide in allergic airway disease. J Allergy Clin Immunol 2000; 105(3):438–448.

25. Juniper EF. Measuring health-related quality of life in rhinitis. J Allergy Clin Immunol 1997; 99:S742–S749.

26. Graf P, Hallén H. Effect on the nasal mucosa of long-term treatment with oxymetazoline, benzalkonium chloride and placebo nasal sprays. Laryngoscope 1996; 106:605–609.

27. Mabry RL. Intranasal steroid injection during pregnancy. South Med J 1980; 73:1176–1179.

28. Toppozada H, Michaels L, Toppozada M, et al. The human respiratory nasal mucosa in pregnancy. J Laryngol Otol 1982; 96:613–626.

29. Bende M, Hallgårde U, Sjögren C. Occurrence of nasal congestion during pregnancy. Am J Rhinol 1989; 3:217–219.
30. Ellegård E, Karlsson G. Nasal congestion during pregnancy. Clin Otolaryngol 1999; 24:307–311.
31. Ellegård E. Clinical and pathogenetic characteristics of pregnancy rhinitis. Clin Rev Allergy Immunol 2004; 26:149–159.
32. Ellegård EK, Karlsson NG. Nasal mucociliary transport in pregnancy. Am J Rhinol 2000; 14(6):375–378.
33. Hellin M, Ruiz CV, Ruiz FM. The influence of pregnancy on mucociliary nasal transport. An Otorrinolaringol Ibero Am 1994; 21(6):595–601.
34. Philpott CM, Conboy P, Al-Azzawi F, et al. Nasal physiological changes during pregnancy. Clin Otolaryngol 2004; 29(4):343–351.
35. Graf P, Juto J-E. Decongestion effect and rebound swelling of the nasal mucosa during 4-week use of oxymetazoline. ORL 1994; 56:157–160.
36. Berg O, Carenfelt C. Analysis of symptoms and clinical signs in the maxillary sinus empyema. Acta Otolaryngol 1988; 105(3–4):343–349.
37. Lindbaek M. Acute sinusitis: guide to selection of antibacterial therapy. Drugs 2004; 64(8):805–819.
38. Sorri M, Hartikainen-Sorri A, Kärjä J. Rhinitis during pregnancy. Rhinology 1980; 18:83–86.
39. Park YW. Nasal granuloma gravidarum. Otolaryngol Head Neck Surg 2002; 126(5): 591–592.
40. Rambur B. Pregnancy rhinitis and rhinitis medicamentosa. J Am Acad Nurse Pract 2002; 14(12):527–530.
41. Stroud RH, Wright ST, Calhoun KH. Nocturnal nasal congestion and nasal resistance. Laryngoscope 1999; 109(9):1450–1453.
42. Turnbull GL, Rundell OH, Rayburn WF, et al. Managing pregnancy-related nocturnal nasal congestion. The external nasal dilator. J Reprod Med 1996; 41(12):897–902.
43. Löth S, Petruson B. Improved nasal breathing reduces snoring and morning tiredness. Arch Otolaryngol Head Neck Surg 1996; 122:1337–1340.
44. Lorino AM, Lofaso F, Drogou I, et al. Effects of different mechanical treatments on nasal resistance assessed by rhinometry. Chest 1998; 114(1):166–170.
45. Vaiman M, Eviatar E, Segal S. Muscle-building therapy in treatment of nasal valve collapse. Rhinology 2004; 42(3):145–152.
46. Eccles R. Nasal air flow in health and disease. Acta Otolaryngol (Stockh) 2000; 120:580–595.
47. Graf P. Rhinitis medicamentosa: a review of causes and treatment. Treat Respir Med 2005; 4(1):21–29.
48. Graf P, Hallen H, Juto J-E. Four-week use of oxymetazoline nasal spray (Nezeril ^R) once daily at night induces rebound swelling and nasal hyperreactivity. Acta Otolaryngol (Stockh) 1995; 115:71–75.
49. Schatz M, Zeiger RS. Asthma and allergy in pregnancy. Clin Perinatol 1997; 24:407–432.
50. Lekas MD. Rhinitis during pregnancy and rhinitis medicamentosa. Otolaryngol Head Neck Surg 1992; 107:845–849.
51. Werler MM, Sheehan JE, Mitchell AA. Maternal medication use and risks of gastroschisis and small intestinal atresia. Am J Epidemiol 2002; 155(1):26–31.
52. Onrust SV, Lamb HM. Mometasone furoate. A review of its intranasal use in allergic rhinitis. Drugs 1998; 56(4):725–745.
53. Storms WW. Risk-benefit assessment of fluticasone propionate in the treatment of asthma and allergic rhinitis. J Asthma 1998; 35(4):313–336.
54. Scadding GK, Lund VJ, Jacques LA, et al. A placebo-controlled study of fluticasone propionate aqueous nasal spray and beclomethasone dipropionate in perennial rhinitis: efficacy in allergic and non-allergic perennial rhinitis. Clin Exp Allergy 1995; 25(8):737–743.
55. Hallen H, Enerdal J, Graf P. Fluticasone propionate nasal spray is more effective and has a faster onset of action than placebo in treatment of rhinitis medicamentosa. Clin Exp Allergy 1997; 27(5):552–558.
56. Lildholdt T, Rundcrantz H, Bende M, et al. Glucocorticoid treatment for nasal polyps. The use of topical budesonide powder, intramuscular betamethasone, and surgical treatment. Arch Otolaryngol Head Neck Surg 1997; 123:595–600.

57. Ellegård EK, Hellgren M, Karlsson NG. Fluticasone propionate aqueous nasal spray in pregnancy rhinitis. Clin Otolaryngol 2001; 26(5):394–400.
58. Källén B, Rydhstroem H, Åberg A. Congenital malformations after the use of inhaled budesonide in early pregnancy. Obstet Gynecol 1999; 93:392–395.
59. Namazy JA, Schatz M. Update in the treatment of asthma during pregnancy. Clin Rev Allergy Immunol 2004; 26(3):139–148.
60. Heikkila A, Erkkola R. Review of beta-lactam antibiotics in pregnancy. The need for adjustment of dosage schedules. Clin Pharmacokinet 1994; 27(1):49–62.
61. Guilleminault C, Kreutzer M, Chang JL. Pregnancy, sleep disordered breathing and treatment with nasal continuous positive airway pressure. Sleep Med 2004; 5(1):43–51.
62. Jackson LE, Koch RJ. Controversies in the management of inferior turbinate hypertrophy: a comprehensive review. Plast Reconstr Surg 1999; 103(1):300–312.
63. Toppozada H, Toppozada M, El-Ghazzawi I, et al. The human respiratory nasal mucosa in females using contraceptive pills. J Laryngol Otol 1984; 98:43–51.
64. Ellegård E, Oscarsson J, Bougoussa M, et al. Serum level of placental growth hormone is raised in pregnancy rhinitis. Arch Otolaryngol Head Neck Surg 1998; 124:439–443.
65. Gluck JC. The change of asthma course during pregnancy. Clin Rev Allergy Immunol 2004; 26(3):171–180.
66. Kircher S, Schatz M, Long L. Variables affecting asthma course during pregnancy. Ann Allergy Asthma Immunol 2002; 89(5):463–466.
67. Boulay ME, Boulet LP. The relationships between atopy, rhinitis and asthma: pathophysiological considerations. Curr Opin Allergy Clin Immunol 2003; 3(1):51–55.
68. Nappi C, Di Spiezio Sardo A, Guerra G, et al. Comparison of intranasal and transdermal estradiol on nasal mucosa in postmenopausal women. Menopause 2004; 11(4):447–455.
69. Skinner DW, Richards SH. Acromegaly—the mucosal changes within the nose and paranasal sinuses. J Laryngol Otol 1988; 102:1107–1110.
70. Fischer A, Wussow A, Cryer A, et al. Neuronal plasticity in persistent perennial allergic rhinitis. J Occup Environ Med 2005; 47(1):20–25.
71. Bende M, Hallgårde U, Sjögren C, et al. Nasal congestion during pregnancy. Clin Otolaryngol 1989; 14:385–387.
72. Eriksson L, Frankenne F, Eden S, et al. Growth hormone 24-h serum profiles during pregnancy—lack of pulsatility for the secretion of the placental variant. Br J Obstet Gynaecol 1989; 96:949–953.
73. Mabry RL. Rhinitis of pregnancy. South Med J 1986; 79:965–971.
74. Sobol SE, Frenkiel S, Nachtigal D, et al. Clinical manifestations of sinonasal pathology during pregnancy. J Otolaryngol 2001; 30(1):24–28.
75. Ellegård E, Hellgren M, Torén K, et al. The incidence of pregnancy rhinitis. Gynecol Obstet Invest 2000; 49:98–101.
76. Bende M, Gredmark T. Nasal stuffiness during pregnancy. Laryngoscope 1999; 109:1108–1110.
77. Ellegård E, Karlsson G. IgE-mediated reactions and hyperreactivity in pregnancy rhinitis. Arch Otolaryngol Head Neck Surg 1999; 125:1121–1125.
78. Ohashi Y, Nakai Y, Tanaka A, et al. Soluble intercellular adhesion molecule-1 level in sera is elevated in perennial allergic rhinitis. Laryngoscope 1997; 107:932–935.
79. Kato M, Hattori T, Matsumoto Y, et al. Dynamics of soluble adhesion molecule levels in patients with pollinosis. Arch Otolaryngol Head Neck Surg 1996; 122:1398–1400.
80. Hallén H, Juto JE. A test for objective diagnosis of nasal hyperreactivity. Rhinology 1993; 31:23–25.
81. Hu FB, Willett WC, Colditz GA, et al. Prospective study of snoring and risk of hypertension in women. Am J Epidemiol 1999; 150(8):806–816.
82. Lundberg JO, Weitzberg E. Nasal nitric oxide in man. Thorax 1999; 54(10), 947–952.
83. Ritter FN. The effects of hypothyroidism upon the ear, nose and throat. Laryngoscope 1967; 77:1427–1479.
84. Proetz AW. Further observations of the effects of thyroid insufficiency on the nasal mucosa. Laryngoscope 1950; 60(7):627–633.
85. Gupta OP, Bhatia PL, Agarwal MK, et al. Nasal, pharyngeal and laryngeal manifestations of hypothyroidism. ENT J 1977; 56:349–356.

86. Beselin O. The nose and acromegaly. Hno 1958; 7(3):84–85.
87. Furlanetto RW. Insulin-like growth factor measurements in the evaluation of growth hormone secretion. Hormone Research 1990; 33(suppl 4):25–30.
88. Petruson B, Hansson H, Petruson K. Insulinlike growth factor I immunoreactivity in nasal polyps. Arch Otolaryngol Head Neck Surg 1988; 114:1272–1275.
89. Fatti LM, Scacchi M, Pincelli AI, et al. Prevalence and pathogenesis of sleep apnea and lung disease in acromegaly. Pituitary 2001; 4(4):259–262.
90. Ellegård E, Ellegård L. Nasal air flow in growth hormone treatment. Rhinology 1998; 36:66–68.
91. Ferguson BJ. Definitions of fungal rhinosinusitis. Otolaryngol Clin North Am 2000; 33(2):227–235.

.

20 Midfacial Segment Pain: Implications for Rhinitis and Rhinosinusitis

Nick S. Jones

Department of Otolaryngology, Head and Neck Surgery, Queen's Medical Center, University Hospital, Nottingham, U.K.

INTRODUCTION

Patients with facial discomfort often make a self-diagnosis of "rhinitis" or "sinusitis" as they know that their sinuses lie within the face. In the medical literature, rhinological causes of facial discomfort include acute infective rhinosinusitis that is typically preceded by an upper respiratory tract infection and responds to antibiotics unless it does not resolve of its own accord. In the past, chronic infective rhinosinusitis has been reported as a common cause of facial pain, but with the advent of nasal endoscopy and computed tomography (CT), this conclusion has been questioned (1). A significant proportion of patients with symptoms of facial discomfort, pressure, heaviness, or blockage and having been treated by endoscopic sinus surgery (ESS) are found to have persistent symptoms after surgery (2–4). It is notable that over 80% of patients with purulent secretions visible at nasal endoscopy have no facial discomfort or pain (3). If patients who have intermittent symptoms of facial discomfort, pressure, heaviness, or blockage believe that it is due to infection, yet when they are seen they have no pain or objective signs of infection, they are asked to return when they are symptomatic. When they do return with symptoms of facial discomfort, many are found not to have any evidence of infection, and another neurological cause for their pain is often responsible (3). In cases of facial discomfort secondary to genuine sinusitis, there are usually endoscopic signs of disease (5), and these patients almost invariably have coexisting symptoms of nasal obstruction, hyposmia, and/or a purulent nasal discharge (6). In patients with genuine sinusitis, ESS has been shown to alleviate their facial discomfort in 75% to 83% of cases (3,7). Other causes of facial discomfort or pain include atypical forms of migraine (8), cluster headache, and paroxysmal hemicrania (9), and atypical facial pain may be responsible among the causes in the differential diagnosis (10).

PROPOSED THEORIES FOR THE ETIOLOGY OF FACIAL DISCOMFORT

Some workers have hypothesized that rhinological causes other than infection can cause facial discomfort, pressure, heaviness, or blockage and these include the presence of contact points or a vacuum in the sinuses.

In 1908, Sluder described "sphenopalatine neuralgia" as a cause of an ipsilateral, boring, burning facial pain beginning along the lateral side of the nose and in the eye, forehead, orbit, temporal, and mastoid regions, constant or paroxysmal, associated with lacrimation, rhinorrhea, and injected conjunctiva, and, sometimes, involving the cheek (11). Since his description, the symptom complex has been categorized as cluster headache (12,13). Sluder also described a different type of frontal pain that he attributed to "vacuum" headaches, which could produce ocular symptoms (14).

The evidence that a vacuum within a blocked sinus can cause protracted discomfort is poor. Transient facial discomfort, pressure, heaviness, or blockage can occur in patients with rhinosinusitis, normally in conjunction with other symptoms and signs. Symptoms are typically worse with pressure changes when flying, diving, or skiing, but this resolves as the pressure within the sinuses equalizes through perfusion with the surrounding vasculature. Silent sinus syndrome due to a blocked sinus with resorption of its contents to the extent that the orbital floor prolapses into the maxillary sinus causes no pain (15–17). Nasal polyposis is likely to block sinus ostia, yet it rarely causes facial discomfort unless there is coexisting infection with a purulent discharge (6).

The theories that implicate contact points as a cause of facial pain originate from McAuliffe who described stimulating various points within the nasal cavity and paranasal sinuses in five individuals and said that both touch and faradic current caused referred pain to areas of the face (18). McAuliffe's work has recently been repeated in a controlled study and was found not to produce the referred pain that he described (19). The prevalence of a contact point has been found to be the same in an asymptomatic population as in a symptomatic population, and when they were present in symptomatic patients with unilateral discomfort, they were present in the contralateral side to the pain in 50% of these patients (20).

Stammberger and Wolf postulated that variations in the anatomy of the nasal cavity result in mucus stasis, infection, and, ultimately, facial pain (21). They also stated that mucosal contact points might result in the release of the neurotransmitter peptide substance P, a recognized neurotransmitter in nociceptive fibers. For contact points to be credible as a cause of facial pain or headache, they should also be a predictor of these facial pains in the whole population (22). Nowhere else in the body does mucosa–mucosa contact causes pain.

Case-controlled studies examining the prevalence of anatomical variations in patients with rhinosinusitis and asymptomatic control groups have shown no significant differences (23–39).

It seems probable that the majority of the case series in the literature that describe a response to surgery for anatomical variations in patients with facial discomfort do so as a result of the effect of cognitive dissonance (40), or from surgery altering neuroplasticity within the brain stem sensory nuclear complex (41–44). This is supported by the finding that the effect of surgery on their discomfort is more often partial than complete, and any response is relatively short lived, lasting no longer than a few weeks or months, and, rarely, as much as one year.

ESS has been advocated by a few workers for facial pain in the absence of endoscopic or CT evidence of sinus disease or anatomical variations (45,46). Boonchoo performed ESS on 16 patients with headache and negative sinus CT scans, and reported total resolution of pain in 10 patients and partial resolution in the other six (46). Cook et al. advocated ESS on patients with facial pain, which also occurred "independently" of episodes of rhinosinusitis, with no CT evidence of sinus pathology (45). Twelve of the eighteen patients who underwent surgery in their series had a significant reduction in their pain severity, yet it is very significant that the authors describe "complete elimination of symptoms was not accomplished in any patient." They had no evidence of osteomeatal obstruction.

If the cause of their pain was due to an anatomical "abnormality" or osteal obstruction, then it might be anticipated that surgery would cure their symptoms of pain. This was not the case as they had residual pain. Similarly Parsons et al. retrospectively described 34 patients with headaches who had contact points removed, and found that, while there was a 91% decrease in intensity and 84% decrease in frequency, 65% had persisting symptoms (47). It is hypothesized that the reason for a temporary or partial reduction in their pain is the effect of surgical trauma on the afferent fibers going to the trigeminal nucleus and this might alter the nucleus and its threshold for spontaneous activity for up to several months as has been found when patients with midfacial segment pain undergo surgery. This will be described later (4).

The evidence to support the theories that either contact points or a blocked sinus on their own in the absence of any infection can cause protracted facial discomfort is poor.

Patients whose primary complaint is headache or facial discomfort are less likely to have evidence of rhinosinusitis than those who have nasal symptoms (48). Patients with facial discomfort or headache without nasal symptoms are very unlikely to be helped by nasal medical or surgical treatment (3).

RECENT ADVANCES IN THE ETIOLOGY OF FACIAL DISCOMFORT

The Copenhagen group has done a great deal to improve our understanding about the possible mechanisms that cause tension-type headache and these can be extrapolated to other types of facial discomfort. These theories expound central sensitization of the trigeminal nucleus from prolonged nociceptive input from a peripheral injury, surgery or inflammation, pericranial myofascial nociceptive input, or psychological or neurological factors that can reduce supraspinal inhibition (41,43,44,49–51). Other researchers have described other mechanisms that can produce central sensitization through neural plasticity and endeavored to explain the phenomenon of hyperalgesia and how pain can persist (42,52).

The characteristics of tension-type headache are as follows:

- A feeling of tightness, pressure, or constriction, which varies in intensity, frequency, and duration and it may be at the vertex or forehead, eyes or temple, and there is often an occipital component.
- Analgesics are of little or no benefit, although many patients continue to take them, often in large quantities. It is usually present on waking.
- The discomfort does not worsen with routine physical activity, and rarely interferes with the patient getting to sleep.
- Hyperesthesia of the skin or muscles of the forehead often occurs.
- The symptom of being worse on leaning forward can occur in this condition.

Midfacial segment pain has all the characteristics of tension-type headache except that it affects the midface. Of relevance is the finding that 60% of patients with midfacial segment pain have some degree of tension-type headache, but they may not initially volunteer these symptoms (it is important to ask open-ended questions in order to avoid pigeonholing them into preconceived diagnoses). Patients describe a feeling of pressure, heaviness, or tightness and they may say that their nose feels blocked when they have no airway obstruction. The symptoms are symmetrical and may involve the nasion, the bridge of the nose, either side of the nose, and the periorbital region, retro-orbitally or across the cheeks (Fig. 1A–F).

(A)

(B)

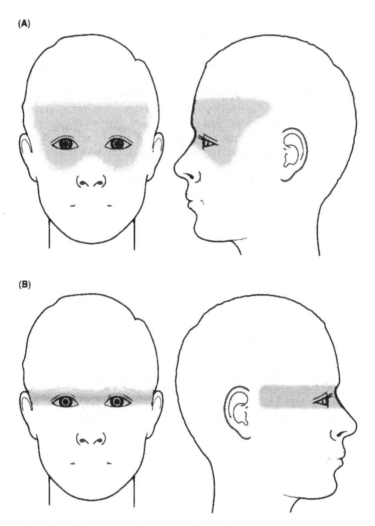

FIGURE 1 (A–F) The variation in the distribution of discomfort in midfacial segment pain. Note that the distribution of facial discomfort is symmetrical, unlike the symptoms associated with infective rhinosinusitis. The distribution of symptoms can occur in any combination of the distributions as shown in the figure. (*Continued on next page*)

There are no consistent exacerbating or relieving factors, and patients often take a range of analgesics, but they have no, or a minimal effect, other than Ibuprofen that may help a few to a minor extent. The symptoms are often initially episodic but are often persistent by the time they are seen in secondary care. Patients may be convinced that their symptoms are due to sinusitis, as they know that their sinuses lie under this area, with the exception of the bridge of the nose. They may have been treated for a long period with antibiotics and topical nasal steroids, and a few patients have had some transient response on occasion that may be related to the placebo effect or cognitive dissonance, but these are inconsistent. Patients'

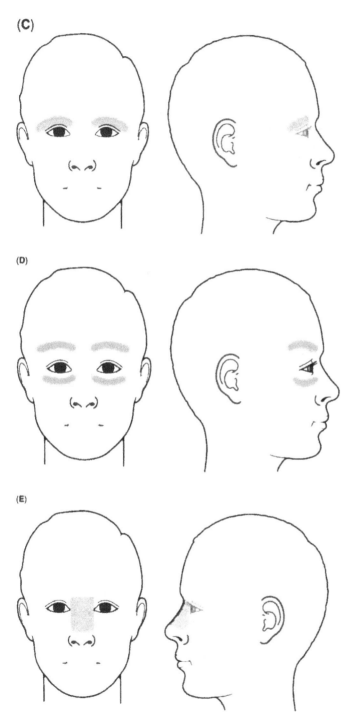

FIGURE 1 (*Continued*)

(F)

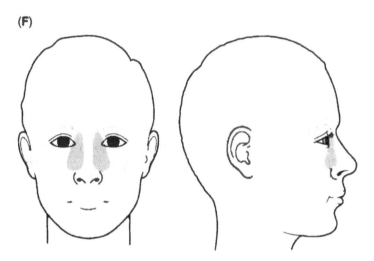

FIGURE 1 (*Continued*)

symptoms are not worse with routine physical activity, and rarely interfere with the patient getting to sleep.

To make matters more complex, the stimulus of a genuine acute sinus infection may exacerbate the symptoms, with a return to the background face ache on resolution of the infection. It is hardly surprising that patients (and doctors) will interpret all their symptoms as being related to their nose or sinuses. Patients often describe tenderness on touching the areas of the forehead or cheeks, leading them to think that there is underlying inflammation of the bone. However, on examination, there is hyperesthesia of the skin and soft tissues in these areas and gently touching these is enough to cause discomfort, and there is no evidence of underlying bony disease. This is similar to the tender areas over the forehead and scalp seen with tension-type headache. Nasal endoscopy is normal. As approximately one in three asymptomatic people have incidental changes on their CT, this may confuse the picture (25). A trial of maximal nasal medical treatment including oral and nasal steroids and a broad-spectrum antibiotic with anaerobic cover fails to help their symptoms, although the transient benefit of a placebo effect needs to be borne in mind and interpreted in the light of clinical findings. The majority of patients with this condition respond to low-dose amitriptyline, but usually require up to six weeks of 10 mg at night and occasionally 20 mg before it works. Amitriptyline should then be continued for six months before stopping it, and in the 20% whose symptoms return when they stop it they need to restart it duplicates. Patients need to be warned of the sedative effects even at this low dose, but they can be reassured that tolerance usually develops in the first few days. It is our practice to inform patients that amitriptyline is also used in higher doses for other conditions such as nocturnal enuresis and depression, but its effectiveness in midfacial segment pain is unrelated to its analgesic properties, which would take effect much more quickly and normally require 75 mg. It is often reassuring for patients to know the dose used for depression is some seven or more times the dose used in tension-type headache or midfacial segment pain. Other serotonin reuptake inhibitors are not effective; again this is akin to tension-type headache.

It is relevant that 10 mg is insufficient to produce any analgesic effect on its own. If amitriptyline fails, then relief may be obtained from neurotonin, propranolol, carbamazepine, and occasionally sodium valproate.

In some patients, there are migrainous features, and a triptan may help acute exacerbations. A higher proportion of these patients have myofascial pain, irritable bowel, and fatigue than is found in the normal population, although many appear to be healthy individuals in all other respects.

It is of interest that if surgery is mistakenly performed as a treatment for midfacial segment pain, the pain may sometimes abate temporarily, only to return after several weeks to months (4). If patients with midfacial segment pain undergo septal or sinus surgery, it makes no difference in approximately a third, in a third it makes their symptoms worse, and in the remaining third, it helps their pain but only for a few weeks and rarely more than a few months. It is as though the surgical stimulus alters the "balance" of neuronal activity in the trigeminal caudal nucleus for a short time. It is possible that the placebo effect or cognitive dissonance may be responsible for a temporary symptomatic improvement. These effects cannot explain the benefit of amitriptyline, as the placebo effect normally subsides within months (40). These theories about the etiology of tension-type headache if extrapolated to midfacial segment pain allow for the superadded potentiation of nociceptors on top of the peripheral/central sensitization, which may sometimes happen in this condition.

The minority whose symptoms were preceded by a peripheral injury or inflammation may have had neuroplastic changes in the trigeminal brain stem sensory nuclear complex to produce central sensitization (42).

The term "midfacial segment pain" avoids the use of the term tension used in tension-type headache that often results in a long and relatively unproductive discussion with the patient, as the term often leads to a misunderstanding about the etiology of their condition.

KEY POINTS

- If facial discomfort and pressure is the *primary* symptom, it is unlikely to be due to sinus disease in the absence of any nasal symptoms or signs.
- If a patient has facial discomfort in addition to nasal obstruction, and a loss of sense of smell, and it is associated with the following symptoms: worse with a cold, flying, or skiing, their symptoms may be helped by nasal medical or surgical treatment.
- In the majority of patients seen in a rhinological clinic with facial discomfort, it is found to be due to causes other than sinusitis (3).
- Patients whose nasal endoscopy is normal are unlikely to have facial discomfort due to rhinosinusitis.
- Patients with a normal CT scan are unlikely to have facial discomfort due to rhinosinusitis. (NB. Approximately a third of asymptomatic patients have incidental mucosal changes on CT, so radiographic changes on their own are not indicative of symptomatic rhinosinusitis).
- Patients with purulent secretions and facial discomfort are likely to benefit from treatment directed at resolving their rhinosinusitis. Paradoxically only a minority of patients with purulent rhinosinusitis at endoscopy have facial discomfort.

- If it is not possible to make a diagnosis at the first consultation, it is often helpful to ask the patient to keep a diary of symptoms and to transmit a trial of medical nasal treatment followed by a review of the patient.
- Surgery done for facial discomfort in patients with no objective signs of paranasal sinus disease has no effect in a third, makes the pain worse in a third, and while it can help reduce the pain of the remaining third, this rarely lasts more than a few months.
- In studies on facial discomfort, it is important to defer assessing the response to treatment until twelve months after treatment. This is because the effect of cognitive dissonance or surgery altering neuroplasticity within the brain stem sensory nuclear complex may have a temporary effect that can last this long (4).

CHARACTERISTICS OF MIDFACIAL SEGMENT PAIN

- A symmetrical sensation of pressure or tightness, although some patients may say that their nose feels blocked when they have no nasal airway obstruction.
- Involve any of the following areas alone or in combination: the nasion, under the bridge of the nose, either side of the nose, the peri- or retro-orbital regions, or across the cheeks. Often the symptoms of tension-type headache coexist.
- There may be hyperesthesia of the skin and soft tissues over the affected area.
- Nasal endoscopy is normal, but as approximately 20% of the population has some form of rhinitis, this can complicate arriving at the correct diagnosis.
- CT of the paranasal sinuses is normal (note a third of asymptomatic patients have incidental mucosal changes on CT, so radiographic changes on their own are not indicative of symptomatic rhinosinusitis).
- These symptoms may be intermittent (<15 days/month) or chronic (>15 days/month).
- There are no consistent exacerbating or relieving factors.
- There are no nasal symptoms (note that approximately 20% of most populations have intermittent or persistent allergic rhinitis and these may occur incidentally in this condition).

THE CHARACTERISTICS OF SYMPTOMS OF FACIAL DISCOMFORT IN RHINOSINUSITIS

Acute sinusitis usually follows an acute upper respiratory tract infection, and symptoms are usually unilateral, intense, associated with pyrexia and unilateral nasal obstruction, and there may be a purulent discharge. In contrast, chronic sinusitis is often painless, with discomfort occurring mainly during acute exacerbations precipitated by an upper respiratory tract infection or when there is an obstruction of the sinus ostia by polyps when pus is present. If there is pain or discomfort, it is often a unilateral dull ache around the medial canthus of the eye, although more severe facial pain can occur, and in maxillary sinusitis, toothache often occurs. An increase in the severity of pain on bending forward is traditionally thought to be the diagnostic of sinusitis, but this is nonspecific, as many types of facial pain and headache are made worse by this action.

The key points in the history of sinogenic pain are an exacerbation of pain during an upper respiratory tract infection, an association with rhinological symptoms and a response to nasal medical treatment. Examination of the face is often normal in patients with chronic sinusitis. Facial swelling is usually due to other pathology such as dental sepsis or malignancy. If a diagnosis of sinusitis has been made and the patient has not responded to treatment, then nasendoscopy is very helpful, if not essential in making the diagnosis of sinusitis. A normal nasal cavity, showing no evidence of middle meatal mucopus or inflammatory changes, makes a diagnosis of sinogenic pain most unlikely, particularly if patients are currently in pain or had pain within the past few days when they are endoscoped. On occasion, it is useful to review patients and repeat the nasendoscopy when they have pain to clarify the diagnosis.

CONCLUSION

The majority of patients who present with facial discomfort believe they have "sinus or nasal trouble." There is an increasing awareness that neurological causes are responsible for a large proportion of patients with headache or facial discomfort (53–55). We believe that patients with facial pain who have no objective evidence of sinus disease (endoscopy negative and CT negative), and whose pain fails to respond to medical antibiotic/steroid therapy aimed at treating sinonasal disease, are very unlikely to be helped by nasal or sinus surgery, particularly in the medium and long term.

A comprehensive examination (including nasendoscopy) is highly desirable if medical nasal treatment has failed to help symptoms of facial discomfort. If a patient has the symptoms of midfacial segment pain with coexisting rhinitis and they have not responded to maximum nasal medical treatment, they should receive medical treatment for midfacial segment pain before surgery is even considered. In the absence of nasal symptoms or signs, they should receive a trial of low-dose amitriptyline in the first instance. Only if there are neurological signs or their discomfort is progressive are further investigations warranted in the first instance. Failure to respond to the treatment for midfacial segment pain should make the physician question the diagnosis, as the treatment is usually successful in the majority of patients with the condition.

REFERENCES

1. Graff-Radford SB. Facial pain. Curr Opin Neurol 2000; 13:291–296.
2. Tarabichi M. Characteristics of sinus-related pain. Otolaryngol Head Neck Surg 2000; 122:84–87.
3. West B, Jones NS. Endoscopy-negative, computed tomography-negative facial pain in a nasal clinic. Laryngoscope 2001; 111:581–586.
4. Jones NS, Cooney TR. Facial pain and sinonasal surgery. Rhinology 2003; 41:193–200.
5. Hughes R, Jones NS. The role of endoscopy in outpatient management. Clin Otolaryngol 1998; 23:224–226.
6. Fahy C, Jones NS. Nasal polyposis and facial pain. Clin Otolaryngology 2001; 26: 510–513.
7. Acquadro MA, Salman SD, Joseph MP. Analysis of pain and endoscopic sinus surgery for sinusitis. Ann Otol Rhinol Laryngol 1997; 106:305–309.
8. Daudia A, Jones NS. Facial migraine in a rhinological setting. Clin Otolaryngol 2002; 27:521–525.
9. Fuad F, Jones NS. Is there an overlap between paroxysmal hemicrania and cluster headache? J Laryngol Otol 2002; 27:472–479.
10. Jones NS. The classification and diagnosis of facial pain. Hosp Med 2001; 62(10): 598–606.

11. Sluder G. The role of the sphenopalatine ganglion in nasal headaches. New York Med J 1908; 87:989–990.
12. The Headache Classification Committee of the International Headache Society. Classification and diagnostic criteria for headache disorders, cranial neuralgia and facial pain. Cephalalgia 1988; 8(7):1–96.
13. Ahamed SH, Jones NS. What is Sluder's neuralgia? J Laryngol Otol 2003; 117:437–443.
14. Sluder G. Headaches and eye disorders of nasal origin. London: Henry Kimpton, 1919:57–85.
15. Montgomery WW. Mucocele of the maxillary sinus causing enophthalmos. Eye Ear Nose Throat Mon 1964; 42:41–44.
16. Eto RT, House JM. Enophthalmos, a sequela of maxillary sinusitis. Am J Neuroradiol 1995; 16:939–941.
17. Raghavan U, Downes R, Jones NS. Spontaneous resolution of eyeball displacement caused by maxillary sinusitis. Br J Ophthalmol 2001; 85(1):118.
18. McAuliffe GW, Goodell H, Wolff HG. Experimental studies on headache: pain from the nasal and paranasal structures. Res Public New York Assoc Res Nerv Mental Dis 1943; 23:185–208.
19. Abu-Bakra M, Jones NS. Does stimulation of the nasal mucosa cause referred pain to the face? Clin Otolaryngol 2001; 26:403–432.
20. Abu-Bakra M, Jones NS. The prevalence of nasal contact points in a population with facial pain and a control population. J Laryngol Otol 2001; 115:629–632.
21. Stammberger H, Wolf G. Headaches and sinus disease: the endoscopic approach. Ann Otol Rhinol Laryngol 1988; 143:3–23.
22. Hennekens CH, Buring JE. Epidemiology in Medicine. In: Mayrent SL, ed. Boston: Little Brown and Company, 1987:294–295.
23. Harar RPS, Chadha NK, Rogers G. The role of septal deviation in adult chronic rhinosinusitis: a study of 500 patients. Rhinology 2004; 42:126–130.
24. Jones NS, Strobl A, Holland I. CT findings in 100 patients with rhinosinusitis and 100 controls. Clin Otolaryngol 1997; 22:47–51.
25. Jones NS. A review of the CT staging systems, the prevalence of anatomical variations, incidence of mucosal findings and their correlation with symptoms, surgical and pathological findings. Clin Otolaryngol 2002; 27:11–17.
26. Basic N, Basic V, Jukic T, Basic M, Jelic M, Hat J. Computed tomographic imaging to determine the frequency of anatomic variations in pneumatization of the ethmoid bone. Eur Arch Otolaryngol 1999; 256:69–71.
27. Arslan H, Aydinhoglu A, Bozkurt M, Egeli E. Anatomic variations of the paranasal sinuses: CT examination for endoscopic sinus surgery. Auris Nasus Larynx 1999; 26:39–48.
28. Danese M, Duvoisin B, Agrifoglio A, Cherpillod J, Krayenbuhl M. Influence of sinonasal variants on recurrent sinusitis of 112 patients. J Radiol 1997; 78:651–657.
29. Perez-Pinas I, Sabate J, Camona A, Catalina-Herrena CJ, Jimenez-Castellanos J. Anatomical variations in the human paranasal sinus region studied by CT. J Anatomy 2000; 197:221–227.
30. Lloyd GA. CT of the paranasal sinuses: study of a control series in relation to endoscopic sinus surgery. J Laryngol Otol 1990; 104(6):477–481.
31. Lloyd GAS, Lund VJ, Scadding GK. CT of the paranasal sinuses and functional endoscopic sinus surgery: a critical analysis of 100 asymptomatic patient. J Laryngol Otol 1991; 105(3):181–185.
32. Clark ST, Babin RW, Salazar J. The incidence of concha bullosa and its relationship to chronic sinonasal disease. Am J Rhinol 1989; 3:11–12.
33. Bolger WE, Butzin CA, Parsons DS. Paranasal sinus bony anatomic variations and mucosal abnormalities: CT analysis for endoscopic sinus surgery. Laryngoscope 1991; 101(1 Pt 1):56–64.
34. Calhoun KH, Waggenspack GA, Simpson CB, Hokanon JA, Bailey BJ. CT evaluation of the paranasal sinuses in symptomatic and asymptomatic populations. Otolaryngol Head Neck Surg 1991; 104:480–483.

35. Willner A, Choi SS, Vezina LG, Lozar RH. Intranasal anatomic variations in pediatric rhinosinusitis. Am J Rhinology 1997; 11(5):355–360.
36. Tonai A, Bala S. Anatomic variations of the bone in sinonasal CT. Acta Otolaryngol Suppl 1996; 525:9–13.
37. Kayalioglu G, Oyar O, Govsa F. Nasal cavity and paranasal sinus bony variations: a computed tomographic study. Rhinology 2000; 38:108–113.
38. Medina J, Tom LWC, Marsh RR, Bilaniuk LT. Development of the paranasal sinuses in children with sinus disease. Am J Rhinol 1999; 13:23–26.
39. Sonkens JW, Harnsberger HR, Blanch GM, Babbel RW, Hunt S. The impact of screening sinus CT on the planning of functional endoscopic sinus surgery. Otolaryngol Head Neck Surg 1991; 105(6):802–813.
40. Homer J, Jones NS, Sheard C, Herbert M. Cognitive dissonance, the placebo effect and the evaluation of surgical results. Clin Otolaryngol 2000; 25:195–199.
41. Olesen J. Clinical and pathophysiological observations in migraine and tension-type headache explained by integration of vascular, supraspinal and myofascial inputs. Pain 1991; 46:125–132.
42. Sessle BJ. Acute and chronic craniofacial pain: brainstem mechanisms and nociceptive transmission and neuroplasticity, and their clinical correlates. Crit Rev Oral Biol Med 2000; 11(1):57–91.
43. Jensen R, Olesen J. Tension-type headache: an update on mechanisms and treatment. Curr Opin Neurol 2000; 13:285–289.
44. Bendtsen L. Central sensitization in tension-type headache—possible pathophysiological mechanisms. Cephalalgia 2000; 20:486–508.
45. Cook PR, Nishioka GJ, Davis WE, McKinsey JP. Functional endoscopic sinus surgery in patients with normal computed tomography scans. Otolaryngol Head Neck Surg 1994; 110:505–509.
46. Boonchoo R. Functional endoscopic sinus surgery in patients with sinugenic headache. J Med Assoc Thai 1997; 80:521–526.
47. Parsons DS, Batra PS. Functional endoscopic sinus surgical outcomes for contact point headaches. Laryngoscope 1998; 108:696–702.
48. Rosbe KW, Jones KR. Usefulness of patient symptoms and nasal endoscopy in the diagnosis of chronic sinusitis. Am J Rhinol 1998; 12:167–171.
49. Bendtsen L, Jensen R, Olesen J. Qualitatively altered nociception in chronic myofascial pain. Pain 1996; 65:259–264.
50. Jensen R. Pathophysiological mechanisms of tension-type headache: a review of epidemiological and experimental studies. Cephalalgia 1999; 19:602–621.
51. Olesen J, Rasmussen BK. Classification of primary headaches. Biomed Pharmacother 1995; 49:446–451.
52. Ren K, Dubner R. Central nervous system plasticity and persistent pain. J Orofac Pain 1999; 13:155–163.
53. Acquadro MA, Salman SD, Joseph MP. Analysis of pain and endoscopic sinus surgery for sinusitis. Ann Otol Rhinol Laryngol 1997; 106(4):305–309.
54. Salman SD. Questions awaiting answers. Curr Opin Otolaryngol Head Neck Surg 1999; 7:1.
55. Ruoff GE. When sinus headache isn't sinus headache. Headache Quart 1997;8:22–31.

Clinical Approach to Diagnosis and Treatment of Nonallergic Rhinitis

Mark S. Dykewicz

Department of Internal Medicine, Division of Allergy and Immunology,
St. Louis University School of Medicine, St. Louis, Missouri, U.S.A.

INTRODUCTION

While the diagnosis and management of nonallergic rhinitis (NAR) sometimes may be relatively straightforward, there are many cases that can be challenging if not vexing. This discussion will provide a practical, logical clinical approach to the diagnosis and management of NAR, including subtleties of diagnosis that are sometimes neglected and considerations that may assist in more appropriate selection of treatments from the available array of standard and alternative treatment options.

Before seeking medical advice, patients with nasal complaints often have used nonprescription, over-the-counter medications such as antihistamines, oral decongestants, or nasal decongestant sprays and have found such treatments unsatisfactory. Subsequently, upon seeking advice from medical practitioners who do not specialize in rhinitis treatment, patients frequently are prescribed medications such as less-sedating or nonsedating antihistamines and/or nasal corticosteroids on an empiric basis without much diagnostic effort to distinguish between allergic or different forms of NAR. Often, it is only when such initial prescription measures fail that further workup for the diagnostic basis of rhinitis complaints is actively pursued.

NOMENCLATURE AND CLINICAL FEATURES OF MAJOR NAR SUBSETS

Although a complete review of the presentation of all forms of NAR is beyond the scope of this review, we will first discuss major clinical features of the most common types of NAR. Before presenting a clinical approach to diagnosis and management, it is necessary to discuss definitions of several major subcategories of NAR, because diagnostic terms are sometimes applied differently by different authors, and several terms may be used to refer to the same set of NAR patients. This is of additional importance in understanding the discussion to follow, because there is some unavoidable inconsistency in the use of some terms when published citations are being discussed, which have used one term or another.

The terms "perennial NAR," "nonallergic, noninfectious rhinitis," nonallergic noninfectious perennial rhinitis, and "idiopathic rhinitis" are general terms that are used to refer to the group of patients who have no immunoglobulin (Ig)E-mediated basis for their rhinitis and typically experience some rhinitis symptoms year round (1–4). "Vasomotor rhinitis" (VMR) is a term that has been used synonymously with these other general terms, but sometimes is used in a somewhat more restricted sense to refer only to a subset of patients who must have their symptoms provoked or aggravated by nonimmunogenic chemical stimuli such as airborne irritants (e.g., perfumes, paint fumes, and cigarette smoke); physical environmental factors such as temperature, changes in barometric pressure, or bright lights; emotions; or alcohol ingestion. Whatever the term used, this is a diagnosis of exclusion, with no generally accepted definition or diagnostic criteria, and comprises several subgroups with ill-defined pathomechanisms (3). Patients have traditionally been classified as "runners" (those with predominantly rhinorrhea), "blockers" (those with predominantly nasal congestion and blockage), or "sneezers" (when sneezing is the predominant symptom) (1,2,5). However, this subdivision of patients has limitations because many patients suffer from more than one type of these symptoms, and sometimes an individual's predominant symptoms might vary under different circumstances.

A better-defined subset of NAR is the NAR with eosinophilia syndrome (NARES). Characterized by prominent eosinophilic infiltrates of the nasal mucosa, patients lack evidence of allergic disease as demonstrated by lack of clinically significant positive skin tests and/or specific IgE antibodies in the serum (6,7). Typically middle-aged patients with NARES experience perennial symptoms of sneezing paroxysms, profuse watery rhinorrhea, nasal congestion, nasal pruritus, and occasional loss of smell. NARES patients tend to have more pronounced nasal symptoms than patients with either VMR or allergic rhinitis (8).

In many patients, there may be coexisting allergic and NAR or "mixed rhinitis." In a retrospective analysis of allergy specialty practices, 43% of patients were classified as having pure allergic rhinitis, 23% as having pure NAR, and 34% as having mixed rhinitis (4).

DIAGNOSIS

When a patient presents with nasal complaints—particularly when refractory to initial attempts at therapy—the diagnostic process may need to not only identify and distinguish allergic rhinitis from NAR, but different diagnostic categories of NAR, common differential considerations such as sinusitis, and uncommon if not rare conditions such as cerebrospinal fluid (CSF) leak and granulomatous disease of the upper airway (Table 1). As with many medical conditions, arriving at the correct diagnosis may require a combined approach of using patient history, physical examination, and diagnostic testing. Unlike allergic rhinitis in which there are specific diagnostic tests to confirm the diagnosis, there are no specific diagnostic tests for NAR, and diagnosis is primarily made on the basis of rhinitis symptoms in the absence of identifiable allergy (by allergy testing), structural abnormality, immune deviation, or sinus disease (1–3).

History
Although a clearly established seasonal history of rhinoconjunctivitis symptoms can help identify patients who are more likely to have an allergic basis, it is not possible to reliably distinguish allergic rhinitis from NAR on the basis of history alone when perennial or persistent symptoms are present (2,9). Compared to perennial allergic rhinitis, one study found that NAR was associated with fewer sneezes and conjunctival symptoms, but rhinorrhea and congestion were of similar prominence (10). While another study also found that VMR patients were less

TABLE 1 Differential Diagnosis of Nasal Symptoms

Allergic rhinitis
NAR
Infectious
    Acute
    Chronic
Perennial NAR/noninfectious NAR/vasomotor rhinitis/idiopathic rhinitis
    Airborne irritants, temperature extremes, or changes
NAR with eosinophilia syndrome
Basophilic/metachromatic cell nasal disease or nasal mastocytosis

Other rhinitis syndromes
Ciliary dyskinesia syndrome
Atrophic rhinitis
Hormonally induced
  Hypothyroidism
  Pregnancy
  Oral contraceptives
  Menstrual cycle–related
Exercise
Drug-induced
  Rhinitis medicamentosa
  Oral contraceptives
  ACE-I and antihypertensive therapy
  cGMP specific PDE5 inhibitors for erectile dysfunction
  Aspirin/nonsteroidal anti-inflammatory
Reflex-induced
  Gustatory (food-related cholinergic) rhinitis
  Airborne chemical or irritant-induced
  Posture reflexes
Occupational (may be allergic or nonallergic)

Conditions that may mimic or aggravate symptoms of rhinitis
Sinusitis
Nasal polyposis
Gastroesophageal reflux
Other structural/mechanical factors
  Deviated septum/septal wall anomalies
  Hypertrophic turbinates
  Adenoidal hypertrophy (particularly in children)
  Foreign bodies
  Nasal tumors
    Benign
    Malignant
  Choanal atresia
Inflammatory/immunologic
  Wegener's granulomatosis
  Sarcoidosis
  Midline granuloma
  Relapsing polychondritis
  Systemic lupus erythematosus
  Sjogren's syndrome (rhinitis sicca)
Cerebrospinal fluid rhinorrhea

Abbreviations: NAR, nonallergic rhinitis; ACE, angiotensin-converting enzyme; cGMP, cyclic guanosine monophosphate; PDE, phosphodiesterase.
Source: From Ref. 1.

likely to experience sneezes and eye irritation, nasal blockage was found to be the predominant symptom in patients with VMR (11). Nonetheless, history may be of value in identifying some types of NAR, nonallergic triggers that should be avoided, systemic factors that may be impacting the nose, and conditions other than rhinitis, which may be causing nasal symptoms (Table 2). As discussed later, identifying symptoms of greatest prominence in a patient with NAR may also guide selection of treatments.

Physical Examination

Examination of the nose is required in all cases of rhinitis (Table 3) (1,2). This may be performed with a nasal speculum with appropriate lighting, otoscope with nasal adapter, or flexible nasopharyngoscope (see section "Other Diagnostic Testing"). With use of the nasal speculum or otoscope with nasal adapter, elevating the end of the nose with the other hand provides a improved view of the nasal passage. The classical appearance of mucosa of allergic rhinitis is pale and swollen, with a bluish-gray appearance when the mucosal edema is severe, but the mucosa can also be hyperemic. Mucosal appearance may not distinguish between allergic and NAR, because NAR may also present with mucosal pallor, edema, or hyperemia (12). Mucosa that is markedly erythematous, congested, and granular, sometimes with areas of punctate bleeding, suggests rhinitis medicamentosa or cocaine abuse. The mucosa is usually erythematous in acute infections, and is typically erythematous, edematous, and occasionally friable in rhinitis medicamentosa or cocaine abuse (13). The quantity and quality of nasal secretions should be noted, but may not differ between allergic and NAR. Purulent drainage may be suggestive of sinusitis, and would raise consideration of treatment of sinusitis or further investigation. However, purulence does not by itself reliably indicate that bacterial infection is present.

It is often possible to appreciate whether significant septal deviation that could explain nasal obstructive symptoms is present, but rhinoscopy or computed tomography (CT) scanning may be necessary to assess whether nasal septal deviation is present beyond the view of the speculum. Nasal polyps, with their pale gray to yellow translucent, gelatinous appearance, may often be visualized by examination, but rhinoscopy or CT scanning also may be needed to detect them. Nasal polyps may be differentiated from edematous mucosa by applying a topical vasoconstrictor and reexamining the mucosa 5 to 10 minutes later; edematous mucosa will shrink in size, whereas nasal polyps will not. Crusting on an inflamed mucosa may suggest atrophic rhinitis or a systemic disease such as sarcoidosis. The presence of a septal perforation should raise the possibility of cocaine abuse, previous surgery, or systemic granulomatous diseases.

In anticipation of prescribing nasal sprays, it is very important to visualize the nares to assure that they are sufficiently patent to permit adequate delivery of nasal sprays to more superior regions of the nares. If the nares are not patent because of marked mucosal edema, short-term use (e.g. five days) of a nasal decongestant spray 15 minutes prior to administration of another nasal agent (e.g., nasal corticosteroid) may redindant reduce edema such that the second agent may then be successfully administered after discontinuing the nasal decongestant spray. Another option is to administer a short (five- to seven-day) burst of short-acting oral corticosteroids such as prednisone or methylprednisolone (1). When nasal sprays are prescribed, reexamination of the nose is important to not only assess treatment benefit, but also assure that there has not been any development of

TABLE 2 Some Useful Historical Questions About Rhinitis and Their Importance

History of illness
  Age of onset?
    If during childhood, allergy more likely
    Over the age of 60–70, new onset rhinitis likely nonallergic
  Prominent rhinorrhea, congestion, sneezing, and pruritus?
    If pruritus, suggests allergy. If certain symptoms predominate, can direct
      symptom-based therapy
  If rhinorrhea prominent, description?
    If persistent and generally purulent, suggests sinusitis
    If clear, nonmucoid, consider CSF fluid leak, especially if onset
      after head trauma
  Unilateral symptoms?
    Suggest anatomic causes (e.g., nasal septal deviation)
    In small children, particularly with purulent drainage, consider the presence
      of a foreign body in the nose
  Seasonal or perennial?
    Seasonal, more likely allergic; perennial symptoms may be allergic or
      nonallergic
  Intermittent or persistent?
    May be useful in choosing medications more suited for intermittent use
  Relation to acute allergen exposure (e.g., pets and house dust)?
    To identify suspect allergen
  Relation to acute nonallergic triggers (e.g., airborne irritants, temperature
    extremes, or changes)
    Consistent with pure NAR (e.g., irritant rhinitis), or with mixed allergic
      rhinitis/NAR
  Relation to food ingestion
    Gustatory rhinitis suggested, implications for choosing among therapies
  Worse indoors or outdoors or with work or school?
    May aid in identifying suspect allergen
  Duration, course
    If acute onset after acute respiratory infection, persistent symptoms suggest
      sinusitis
  Past history of nasal or head trauma
    Consider anatomic disease (past nasal septal fracture with altered architecture
      after healing) or if thin, clear rhinorrhea, CSF leak

Medication history (current and past)
  History of poor response to medications taken for nasal symptoms?
    Directs subsequent choice of empiric therapy
    Was patient sufficiently compliant to expect treatment effect from the drug?
    If nasal sprays had been taken for sufficient duration to have treatment effect?
    If nasal sprays used, and congestion is a prominent symptom, severe mucosal edema
      may have blocked effective distribution to more superior regions of the nose
  Chronic use of nasal decongestant sprays?
    Suggests rhinitis medicamentosa
  Nasal cocaine use?
    Causes rhinitis similar to that caused by nasal decongestant spray
  Taking systemic drugs that may cause rhinitis (e.g., ACE inhibitors,
    antihypertensives, oral contraceptives, and cGMP–specific PDE5 inhibitors for
    erectile dysfunction)?
    Changing drug regimen to alternate classes or treatments may eliminate or
      improve rhinitis. For ACE inhibitors, rhinitis symptoms may develop well after
      onset of medication use, and associated cough may or may not be present

(Continued)

TABLE 2 Some Useful Historical Questions About Rhinitis and Their Importance (*Continued*)

If aspirin or nonsteroidal anti-inflammatories are used, do these aggravate respiratory symptoms?
    Suggests NAR with eosinophilia syndrome or nasal polyps, may be associated with asthma

Review of systems/past history
    Weight gain, lethargy, or changes in skin or bowel habits?
        Consider hypothyroidism, check TSH level
    Symptoms of GE reflux or cough, uncontrolled?
        Supraesophageal effects of reflux may aggravate or cause rhinitis; treat GE reflux as well as rhinitis
    Pulmonary complaints (dyspnea, cough)
        Consider asthma, GE reflux, or rarely, multiorgan disease such as Wegener's granulomatosis and sarcoidosis
    Halitosis?
        Suggests sinusitis
    Frequent documented infections (e.g., pneumonia with recurrent chronic sinusitis)?
        Possible immune deficiency, ciliary dyskinesia, cystic fibrosis; consider immune workup
    If adult male, and childless with chronic sinusitis?
        Possible ciliary dyskinesia syndrome
    Prominent musculoskeletal complaints?
        Possible underlying connective tissue disease
        Midline granuloma
        Relapsing polychondritis
        Systemic lupus erythematosus
        Sjogren's syndrome (rhinitis sicca)

Abbreviations: CSF, cerebrospinal fluid; NAR, nonallergic rhinitis; ACE, angiotensin-converting enzyme; GE, gastroesophageal; TSH, thyroid stimulating hormone; cGMP, cyclic guanosine monophosphate.

TABLE 3 Elements of Physical Examination and Procedures to Consider in Patients with Rhinitis

General observations: "allergic shiners" (may be present in allergic rhinitis or NAR), mouth breathing, and nasal crease, evidence of systemic disease (e.g., nail clubbing suggests need for pulmonary and possibly additional investigation)
Growth percentiles for children
Eyes: evidence for allergic conjunctivitis (suggests allergic rhinitis rather than NAR)
Nose: presence or absence of external deformity (suggests anatomic abnormality, saddle nose suggests multisystem disease such as Wegener's granulomatosis), nasal mucosa [appearance, degree of swelling, nasal polyps, deviated septum, septal perforation, discharge (noting color and consistency)], and blood
Ears: abnormalities of associated middle ear disease: tympanic membranes—abnormal mobility patterns, retraction, air–fluid levels, bubbles behind tympanic membrane; consider tympanometry to confirm the presence or absence of effusion and middle ear under- or overpressures
Mouth: Observe for malocclusion or high arched palate associated with chronic mouth breathing, tonsilar hypertrophy, lymphoid "streaking" in the oropharynx, pharyngeal postnasal discharge, and halitosis
Neck: Lymphadenopathy and thyroid enlargement
Chest: Signs of asthma (may be associated with allergic rhinitis or NAR)
Skin: Eczema (associated with allergic rhinitis) and generalized skin dryness (consider hypothyroidism)

Abbreviation: NAR, nonallergic rhinitis.
Source: From Ref. 1.

mucosal erosions because of use of the prescribed spray. In particular, the nasal septum should be examined to assure that there are no erosions or ulcerations of the mucosa, which may precede development of nasal septal perforation.

Diagnostic Testing

Unlike allergic rhinitis in which the diagnosis can be readily supported by tests for specific IgE, there are no specific diagnostic tests per se for NAR. However, diagnostic testing may be useful in distinguishing some types of NAR from others, and for identifying sinusitis and structural and other disorders that can mimic rhinitis. Certainly in a patient who is not responding well to empiric treatment, further diagnostic testing should be considered.

Testing for Specific IgE

At an early point in the diagnostic process for rhinitis, and particularly if initial therapeutic measures fail, there should be assessment of whether specific IgE antibodies to relevant aeroallergens are present (1,2). With few exceptions, if specific IgE antibodies are absent, it can be generally assumed that a patient's upper airway problems are not allergic and NAR is likely (14,15). Whether determined by skin testing or in vitro testing, positive results for specific IgE must be correlated with history to determine clinical relevance. Percutaneous skin testing has much better negative and positive predictive value for the presence of an allergic component than does intradermal skin testing (16–22). It is also important to consider that positive skin tests or in vitro tests for specific IgE may be present in NAR, yet not be clinically relevant. Supportive of this principle is the finding that the incidence of positive skin tests to inhalant allergens is far greater than the incidence of rhinitis symptoms in large cross-sectional epidemiological studies, suggesting that both allergic and NAR patients are capable of demonstrating skin test positivity (3). This also suggests that rhinitis symptoms in a patient with a positive skin test are not necessarily caused by the allergen and that the contribution of NAR to the total population of rhinitis patients may be substantially greater than previously estimated (3).

Other Diagnostic Testing

After assessment of the presence or absence of allergies, many physicians including rhinitis specialists will proceed to the selection of therapy (see discussion below) without additional diagnostic testing. However, further diagnostic testing to better define the basis of a patient's problems may be pursued early on after failure of initial therapy, particularly if a patient's symptoms are severe. In other cases, a physician should certainly consider additional diagnostic testing when additional therapies have been administered and a patient continues to have suboptimal results. What follows is a discussion of additional diagnostic testing that may be considered, with a discussion of the advantages and limitations of the tests.

Upper Airway Endoscopy

Upper airway endoscopy (rhinolaryngoscopy) is the most useful procedure in an evaluation for anatomic factors causing upper airway symptoms and should be performed when medical treatment of rhinitis is unsatisfactory. Because, at best, nasal examination with a nasal speculum or otoscope visualizes only approximately one-third of the nasal cavity. In contrast, rhinolaryngoscopy can readily identify nasal septal deviation or nasal polyps that are missed with standard nasal examination. Endoscopy provides a clear view of the nasal cavity and allows for detailed examination of the nasal septum, middle meatus, superior meatus, sphenoethmoidal recess, and posterior nasopharynx, as well as structures of the oropharynx and larynx (23–25).

If possible, the middle meatus should be examined to evaluate bony or mucosal crowding with obstruction of the sinus ostia, which would predispose to sinusitis. Mucopurulent material in this region is suggestive of sinusitis.

Nasal Smears and Scrapings for Cytology

Nasal cytology obtained from nasal smears or scrapings may aid in differentiating allergic rhinitis and NARES from other forms of rhinitis (e.g., VMR and infectious rhinitis), if the correct procedure is followed and the appropriate stains are utilized (1,2). There is lack of expert consensus about whether nasal cytology should be routinely performed in the clinical evaluation of rhinitis (1), but some might argue that nasal cytology may be of particular value when patients are refractory to initial treatment. In controlled studies of NAR patients, nasal cytology is typically performed to better characterize patient subsets.

Visualization of large numbers of eosinophils, characteristic of allergic rhinitis and NARES, may be helpful in narrowing the differential diagnosis between these forms of rhinitis and other types of rhinitis (14,26,27). Nasal smears from secretions and nasal scrapings are easily obtained, but nasal biopsy has been reported to be superior to nasal smear for finding eosinophils in NAR (28). In allergic rhinitis, investigations have suggested that nasal secretions, obtained by lavage or scraping, and the nasal submucosa, sampled by biopsy, are different with respect to the patterns of cellular accumulation and act as two distinct compartments (29–31).

One argument for the use of nasal cytology is that the presence of eosinophils would help identify patients more likely to respond to nasal corticosteroids (4), but this may be incorrect. In reviewing data of 983 patients in three randomized, double-blind, placebo-controlled trials of perennial NAR, patients with NARES and non-NARES had similar statistical improvement with fluticasone propionate nasal treatment (32). Although histologic findings of eosinophilic inflammation are a characteristic feature of allergic rhinitis and NARES, there is controversy about whether inflammation is present in other forms of NAR. Some studies have suggested that the absence of inflammatory cytology is indicative of non-NARES NAR (2), whereas other studies have reported that most of the non-NARES NAR patients have some degree of inflammation (33,34).

The presence of neutrophils may support a diagnosis of infectious bacterial rhinitis or sinusitis, especially when humoral immunodeficiency or ciliary dysmotility are present. However, some level of secretion neutrophilia is not uncommon in apparently normal subjects (1). In a study of 315 university students, 319 school children, and 60 normal infants, nasal secretion neutrophilia occurred in 47% of the students, 79% of the school children, and 97% of the infants (35).

Radiologic Imaging

Radiologic imaging of the upper airway should be considered when empiric treatment has failed, which should elicit consideration of anatomic disease or sinus disease (36).

Standard radiographs are not indicated in the evaluation of patients with uncomplicated rhinitis (1). The Caldwell (anterior–posterior), Waters, and lateral views may have limited value in the imaging of the sinuses but are not useful for demonstration of structures of the nasal cavity and are of limited use in demonstration of structures of the nasopharynx, oropharynx, and larynx. Lateral views may assist in evaluation of the soft tissues of the nasopharynx, adenoids, oropharynx, and larynx, but are generally not needed when endoscopy is available.

CT scanning and magnetic resonance imaging (MRI) using coronal sections for imaging of sinuses frequently identify turbinate congestion, concha bullosa, polyps, and septal deviation as causes of nasal airway obstruction (1,2). High-resolution CT can demonstrate sinus disease that is not shown on routine X-ray films and anatomic structures inaccessible by physical examination or endoscopy. The principal indications for the CT are suspected chronic sinusitis not responding to appropriate medical therapy, acute recurrent sinusitis, abnormal diagnostic nasal endoscopic examination, and persistent facial pain (37). In some hospitals, a limited CT study of only four to five coronal views may be available as a cost-effective alternative to sinus radiographs.

MRI is superior to CT for soft-tissue imaging of the upper airway, but it is less suited for imaging of the bony anatomy. Because bone and air yield similar signal intensities on MRI, precise definition of the ostiomeatal complex is problematic. The signal intensity of extensive inflammatory disease is indistinguishable from normal mucosa in the edematous phase of the nasal cycle. MRI may be useful in the evaluation of upper airway malignancies.

Nasal Glucose and β_2-Transferrin

As discussed earlier, CSF leak should be considered when thin rhinorrhea develops after trauma, although this may also occur as a complication of surgery or spontaneously (38,39). Nasal mucus does not contain significant amounts of glucose, whereas CSF does; so quantitative testing for glucose in nasal drainage (more than 30 mg/100 mL glucose) supports the diagnosis. β_2-transferrin is a more specific test for CSF rhinorrhea (40). Thin slice coronal CT, magnetic resonance cisternography, or radionuclide cisternography can be used to localize the site of CSF leakage (41).

PHARMACOLOGIC TREATMENT

Compared to the large number of randomized, placebo-controlled clinical studies of the efficacy of medications in allergic rhinitis, far fewer placebo-controlled efficacy studies for NAR have been conducted, and even fewer studies have made head-to-head comparisons of active treatments for NAR (42).

Accordingly, it is difficult to state a preferred, universally applicable hierarchy of treatments for NAR, although one can consider the theoretical advantages and disadvantages of different available medications in choosing them for treatment. In the discussion that follows, various pharmacologic treatment options for NAR will be discussed, with a review of evidence for efficacy (or lack thereof) in NAR. This will be followed by a tabular summary of the relative advantages and disadvantages of therapeutic agents, considered from the perspective of treating patient subsets with differing predominant symptoms.

Before discussing individual agents, a general comment about administration of nasal sprays is in order. Most nasal sprays appropriate for treatment of NAR are not absorbed systemically to any substantial amount, and their clinical benefit is almost wholly dependent on direct topical effects on the nasal mucosa. Accordingly, if the nares are significantly obstructed inferiorly (e.g., because of extreme edema of the inferior turbinates—something that can be easily assessed by physical examination), nasal sprays may not be delivered successfully to large areas of the nasal mucosa, leading to diminished effectiveness. Accordingly, when nasal mucosal edema is so severe that there is very limited patency of the nasal vault, the edema should be reduced during initiation of a treatment course of a nondecongestant nose spray. One approach is to use a topical nasal decongestant spray 15 to 20 minutes prior to the use of a nondecongestant nasal spray, during the first five days of administration of the nondecongestant spray. For agents such as nasal corticosteroids that have an anti-inflammatory effect, edema can be reduced with their continued administration so that the nasal decongestant spray is no longer needed. Another approach is to administer a short course of oral corticosteroids (prednisone 40 mg q.d. for one week in an adult) to reduce nasal edema as a treatment course of the nondecongestant nose spray is begun (1).

Pharmacologic Agents

The discussion that immediately follows reviews key information about the principal treatments used for NAR. Although the literature is generally limited to studies of individual therapies, in clinical practice it is not unusual for several therapies to be used concomitantly in an effort to achieve additive or complementary effects. Following discussion of individual agents, these drugs are reviewed in table format, focused on their use in symptom-directed treatment (Table 4).

Intranasal Corticosteroids

Compared to an extensive number of trials demonstrating the effectiveness of internasal corticosteroids in allergic rhinitis, a relatively smaller number of studies have demonstrated the benefit of these agents in NAR. Several nasal corticosteroids have been approved by the U.S. Food and Drug Administration (FDA) for the treatment of symptoms of NAR/VMR: beclomethasone aqueous preparation, budesonide aerosol preparation (now removed from the U.S. market because of its fluorocarbon propellant), and fluticasone proprionate aqueous preparation. Although one study of budesonide found significant improvement in the symptom of nasal obstruction but no improvement in other symptoms (43), other studies of nasal steroids have found broader benefit including improvement in rhinorrhea and sneezing (44–47). As mentioned earlier, it had been proposed that nasal steroids would have a greater benefit when eosinophilic nasal mucosal inflammation is present. However, in randomized, double-blind, placebo-controlled trials of perennial NAR, patients with NARES and non-NARES had similar statistical improvement with fluticasone proprionate nasal treatment (32). Accordingly, nasal corticosteroids can be considered for general use in NAR.

In general, the drugs have an excellent safety profile, with the major concern being local side effects such as stinging, epistaxis, and rarely nasal septal perforation. For the latter reason, patients should be instructed on use of the nasal devices so that they direct the spray nozzles away from the septum and have periodic nasal examinations to detect mucosal erosions that may precede the

TABLE 4 Selection of Medical Treatment for Nonallergic Rhinitis Based upon Symptoms

Congestion predominating
  Nasal corticosteroids
    Pro: benefit in controlled studies
    Con: local side effects (epistaxis)
  Oral decongestants
    Pro: focused treatment for congestion
    Con: adverse effects (e.g., insomnia, tachycardia, and hypertension)
  Nasal azelastine
    Pro: benefit vs. placebo
    Con: adverse taste and occasional sedation

Rhinorrhea predominating
  Ipratropium bromide
    Pro: topical anticholinergic effects on mucus reduction, no significant systemic
      anticholinergic effects, and quick onset of action (within 30 minutes)
    Con: no relief of other symptoms (e.g., congestion) if present; dosing t.i.d.–q.i.d.
  Nasal steroids
    Pro: can reduce rhinitis symptoms other than rhinorrhea; considered drug of
      choice for NARES; can reduce rhinorrhea from non-NARES/nonallergic
      rhinitis, even if eosinophilic cytology is absent
    Con: for rhinorrhea as predominant symptom, less focused therapy than nasal
      ipratropium
  Nasal azelastine
    Pro: benefit in rhinorrhea in controlled trials
    Con: adverse taste and occasional sedation
  Sedating antihistamines
    Pro: anticholinergic effects might reduce rhinorrhea?
    Con: adverse effects (sedation and systemic anticholinergic effects)
  Oral decongestants
    Pro: may have mild effects to reduce rhinorrhea
    Con: minimal controlled studies; adverse effects (insomnia, tachycardia, etc.)
  Oral methscopolamine
    Pro: anticholinergic effects can reduce rhinorrhea
    Con: only available in combination preparations (e.g., with sedating
      antihistamines), frequent systemic anticholinergic adverse effects

development of nasal septal perforations. Adverse effects on children's growth have been detected with beclomethasone nasal (48), making other nasal steroids that do not have this effect preferred for pediatric use.

Nasal Antihistamines
Azelastine nasal spray has been approved by the FDA for the treatment of the symptoms of VMR, although its mechanism of action in NAR is unclear. In clinical trials of VMR, it has been demonstrated to cause broad-based improvement in all principal symptoms (congestion, rhinorrhea, postnasal drip, and sneezing) (49,50). In dose-ranging trials, azelastine nasal compared to saline spray resulted in a statistically greater reduction in symptoms within three hours of initial dosing (4). There are no direct comparison studies between intranasal steroids and nasal azelastine. The principal adverse effects of nasal azelastine are taste perversion and occasional sedation.

Oral Antihistamines
Theoretically, first-generation antihistamines might be of benefit for rhinorrhea of NAR, because of their anticholinergic, drying effect on nasal mucosa. It has been

suggested that antihistamines might also benefit sneezing from NAR (2). However, only one well-controlled study has studied the potential benefit of a first-generation antihistamine in NAR (51). In this study, the antihistamine brompheniramine was used as part of antihistamine–decongestant combination product, and accordingly, outcomes related to the antihistamine component of this drug cannot be separately identified.

First-generation oral antihistamines may not be well tolerated because of their sedation and systemic anticholinergic effects. Accordingly, oral first-generation antihistamines would not be a preferred class for empiric attempts to treat NAR. Nonsedating or less-sedating second-generation antihistamines, possessing no significant anticholinergic drying effects, would not be expected to benefit rhinorrhea in NAR, and there are no published trials of their use for NAR. For the treatment of rhinorrhea from NAR, nasal ipratropium would be a preferred agent.

Ipratropium Nasal

Ipratropium nasal spray has been approved by the U.S. FDA for the indications of "rhinorrhea associated with allergic and nonallergic perennial rhinitis" (for 0.03% concentration), or rhinorrhea associated with "acute viral rhinitis" (for 0.06% concentration). This anticholinergic agent has been demonstrated to reduce nasal blowing and rhinorrhea in NAR (52–56), and accordingly is well suited for the treatment of NAR when rhinorrhea is the predominant symptom. For this reason, it has a favored position in gustatory rhinitis in which rhinorrhea is a prominent symptom. Although it may have topical side effects such as infrequent episodes of nasal dryness and minor epistaxis, intranasal ipratropium bromide is well tolerated with no associated systemic anticholinergic adverse effects (57,58).

Comparisons of nasal corticosteroids and ipratropium in NAR yield conflicting results (42). One study found that compared to ipratropium, there was a superior effect for budesonide with respect to symptoms of nasal secretion and sneezing (59). In another double blind, randomized controlled trial in NAR characterized by hypersecretion, there was no observed difference in efficacy of the two medications, although conclusions are qualified because there was no placebo control (60).

Decongestants

Although not subjected to extensive clinical trials in NAR, oral and nasal decongestants are considered first-line agents for the treatment of nasal congestion of NAR. Nasal decongestant sprays may be used for short periods (e.g., three to five days) without significant risk for rebound congestion.

Nasal Saline

Topical saline administered by nasal spray or by irrigation devices is used to reduce postnasal drip, sneezing, and congestion and is considered a useful adjunctive measure for the treatment of NAR (1,4).

Other Agents

There is a natural interest in using medications known to benefit allergic rhinitis in NAR. Intranasal cromolyn (delivered as an inhaled powder) was examined in one double-blind crossover study of VMR, but there was no significant difference between the outcomes of variables measured (61). There is little rationale for the use of oral antileukotriene agents in NAR, although there is rationale for using these drugs in the treatment of nasal polyp disease because leukotrienes are prominently present in polyp tissue.

SELECTION OF THERAPEUTIC AGENTS FOR TREATMENT

Because treatment for NAR is often empiric, two basic strategies may be used in selecting medications. One approach is to direct treatment at a patient's predominant symptoms. As mentioned previously, patients with nonallergic (vasomotor) rhinitis often fall into groups in which the predominant nasal symptom is rhinorrhea (runners) or congestion (blockers) (5). Using this paradigm, agents can be selected on the basis of their likelihood to positively impact these symptoms (Table 4).

Alternatively, another treatment approach is to select "broad-based," nonspecific therapy such topical steroids or topical azelastine, because such agents can address multiple symptoms if present. One advantage of this nonspecific approach is that over time, symptoms of NAR in an individual can alternate from congestion to rhinorrhea (4). Another advantage to this nonspecific approach is that if a patient has an allergic component or mixed rhinitis, both of these types of agents can address the allergic and nonallergic components.

Ultimately, the decision to choose particular therapies must be based upon a combination of factors that include not only the likely clinical effectiveness and side-effect profile of therapies, but also patient preference, willingness to be compliant with the treatment, and cost.

SURGERY

When medical measures fail, there are unusual cases when surgical intervention may be considered for NAR. Specifically, patients who suffer from perennial allergic rhinitis or NAR may develop a severe drug-resistant hypertrophy of the inferior turbinates, leading to constant nasal obstruction and watery secretion due to an increase in glandular structures (2). Limited surgical reduction of the inferior turbinate body and mucosal surface using several techniques can reduce nasal obstruction and secretion, although radical turbinectomy may inhibit the ability of nasal mucosa to return to normal functioning (62–64).

There are other surgical techniques, such as vidian neurectomy, that have been developed to denervate the nose of its autonomic supply, primarily in an effort to reduce excessive secretion. However, re-enervation may occur over time with consequent loss of benefit, and because of complications (65–67), vidian neurectomy is not recommended for rhinitis (2).

There are also surgical procedures that may be useful to treat certain other diseases or abnormalities of the upper airways that may accompany NAR. These include anatomical variations of the septum with functional relevance, secondary or independently developing chronic sinusitis, allergic fungal sinusitis, nasal polyposis, or CSF leak (1,2).

REFERENCES

1. Dykewicz MS, Fineman S, Skoner DP, et al. Diagnosis and management of rhinitis: complete guidelines of the Joint Task Force on Practice Parameters in Allergy, Asthma, and Immunology. Ann Allergy Asthma Immunol 1998; 81(5 pt 2):478–518.

2. Bousquet J, van Cauwenberge P, Khaltaev N. The ARIA Workshop Group. Allergic rhinitis and its impact on asthma—ARIA workshop report. J Allergy Clin Immunol 2001; 108:S147–S333.
3. Bachert C. Persistent rhinitis—allergic or nonallergic? Allergy 2004; 59(suppl 76):11–15.
4. Settipane RA, Lieberman P. Update on nonallergic rhinitis. Ann Allergy Asthma Immunol 2001; 86(5):494–507.
5. Mygind N, Naclerio RM, eds. Allergic and nonallergic rhinitis. Philadelphia, PA: 1993.
6. Jacobs RL, Freedman PM, Boswell RN. Non-allergic rhinitis with eosinophilia (NARES syndrome): clinical and immunologic presentation. J Allergy Clin Immunol 1981; 67:253.
7. Mullarkey MF. Eosinophilic nonallergic rhinitis. J Allergy Clin Immunol 1988; 82:941–949.
8. Moneret-Vautrin DA, Shieh V, Wayoff M. Non-allergic rhinitis with eosinophilia syndrome (NARES)—a precursor of the triad. Ann Allergy 1990; 64:513–518.
9. Settipane RA. Rhinitis: a dose of epidemiological reality. Allergy Asthma Proc 2003; 24(3):147–154.
10. Togias A. Age relationships and clinical features of nonallergic rhinitis. JACI 1990; 85:182.
11. Lindberg S, Malm L. Comparison of allergic rhinitis and vasomotor rhinitis patients on the basis of a computer questionnaire. Allergy 1993; 48:602–607.
12. deShazo RD, Kemp SF. Rhinosinusitis. South Med J 2003; 96:1055–1060.
13. Graf P, Hallen H, Juto JE. The pathophysiology and treatment of rhinitis medicamentosa. Clin Otolaryngol 1995; 20:224–229.
14. Romero JN, Scadding GK. Eosinophilia in nasal secretions compared to skin prick test and nasal challenge test in the diagnosis of nasal allergy. Rhinology 1992; 30:169–175.
15. Huggins KG, Brostoff J. Local production of specific IgE antibodies in allergic-rhinitis patients with negative skin prick tests. Lancet 1976; 7926:148–150.
16. Nelson HS, Oppenheimer J, Buchmeier A, et al. An assessment of the role of intradermal skin testing in the diagnosis of clinically relevant allergy to timothy grass. J Allergy Clin Immunol 1996; 97:1193–1201.
17. Reddy PM, Nagaya H, Pascual HC, et al. Reappraisal of intracutaneous tests in the diagnosis of reaginic allergy. J Allergy Clin Immunol 1978; 61:36–41.
18. Brown WG, Halonen MJ, Kaltenborn WT, Barbee RA. The relationship of respiratory allergy, skin test reactivity, and serum IgE in a community population sample. J Allergy Clin Immunol 1979; 63:328–335.
19. Wood RA, Phipatanakul W, Hamilton RG, et al. A comparison of skin prick tests, intradermal skin tests, and RASTs in the diagnosis of cat allergy. J Allergy Clin Immunol 1999; 103:773–779.
20. Mènardo JL, Bousquet J, Michel FB. Comparison of three prick test methods with the intradermal test and with the RAST in the diagnosis of mite allergy. Ann Allergy 1982; 48:235–239.
21. Gendo K, Larson EB. Evidence-based diagnostic strategies for evaluating suspected allergic rhinitis. Ann Intern Med 2004; 140:278–289.
22. Schwindt CD, Hutcheson PS, Leu SY, Dykewicz MS. Role of intradermal skin tests in the evaluation of clinically relevant respiratory allergy assessed using patient history and nasal challenges. Ann Allergy Asthma Immunol 2005; 94:627–633.
23. Rohr A, Hassner A, Saxon A. Rhinopharyngoscopy for the evaluation of allergic-immunologic disorders. Ann Allergy 1983; 50:380–384.
24. Stafford CT. The clinician's view of sinusitis. Otolaryngol Head Neck Surg 1990; 103:870–875.
25. Dolen WK, Selner JC. Endoscopy of the upper airway. In: Middleton E, Reed CE, Ellis EF, eds. Allergy Principles Practice. 5th eds. St. Louis: Mosby-Year Book, 1998:1017–1023.
26. Crobach M, Hermans J, Kaptein A, Ridderikhoff J, Mulder J. Nasal smear eosinophilia for the diagnosis of allergic rhinitis and eosinophilic non-allergic rhinitis. Scand J Prim Health Care 1996; 14:116–121.

27. Meltzer E, Orgel H, Jalowaski A. Nasal cytology. In: Naclerio R, Durham S, Mygind N, eds. Rhinitis: Mechanisms and Management. New York: Marcel Dekker, 1999:175–202.
28. Ingels K, Durdurez JP, Cuvelier C, van Cauwenberge P. Nasal biopsy is superior to nasal smear for finding eosinophils in nonallergic rhinitis. Allergy 1997; 52:338–341.
29. Lim-Mombay M, Baroody F, Taylor R, Naclerio R. Mucosal cellular changes after nasal antigen challenge abstr. J Allergy Clin Immunol 1992; 89:A205.
30. Durham SR, Ying S, Varney VA, et al. Cytokine messenger RNA expression for IL-3, IL-4, IL-5, and granulocyte/macrophage-colony-stimulating factor in the nasal mucosa after local allergen provocation: relationship to tissue eosinophilia. J Immunol 1992; 148:2390–2394.
31. Baroody FM, Rouadi P, Driscoll PV, Bochner BS, Naclerio RM. Intranasal beclomethasone reduces allergen-induced symptoms and superficial mucosal eosinophilia without affecting submucosal inflammation. Am J Respir Crit Care Med 1998; 157:899–906.
32. Webb DR, Meltzer EO, Finn AF Jr., et al. Intranasal fluticasone propionate is effective for perennial nonallergic rhinitis with or without eosinophilia. Ann Allergy Asthma Immunol 2002; 88:385–390.
33. Fokkens WJ. Thoughts on the pathophysiology of nonallergic rhinitis. Curr Allergy Asthma Rep 2002; 2:203–209.
34. Powe DG, Huskisson RS, Carney AS, Jenkins D, Jones NS. Evidence for an inflammatory pathophysiology in idiopathic rhinitis. Clin Exp Allergy 2001; 31:864–872.
35. Malmberg H. Symptoms of chronic and allergic rhinitis and occurrence of nasal secretion granulocytes in university students, school children and infants. Allergy 1979; 34:389–394.
36. Zinreich SJ. Radiologic diagnosis of the nasal cavity and paranasal sinuses. In: Druce HM, ed. Sinusitis: Pathophysiology and Treatment. New York: Marcel Dekker, 1993.
37. Bingham B, Shankar L, Hawke M. Pitfalls in computed tomography of the paranasal sinuses. J Otolaryngol 1991; 20:414–418.
38. Zlab MK, Moore GF, Daly DT, Yonkers AJ. Cerebrospinal fluid rhinorrhea: a review of the literature. Ear Nose Throat J 1992; 71:314–317.
39. Ricketti AJ, Cleri DJ, Porwancher RB, Panesar M, Villota FJ, Seelagy MM. Cerebrospinal fluid leak mimicking allergic rhinitis. Allergy Asthma Proc 2005; 26(2):125–128.
40. Skedros DG, Cass SP, Hirsch BE, Kelly RH. Beta-2 transferrin assay in clinical management of cerebral spinal fluid and perilymphatic fluid leaks. J Otolaryngol 1993; 22:341–344.
41. Sillers MJ, Morgan CE, el-Gammal T. Magnetic resonance cisternography and thin coronal computerized tomography in the evaluation of cerebrospinal fluid rhinorrhea. Am J Rhinol 1997; 11:387–392.
42. Long A, McFadden C, DeVine D, et al. Management of allergic and nonallergic rhinitis. New England Medical Center Evidence-based Practice Center under Contract No. 290–97–0019. Evidence Report/Technology Assessment No. 54. AHRQ Pub. No. 02-E024. Rockville, MD: Agency for Healthcare Research and Quality, May 2002.
43. Wight RG, Jones AS, Beckingham E, et al. A double blind comparison of intranasal budesonide 400 micrograms and 800 micrograms in perennial rhinitis. Clin Otolaryngol 1992; 17:354–358.
44. Malm L, Wihl JA. Intra-nasal beclomethasone diproprionate in vasomotor rhinitis. Acta Allergol 1976; 31:245–253.
45. Small P, Black M, Frenkiel S. Effects of treatment with beclomethasone dipropionate in subpopulations of perennial rhinitis patients. J Allergy Clin Immunol 1982; 70:178–182.
46. Kondo H, Nachtigal D, Frenkiel S, et al. Effect of steroids on nasal inflammatory cells and cytokine profile. Laryngoscope 1999; 109:91–97.
47. Wiseman LR, Benfield P. Intranasal fluticasone propionate. A reappraisal of its pharmacology and clinical efficacy in the treatment of rhinitis. Drugs 1997; 53:885–907.
48. Skoner D, Rachelefsky G, Meltzer E, et al. Detection of growth suppression in children during treatment with intranasal belcomethasone dipropionate. Pediatrics 2000; 105:E23.

49. Banov C, Laforce C, Lieberman P. Double-blind trial of Astelin nasal spray in the treatment of vasomotor rhinitis. Ann Allergy Asthma Immunol 2000; 84:138.
50. Banov CH, Lieberman P, Vasomotor Rhinitis Study Groups. Efficacy of azelastine nasal spray in the treatment of vasomotor (perennial nonallergic) rhinitis. Ann Allergy Asthma Immunol 2001; 86:28–35.
51. Broms P, Malm L. Oral vasoconstrictors in perennial non-allergic rhinitis. Allergy 1982; 37:67–74.
52. Sjogren I, Jonsson L, Koling A, et al. The effect of ipratropium bromide on nasal hypersecretion induced by methacholine in patients with vasomotor rhinitis. A double-blind, cross-over, placebo-controlled and randomized dose-response study. Acta Otolaryngol 1988; 106(5–6):453–459.
53. Grossman J, Banov C, Boggs P, et al. Use of ipratropium bromide nasal spray in chronic treatment of nonallergic perennial rhinitis, alone and in combination with other perennial rhinitis medications. J Allergy Clin Immunol 1995; 95:1123–1127.
54. Kirkegaard J, Mygind N, Molgaard F, et al. Ipratropium treatment of rhinorrhea in perennial nonallergic rhinitis. A Nordic multicenter study. Acta Otolaryngol Suppl 1988; 449:93–95.
55. Kirkegaard J, Mygind N, Molgaard F, et al. Ordinary and high-dose ipratropium in perennial nonallergic rhinitis. J Allergy Clin Immunol 1987; 79:585–590.
56. Jokinen K, Sipila P. Intranasal ipratropium in the treatment of vasomotor rhinitis. Rhinology 1983; 21:341–345.
57. Wood CC, Fireman P, Grossman J, Wecker M, MacGregor T. Product characteristics and pharmacokinetics of intranasal ipratropium bromide. J Allergy Clin Immunol 1995; 95:1111–1116.
58. Bronsky EA, Druce H, Findlay SR, Hampel FC. A clinical trial of ipratropium bromide nasal spray in patients with perennial nonallergic rhinitis. J Allergy Clin Immunol 1995; 95:1117–1122.
59. Bende M, Rundcrantz H. Treatment of perennial secretory rhinitis. ORL J Otorhinolaryngol Relat Spec 1985; 47(6):303–306.
60. Jessen M, Bylander A. Treatment of non-allergic nasal hypersecretion with ipratropium and beclomethasone. Rhinology 1990; 28:77–81.
61. Lofkvist T, Rundcrantz H, Svensson G. Treatment of vasomotor rhinitis with intranasal disodium cromoglycate (SCG). Results from a double-blind cross-over study. Acta Allergol 1977; 32(1):35–43.
62. Mori S, Fujieda S, Igarashi M, Fan GK, Saito H. Submucous turbinectomy decreases not only nasal stiffness but also sneezing and rhinorrhea in patients with perennial allergic rhinitis. Clin Exp Allergy 1999; 29:1542–1548.
63. Inouye T, Tanabe T, Nakanoboh M, Ogura M. Laser surgery for allergic and hypertrophic rhinitis. Ann Otol Rhinol Laryngol Suppl 1999; 180:3–19.
64. Mladina R, Risavi R, Subaric M. CO_2 laser anterior turbinectomy in the treatment of non-allergic vasomotor rhinopathia. A prospective study upon 78 patients. Rhinology 1991; 29:267–271.
65. Golding-Wood PH. Vidian neurectomy: its results and complications. Laryngoscope 1973; 83:1673–1683.
66. Grote JJ. The Autonomic Innervation of the Nasal Mucosa. Nijmegen, The Netherlands: University of Nijmegen, 1974.
67. Sadanaga M. Clinical evaluation of vidian neurectomy for nasal allergy. Auris Nasus Larynx 1989; 16(suppl 1):S53–S57.

The Treatment of Vasomotor Nonallergic Rhinitis

Michael A. Kaliner

Institute for Asthma and Allergy, Chevy Chase, Maryland, and George Washington University School of Medicine, Washington, D.C., U.S.A.

INTRODUCTION

Rhinitis, which can be classified as allergic or nonallergic, is an exceptionally common disorder characterized by inflammation of the mucous membranes lining the nasal passages. The symptoms of allergic rhinitis (AR), which can be difficult to accurately distinguish from those of non-AR (NAR), typically include sneezing, nasal itch, rhinorrhea, nasal obstruction, and postnasal drip. Based on timing or periodicity of symptoms, AR may be classified as either seasonal or perennial (1). An alternative classification presented in the World Health Organization's Allergic Rhinitis and Its Impact on Asthma guidelines utilizes a combination of severity (mild or moderately severe) and persistence (intermittent or persistent) (2). In the United States, "seasonal" and "perennial" remain the classification scheme most frequently employed.

CLASSIFYING NAR

NAR can be classified into seven subtypes: drug-induced rhinitis, gustatory rhinitis, hormonal rhinitis, infectious rhinitis, NAR with eosinophilia syndrome (NARES), occupational rhinitis, and vasomotor rhinitis (VMR) (3,4). VMR is also known as perennial NAR and may have other acceptable names, including idiopathic rhinitis. VMR is the most common type of NAR encountered in clinical practice. VMR is thought to affect approximately 5% to 10% of the population, with a higher prevalence in females (5). The symptoms of VMR—including rhinorrhea, nasal congestion, and postnasal drip—can be provoked by stimuli such as changes in temperature, barometric pressure, and humidity; strong odors (perfume, paint, and tobacco smoke) and other respiratory irritants; emotional stress; and spicy foods and alcoholic beverages. A family history of allergy or allergic symptoms is uncommon. Patients with VMR may be further subdivided into two groups: "runners," patients with rhinorrhea, and "blockers," patients with nasal obstruction and airflow resistance but minimal rhinorrhea (6). VMR is believed to result from an autonomic nervous system dysfunction that is characterized by domination of the parasympathetic system, resulting in secretions, vasodilatation, and edema of the nasal vasculature (7,8). Other possibilities include a hyperreactive sensory nervous response with the release of neuropeptides, which cause the symptoms typically found in VMR. Recent studies by Jaradeh et al. (9) and Loehrl et al. (10) have postulated that VMR may also be influenced by a hypoactive sympathetic nervous system rather than a hyperactive parasympathetic system, while Terrahe has suggested a role for mast cell degranulation (11). One experiment on cold air–induced rhinorrhea demonstrated histamine release, suggesting a link between the VMR and mast cell activation (12), but other studies have failed to confirm mast cell activation in VMR.

While the presenting symptoms of VMR may resemble those of AR, both the elucidation of environmental triggers in VMR by history and the negative relevant allergy skin tests to local seasonal and perennial allergens differentiate VMR from AR and confirm the diagnosis (13). On physical examination, patients with VMR are likely to exhibit a normal exam or slightly erythematous and boggy turbinates rather than the pale bluish hue found in AR (14).

Infectious Rhinitis

Infectious rhinitis is usually caused by an upper respiratory tract infection of either viral or bacterial origin. While most viral infections resolve within 7 to 10 days, bacterial infections may require antibiotics for resolution. Infectious rhinitis presents with congestion, secretions (which may be purulent), and associated pain and pressure felt in and around the eyes. There is a population of patients who present with symptoms resembling sinusitis—congestion, rhinorrhea, postnasal drip, pain and pressure, and purulent drainage—but who retain their sense of smell and have normal computed tomography scans of the sinuses. Cultures of the nasal passage reveal staphylococcal species. Such patients may have "bacterial rhinitis," indicating a local staphlococcal infection of the nasal passage but not the sinuses, and are treated with topical, nasal antibiotics.

Drug-Induced Rhinitis

Several medications have been implicated in the development of "drug-induced rhinitis," including angiotensin-converting enzyme inhibitors, reserpine, guanethidine, phentolamine, methyldopa, beta-blockers, chlorpromazine, gabapentin, penicillamine, aspirin, nonsteroidal anti-inflammatory drugs, exogenous estrogens, and oral contraceptives. "Rhinitis medicamentosa" is a type of drug-induced rhinitis, and is caused by prolonged topical use of local decongestants. Nasal stuffiness usually responds to topical decongestants with immediate relief. However, because decongestants are used repeatedly, a rebound swelling occurs and patients start to use larger or more frequent doses of the decongestants. After a week or two of frequent use of nasal decongestants, patients are addicted to their use and have rhinitis medicamentosa. These patients typically present with extensive nasal congestion and rhinorrhea, resulting from loss of adrenergic tone rather than the original cause of the rhinitis. Treatment involves use of topical nasal corticosteroids (NCS) and gradual withdrawal of nasal decongestants. Abuse of nasal decongestants for more than 5 to 10 days is usually necessary before rhinitis medicamentosa develops. Therefore, patients should limit their use of nasal decongestants to three days out of any week. Normal nasal function usually resumes within 7 to 21 days after cessation of decongestants (15).

Gustatory Rhinitis

Gustatory rhinitis typically follows consumption of foods that are hot and spicy. Watery rhinorrhea after eating is secondary to nasal cholinergic discharge with stimulation of secretions. Gustatory rhinitis occurs in response to stimulation of sensory nerves in the mouth and pharynx during eating. Most commonly, hot and spicy foods trigger these responses. Symptoms develop within a few minutes of eating and may include sweating (particularly on top of the head) and tearing. In some older patients, gustatory rhinitis may occur during the process of eating any food, not just spicy foods. This form of gustatory rhinitis is common in nursing homes, and is a form of senile rhinitis. Treatment of gustatory rhinitis involves nasal ipratropium (Atrovent, 0.03% or 0.06%) before eating, which is usually quite effective.

Some people may experience "hormonal rhinitis" during periods of hormonal imbalances such as pregnancy, in association with the menstrual cycle, in hypothyroid states, at puberty, with oral contraceptive use, or with the use of conjugated estrogens. Primary presenting symptoms are nasal congestion and rhinorrhea (16). Symptoms of "occupational rhinitis" usually occur only in the workplace, as the result of an inhaled irritant such as grains, wood dust chemicals, or laboratory animal antigens (17).

Nonallergic Rhinitis with Eosinophilia Syndrome

NARES accounts for less than 5% to 10% of NAR. The NARES syndrome was originally reported in 1981 by Jacobs et al. (18). They described patients with perennial nasal symptoms including sneezing paroxysms, profuse watery rhinorrhea, and pruritus of the nasopharyngeal mucosa in an "on-again-off-again" symptomatic pattern with a profound eosinophilia in the nasal smear, and no signs of allergy as tested by skin-prick testing or measurement of total and specific immunoglobulin E (IgE). Trigger factors associated by the patients with the acute onset of nasal symptoms were none or unknown (42%), weather changes (31%), odors (15%), and noxious or irritating substances (12%) (16). Some research suggests that NARES is a precursor of aspirin sensitivity (19). The definition of NARES as a subgroup of NAR is relevant for therapy, because there are indications that eosinophilia is in important predictor of the effectiveness of NCS therapy. Patients with eosinophilia are more prone to a positive effect with NCS.

VASOMOTOR RHINITIS

VMR is characterized by persistent nasal symptoms that are triggered by nonallergic events such as changes in temperature, barometric pressure, and/or humidity, strong odors, respiratory irritants, spicy foods, or alcoholic beverages (20). The symptoms are similar to those seen in patients with AR, but with a less prominent nasal itch, sneezing, and conjunctiva irritation. The symptoms of VMR consist primarily of nasal congestion, rhinorrhea, and postnasal drip. The distinction between AR and VMR can be difficult clinically, but separating the two diseases is important for making treatment decisions.

The diagnosis of VMR is made by history taking. Patients who develop nasal symptoms in response to environmental irritants (such as those noted above) have VMR. Such patients may also have AR and, in fact, as many as 60% of patients with AR have a nonallergic component. Such patients have "mixed rhinitis" and it is important for the physician to decide which disease is the predominant cause of rhinitis, because oral antihistamines are ineffective for treating VMR. In the past, VMR was incorrectly diagnosed by exclusion: nasal symptoms plus negative skin tests led to the diagnosis of VMR. We now recognize that elicitation of nasal symptoms by environmental irritants defines VMR and helps determine which patients will respond to treatments aimed at VMR rather than AR.

We are moving to a more generally accepted definition of VMR, employing identification of triggers, age at onset, and pattern of symptoms as key differentiating points. AR has a peak incidence at ages 13 to 30, with a declining incidence thereafter. VMR tends to present at ages 30 to 60 and remains steady thereafter (21).

Females have VMR more than males, with estimates ranging from 58% to 71% (22). In addition to "pure" allergic and NAR, it is estimated that 26 to 40 million people have mixed rhinitis—seasonal or perennial AR with exacerbations from exposure to nonallergic triggers (5,23).

Statistics on the incidence and demographics of NAR are difficult to evaluate. In one national survey of medical practices, the classification of patients with rhinitis was 43% "pure" AR, 23% "pure" NAR, and 34% "mixed rhinitis" (24). Thus, in this survey of 50 geographically distributed allergists, nearly one half of the patients with AR had nonallergic triggers. In other studies, the prevalence of NAR has ranged from 17% to 52% of all patients with rhinitis (25–28). Based on these prevalence rates, epidemiologic estimates of the number of people with pure NAR probably exceeds 20 million Americans (29).

TREATING VMR

Although a proper diagnosis should lead to effective therapy for AR, symptoms persist in many patients despite treatment with one or more prescription medications. Ample evidence supports treating AR with a combination of antihistamines (oral or nasal) and topical NCS. However, in a survey conducted by the American College of Allergy, Asthma and Immunology, 52% of allergists and 39% of primary-care physicians reported that they used more than one oral antihistamine to treat patients with rhinitis, and more than 75% of allergists and primary-care physicians cited inadequate symptom relief as the reason for changing medications or implementing combination therapies (30). It seems possible that one of the reasons that so many patients failed to respond to oral antihistamines is that they had a nonallergic component to their disease that was not being adequately treated by oral antihistamines.

A wide variety of etiologies are included under the heading of NAR. Most studies have focused on the most frequent type of NAR, VMR, and that will be the focus hereafter, as well. Treatment strategies for AR have traditionally included attempts at avoidance of allergic triggers that elicit symptoms; however, it is very difficult to avoid the temperature and humidity changes that cause symptoms in VMR. Many agents and procedures have been suggested as effective treatments for VMR, including topical corticosteroids, intranasal antihistamines, intranasal anticholinergics, intranasal saline, and various surgical procedures (13).

Nasal Corticosteroids
Fluticasone propionate, budesonide in its metered dosed inhaled formulation that is no longer sold in the United States, and beclomethasone are the only topical NCS approved by the U.S. Food and Drug Administration (FDA) for the treatment of VMR. NCS are effective in reducing nasal blockage and rhinorrhea in patients with VMR, especially those patients with little watery discharge. It is likely that the anti-inflammatory activities of topical corticosteroids are responsible for their beneficial effect in NAR. When applied unilaterally, fluticasone propionate nasal spray has been shown to decrease the number of CD3+ cells, the amount of major basic protein, and the number of tryptase-positive cells in subjects with VMR (31). NCS have proven safe and effective in treating rhinitis but rarely completely suppress the nasal congestion, rhinorrhea, sneezing, and postnasal drip associated with VMR (16). NCS are effective for the treatment of NARES.

An assessment of three randomized, double-blind studies found that intranasal fluticasone propionate was effective in treatment of NAR with or without eosinophilia (32). The studies included 983 patients classified as NARES or non-NARES based on a five-point nasal eosinophil scoring scale. Patients received a total dose of fluticasone propionate 200 µg ($n = 332$), fluticasone propionate 400 µg ($n = 325$), or placebo ($n = 326$) for 28 days. Patients were 12 years of age or older with perennial rhinitis and had negative skin tests to all allergens relevant to the geographic area. Efficacy of the fluticasone propionate was evaluated by the mean change in total nasal symptom score, comprising patient ratings of nasal obstruction, postnasal drip, and rhinorrhea. Both the NARES and the non-NARES patients in the two fluticasone propionate treatment groups showed significantly nongreater improvement over placebo in nasal symptom scores (31).

A small ($n = 20$), randomized, double-blind study has shown that fluticasone propionate is an effective and rapid treatment for rhinitis medicamentosa when compared with a placebo nasal spray (33). In a double-blind, placebo-controlled trial, Wight et al. (34) showed a significant improvement in the symptom of nasal obstruction with each of two doses of budesonide presourized metered dose nasal inhaler (MDI). No other symptoms were altered, no difference was seen between the two doses, and no significant side effects were recorded.

Nasal Anticholinergics

Five randomized, controlled, clinical trials have addressed the efficacy of anticholinergic agents in the treatment of NAR. Each of these five trials studied intranasal ipratropium bromide, and each documented efficacy for ipratropium in reducing nose-blowing frequency and rhinorrhea. Kirkegaard et al. (35) documented a significant reduction in mean daily episodes of nose blowing by treatment with 80 µg of ipratropium four times per day. Sjogren et al. (36) documented a dose-dependent decrease in methacholine-induced nasal secretions by treatment for one day with doses of ipratropium of 40 µg, 100 µg, and 200 µg. Jokinen and Sipila (37) documented a physician-rated significant reduction in the symptoms on rhinorrhea with ipratropium but no effect on the symptoms of nasal congestion, sneezing, or nasal itching. In a second study, Kirkegaard et al. (38) compared two doses of ipratropium (80 µg four times/day vs. 400 µg four times/day) to placebo. Both doses resulted in a significantly decreased mean daily number of nose-blowing episodes compared to placebo, with 400 µg four times daily being significantly more effective than 80 µg four times daily. No effect was observed on symptoms of nasal congestion or sneezing. Malmberg et al. (39) also documented a significant reduction in the number of nose-blowing episodes as well as in the symptoms of rhinorrhea with ipratropium compared to placebo. No effect was seen on nasal congestion.

Anticholinergic agents are useful for those patients whose symptoms are predominantly secretory, i.e., rhinorrhea. The only intranasal anticholinergic drug approved for use in the United States is ipratropium bromide (Atrovent), which is available in 0.03% and 0.06% solutions. Ipratropium may be used alone or in combination with corticosteroid sprays or azelastine nasal spray. In a large, double-blind, controlled, randomized clinical trial (40), the combined use of ipratropium and beclomethasone nasal sprays was found to be more effective than either agent alone for the treatment of rhinorrhea from perennial rhinitis, and did not cause any increase in adverse reactions. This study further proposed that ipratropium alone be used for patients in whom rhinorrhea is the primary symptom, and in combination with an NCS for patients with several symptoms or symptoms resistant to ipratropium treatment.

Comparisons of NCS and ipratropium in NAR yield conflicting results. Bende and Rundcantz (41) compared budesonide MDI with ipratropium nasal sprays and showed a superior effect for budesonide with respect to symptoms of nasal secretion and sneezing. Jessen and Bylander (42) report a double-blind, randomized, control trial comparing ipratropium and beclomethasone in 24 patients with NAR characterized by hypersecretion. No difference was identifiable between the efficacy of the two medications.

Antihistamines

Oral antihistamines, which are used effectively in the treatment of AR, have produced inconsistent results when used in the treatment of NAR. The majority of antihistamines are considered to have little or no benefit in the treatment of NAR, with the exception of topically applied azelastine hydrochloride, a pharmacologically distinct H_1-receptor antagonist with a broad spectrum of antiallergic and anti-inflammatory activities (43).

There is a paucity of data relative to the use of oral antihistamines in the treatment of NAR. Broms and Malm evaluated nasal airway resistance and nasal symptoms in patients with NAR using phenylpropanolamine (PPA) in combination with an oral antihistamine or PPA alone. Decreased nasal airway resistance was noted with PPA in a dose of 100 mg sustained release, while PPA in a dose of 50 mg combined with an antihistamine had no decongesting effect (44). Mullarkey noted that in a cohort of patients with NARES, response was better to topical corticosteroids than to oral antihistamines (45). Rinne et al. (46) investigated whether long-term daily steroid treatment or an oral antihistamine would have a positive effect on the clinical outcome of 143 patients with AR and NARES. The patients were randomized to receive either 400 mg budesonide dry powder intranasally or cetirizine 10 mg orally for one year. At the end of the double-blind treatment period, medication was stopped and patients were followed up for another year, during which time they could use 14-day courses of budesonide as needed to control relapses. After discontinuation of the randomized treatment, 38% of patients treated with budesonide and 56% of those who received cetirizine had a relapse within the first month ($p = 0.04$). The authors concluded that budesonide was significantly more effective than cetirizine in controlling the symptoms of AR or NARES.

Azelastine nasal spray is approved in the United States for the treatment of both AR and VMR. The efficacy and safety of azelastine nasal spray in the treatment of VMR is based on two multicenter, randomized, double-blind, placebo-controlled, clinical trials to determine whether patients with symptoms of VMR could be effectively treated with azelastine nasal spray (47). In the first study, 223 patients were randomized to double-blind treatment; 203 patients were randomized to double-blind treatment in the second study. All participants were aged 12 or older; had a history of chronic rhinitis symptoms for one year or more and a diagnosis of VMR; had a positive histamine epicutaneous skin test; had negative skin tests to a mixed panel of common household allergens; had nasal cytology negative for eosinophils; had a normal sinus X ray; and had no clinically significant nasal anatomical deformities. After a one-week, single-blind, placebo lead-in period, patients were randomized to receive either azelastine nasal spray (two sprays per nostril twice daily, 1.1 mg/day) or placebo nasal spray for 21 days. Patients self-recorded their symptoms each morning and night using a four-point rating system. The primary outcome variable was the overall reduction from baseline when compared with placebo over the 21-day, double-blind treatment period. In both studies, azelastine nasal spray significantly (study 1, $p = 0.002$; study 2, $p = 0.005$) reduced the nasal symptoms from baseline when compared with placebo. In both studies, treatment with azelastine resulted in clinical improvement in all of the individual symptoms of the symptom complex.

In the first study, azelastine significantly improved rhinorrhea ($p = 0.009$), sneezes ($p < 0.001$), nasal congestion ($p = 0.036$), and postnasal drip ($p = 0.038$) when compared to placebo. In the second study, there was statistically significant improvement in rhinorrhea ($p = 0.003$) and postnasal drip ($p = 0.019$) versus placebo. No serious or unexpected adverse events were reported in either group, although there was a significantly greater incidence of bitter taste in the azelastine group than in the placebo group ($p < 0.05$). It is important to note that the placebo rating in these two studies was very high, likely due to the fact that the saline nasal spray used as a "placebo" is also known to be beneficial in this disorder (48).

In another multicenter, randomized, double-blind, parallel-group study, Gehanno et al. (49) treated 89 adult patients with a history of VMR. Following a wash-out period, patients were treated for 15 days with one puff of azelastine three times per day ($n = 44$) or placebo saline nasal spray ($n = 45$). Efficacy was determined by rhinoscopy and by reduction of symptoms, including nasal obstruction, rhinorrhea, sneezing, anosmia, and olfactometry. The study demonstrated that by the end of the treatment period, azelastine significantly improved nasal obstruction and rhinorrhea ($p = 0.017$ and $p = 0.023$, respectively) compared to placebo, as well as significantly reducing edema and inflammation of the nasal mucosa ($p = 0.03$ and $p = 0.02$, respectively). Assessment by both the physician and the patient demonstrated that azelastine was well tolerated (47).

Another study evaluated the effectiveness of azelastine nasal spray in the treatment of seasonal AR, mixed rhinitis, and VMR (50). A total of 2343 primary-care physicians, allergists, ear, nose, and throat specialists, and other health professionals participated in this two-week, open-label evaluation of azelastine nasal spray. Data were collected through a physician questionnaire that included patient demographics, rhinitis diagnosis, medication history, and inclusion or exclusion criteria; and two patient questionnaires that included symptom history, response to previous rhinitis medications, symptom control, and level of satisfaction with azelastine nasal spray. A completed physician questionnaire and two completed patient questionnaires were required for each patient to be included in the analysis. Patients who qualified for enrollment were given open-label azelastine nasal spray and instructed to administer two sprays per nostril twice daily for two weeks.

A total of 1225 health professionals enrolled 7864 patients in the study. Completed physician and patient questionnaires were returned by 1081 health professionals and 5073 patients, 4364 of whom used azelastine nasal spray as their only rhinitis medication during the two-week study period. The patients were predominantly Caucasian (82.6%) and female (61.1%), with a mean age of 50. The majority had a diagnosis of mixed rhinitis (51.5%), followed by seasonal AR (32.3%), and VMR (16.2%). After two weeks of treatment, the percentage of patients reporting some control or complete control of individual symptoms ranged from 78% for postnasal drip in patients with VMR to 90% for sneezing in patients with seasonal AR. More than 85% of patients who reported difficulty in sleeping or impairment of daytime activities due to rhinitis symptoms had improvement in these parameters. Azelastine nasal spray was well tolerated, with a discontinuation rate due to adverse events of 2.3%. Regression analysis identified patients with seasonal AR and seasonal AR plus nonallergic triggers as most likely to respond to azelastine nasal spray (48).

The high incidence of mixed rhinitis (20) suggests that empiric treatment should include agents that are effective in both AR and NAR when there is any indication of a nonallergic component to the rhinitis. Intranasal azelastine is the only antihistamine therapy currently approved by the U.S. FDA for both AR and NAR. For patients with NAR who present with blockage or congestion symptoms and little rhinorrhea or sneezing, oral or topical decongestants can be helpful. However, the side effects of oral decongestants (e.g., insomnia, nervousness, loss of appetite, and hypertension) restrict their long-term use (51). The use of decongestant nasal sprays should be limited to a maximum of 3 to 10 days because of the risk of developing rhinitis medicamentosa. Both azelastine and topical NCS sprays reduce nasal congestion with few side effects. A saline nasal spray may also be useful for relieving sneezing, congestion, rhinorrhea, and postnasal drip in patients with VMR (47).

THE TREATMENT OF VMR

In practice, most (>90%) patients respond well to a combination of nasal saline, NCS, and azelastine nasal sprays. Each of these treatments works uniquely and the combination appears anecdotally to be more effective than the individual components, although no clinical trials have measured these observations objectively. The major side effect of azelastine is a bitter taste; in order to reduce this problem, azelastine may be used as one spray per nostril twice a day. When the combination of azelastine and NCS is used together, each medication is administered as a single spray twice daily. Several recent studies have confirmed the efficacy of azelastine versus three different oral antihistamines in treating the symptoms of AR; however, these studies did not include patients with VMR (52–54). Studies confirming the effectiveness of azelastine one spray each nostril BID are under review by the FDA for approval. One spray of azelastine two times daily is associated with fewer side effects, and will likely lead to increased compliance.

VMR is not a life-threatening disease. While patients' quality of life may be affected by the symptoms of VMR, treatment should be aimed at relieving symptoms without incurring any risks. Once patients respond to treatment, use of a minimally effective dose is appropriate. Thus, in practice, we usually start patients with a combination of azelastine nasal spray and NCS, one spray of each product in each nostril twice daily. However, they are instructed to use the medications at the lowest dose that works for them. Thus, many patients end up using one or the other spray and may only need the medication once a day for adequate symptom control. For persistent congestion, an oral decongestant can be added to this treatment and used as needed. For rhinorrhea, nasal ipratropium can be tried. For persistent postnasal drip, an oral anticholinergic can be added.

In patients with AR and concomitant VMR triggers (mixed rhinitis), use of the combination of NCS and azelastine makes sense, because both treatment modalities are effective in both disorders. Thus, wider use of nasal azelastine should result in fewer treatment failures because of the broad efficacy of this product.

TABLE 1 Differential Diagnosis of Allergic, Mixed, and Vasomotor Rhinitis

Characteristic		Seasonal or perennial allergic rhinitis	Mixed vasomotor and allergic rhinitis[a]	Vasomotor, nonallergic rhinitis
Pattern	Seasonal	Seasonal	Year-round	Year-round
	Perennial	Perennial		
Symptoms	Congestion	Yes	Yes	Yes
	Rhinorrhea	Yes	Yes	Yes
	Sneezes	Yes	Can be yes	Some
	Itch	Yes	Can be yes	Some
	Postnasal drip	some	Likely	Likely
Triggers—allergens	Indoor Allergens	Perennial, yes	Yes	No
	Pollens	Seasonal, yes	Can be yes	No
Triggers—environmental	Smells	No	Yes[b]	Yes[b]
	Temperature changes	No	Yes[b]	Yes[b]
	Humidity barometric pressure changes	No	Yes[b]	Yes[b]
	Alcohol ingestion	No	Yes[b]	Yes[b]
	Emotions, stress	No	Yes[b]	Yes[b]
Skin tests	Positive	Yes	Yes	No (or irrelevant)
	Negative or irrelevant	No	Can be yes	Yes
Treatments	Allergen avoidance	Yes	Yes	No
	Antihistamine Oral	Yes	No	No
	Antihistamine Nasal	Yes	Yes	Yes
	Nasal corticosteroid	Yes	Yes	Yes
	Immunotherapy	Consider	Consider	No

[a]Patients with mixed rhinitis can have predominantly vasomotor triggers and some allergies; they may have equal parts of allergic and vasomotor triggers; or they can have allergic triggers upon which some environmental triggers are superimposed.
[b]Vasomotor rhinitis is triggered by environmental irritants. Some patients respond to only one stimulus, while others respond to multiple irritating conditions.

CLINICAL PEARLS

- NAR is a perennial, non–IgE-mediated condition characterized by congestion, rhinorrhea, and postnasal drip, but not by itching or sneezing.
- Epidemiologic estimates of the number of Americans with pure NAR probably exceed 20 million.
- There are no characteristic physical findings and diagnosis is based primarily on the symptom complex, identification of environmental triggers, age of onset, and pattern of symptoms.
- While the distinction between allergic and NAR can be difficult to determine clinically, the differentiation may be important for prognosis and treatment decisions. In mixed rhinitis, the most important decision is which disease predominates, because oral histamines are ineffective in managing VMR.
- Topical NCS and azelastine nasal spray have both produced favorable results in patients with NAR (as well as AR). However, azelastine has broader efficacy in treating the range of symptoms associated with VMR. Using both agents concomitantly may be more effective than using either alone.
- Treatment of VMR should be broad based and include the use of both topical corticosteroids and/or azelastine.
- Adjunctive treatment can also be directed to specific symptoms. For example, patients with rhinorrhea may respond to ipratropium bromide or topical nasal saline sprays. Patients with congestion may require oral or topical decongestants on an as-needed basis, and patients with persistent postnasal drip may require oral anticholinergic agents.

ACKNOWLEDGMENT

The authors gratefully acknowledge the contribution of Jill M. Shuman, MS, ELS in the preparation of this manuscript.

REFERENCES

1. Management of allergic and nonallergic rhinitis. Agency for Healthcare Research and Quality. Evid Rep/Tech Assessment #54. US Dept of Health and Human Services. Pub #02-E203, May 2002.
2. Allergic Rhinitis and its Impact on Asthma. ARIA guidelines. 1999. Available at: http://www.whiar.com. Accessed Dec 16, 2005.
3. Dykewicz MS, Fineman S, Skoner DP, et al. Diagnosis and management of rhinitis: complete guidelines of the joint task force on practice parameters in allergy, asthma, and immunology. Ann Allergy Asthma Immun 1998; 81(5 pt 2):478–518.
4. Economides A, Kaliner MA. Vasomotor rhinitis: making the diagnosis and determining therapy. J Respir Dis 1999; 20:463–464.
5. Settipane RA, Lieberman P. Update on nonallergic rhinitis. Ann Allergy Asthma Immunol 2001; 86:494–508.
6. Wheeler P, Wheeler S. Vasomotor rhinitis. Am Family Physician 2005; 72:1057–1062.
7. Canning BJ. Neurology of allergic inflammation and rhinitis. Curr Allergy Asthma Rep 2002; 3:210–215.
8. Garay R. Mechanisms of vasomotor rhinitis. Allergy 2004; 59(suppl 76):4–10.
9. Jaradeh SS, Smith TL, Torrico L, et al. Autonomic nervous system evaluation of patients with vasomotor rhinitis. Laryngoscope 2000; 110:1828–1831.
10. Loehrl TA, Smith TL, Darling RJ, et al. Autonomic dysfunction, vasomotor rhinitis, and extraesophageal manifestations of gastroesophageal reflux. Otolaryngol Head Neck Surg 2002; 126:382–387.

11. Terrahe K. Hyperreflectoric rhinopathy. HNO 1985; 33:51–57.
12. Togias AG, Proud D, Lichtenstein LM, et al. The osmolality of nasal secretions increases when inflammatory mediators are released in response to inhalation of cold, dry air. Am Rev Respir Dis 1988; 137(3):625–629.
13. Settipane RA, Settipane GA. Nonallergic rhinitis. In: Kaliner MA, ed. Current Review of Allergic Diseases. Boston: Blackwell Science, 1998:101–112.
14. deShazo RD, Kemp SF. Rhinosinusitis. South Med J 2003; 96:1055–1060.
15. Graf P. Rhinitis medicamentosa: a review of causes and treatment. Treat Resp Med 2005; 41:21–29.
16. Mabry RL. Rhinitis of pregnancy. South Med J 1986; 79:965–971.
17. Slavin RG. Occupational rhinitis. Ann Allergy Asthma Immunol 1999; 83:597–601.
18. Jacobs RL, Freedman PM, Boswell RN. Nonallergic rhinitis with eosinophilia (NARES syndrome). Clinical and immunologic presentation. J Allergy Clin Immunol 1981; 67:253–262.
19. Moneret-Vautrin DA, Hsieh V, Wayoff M, Guyot JL, Mouton C, Maria Y. Nonallergic rhinitis with eosinophilia syndrome a precursor of the triad: nasal polyposis, intrinsic asthma, and intolerance to aspirin. Ann Allergy 1990; 64:513–518.
20. Druce HM. Allergic and nonallergic rhinitis. In: Middleton E, Reed CE, Ellis EF, eds. Allergy Principles Practice. 5th ed. St Louis: Mosby-Year Book, Inc., 1999:1005–1016.
21. Settipane RA. Demographics and epidemiology of allergic and nonallergic rhinitis. Allergy Asthma Proc 2001; 22:185–189.
22. Settipane RA, Klein DE. Non-allergic rhinitis: demography of eosinophils in nasal smear, blood total eosinophil counts, and IgE levels. N Engl Reg Allergy Proc 1985; 6:363–366.
23. Kaliner MA, Lieberman P. Incidence of allergic, nonallergic and mixed rhinitis in clinical practice. Annual Meeting of the American Academy of Otolaryngology-Head and Neck Surgery Foundation, Sept 24–27, 2000, Poster PO75.
24. Mullarkey MF, Hill JS, Webb DR. Allergic and nonallergic rhinitis: their characterization with attention to the meaning of nasal eosinophilia. J Allergy Clin Immun 1980; 65: 122–126.
25. Enberg RN. Perennial nonallergic rhinitis: a retrospective review. Ann Allergy Asthma Immunol 1989; 63:513–516.
26. Togias A. Age relationships and clinical features of nonallergic rhinitis. J Allergy Clin Immunol 1990; 85:182–187.
27. The National Rhinitis Classification Task Force. The Broad Spectrum of Rhinitis: Etiology, Diagnosis, and Advances in Treatment. The meeting of the National Allergy Advisory Council (NAAC), St. Thomas, US Virgin Islands, Oct 16, 1999.
28. Leynaert B, Bousquet J, Neukirch C, Liard R, Neukirch F. Perennial rhinitis: an independent risk factor for asthma in nonatopic subjects. Results from the European Community Respiratory Health Survey. J Allergy Clin Immunol 1999; 104:301–304.
29. Lieberman P. Treatment update: nonallergic rhinitis. Allergy Asthma Proc 2001; 22: 199–202.
30. Physician Survey sponsored by the American College of Allergy, Asthma and Immunology. Rochester, NY: Harris Interactive, Inc., 2001.
31. Kondo H, Nachtigal D, Frenkiel S, Schotman E, Hamid Q. Effect of steroids on nasal inflammatory cells and cytokine profile. Laryngoscope 1999; 109:91–97.
32. Webb DR, Meltzer EO, Finn AF, et al. Intranasal fluticasone propionate is effective for perennial nonallergic rhinitis with or without eosinophilia. Ann Allergy Asthma Immunol 2002; 88:385–390.
33. Hallen H, Enerdal J, Graf P. Fluticasone propionate nasal spray is more effective and has a faster onset of action than placebo in the treatment of rhinitis medicamentosa. Clin Exp Allergy 1997; 27:552–558.
34. Wight RG, Jones AS, Beckingham E, Andersson B, Ek L. A double blind comparison of intranasal budesonide 400 micrograms and 800 micrograms in perennial rhinitis. Clin Otolaryngol 1992; 17(4):354–358.
35. Kirkegaard J, Mygind N, Molgaard F, et al. Ipratropium treatment of rhinorrhea in perennial nonallergic rhinitis. A Nordic multicenter study. Acta Otolaryngol Suppl 1988; 449:93–95.

36. Sjogren I, Jonsson L, Koling A, Jansson C, Osterman K, Hakansson B. The effect of ipra-
    tropium bromide on nasal hypersecretion induced by methacholine in patients with
    vasomotor rhinitis. A double-blind, cross-over, placebo-controlled and randomized
    dose-response study. Acta Otolaryngol 1988; 106:453–459.
37. Jokinen K, Sipila P. Intranasal ipratropium in the treatment of vasomotor rhinitis. Rhi-
    nology 1983; 21:341–345.
38. Kirkegaard J, Mygind N, Molgaard F, et al. Ordinary and high-dose ipratropium in per-
    ennial nonallergic rhinitis. J Allergy Clin Immunol 1987; 4:585–590.
39. Malmberg H, Grahne B, Holopainen E, Binder E. Ipratropium (Atrovent) in the treat-
    ment of vasomotor rhinitis of elderly patients. Clin Otolaryngol 1983; 8:273–276.
40. Dockhorn R, Aaronson D, Bronsky E, et al. Ipratropium bromide nasal spray 0.03% and
    beclomethasone nasal spray alone and in combination for the treatment of rhinorrhea in
    perennial rhinitis. Ann Allergy Asthma Immunol 1999; 82:349–359.
41. Bende M, Rundcantz H. Treatment of perennial secretory rhinitis. J Otorhinolaryngol
    Relat Spec 1985; 47:303–306.
42. Jessen M, Bylander A. Treatment of non-allergic nasal hypersecretion with ipratropium
    and beclomethasone. Rhinology 1990; 28:77–81.
43. Lieberman PL, Settipane RA. Azelastine nasal spray: a review of pharmacology and
    clinical efficacy in allergic and nonallergic rhinitis. Allergy Asthma Proc 2003; 24:
    95–105.
44. Broms P, Malm L. Oral vasoconstrictors in perennial non-allergic rhinitis. Allergy 1982;
    37:67–74.
45. Mullarkey MF. Eosinophilic nonallergic rhinitis. J Allergy Clin Immunol 1988; 82(5 Pt 2):
    941–949.
46. Rinne J, Simola M, Malmberg H, Haahtela T. Early treatment of perennial rhinitis with
    budesonide or cetirizine and its effect on long-term outcome. J Allergy Clin Immunol
    2002; 109:426–432.
47. Banov CH, Lieberman P. Efficacy of azelastine nasal spray in the treatment of vaso-
    motor (perennial nonallergic) rhinitis. Ann Allergy Asthma Immunol 2001; 86:28–35.
48. Lieberman P. Nonallergic rhinitis. In: Rakel RE, Bope ET, eds. Latest Approved Methods
    of Treatment for the Practicing Physician. Philadelphia, PA: WB Saunders, 2002:235–238.
49. Gehanno P, Deschamps E, Garay E, Baehre M, Garay RP. Vasomotor rhinitis: clinical
    efficacy of azelastine nasal spray in comparison with placebo. ORL 2001; 63:76–81.
50. Lieberman P, Kaliner MA, Wheeler WJ. Open-label evaluations of azelastine nasal spray
    in patients with seasonal allergic rhinitis and nonallergic vasomotor rhinitis. Curr Med
    Res Opin 2005; 21:611–618.
51. Kaliner M. Progressive management strategies in the treatment of rhinitis. Allergy
    Asthma Proc 2003; 24:163–169.
52. Corren J, Storms W, Bernstein J, Berger W, Nayak A, Sacks H. Effectiveness of azelastine
    nasal spray compared with oral cetirizine with seasonal allergic rhinitis. Clin Ther 2005;
    27:545–553.
53. LaForce CF, Corren J, Wheeler WJ, Berger WE, Rhinitis Study Group. The treatment of
    vasomotor nonallergic rhinitis. Ann AllergyAsthma Immunol 2004; 93:154–159.
54. Berger WE, White MV, Rhinitis Study Group. Efficacy of azelastine nasal spray in pati-
    ents with an unsatisfactory response to loratadine. Ann Allergy Asthma Immunol 2003;
    91:205–211.

23 Outpatient Therapy for Nonallergic Rhinitis

Wytske Fokkens

Academic Medical Centre, Amsterdam, The Netherlands

INTRODUCTION

Rhinitis is a very common and well-known disorder. Chronic rhinitis affects up to 20% of the general population (1) and can be due to common factors such as allergy or smoking, or less common factors such as xylometazoline abuse or cystic fibrosis. Rhinitis means inflammation of the nasal mucosal membrane. However, markers of inflammation are not examined in routine clinical work. The term "rhinitis" is therefore used in daily practice for nasal dysfunction causing symptoms like nasal itching, sneezing, rhinorrhea, and/or nasal blockage (1).

When allergy, mechanical obstruction, and infections have been excluded as the cause of rhinitis, a number of poorly defined nasal conditions of partly unknown etiology and pathophysiology remain. The differential diagnosis of nonallergic noninfectious rhinitis is extensive (Table 1) (1,2). The mechanisms have only partly been unraveled. If the pathophysiology is unknown, the term idiopathic rhinitis (IR) is used (1).

Disease treatment should target the pathophysiology as much as possible. However, our knowledge of the pathophysiology of nonallergic rhinitis (NAR) and the effect of treatment on different pathophysiological entities is very limited. This chapter on outpatient treatment (excluding surgery) will describe the various treatment options. Where specific knowledge concerning subgroups of NAR is available, this will be indicated.

TREATMENT OF NAR

In general, the less is known about a disease (and its underlying pathophysiology), the more treatment options are available. This is particularly true of IR, where partial success is claimed for a wide range of available therapies, both surgical and pharmacotherapeutical. With the exception of rhinitis of the elderly, where ipratropium bromide is the obvious first treatment of choice, there is no obvious best treatment or first treatment for nonallergic noninfectious rhinitis.

TREATMENT OPTIONS

Avoidance of Environmental Factors

Although avoidance of environmental factors, including smoking, is widely recommended, there is no actual data demonstrating efficacy. Smoke, in particular cigarette smoke, is known for its irritative effect on the mucosa of the respiratory tract. A mucosal cellular infiltration with T helper-2 cell (Th2)-like profile including eosinophils, increased immunoglobulin E–positive cells, and increased interleukin-4 is found in passive smoking, nonallergic children and in smoking adults (3,4). Smoking results in many individuals with the same clinical picture of rhinitis with

TABLE 1 The Differential Diagnosis of Nonallergic Noninfectious Rhinitis

Occupational (irritant)
Drug-induced:
  Rhinitis medicamentosa (topical vasoconstrictive α-adrenoceptor
  agonists)
    Other drugs
Hormonal
Rhinitis of the elderly
Nonallergic rhinitis with eosinophilia
Smoking
Idiopathic rhinitis (of unknown cause)

Source: From Ref. 1.

rhinorrhea and nasal obstruction, and so it has to be viewed as a cause of rhinitis in its own right. It might even be that a proportion of the NAR with eosinophilia (NARES) type of NAR is caused by smoking or passive smoking, inducing an "allergy-like" inflammatory response (3,4). Most doctors strongly advise patients with NAR to stop smoking. Although there are some data showing an increased prevalence of NAR in smokers (5), there are no data demonstrating that stopping smoking is effective. However, in lower airway disease, there are sufficient data to demonstrate that cutting down or stopping smoking is effective in improving lung function, quality of life, and mortality (6,7). There are no data available about the effect of avoiding factors other than smoking—such as environmental tobacco smoke or pollutants—on symptoms in NAR patients. However, cold dry air is used to characterize and assess the presence and degree of nasal reactivity in NAR patients (8,9). Moreover, it has been shown that even minor pollution and meteorological disturbances result in substantial changes in nasal symptoms in NAR but not in controls (10). In conclusion, there are data indicating that environmental factors have negative effects on the symptoms of patients with NAR. However, the logical conclusion that avoidance of these factors may decrease symptomatology remains unproven.

Local Corticosteroids

Topical corticosteroids are widely used in the treatment of NAR. By contrast with allergic rhinitis, the studies supporting this regime are limited and inconclusive.

TABLE 2 Level of Evidence for Treatment of Nonallergic Rhinitis

Therapy	Level of evidence	Reduction in
Avoidance of environmental factors	IV	Overall symptoms
Local corticosteroid	1b	Overall symptoms
Decongestants	1b	Nasal blockage, rhinorrhea
Ipratropium bromide	1b	Rhinorrhea
Capsaicin	1b	Overall symptoms
Antihistamines (azetelastine)	1b	Overall symptoms
Botulin toxin	III	Rhinorrhea
Silver nitrate	IIa	Overall symptoms
Outpatient inferior turbinate reduction	1b	Nasal blockage
Vidian neurectomy	III	Sneezing, rhinorrhea

In general, there is a considerable placebo effect, possibly because of the positive effect of nasal douching with the nasal spray (11,12). The first study showed a significant improvement in nasal symptomatology in 21 patients with NAR after the use of local beclomethasone (13). Some studies have examined mixed populations of allergic and nonallergic patients, making it less possible to determine efficacy in patients with NAR (11,14). Lundblad et al.'s study is the largest and most convincing, showing efficacy in 56% of the patients treated with mometasone and in 49% in the placebo group. Some studies found no effect compared to placebo (15). The differences in these studies might well be explained by the wastebasket problem: NAR is most likely a combination of a number of pathophysiological entities. One might expect an anti-inflammatory drug to be effective in situations where inflammation is found (16), as in NARES (17,18). However, in populations of patients with NAR where inflammation does not play a role (19–21), it is understandable that corticosteroids are not effective. It is interesting to see that, in this noninflammatory population, local corticosteroids do have an effect on the inflammatory cells in the nasal mucosa but not on the symptoms (15). Keeping the relatively small effect in mind, we still believe that a topical steroid aqueous spray once or twice daily, preferably combined with nasal 0.9% saline douches, is the treatment of first choice in NAR. It should be tried for a minimum period of six weeks before treatment evaluation takes place, because it can take a few weeks before the maximum treatment effect is reached. Often, IR patients referred by the general practitioner to hospitals or specialist centers due to treatment failure after a short period of use of a topical steroid spray still react favorably to a topical steroid spray used over a longer period (personal observation).

Decongestants

Decongestants generally serve as the first-line treatment of nasal obstruction. They can be given topically or orally. Topical vasoconstrictors are divided into two categories: the sympatomemitic amines (ephedrine/phenylephrine) and their imidazoline derivates (xylomethazoline, oxymetazoline, and naphazoline). A topical sympathicomimetic provides instant relief but only for a short period. Topical sympathicomimetics (xylomethazoline) are more effective than oral decongestants (oral pseudoephedrine) (22). They should not be used for more than one week in view of the risk of rhinitis medicamentosa (23). However, there is one paper showing that the use of oxymetazoline nasal spray for four weeks did not cause rebound congestion or tachyphylaxis (24).

Rhinitis Medicamentosa

Rhinitis medicamentosa can be defined as a condition of nasal hyperreactivity, mucosal swelling, and rebound nasal congestion, and tolerance that is induced, or aggravated, by the overuse of topical vasoconstrictors with or without a preservative (23–27). The effects are mostly dose independent (28). Weaning patients off a topical vasoconstrictor can be difficult. Patients can be advised to stop using the vasoconstrictor in one nostril for a period of weeks or months until this nostril remains open, and then stop with the second nostril. A topical corticosteroid spray may be prescribed to alleviate the withdrawal process (29–31). After successful vasoconstrictor withdrawal, any possible remaining nasal disorder can be treated. Given this, vasoconstrictors have only a very limited role in the therapeutic arsenal of chronic NAR. Systemic sympathicomimetics are effective in treating nasal blockage in NAR (32). They are not known to cause rhinitis medicamentosa. A combination of systemic antihistamine and a sympathicomimetics has proven effective for allergic rhinitis (33–35). In some countries, systemic sympathicomimetics are not allowed because of the risk of cardiovascular side effects (36).

Ipratropium Bromide

Ipratropium bromide is an anticholinergic drug used mainly in the treatment of asthma. Clinical studies using this drug as a nasal spray have shown it to be effective in reducing the severity and duration of rhinorrhea in NAR, especially in rhinitis of the elderly (37–39). It is therefore the first treatment option in rhinitis of the elderly. Ipratropium bromide is usually administered as a 0.03% spray. The dosage necessary to achieve the optimal effect may vary considerably. It is advised to start with 80 to 100 µg twice daily, but some patients need higher dosages and dosage can usually be safely increased to 400 µg four times daily (40–42).

Capsaicin

An imbalance in the nonadrenergic, noncholinergic peptidergic neuronal system has been proposed as the underlying mechanism of IR (43). Treatment with capsaicin may fit in with this hypothesis (44). Neuropeptides [calcitonin gene related peptide (CGRP), substance P (SP), etc.] are released from peptidergic neurons in the nasal mucosa after activation by unspecific stimuli, and can be responsible for the symptoms of IR (44). Several studies have been published showing a therapeutic effect in IR patients for repeated topical applications of capsaicin (0.1 mmol/l) (21,45,46). The treatment effect lasts for at least one year and can easily be repeated (44). Capsaicin, the pungent agent in hot pepper, is known for its degeneration or desensitization effect on peptidergic sensory C-fibers, possibly explaining its therapeutic effect (44). Several treatment regimes have been tried out. The most efficient is spraying with capsaicin five times in a single day at intervals of one hour (45). This approach has been shown to be at least as effective as capsaicin treatment once every second or third day (45). Capsaicin treatment has been shown to be safe: blood pressure, heart rate, olfactory function, and mucosal sensibility are not affected by the treatment (45).

Antihistamines

There is a general lack of data about the effect of antihistamines in NAR. There is one exception—the intranasal antihistamine azelastine. A number of studies have shown that intranasal azelastine significantly reduces total symptoms and individual symptom scores, including nasal obstruction in patients with NAR. The studies are all relatively short (2–3 weeks). Only one study has been published with the other nasal antihistamine, Levocabastine. It looked at efficacy in a small mixed group of allergic and nonallergic patients and lacked sufficient power to show differences between the two groups (47). No studies could be found on the effect of oral antihistamines in NAR.

Azelastine has been shown to have anti-inflammatory effects that are independent of H-1 receptor inhibition, including inhibitory effects on the synthesis of leukotrienes, kinins, and cytokines. It also inhibits the generation of superoxide free radicals and the expression of intercellular adhesion molecules. The antihistaminic effect reduces mucosal edema, prostaglandin production, and the stimulation of irritant receptors. The limited number of immunohistological studies of the nasal mucosa of well-characterized nonallergic patients has shown differences that have so far remained unexplained (16,19,44). The inflammation of the nasal mucosa in IR is less pronounced than in allergic rhinitis (16) and it has even been found to be non-existent (19,44). It is still not known whether the anti-inflammatory effects explain the efficacy of azelastine or whether there is another, unknown, mechanism.

Botulin Toxin

Botulin toxin is a neurotoxin that inhibits the release of acetylcholine from the pre-synaptic nerve terminal. After intramuscular injection, its paralytic effects last between two and six months. Apart from its anticholinergic effects on motor nerves, botulin toxin also blocks the parasympathetic nerve supply to the salivary glands in dogs (48). Because the serous secretion of vasomotor rhinitis is under parasympathetic control, it might also be sensitive to botulin toxin. There is one Chinese study showing the effect of botulin toxin A on patients with NAR. This non–placebo-controlled study showed that there was a reduction in rhinorrhea for six weeks, but no effect on nasal blockage or sneezing (49). In a parallel study in guinea pigs, it was shown that botulin toxin induced the degeneration of glandular cells in nasal mucosa (49). The intranasal application of botulin toxin could therefore be an effective long-term therapy for vasomotor rhinitis.

Silver Nitrate

Application of silver nitrate to the anterior portion of both the inferior turbinates and the anterior part of the nasal septum has been reported to be an effective treatment for NAR, especially for the symptoms of rhinorrhea and sneezing. The most effective regime and concentration were five applications weekly of a silver nitrate concentration of 15% (50–52).

THE NASAL VALVE

The nasal valve is the narrowest portion of the nasal cavity. The internal nasal valve comprises the caudal end of the upper lateral cartilage and the nasal septum, whereas the internal nasal valve area or external nasal valve contains additional anatomic components such as the lower lateral (alar) cartilage, the anterior head of the inferior turbinate, and the inferior rim of the piriform aperture (53). The cross-sectional area of the nasal valve determines nasal airway resistance. Nasal valve instability can be a reason for nasal blockage on its own. However, in patients with congestion because of rhinitis, the nasal valve also tends to collapse more often than in controls. Different components of the nasal valve can be treated to improve airflow, the most important being the head of the inferior turbinate and the lower lateral alar cartilage. To determine whether nasal valve collapse plays a role in symptoms of nasal obstruction, the Cottle maneuver can be performed. The Cottle maneuver is considered positive (indicative of nasal valve obstruction), if the patient senses improved airflow with gentle superior lateral displacement of the valve area (Fig. 1).

Nasal Dilators

In addition to surgery, nonsurgical techniques can also be used to improve nasal breathing. Nasal dilators like the Breath Right (CNS, Inc., Chanhassen, Minnesota,

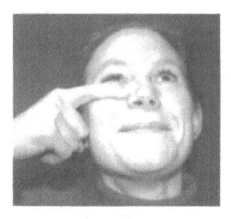

FIGURE 1 Cottle maneuver.

U.S.A.), The Side Strip (SS) Nasal Dilator (BRS Enterprises Pty. Ltd., Mount George, South Australia), or the Nozovent (Scandinavian Formulas, Sellersville, U.S.A.) stabilize the lateral wall of the nasal valve and are therefore effective in increasing nasal flow (54–58). They are particularly effective in reducing the amount of snoring in patients with chronic rhinitis (59,60).

Surgery

Most authors feel that surgical therapy should only be considered for those patients who fail to obtain symptomatic relief with medical therapy (44,61,62). Surgical procedures for nonallergic noninfectious rhinitis aim either to modify the size of the nasal valve or the rest of the inferior turbinate, or to denervate the nose of its autonomic supply. Turbinate reduction can be a valuable alternative when medical therapy fails. The use of surgical scalpel, chemical sclerosing solutions, and snake venom, electrocautery, cryosurgery, and laser surgery have all been found to diminish obstruction complaints (50,63–67). The duration of effectiveness reported varies from six months to several years (68,69). Here, I will only discuss the techniques that can be performed in an outpatient setting.

OUTPATIENT INFERIOR TURBINATE REDUCTION

After optimal medical therapy, some patients with NAR still have nasal obstruction caused by inferior turbinate hypertrophy. There is a large range of techniques for reducing the inferior turbinate. Although hundreds of papers have been written describing these techniques, very few describe prospective, randomized, controlled trials (64–67,70). The ideal turbinate reduction procedure would be one that effectively reduces the turbinate volume, preserves physiological function, and avoids complications (68). Techniques can be broken down into submucosal techniques that are intended to preserve the epithelium as much as possible and more aggressive techniques that partly destroy the covering nasal epithelium There is a tendency toward less aggressive methods for the reduction of the turbinate, partly because of the new instruments that have recently become available (69). The submucosal techniques rely on postoperative wound contracture and fibrosis to induce tissue volume reduction. Most of these techniques can be used in an outpatient setting; they include electrocautery, cryotherapy, and tissue reduction with radiofrequency (68,71).

VIDIAN NEURECTOMY

The effect of vidian neurectomy in vasomotor rhinitis was described as early as in 1970 (72,73). This procedure is effective in relieving excessive secretion but not as effective for the obstruction. Both preganglionic parasympathetic and sympathetic fibers are interrupted.

However, not all authors are very convinced about the long-term results, probably because re-enervation can occur (74–76).

CONCLUSION

Although the percentage of patients with nonallergic noninfectious rhinitis with a known cause have increased in recent decades, about 50% of patients with a non-allergic noninfectious rhinitis still have to be classified as suffering from IR. It is to be expected that, in the near future, some more explanatory pathophysiologic mechanisms for nonallergic noninfectious rhinitis will be found, doing justice to the idea that the diagnosis of IR is still a "melting pot" of several pathophysiologic conditions. It is to be hoped that the future unraveling of this intriguing disease will lead to more specific—and possibly improved—treatment options. Fortunately, progress has been made recently in therapy for IR patients who do not react to topical steroids, with the improved and patient- (and physician-) friendly treatment of five intranasal capsaicin applications in a single day at one-hour intervals (after local anesthesia). It is hoped that capsaicin treatment will be corroborated in many centers in the near future.

REFERENCES

1. Bousquet J, Van Cauwenberge P, Khaltaev N. Allergic rhinitis and its impact on asthma. J Allergy Clin Immunol 2001; 108(5 Part 2):S147–S334.
2. Bachert C. Persistent rhinitis—allergic or nonallergic? Allergy 2004; 59 (Suppl 76):11–15; discussion 5.
3. Villar MT, Holgate ST. IgE, smoking and lung function. Clin Exp Allergy 1995; 25(3):206–209.
4. Vinke JG, KleinJan A, Severijnen LW, Fokkens WJ. Passive smoking causes an "allergic" cell infiltrate in the nasal mucosa of non-atopic children. Int J Pediatr Otorhinolaryngol 1999; 51(2):73–81.
5. Hellgren J, Lillienberg L, Jarlstedt J, Karlsson G, Toren K. Population-based study of non-infectious rhinitis in relation to occupational exposure, age, sex, and smoking. Am J Ind Med 2002; 42(1):23–28.
6. Stein MD, Weinstock MC, Herman DS, Anderson BJ. Respiratory symptom relief related to reduction in cigarette use. J Gen Intern Med 2005; 20(10):889–894.
7. Scanlon PD, Connett JE, Waller LA, Altose MD, Bailey WC, Buist AS. Smoking cessation and lung function in mild-to-moderate chronic obstructive pulmonary disease. The lung health study. Am J Respir Crit Care Med 2000; 161(2 Pt 1):381–390.
8. Braat JP, Mulder PG, Fokkens WJ, van Wijk RG, Rijntjes E. Intranasal cold dry air is superior to histamine challenge in determining the presence and degree of nasal hyper-reactivity in nonallergic noninfectious perennial rhinitis. Am J Respir Crit Care Med 1998; 157(6 Pt 1):1748–1755.
9. Naclerio RM, Proud D, Kagey-Sobotka A, Lichtenstein LM, Thompson M, Togias A. Cold dry air-induced rhinitis: effect of inhalation and exhalation through the nose. J Appl Physiol 1995; 79(2):467–471.
10. Braat JP, Mulder PG, Duivenvoorden HJ, Gerth Van Wijk R, Rijntjes E, Fokkens WJ. Pollutional and meteorological factors are closely related to complaints of non-allergic,

non-infectious perennial rhinitis patients: a time series model. Clin Exp Allergy 2002; 32(5):690–697.

11. Scadding GK, Lund VJ, Jacques LA, Richards DH. A placebo-controlled study of fluticasone propionate aqueous nasal spray and beclomethasone dipropionate in perennial rhinitis: efficacy in allergic and non-allergic perennial rhinitis. Clin Exp Allergy 1995; 25(8):737–743.

12. Lundblad L, Sipila P, Farstad T, Drozdziewicz D. Mometasone furoate nasal spray in the treatment of perennial non-allergic rhinitis: a nordic, multicenter, randomized, double-blind, placebo-controlled study. Acta Otolaryngol 2001; 121(4):505–509.

13. Malm L, Wihl JA. Intra-nasal beclomethasone dipropionate in vasomotor rhinitis. Acta Allergol 1976; 31(3):245–253.

14. Bende M, Lindqvist N, Pipkorn U. Effect of a topical glucocorticoid, budesonide, on nasal mucosal blood flow as measured with 133Xe wash-out technique. Allergy 1983; 38(7):461–464.

15. Blom HM, Godthelp T, Fokkens WJ, KleinJan A, Mulder PG, Rijntjes E. The effect of nasal steroid aqueous spray on nasal complaint scores and cellular infiltrates in the nasal mucosa of patients with nonallergic, noninfectious perennial rhinitis. J Allergy Clin Immunol 1997; 100(6 Pt 1):739–747.

16. Powe DG, Huskisson RS, Carney AS, Jenkins D, Jones NS. Evidence for an inflammatory pathophysiology in idiopathic rhinitis. Clin Exp Allergy 2001; 31(6):864–872.

17. Moneret-Vautrin DA, Hsieh V, Wayoff M, Guyot JL, Mouton C, Maria Y. Nonallergic rhinitis with eosinophilia syndrome a precursor of the triad: nasal polyposis, intrinsic asthma, and intolerance to aspirin. Ann Allergy 1990; 64(6):513–518.

18. Purello-D'Ambrosio F, Isola S, Ricciardi L, Gangemi S, Barresi L, Bagnato GF. A controlled study on the effectiveness of loratadine in combination with flunisolide in the treatment of nonallergic rhinitis with eosinophilia (NARES). Clin Exp Allergy 1999; 29(8):1143–1147.

19. van Rijswijk JB, Blom HM, KleinJan A, Mulder PG, Rijntjes E, Fokkens WJ. Inflammatory cells seem not to be involved in idiopathic rhinitis. Rhinology 2003; 41(1):25–30.

20. Blom H, Godthelp T, Fokkens W, et al. Mast cells, eosinophils and IgE-positive cells in the nasal mucosa of patients with vasomotor rhinitis. An immunohistochemical study. Eur Arch Otorhinolaryngolgoy 1995; 252(Suppl 1):S33–S39.

21. Blom HM, Van Rijswijk JB, Garrelds IM, Mulder PG, Timmermans T, Gerth van Wijk R. Intranasal capsaicin is efficacious in non-allergic, non-infectious perennial rhinitis. A placebo-controlled study. Clin Exp Allergy 1997; 27(7):796–801.

22. Caenen M, Hamels K, Deron P, Clement P. Comparison of decongestive capacity of xylometazoline and pseudoephedrine with rhinomanometry and MRI. Rhinology 2005; 43(3):205–209.

23. Graf P. Rhinitis medicamentosa: a review of causes and treatment. Treat Respir Med 2005; 4(1):21–29.

24. Watanabe H, Foo TH, Djazaeri B, Duncombe P, Mackay IS, Durham SR. Oxymetazoline nasal spray three times daily for four weeks in normal subjects is not associated with rebound congestion or tachyphylaxis. Rhinology 2003; 41(3):167–174.

25. Graf P, Juto JE. Decongestion effect and rebound swelling of the nasal mucosa during 4-week use of oxymetazoline. ORL J Otorhinolaryngol Relat Spec 1994; 56(3):157–160.

26. Graf PM, Hallen H. One year follow-up of patients with rhinitis medicamentosa after vasoconstrictor withdrawal. Am J Rhinol 1997; 11(1):67–72.

27. Graf P, Enerdal J, Hallen H. Ten days' use of oxymetazoline nasal spray with or without benzalkonium chloride in patients with vasomotor rhinitis. Arch Otolaryngol Head Neck Surg 1999; 125(10):1128–1132.

28. Graf P, Hallen H, Juto JE. Four-week use of oxymetazoline nasal spray (Nezeril) once daily at night induces rebound swelling and nasal hyperreactivity. Acta Otolaryngol 1995; 115(1):71–75.

29. Ferguson BJ, Paramaesvaran S, Rubinstein E. A study of the effect of nasal steroid sprays in perennial allergic rhinitis patients with rhinitis medicamentosa. Otolaryngol Head Neck Surg 2001; 125(3):253–260.

30. Graf PM, Hallen H. Changes in nasal reactivity in patients with rhinitis medicamentosa after treatment with fluticasone propionate and placebo nasal spray. ORL J Otorhinolaryngol Relat Spec 1998; 60(6):334–338.
31. Hallen H, Enerdal J, Graf P. Fluticasone propionate nasal spray is more effective and has a faster onset of action than placebo in treatment of rhinitis medicamentosa. Clin Exp Allergy 1997; 27(5):552–558.
32. Lofkvist T. A comparative evaluation of oral decongestants in the treatment of vasomotor rhinitis. J Int Med Res 1978; 6(1):56–60.
33. Meltzer EO, Casale TB, Gold MS, et al. Efficacy and safety of clemastine-pseudoephedrine-acetaminophen versus pseudoephedrine-acetaminophen in the treatment of seasonal allergic rhinitis in a 1-day, placebo-controlled park study. Ann Allergy Asthma Immunol 2003; 90(1):79–86.
34. Berkowitz RB, McCafferty F, Lutz C, et al. Fexofenadine HCl 60 mg/pseudoephedrine HCl 120 mg has a 60-minute onset of action in the treatment of seasonal allergic rhinitis symptoms, as assessed in an allergen exposure unit. Allergy Asthma Proc 2004; 25(5): 335–343.
35. Pleskow W, Grubbe R, Weiss S,.Lutsky B. Efficacy and safety of an extended-release formulation of desloratadine and pseudoephedrine vs the individual components in the treatment of seasonal allergic rhinitis. Ann Allergy Asthma Immunol 2005; 94(3):348–354.
36. Salerno SM, Jackson JL, Berbano EP. Effect of oral pseudoephedrine on blood pressure and heart rate: a meta-analysis. Arch Intern Med 2005; 165(15):1686–1694.
37. Jokinen K, Sipila P. Intranasal ipratropium in the treatment of vasomotor rhinitis. Rhinology 1983; 21(4):341–345.
38. Malmberg H, Grahne B, Holopainen E, Binder E. Ipratropium (Atrovent) in the treatment of vasomotor rhinitis of elderly patients. Clin Otolaryngol Allied Sci 1983; 8(4): 273–276.
39. Knight A, Kazim F, Salvatori VA. A trial of intranasal Atrovent versus placebo in the treatment of vasomotor rhinitis. Ann Allergy 1986; 57(5):348–354.
40. Assanasen P, Baroody FM, Rouadi P, Naureckas E, Solway J, Naclerio RM. Ipratropium bromide increases the ability of the nose to warm and humidify air. Am J Respir Crit Care Med 2000; 162(3 Pt 1):1031–1037.
41. Ostberg B, Winther B, Borum P, Mygind N. Common cold and high-dose ipratropium bromide: use of anticholinergic medication as an indicator of reflex-mediated hypersecretion. Rhinology 1997; 35(2):58–62.
42. Becker B, Borum S, Nielsen K, Mygind N, Borum P. A time-dose study of the effect of topical ipratropium bromide on methacholine-induced rhinorrhoea in patients with perennial non-allergic rhinitis. Clin Otolaryngol Allied Sci 1997; 22(2):132–134.
43. Baraniuk JN. Sensory, parasympathetic, and sympathetic neural influences in the nasal mucosa. J Allergy Clin Immunol 1992; 90(6 Pt 2):1045–1050.
44. van Rijswijk JB, Blom HM, Fokkens WJ. Idiopathic rhinitis, the ongoing quest. Allergy 2005; 60(12):1471–1481.
45. van Rijswijk JB, Boeke EL, Keizer JM, Mulder PG, Blom HM, Fokkens WJ. Intranasal capsaicin reduces nasal hyperreactivity in idiopathic rhinitis: a double-blind randomized application regimen study. Allergy 2003; 58(8):754–761.
46. Wolf G. New aspects in the pathogenesis and therapy of hyperreflexive rhinopathy. Laryngol Rhinol Otol (Stuttg) 1988; 67(9):438–445.
47. van de Heyning PH, van Haesendonck J, Creten W, Rombaut N. Effect of topical levocabastine on allergic and non-allergic perennial rhinitis. A double-blind study, levocabastine vs. placebo, followed by an open, prospective, single-blind study on beclomethasone. Allergy 1988; 43(5):386–391.
48. Shaari CM, Sanders I, Wu BL, Biller HF. Rhinorrhea is decreased in dogs after nasal application of botulinum toxin. Otolaryngol Head Neck Surg 1995; 112(4):566–571.
49. Wang J, Chen F, Meng M, et al. The influence of botulinum toxin type A on vasomotor rhinitis and morphological study. Lin Chuang Er Bi Yan Hou Ke Za Zhi 2003; 17(11): 643–645.

50. Bhargava KB, Shirali GN, Abhyankar US, Gadre KC. Treatment of allergic and vaso-
    motor rhinitis by the local application of different concentrations of silver nitrate.
    J Laryngol Otol 1992; 106(8):699–701.
51. al-Samarrae SM. Treatment of "vasomotor rhinitis" by the local application of silver
    nitrate. J Laryngol Otol 1991; 105(4):285–287.
52. Bhargava KB, Abhyankar US, Shah TM. Treatment of allergic and vasomotor rhinitis by
    the local application of silver nitrate. J Laryngol Otol 1980; 94(9):1025–1036.
53. Wexler DB, Davidson TM. The nasal valve: a review of the anatomy, imaging, and
    physiology. Am J Rhinol 2004; 18(3):143–150.
54. Latte J, Taverner D. Opening the nasal valve with external dilators reduces congestive
    symptoms in normal subjects. Am J Rhinol 2005; 19(2):215–219.
55. Di Somma EM, West SN, Wheatley JR, Amis TC. Nasal dilator strips increase
    maximum inspiratory flow via nasal wall stabilization. Laryngoscope 1999; 109(5):
    780–784.
56. Ng BA, Mamikoglu B, Ahmed MS, Corey JP. The effect of external nasal dilators as
    measured by acoustic rhinometry. Ear Nose Throat J 1998; 77(10):840–844.
57. Petruson B. Increased nasal breathing decreases snoring and improves oxygen
    saturation during sleep apnoea. Rhinology 1994; 32(2):87–89.
58. Awan MS, Ali MM, Ahmed M, Iqbal A, Aslam MJ. Clinical study on the use of nozovent
    in a tertiary care setting. J Pak Med Assoc 2004; 54(12):614–617.
59. Petruson B, Theman K. Clinical evaluation of the nasal dilator nozovent. The effect on
    snoring and dryness of the mouth. Rhinology 1992; 30(4):283–287.
60. Pevernagie D, Hamans E, Van Cauwenberge P, Pauwels R. External nasal dilation
    reduces snoring in chronic rhinitis patients: a randomized controlled trial. Eur Respir
    J 2000; 15(6):996–1000.
61. Jones AS, Lancer JM. Vasomotor rhinitis. Br Med J (Clin Res Ed) 1987; 294(6586):
    1505–1506.
62. Lieberman P. Treatment update: nonallergic rhinitis. Allergy Asthma Proc 2001;
    22(4):199–202.
63. Ibragimov GT, Rasunova AK. Treatment of patients with vasomotor rhinitis using snake
    venom. Vestn Otorinolaringol 1987(1):39–41.
64. Nunez DA, Bradley PJ. A randomised clinical trial of turbinectomy for compensatory
    turbinate hypertrophy in patients with anterior septal deviations. Clin Otolaryngol
    Allied Sci 2000; 25(6):495–498.
65. Sapci T, Sahin B, Karavus A, Akbulut UG. Comparison of the effects of radiofrequency
    tissue ablation, CO_2 laser ablation, and partial turbinectomy applications on nasal
    mucociliary functions. Laryngoscope 2003; 113(3):514–519.
66. Passali D, Passali FM, Damiani V, Passali GC, Bellussi L. Treatment of inferior turbinate
    hypertrophy: a randomized clinical trial. Ann Otol Rhinol Laryngol 2003; 112(8):
    683–688.
67. Nease CJ, Krempl GA. Radiofrequency treatment of turbinate hypertrophy: a random-
    ized, blinded, placebo-controlled clinical trial. Otolaryngol Head Neck Surg 2004;
    130(3):291–299.
68. Chang CW, Ries WR. Surgical treatment of the inferior turbinate: new techniques. Curr
    Opin Otolaryngol Head Neck Surg 2004; 12(1):53–57.
69. Clement WA, White PS. Trends in turbinate surgery literature: a 35-year review. Clin
    Otolaryngol Allied Sci 2001; 26(2):124–128.
70. Passali D, Lauriello M, Anselmi M, Bellussi L. Treatment of hypertrophy of the inferior
    turbinate: long–term results in 382 patients randomly assigned to therapy. Ann Otol
    Rhinol Laryngol 1999; 108(6):569–575.
71. Corey JP, Houser SM, Ng BA. Nasal congestion: a review of its etiology, evaluation, and
    treatment. Ear Nose Throat J 2000; 79(9):690–693, 696, 698 passim.
72. Golding-Wood PH. Vidian neurectomy: its results and complications. Laryngoscope
    1973; 83(10):1673–1683.
73. Chasin WD, Lofgren RH. Vidian nerve section for vasomotor rhinitis. Arch Otolaryngol
    1967; 86(1):103–109.

74. Ogale SB, Shah A, Rao SC, Shah KL. Is vidian neurectomy worthwhile? J Laryngol Otol 1988; 102(1):62–63.
75. Patel KH, Gaikwad GA. Bilateral transnasal cauterization of the vidian nerve in vasomotor rhinitis. J Laryngol Otol 1975; 89(12):1291–1296.
76. Krant JN, Wildervanck de Blecourt P, Dieges PH, de Heer LJ. Long-term results of vidian neurectomy. Rhinology 1979; 17(4):231–235.

24 Surgical Management of Inferior Turbinate Hypertrophy in Nonallergic Rhinitis

Mohamed M. Nagi and Martin Desrosiers

Department of Otolaryngology, McGill University, Montreal, Quebec, Canada

INTRODUCTION

The surgical management of inferior turbinate (IT) hypertrophy is directed toward improving nasal airflow without adversely interfering with the normal physiology of the nose. The central strategy common to all surgical procedures discussed below is volume reduction of the IT, particularly its anterior portion, which, as a component of the internal nasal valve, is the most resistive segment of the upper airway.

Surgical options to shrink the IT range from nondestructive procedures to complete turbinate excision. Despite the frequency of the disorder and the number of surgical procedures performed yearly, the surgical literature provides scant evidence-based support for the primacy of any particular treatment method. The selection of concurrently available surgical techniques is vast, attesting to the fact that none of these procedures is ideal. Each is associated with varying complications and degrees of success. A lack of consensus as to their respective merits effectively means that the surgeon's attitudes and experience will determine which procedure is chosen.

The exact function of the turbinates remains to be fully elucidated, but it includes filtration and conditioning of inspired air. The IT plays an important role in regulating the aerodynamic flow of inspired air, which is necessary for the subjective feeling of comfortable breathing as well as for optimal olfactory function. The presence of IgA secretory antibodies on the mucosal surface of the IT, along with the beating of its ciliated epithelium, plays a role in protecting the host from environmental pathogens and toxins.

Transient *asymmetric* bilateral congestion of the mucosa increases IT volume, and is responsible for generating the physiologic nasal cycle. Similarly, *symmetric* congestion in response to various stimuli acts to warm, humidify, and filter inspired air before it reaches the lower airway. Therefore, the ideal turbinate reduction procedure should reduce IT volume, and preserve overall turbinate shape and physiologic functions, while minimizing iatrogenic complications.

INJECTION

Intraturbinal injection of corticosteroids was first used in the 1950s. It was shown to be effective in the temporary improvement of nasal obstruction, but only secondary to IT hypertrophy. The procedure is minimally invasive and is performed in the clinic. Disadvantages include the transient nature of the treatment and the need for repeated injections. Side effects include facial flushing and, rarely, transient or permanent visual loss. This is thought to occur from retrograde embolization of injected material into the retinal circulation, and may be prone to occur with large molecular size corticosteroids. Although extremely rare with an incidence of 0.006% (1), this complication has undoubtedly curtailed the widespread use of intraturbinal corticosteroid injection.

TURBINATE RESECTION PROCEDURES

Resection of hypertrophic IT (turbinectomy) has historically been the mainstay of surgical treatment. It involves partial or complete removal of the IT and may be performed under general or local anesthesia. Resection procedures are very effective in alleviating the symptoms of nasal obstruction (2,3). However, these procedures may be associated with comparatively increased morbidity, which is directly related to the extent of the resection. A summary of available treatment options is presented in Table 1.

Total IT Resection

Total turbinectomy was one of the first methods introduced for surgical reduction of the ITs. It falls at the extreme of the turbinate resection continuum and involves a high risk of complications. Prima facie, it is a simple and effective method to improve nasal airflow. However, it has the potential of affecting several of the patient's physiologic, albeit poorly understood, functions. Indeed, complete resection of the IT increases turbulent airflow, misdirecting the airstream away from the olfactory epithelium. It is associated with a high risk of bleeding, which necessitates postoperative nasal packing, causing discomfort to the patient. Morbidity includes prolonged nasal crusting, synechiae, nasal and pharyngeal dryness, intolerance to cold air, olfactory dysfunction, and a paradoxical sensation of nasal obstruction, the so-called "empty nose syndrome." Complete IT resection has also been associated with atrophic rhinitis (rhinitis sicca and ozena), though an incontrovertible causal link is lacking (4–7). These effects may be more pronounced in individuals living in dry climates or environments. It is thus not surprising that this procedure has been falling out of favor among most surgeons, who now tend to be more conservative as to the extent of turbinate resection.

Partial IT Resection

This procedure involves a more limited resection of the IT to preserve its normal physiologic function. It aims to maximize results by limiting resection to the nasal valve region, the most critical determinant of nasal airway resistance. Many variations of this technique exist, depending on the extent of the resection. Overall, the benefits of partial IT resection are comparable to total turbinectomy (8,9). Likewise, complications are similar. Synechiae occur in up to 10% of patients, but the risk of bleeding is decreased when compared to total turbinectomy (0.9% vs. 5.8%) (10). Anecdotally, the incidence of atrophic rhinitis is also lesser.

Submucous Resection of the IT

Partial resection of the IT (as well as most of the reduction techniques discussed below) may change the histological architecture of the turbinate mucosa, affecting normal mucociliary clearance. Submucous resection addresses this issue by preserving the mucosal covering of the IT. Pathologically redundant submucosal tissue is resected selectively in an attempt to mitigate the outcome of tampering with the mucosa or changing the shape of the IT. In practice, it is not clear whether this logic

TABLE 1 Surgical Management of Inferior Turbinate Hypertrophy in Nonallergic Rhinitis

Technique	Advantages	Disadvantages
Steroid injection	Minimally invasive	Brief duration, rare reports of visual loss
Turbinate outfracture	Minimal risk	Minor relief, of brief duration
	No mucosal damage	Does not address mucosa
	Can be combined with other procedures	
Electrocautery	Simple	Effect of short duration
	Local or general anesthesia	
	Crusting	
		Adhesions
		Risk of bone necrosis
		Delayed hemorrhage
		Does not address bony hypertrophy
Laser reduction	Local or general anesthesia	Expensive equipment
	Good hemostasis	Expertise
	Duration >2 yr	Does not address bony hypertrophy
	Local or general anesthesia	
Partial resection	Easy to perform	Crusting
	Durable efficacy	Adhesions
	Addresses bone and mucosa	Hemorrhage
Total turbinectomy	Durable efficacy	Crusting
	Addresses bone and mucosa	Adhesions
		Hemorrhage
		Possibility of atrophic rhinitis
Submucous resection	Preserves mucosal integrity and function	Technically more difficult
	Can address bone	Recurrence 25%
	Minimal crusting	
	Minimal hemorrhage	
Microdebrider-surface	Similar to partial resection	Similar to partial resection
Microdebrider-submucous	No crusting	Mucosal tear in inexperienced hands
	Preserves mucosal integrity and function	
	Addresses bone and mucosa	
	Minimal bleeding	
Radiofrequency ablation	Preserves mucosal integrity and function	Does not address bony hypertrophy
	Local anesthesia	Cost
		Duration

translates into clear benefits for the patient. Moreover, this procedure is technically more demanding. Persistence or recurrence of symptoms is also a concern and can be observed in as much as 25% of patients up to five years postoperatively (11,12). Thus, even though the associated crusting and potential for bleeding is minimized, thanks to reduced mucosal disruption (13), this procedure is not widely utilized.

Inferior turbinoplasty, a variation on the same theme, involves creating an incision along the anterior edge of the IT, lifting mucosa off the IT bone, removing a wedge of inferior and anterior turbinate mucosa along with bone, and then laying the mucosa back down. This is presumably most effective for cases of hypertrophy of the bony turbinate. Complications include crusting in up to 15% of patients up to one year postoperatively (12).

TURBINATE OUTFRACTURE

This procedure consists of fracturing the turbinate bone in a lateral direction to improve the nasal airway. The IT is typically outfractured in a single piece by pushing it toward the lateral nasal wall. Alternatively, some surgeons create a submucosal tunnel and outfracture the IT into several small fragments in an anterior-to-posterior direction. This procedure is easy to perform and is associated with minimal morbidity. However, because it does not address the hypertrophied mucosa per se, and because the turbinates have a tendency to spring back (especially when fractured in a single fragment), this procedure is associated with modest improvement in symptoms when used by itself. It is thus often combined with the other techniques described in this chapter.

MICRODEBRIDER SUBMUCOSAL REDUCTION OF THE IT

The microdebrider is an instrument that uses a rotating burr with an associated suction to remove tissue in a controlled fashion. There are two variations of this technique: surface reduction and submucosal reduction. The former was associated with bleeding in up to 23% of patients in one study (14), the latter was associated with a 1.6% incidence of bleeding (15). The reduced risk of bleeding and potential for its performance under local anesthesia make this an attractive option for selected patients with obstructive sleep apnea.

IT REDUCTION PROCEDURES

These procedures target the IT mucosal surface. Generally, these procedures produce transient outcomes and are to be repeated as needed. The rationale behind choosing a reduction procedure is threefold: preserving the IT architecture responsible for shaping an aerodynamic airstream, minimizing the impact on normal nasal physiology, and minimizing iatrogenic sequelae.

Some of the procedures described below are effective for periods of varying duration. Recurrence of symptoms is thought to be caused by regrowth of turbinate soft tissue, but the processes underlying turbinate healing remain to be fully elucidated (14).

Electrocautery

This procedure involves applying electrocautery either to the surface of the IT or submucosally. Electrocautery causes heat destruction of the hypertrophied tissue along with vessel thrombosis, which prevents the venous sinusoids in the turbinate mucosa from engorging. Electrocautery of the IT is simple to perform and can be carried out in the clinic under local anesthesia. Results usually last months to years. Surface electrocautery is associated with adhesions and crusting for up to six weeks after the procedure, which can exacerbate symptoms of nasal obstruction. Cautery of the bone must be avoided to prevent bony necrosis, which is associated with prolonged edema and discomfort. Rarely, electrocautery is associated with hemorrhage that lasts up to 10 days after the procedure (16).

Cryosurgery

In this procedure, a cold probe ($\sim$70°C) is placed along the anterior and medial surface of the IT for various intervals ranging from seconds to minutes. The mechanism is similar to electrocautery, but uses cold instead of heat. This easy-to-perform procedure can be done under local anesthesia in the clinic and is associated with minimal complications. The duration of results is variable, lasting at least a year or longer (17,18). Cryosurgery equipment is, however, less readily available compared to electrocautery, limiting its widespread use and increasing its cost. This technique is now only infrequently performed.

Laser Reduction

Laser reduction of the IT can be performed in the clinic under local anesthesia. Several laser systems are used in the treatment of IT hypertrophy. Postoperative complications are minimal (19). Generally, the laser is applied in a linear fashion along the entire length of the turbinate or along its inferior edge. Some authors additionally deliver the laser to the anterior aspect of the IT to improve airflow in the internal valve area. Many publications reported good results with laser treatment of hypertrophied IT (20,21). Disadvantages include considerable crusting, which may be bothersome to patients. Furthermore, the equipment's cost and added expertise required to operate it increase the cost of the procedure.

Radiofrequency

This is the most recent addition to the list of procedures used for IT reduction. It is most similar in mechanism to electrocautery: a probe is inserted submucosally to deliver low-frequency energy that causes a localized rise in temperature, resulting in soft tissue reduction. Ensuing postoperative fibrosis of the IT limits swelling. The procedure is performed in the clinic under local anesthesia. It is well tolerated, as it is associated with minimal postoperative pain, crusting, or bleeding (22). It is not associated with any detectable respiratory epithelial damage and has no effect on mucociliary clearance.

Coblation[R]

Coblation, short for controlled ablation, is a patented process that uses radiofrequency energy to ablate soft tissue. Although it uses a bipolar radiofrequency reduction technique through thermal ablation of the tissue, it is touted as a technique that has minimal thermal effect and is marketed as a device that dissolves tissue without being heat driven (23). It is fast, taking only 20 to 30 seconds per nostril (24). The main drawback of this procedure is crusting, which is observed transiently in 16% of patients (24). As this is a new procedure, long-term effectiveness remains to be evaluated.

COMPARISON STUDIES

Most studies analyzing the various methods of IT reduction are prospective in nature, with short-term follow-up periods. Few studies use a control, and even fewer are randomized. Passali et al. conducted a randomized clinical trial comparing total turbinectomy, CO_2 laser resection, electrocautery, cryotherapy, and submucosal resection over a six-year follow-up period (25). Their results are summarized in

TABLE 2 A Comparative Analysis of the Surgical Methods Addressing Inferior Turbinate Hypertrophy

Procedure	n	Chronic crusting	Synechiae	Bleeding	Atrophy
Total turbinectomy	45	34	14	25	10
CO_2 laser resection	54	40	4	0	6
Electrocautery	62	39	21	0	2
Cryotherapy	58	40	8	0	3
Submucous resection	69	7	2	10	0

Table 2. Sapci et al. compared the efficacy and the effects of radiofrequency ablation, laser reduction, and partial turbinectomy on mucociliary clearance (26). They concluded that although all these methods had comparable efficacy, mucociliary function was most disrupted by laser reduction, whereas radiofrequency ablation had a minimal impact.

CONCLUSION

Treatment strategies are based on the assumption that decreasing airflow resistance will lead to an improvement in symptoms of nasal obstruction. However, it is prudent to bear in mind normal nasal physiology, as it relates to inspired airflow and the subjective feeling of unimpeded, comfortable nasal breathing, which remains poorly understood. Undoubtedly, all types of turbinate surgery affect nasal physiology to varying degrees. Some of the procedures discussed above, although effective in relieving symptoms of nasal obstruction, can have undesirable consequences related to increased turbulent airflow, and altered airstream. Indeed, extensive IT resection leads to excessive nasal and pharyngeal dryness, crust formation, decreased efficiency of mucociliary transport, and a reduction in IgA production (25). Thus, the conservative tendencies of most surgeons today are wise, given our incomplete understanding of turbinate physiology.

The concurrent utilization of multiple surgical procedures to treat IT hypertrophy betrays the lack of a differentially superior method. Even though there exists no ideal surgical procedure to address IT hypertrophy, all methods referred to in this chapter are effective for the symptomatic relief of IT hypertrophy. Treatment methods have differing efficacy and variable duration of effect. As such, each procedure should be weighed against its inherent risks of complication and morbidity. In general, procedures with the greatest duration of effect tend to be those that physically remove tissue, bone, or both (27). However, the risk of postoperative morbidity increases with the extent of the procedure (28). Consequently, selecting and recommending a technique for the relief of nasal obstruction remains an imperfect process, based on perceived patient characteristics and physician judgment and experience.

REFERENCES

1. Mabry RL. Intranasal steroids in rhinology: the changing role of intraturbinal injection. Ear Nose Throat J 1994; 73:24–26.
2. Courtiss EH, Goldwyn RM. Resection of obstructing inferior nasal turbinates: a 10-year follow-up. Plast Reconstr Surg 1990; 86:152–154.

3. Fanous N. Anterior turbinectomy. A new surgical approach to turbinate hypertrophy: a review of 220 cases. Arch Otolaryngol Head Neck Surg 1986; 112:850–852.
4. Fry H. Long-term follow-up of the effectiveness and safety of inferior turbinectomy [Discussion]. Plast Reconstr Surg 1992; 90:985.
5. Moore GF, Freeman TJ, Ogren FP, Yonkers AJ. Extended follow-up of total inferior turbinate resection for relief of chronic nasal obstruction. Laryngoscope 1985; 95:1095–1099.
6. Ophir D. Resection of obstructing inferior turbinates following rhinoplasty. Plast Reconstr Surg 1990; 85:724–727.
7. Ophir D, Shapira A, Marshak G. Total inferior turbinectomy for nasal airway obstruction. Arch Otolaryngol 1985; 111:93–95.
8. Ophir D, Schindel D, Halperin D, Marshak G. Long-term follow-up of the effectiveness and safety of inferior turbinectomy. Plast Reconstr Surg 1992; 90:980–984.
9. Wight RG, Jones AS, Clegg RT. A comparison of anterior and radical trimming of the inferior nasal turbinates and the effects on nasal resistance to airflow. Clin Otolaryngol 1988; 13:223–226.
10. Garth RJ, Cox HJ, Thomas MR. Haemorrhage as a complication of inferior turbinectomy: a comparison of anterior and radical trimming. Clin Otolaryngol 1995; 20:236–238.
11. Katz S, Schmelzer B, Cammaert T, Della Faille D, Leirens J. Our technique of partial inferior turbinoplasty: long-term results evaluated by rhinomanometry. Acta Otorhinolaryngol Belg 1996; 50:13–18.
12. Mabry RL. Inferior turbinoplasty: patient selection, technique, and long-term consequences. Otolaryngol Head Neck Surg 1988; 98:60–66.
13. King HC, Mabry RL. A Practical Guide to the Management of Nasal and Sinus Disorders. New York: Thieme Medical Publishers, Inc.,, 1993:94–118.
14. Wexler D, Braverman I. Partial inferior turbinectomy using the microdebrider. J Otolaryngol 2005; 34(3):189–193.
15. Friedman M, Tanyeri H, Lim J, et al. A safe alternative technique for inferior turbinate reduction. Laryngoscope 1999; 109:1834–1837.
16. Meredith GM Jr. Surgical reduction of hypertrophied inferior turbinates: a comparison of electrofulguration and partial resection. Plast Reconstr Surg 1988; 81:891–899.
17. Chiossone E, Guitierrez JR, Emmanuelli JL. Cryosurgery of the inferior turbinates. Auris Nasus Larynx 1990; 17:87–93.
18. Rakover Y, Rosen G. A comparison of partial inferior turbinectomy and cryosurgery for hypertrophic inferior turbinates. J Laryngol Otol 1996; 110:732–735.
19. Lippert BM, Werner JA. CO_2 laser surgery of hypertrophied inferior turbinates. Rhinology 1997; 35:33–36.
20. Kawamura S, Fukutake T, Kubo N, Yamashita T, Kumazawa T. Subjective results of laser surgery for allergic rhinitis. Acta Otolaryngol Suppl (Stockh) 1993; 500:109–112.
21. Lippert BM, Werner JA. Reduction of hyperplastic turbinates with CO_2 laser. Adv Otorhinolaryngol 1995; 49:119–121.
22. Coste A, Laurent Y, Blumen M, et al. Radiofrequency is a safe and effective treatment of turbinate hypertrophy. The Laryngoscope 2001; 111:894–899.
23. Chang D, Ries R. Surgical treatment of the inferior turbinate: new techniques. Curr Opin Otolaryngol Head Neck Surg 2004; 12(1):53–57.
24. Bhattacharyya N, Kepnes L. Clinical effectiveness of coblation inferior turbinate reduction. Otolaryngol Head Neck Surg 2003; 129(4):365–371.
25. Passali D, Passali FM, Damiani V, Passali GC, Bellussi L. Treatment of inferior turbinate hypertrophy: a randomized clinical trial. [Clinical Trial. Journal Article. Randomized Controlled Trial]. Ann Otol Rhinol Laryngol 2003; 112(8):683–688.
26. Sapci T, Sahin B, Karavus A, Akbulut U. Comparison of the effects of radiofrequency tissue ablation, CO_2 laser ablation, and partial turbinectomy applications on nasal mucociliary functions. Laryngoscope 2003; 113(3):514–519.
27. Hol MK, Huizing EH. Treatment of inferior turbinate pathology: a review and critical evaluation of the different techniques. Rhinology 2000; 38(4):157–166.
28. Tomasi M, Charpentier P, Lombard P, Boulat E, Salgas P. Hemorrhagic complications of lower turbinectomy. Rev Laryngol Otol Rhinol (Bord) 1993; 114:63–66.

25 Quality of Life in Nonallergic Rhinitis

Johan Hellgren

Department of Otolaryngology, Head and Neck Surgery, Capio Lundby Hospital, University of Gothenburg, Göteborg, Sweden

INTRODUCTION

Health-related quality-of-life questionnaires are diagnostic tools to evaluate the impact of a disease on daily life and well-being "as perceived by the patient" (1). Measuring health-related quality of life has been described as a structured way of taking a patient history. While the traditional medical history taken by the physician focuses on individual symptoms related to the underlying medical disorder, such as pain related to inflammation or tumor growth, health-related quality of life focuses on the outcomes of these symptoms in terms of function and well-being. This means that a similar level of symptoms can have a different impact on the health-related quality of life of different patients, depending on their individual tolerance of this symptom.

In the study of nonallergic rhinitis, health-related quality of life is a comparatively new measure that has not been widely used so far. Several studies have, however, addressed health-related quality of life in allergic rhinitis and this has contributed significantly to the understanding of rhinitis and its impact on well-being. Because the main symptoms of nonallergic rhinitis and allergic rhinitis are the same, including nasal blockage, secretion, itching, and sneezing, and because the perception of the two diseases has been shown to be similar, this chapter discusses the usefulness of health-related quality of life instruments in the study of nonallergic rhinitis, primarily, on the basis of studies of patients with allergic rhinitis (2). The papers referred to in this chapter are derived from a Pubmed/Medline search including the search terms "health-related quality of life," "rhinitis quality of life," "quality of life," "nonallergic rhinitis," "vasomotor rhinitis," "idiopathic rhinitis," "allergic rhinitis," and "rhinitis."

TYPES OF HEALTH-RELATED QUALITY-OF-LIFE INSTRUMENTS

There two main types of health-related quality-of-life questionnaires, the "generic" and the "disease specific." The generic instrument is not aimed at any specific disease and as a result it can be used in a wide range of conditions, including normal populations. One major advantage of the generic health-related quality-of-life instrument is that the results of studies addressing different diseases can be compared with one another and the relative burden of two conditions, such as rhinitis and asthma, on health-related quality of life can be assessed. The main weakness of the generic health-related quality-of-life instrument is the lack of "depth," which means that aspects of health-related quality of life that are important for a certain group of patients may not be included in the questionnaire; for example, having to carry tissues could be a burden for patients with rhinitis and a runny nose but not for patients who have had a hip replacement (3,4). There are several generic health-related quality-of-life instruments that have been validated. They include the "Sickness Impact Profile," the "Nottingham Health Profile" and the "Medical Outcome Short Form 36" (SF-36) (5–7).

The SF-36 is the most widely used of the generic questionnaires and it consists of 36 questions organized in eight different domains of physical and mental health and a ninth item relating to change in health compared to one year ago. The domains are physical functioning, role physical, bodily pain, general health, vitality, social functioning, role emotional, and mental health. The physical and mental domains are summarized into two summary scores—the physical component summary (first four domains listed above) and the mental component summary (last four domains listed above).

The questions are of the multiple-choice type, such as, "How much bodily pain have you had during the past four weeks?" and the possible answers are no bodily pain, very mild, mild, moderate, severe, and very severe. The results are transformed into a 0 to 100 scale where higher values mean better function or freedom from pain (7).

In a study of 111 patients with perennial allergic rhinitis (PAR) and 116 healthy controls, Bousquet et al. found that the patients with PAR scored significantly lower than the controls in eight domains of the SF-36, but not in change of health (8). In a later study by the same group, 240 subjects with allergic rhinitis (seasonal + PAR) scored significantly lower in all domains apart from physical functioning compared with controls ($n = 349$) (9). Women scored lower than men and the most affected domains were the ones related to mental function and well-being, such as mental health, social functioning and role emotional, which was confirmed by a significantly lower mental component summary. Meltzer studied 312 subjects with allergic rhinitis and found a significant difference in all domains except role emotional and change in health, compared with healthy controls (10). The consistency of these results is further supported by the fact that rhinitis has a similar effect on health-related quality of life when it is studied as a comorbidity in subjects with asthma. In a study of 180 subjects with asthma, our group found that a history of "noninfectious rhinitis" (allergic + nonallergic rhinitis) was associated with a significantly lower mental component summary compared with controls (11). This observation is further supported in the previously mentioned study by Leynaert et al., where coexisting asthma in the subjects with allergic rhinitis did not affect the change in mental quality of life imposed by the allergic rhinitis (9).

In the absence of comprehensive quality-of-life studies on patients with nonallergic rhinitis, the results from studies on patients with allergic rhinitis is the main source of information on health related quality of life in rhinitis. The disease perception between patients with PAR and patients with perennial nonallergic rhinitis (PNR) was compared in a study using in-depth interviews (2). Half of the patients with PNR and a third of the patients with PAR reported that the quality of life had been affected by their nasal symptoms because it prevented them from taking part in activities. About half of the patients in both groups reported being easily irritated because of their symptoms, whereas patients with PNR were more likely to avoid questions about their symptoms than the patients with PAR (44% vs. 7%). The overall conclusion was that disease perception and social behavior was independent of the allergic or nonallergic origin.

DISEASE-SPECIFIC, HEALTH-RELATED QUALITY-OF-LIFE INSTRUMENTS

Disease-specific, health-related quality-of-life instruments are constructed by asking a large number of patients with the disease about the impairments that are most

TABLE 1   Problems Identified Most Frequently by Rhinitis Patients

Problem areas	Limitations
Sleep problems	Daytime fatigue
Non-nasal symptoms	Thirst, poor concentration, headache
Nasal symptoms	Blocked, runny nose, sneezing
Practical problems	Having to carry tissues, blow the nose
Activity limitations	Work impairment, leisure impairment
Emotional problems	Frustration, irritation

Source: From Ref. 3.

important to them. Disease-specific, health-related quality-of-life instruments, therefore, have more "depth" than generic instruments. There are several rhinitis-specific questionnaires, such as the "Rhinosinusitis Outcome Measure," the "Sinonasal Outcome Test," and the "Rhinitis Disability Index" (12,13). The most extensively used rhinitis-specific quality-of-life instrument is the "Rhinitis Quality of Life Questionnaire" (RQLQ) (14). While constructing this instrument, Juniper et al. found that the most frequently identified problems in rhinitis are sleep problems, non-nasal symptoms, nasal symptoms, practical problems, activity limitations, and emotional problems. The limitations imposed by these problems are listed in Table 1 (3).

The RQLQ consists of 28 questions, organized in seven domains including eye symptoms (Table 1). Three functions that have been most affected during the past week due to nose/eye symptoms are selected by the subjects. The impairment is graded from 0 (not troubled) to 6 (extremely troubled). A higher score means poorer quality of life.

The interrelation between the health-related quality of life measured by the SF-36 and by the RQLQ, respectively, was evaluated in 312 patients with allergic rhinitis. They scored significantly lower compared with controls in all seven domains of the RQLQ and in all domains apart from role emotional and change in health in the SF-36 (4). In that study, the generic and the disease-specific questionnaires correlated well. In another study evaluating 160 patients with allergic rhinitis triggered by house-dust mites, the SF-36 domain of vitality showed a good correlation with the RQLQ domain of non-nasal symptoms, but apart from this the correlation between the two questionnaires was weak (15). In a recently published study, the SF-36 and the RQLQ were compared in 43 subjects with allergic rhinitis and 44 controls (16). Both questionnaires showed good discrimination between allergic rhinitis patients and controls. In the Rhinitis Quality of Life Questionnaire, all the items showed a significant difference between allergic rhinitis patients and controls and, in the SF-36, all the domains apart from physical function showed a significant difference. The items in the Rhinitis Quality of Life Questionnaire, however, changed to a greater extent in patients who reported an improvement of their rhinitis in interviews than the domains in the SF-36. The overall conclusion is that these instruments measure different aspects of the disease and should therefore be used in combination, but that the RQLQ is more sensitive to changes (17).

INTERVENTIONAL STUDIES

Several clinical studies have shown a positive effect on health-related quality of life after the treatment of allergic rhinitis with antihistamines and intranasal steroids, but there is a shortage of placebo-controlled studies evaluating the effect of medical intervention on health-related quality of life in nonallergic rhinitis (18). As other measures of treatment effect in general have shown less efficacy in subjects with nonallergic rhinitis when it comes to common medications such as nasal steroids and antihistamines compared with allergic rhinitis, there is a need for quality-of-life assessments in interventional studies of subjects with nonallergic rhinitis (19,20).

SUMMARY

Health-related quality-of-life questionnaires are instruments to assess the burden of a disease as perceived by the patient. Few data are available on the health-related quality of life of patients with nonallergic rhinitis, but data from studies of patients with allergic rhinitis show that rhinitis predominantly affects mental quality of life. This burden of rhinitis is associated with impaired sleep, excessive daytime sleepiness, concentration problems, and increased irritability.

REFERENCES

1. Schipper H, Clinch J, Powell V. Definitions and conceptual issues. In: Spilker B, ed. Quality of Life Assessment in Clinical Trials. New York: Raven Press, 1990:11–24.
2. Rydén O, Anderson B, Andersson M. Disease perception and social behaviour in persistent rhinitis: a comparison between patients with allergic and non-allergic rhinitis. Allergy 2004; 59:461–464.
3. Juniper EF. Measuring health-related quality of life in rhinitis. J Allergy Clin Immunol 1997; 99(2):742–749.
4. Meltzer E. Quality of life in adults and children with allergic rhinitis. J Allergy Clin Immunol 2001; 108(1):45–53.
5. Bergner M, Bobbitt RA, Carter WB, Gilson BS. The sickness impact profile: development and final revision of a health status measure. Med Care 1981; 19:787–805.
6. Hunt SM, McEwan J, McKenna SP. Measuring Health Status. Beckenham: Croom Helm, 1986.
7. Ware JE Jr., Sherbourne CD. The MOS 36-item short-form health survey (SF-36). I. Conceptual framework and item selection. Med Care 1992; 30(6):473–483.
8. Bousquet J, Bullinger M, Fayol C, Marquis P, Valentin B, Burtin B. Assessment of quality of life in patients with perennial allergic rhinitis with the French version of the SF-36 health status questionnaire. J Allergy Clin Immunol 1994; 94(2 Pt 1):182–188.
9. Leynaert B, Neukirch C, Liard R, Bousquet J, Neukirch F. Quality of life in allergic rhinitis and asthma. A population-based study of young adults. Am J Respir Crit Care Med 2000; 162(4 Pt 1):1391–1396.
10. Meltzer EO. The prevalence and medical and economic impact of allergic rhinitis in the United States. J Allergy Clin Immunol 1997; 99:805–828.
11. Hellgren J, Balder B, Palmqvist M, et al. Quality of life in non-infectious rhinitis and asthma. Rhinology 2004; 42:183–188.
12. Piccrillo J, Edwards D, Haiduk A, Yonan C, Thawley S. Psychometric and clinimetric validity of the 31-item rhinosinusitis outcome measure (RSOM-31). Am J Rhinol 1995; 9:297–306.
13. Benninger M. The development of the Rhinosinusitis Disability Index (RSDI). Arch Otolaryngol 1997; 123:1175–1179.
14. Juniper E, Guyatt G. Development and testing of a new measure of health status for clinical trials in rhinoconjunctivitis. Clin Exp Allergy 1991; 21:77–83.
15. Terreehorst I, Duivenvoorden HJ, Temples-Pavlica Z, et al. Comparison of a generic and a rhinitis-specific quality-of-life (QOL) instrument in patients with house dust mite

allergy: relationship between the SF-36 and rhinitis QOL questionnaire. Clin Exp Allergy 2004; 34:1673–1677.
16. Leong K, Yeak S, Saurajen A, Mok P, Earnest A, et al. Why generic and disease-specific quality-of-life instruments should be used together in the evaluation of patients with persistent allergic rhinitis. Clin Exp Allergy 2005; 35:288–298.
17. Juniper E, Ståhl E, Doty R, Simmons E, Allen D, Howarth P. Clinical outcomes and adverse effect monitoring in allergic rhinitis. J Allergy Clin Immunol 2005; 115:390–400.
18. Tripathi A, Patterson R. Impact of allergic rhinitis treatment on quality of life. Pharmacoeconomics 2001; 19:891–899.
19. Ciprandi G. Treatment of non-allergic perennial rhinitis. Allergy 2004; 59(suppl 76): 16–23.
20. Dockhorn R, Aaronson D, Bronsky E, Chervinsky P, et al. Ipratroprium bromide nasal spray 0.03% and beclomethasone nasal spray alone and in combination for the treatment of rhinorrhea in perennial rhinitis. Ann Allergy 1999; 82:349–359.

26

Impact of Nonallergic Rhinitis on Chemosensory Function

Thomas Hummel, Mandy Scheibe, and Thomas Zahnert
Department of Otolaryngology, Smell and Taste Clinic, University of Dresden Medical School ("Technische Universität Dresden"), Dresden, Germany

Basile N. Landis
Department of Otolaryngology, University of Geneva, Geneva, Switzerland

INTRODUCTION

Disturbances of the chemical senses are frequent. It has been estimated that hundreds of thousands of patients present to medical practitioners each year with complaints of smell dysfunction (1–4). The high prevalence of olfactory disorders becomes clearer from results of population-based studies. In one such investigation, 24% of individuals aged 53 to 97 were found to have impaired olfactory function (5), whereas another such study showed a prevalence of 19% among individuals aged 20 and older (6). Other work indicates that at least 5% of the general population has a severe olfactory deficit in the sense of anosmia (Table 1) (7).

Apart from aging, which is the most significant cause of olfactory loss (10,11), the three other major causes of olfactory disorders are (i) head trauma, (ii) infections of the upper respiratory tract (URTI), and (iii) sinunasal disease (SND). Major characteristics of these three causes are summarized in Table 2. Among patients who present themselves with chemosensory disorders to specialized centers, these three etiologies account for approximately 60% to 80% of the underlying causes (12–15), with each of the three different etiologies contributing approximately 20% to 30% to that percentage. However, among patients who are referred to otorhinolaryngological outpatient clinics (4), these figures are 72% for SND-related olfactory loss, 11% for post-URTI olfactory dysfunction, and 5% for olfactory loss following head trauma, suggesting that SND-related olfactory loss is most significant. In fact, it has been suggested that one-third of patients with chronic rhinosinusitis exhibit severe olfactory dysfunction and that another one-third have moderate olfactory loss (16) [compare also (17)]. However, the likelihood of a severe olfactory impairment is strongly related to the type of SND. According to the recent publication of the European Academy of Allergology and Clinical Immunology (18), SND has different presentations. Further, chronic SND can be divided into chronic SND with and without nasal polyps. The presence of polyps significantly raises the chance of severe hyposmia or even anosmia, whereas mild forms of chronic SND are rarely associated with anosmia.

Why is it important to have normal olfactory function? When the sense of smell is lost, our appreciation of foods and drinks is seriously compromised. In addition, we are deprived of a warning system that alerts us to dangers from fire or spoiled foods (19–23). Olfactory function also plays a significant role in interpersonal relations (24–27). However, it is probably the inability to enjoy foods or drinks that is the top complaint when the sense of smell has been lost (8,13,22,28).

TABLE 1 Definitions of Terms Related to Olfactory Loss

Category of olfactory dysfunction	Term	Definition
Quantitative olfactory dysfunction	Anosmia	Complete loss of olfactory function
	Functional anosmia	Diagnosed on the basis of psycho-physical tests; subjects score in the range compatible with anosmia; however, some olfactory function may still be present
	Hyposmia	Decreased olfactory sensitivity
	Hyperosmia	Increased olfactory sensitivity
Qualitative olfactory dysfunction	Parosmia/troposmia	Distorted perception of odors in the presence of an odor source
	Phantosmia	Perception of odors in the absence of an odor source, "odor phantoms"

Source: From Refs. 8 and 9.

In this context, it appears to be important to mention that olfactory loss typically also produces a decrease in intranasal trigeminal sensitivity (29–32), at least temporarily, meaning that the perception of stinging, tickling, burning, etc., decreases. On the other hand, inflammatory conditions may also produce an

TABLE 2 Olfactory Dysfunction in Relation to Its Three Major Causes

	Head trauma	Upper respiratory tract infection	Sinunasal disease
Assumed cause	Shearing of axons from olfactory receptor neurons at the level of the cribriform plate	Destruction of olfactory epithelium, either directly through microbiological agent or following autoimmune responses	Mechanical obstruction of olfactory cleft; secondary edema due to local inflammatory processes; and functional disruption of olfactory receptor neuron action
Epithelial findings	Degeneration	Metaplasia, defective development of olfactory receptor neurons	Mostly normal; often influx of lymphocytes, macrophages, and eosinophils
Occurrence of olfactory disturbances	≤5%	≤1%	Frequent
Approximate age	All ages	Older than 50 yr	20–70 yr
Rapid onset of olfactory dysfunction	+++	+++	−
Degree of olfactory loss	+++	++	+
Occurrence of parosmia	++	+++	−
Recovery possible	+	++	+++
	Improvement mostly in hyposmic patients, mostly within 2 years following the trauma	Improvement in more than 60%, even over a period of several years	Responsive to surgical therapy or anti-inflammatory treatment, e.g., with corticosteroids

Note: −, not true; +, sometimes the case; ++, frequently so; +++, mostly the case.

increased responsiveness to intranasal trigeminal stimuli (33,34), in the sense that people react more strongly to irritants. Although the evidence for an increased trigeminal sensitivity is largely based upon work in allergic rhinitis, this effect may be found to extrapolate to nonallergic rhinitis in the future.

HOW TO ASSESS OLFACTORY FUNCTION

Testing of olfactory function is necessary because the subjects' self ratings of olfactory function are unreliable (35). Although there are numerous ways of addressing this issue in the clinical context, it is the psychophysical tests that are most frequently used, simply because they are relatively straightforward. A differentiation should be made between quick screening tests (e.g., 36,39) and more extensive, validated tests that allow for the detailed diagnosis of patients (e.g., 10,15,40–43). The best validated olfactory tests include the University of Pennsylvania Smell Identification Test [a test based on the forced choice identification of odors (10)], the Connecticut Chemosensory Clinical Research Center test [a test combining a measure for odor thresholds and odor identification (15)], and the "Sniffin' Sticks" (a test combining measures for odor threshold, odor identification, and odor discrimination) (41,42). Generally, identification and discrimination tests are believed to reflect central olfactory processing while thresholds are thought to reflect peripheral function to a stronger degree (44–49). Although this idea of a certain pattern pathognomonic for "central" olfactory disturbances seems attractive, the vast majority of studies have as yet failed to confirm such typical pathology-associated patterns (50,51).

In addition, olfactory function may be assessed using olfactory event-related potentials (ERP), which are extracted from the electroencephalogram (52). Olfactory ERP (i) are direct correlates of neuronal activation, (ii) have a high temporal resolution, (iii) allow the investigation of the sequential processing of olfactory information, and (iv) can be obtained independently of the subject's response bias. Based on a system developed by Kobal (53,54), odors are applied intranasally. Earlier peaks of the olfactory ERP are more related to the encoding of stimulus intensity or stimulus quality, whereas later components are more related to the frequency or the salience of the stimulus (55–58). Results from ERP investigations provide significant information in the testing of malingering patients.

In addition, olfactory activation can be assessed through functional imaging (59–61), e.g., positron emission tomography, functional magnetic resonance imaging, or magnetic source imaging based on magnetoencephalography. However, in order to become relevant for routine clinical investigations (62), these techniques await standardization and validation.

OLFACTORY LOSS FOLLOWING INFECTIONS OF THE URTI

Olfactory loss following URTI typically starts with an episode of a cold during which the sense of smell is lost (63). Few studies have investigated the epidemiology and/or prognostic outcome of post-URTI olfactory loss (64–67). While the agent leading to olfactory loss remains unknown, it has been suggested that influenza and parainfluenza viruses play a dominant role (68) [compare (65)]. Interestingly, decreased olfactory function during the course of a cold has been observed in the absence of signs of nasal congestion (63), while there was little or no change in trigeminal function (69). Women above the age of 50 seem to be particularly prone to acquire post-URTI olfactory loss (65,70,71). Clinically, it is important to inform patients with post-URTI olfactory loss about the possibility of parosmia, which is frequently found during the recovery period (see below) (72,73).

Prognosis and Treatment of Post-URTI Olfactory Loss

Several authors described recovery rates for post-URTI disorders to be highest within the first year (66,74,75). In approximately 5% to 10% of the cases, total recovery can be observed, while up to 60% of all patients experience partial recovery of some olfactory function over the following years. This recovery is probably based on the ability of olfactory receptor neurons to regenerate (76,77). Younger patients seem to exhibit a higher recovery rate than older ones (71,78). Other than quantitative olfactory loss, qualitative disorders have a better prognosis. Parosmias tend to disappear/decrease to a bearable level after one to two years (8,72).

No pharmacological therapy has been established for post-URTI olfactory loss (79–81). In some patients with parosmia, surgical removal of the olfactory epithelium may be considered as a cure (82).

Studies on treating olfactory dysfunction with zinc produced negative results (70,79,83). Similarly, estrogens are probably ineffective in the treatment of olfactory loss (7,12,84,85). Candidates for the pharmacological treatment of olfactory dysfunction include caroverine (70), vitamin A (80,86), and minocycline (87). Nonpharmacological treatments include, for example, olfactory training (88).

SND–RELATED OLFACTORY LOSS

SND has been known for a long time to decrease olfactory abilities due to the mechanical obstruction of nasal cavity and thereby restricting the airflow to the olfactory cleft (89–93). During the last two decades and especially due to standardization of olfactory tests (10,93), mild olfactory impairments could also be identified in other groups of patients, such as uncomplicated chronic rhinitis or allergies (94–98). The diagnosis of SND-related olfactory is based on a thorough history (Table 2), nasal endoscopy, structured olfactory testing, a computed tomography scan/magnetic resonance imaging of the nasal cavities, and, possibly, the results from a therapeutic trial of systemic corticosteroids (93). SND may be of allergic or nonallergic origin [roughly one-quarter of patients with sinus disease are nonatopic (99) and approximately one-third of patients with polyps are nonallergic (100)], but the etiology will not be discussed in detail (90,94–98,101). However, it appears to be of interest to mention that nasal allergies may also produce an increased responsiveness to trigeminal stimuli (33,34).

Surgical Treatment

When SND patients do not experience improvement by conservative treatment (see below), endoscopic sinus surgery (ESS) should be considered. Preoperative assessment of olfactory function is important because (i) patients with SND are frequently unaware of their olfactory loss and (ii) occurrence of olfactory loss after endonasal surgery has been reported to be as high as 1% (102,103), although these estimates may exaggerate the potential risk (104–106).

In most cases, ESS is associated with significant improvement of olfactory function (104,105). Specifically, most successful outcomes have been described for radical ethmoidectomy with middle turbinate resection (107). However, absence or deterioration of olfactory detection thresholds in SND patients following ESS has been reported (108,109). Post-ESS olfactory dysfunction could be due to several mechanisms with persistent mucosal inflammation/edema in the region of the olfactory epithelium being one possible explanation (110). In addition to postoperative edema, recurrence of polyps, scar tissue, or granulation may contribute to failure of surgery in terms of the sense of smell (111). Furthermore, there is a certain risk of iatrogenic injuries to the olfactory epithelium, associated with extensive ethmoidectomy (112). So far there is no study investigating the exact indication for surgery in order to improve olfactory function. Having said this, the surgical indication is usually based on sinunasal symptoms such as nasal obstruction, rhinorrhea, or facial pain, and postoperative improvement of olfactory function is typically regarded as a "beneficial side effect." Based on the current literature, it is difficult if not impossible to predict the extent of post-ESS olfactory improvement.

Conservative Therapy

Bacteria involved in purulent acute sinusitis are relatively sensitive to antibiotic therapy, although *Staphylococcus aureus* and *Pseudomonas aeruginosa* can exhibit antibiotic resistance. Recently, minocycline has been proposed for the treatment of SND-related olfactory loss (87), partly also because of its possible antiapoptotic effects on olfactory receptor neurons.

Among other effects, corticosteroids act as anti-inflammatory drugs (113). They reduce submucosal edema and mucosal hypersecretion and thereby increase nasal patency. Systemically administered steroids are of help in many SND patients (93,114–117). In addition to their anti-inflammatory activity, corticosteroids may also have a direct effect on olfactory function (94,118) by modulating the function of olfactory receptor neurons through effects on olfactory Na–K–ATPase (113). In fact, systemic steroids are often helpful in patients without mechanical obstruction due to polyps or obvious inflammatory changes [compare (93,117,119)]. In these cases, steroids are believed to be helpful in the diagnosis of cryptogenic SND-associated olfactory loss (120).

Systemic administration of corticosteroids is frequently employed for diagnostic purposes (120). In those cases in which a patients' sense of smell improves in response to systemic steroids, treatment is typically continued with locally administered steroids. Although systemic steroids are more effective than locally administered steroids (118,121), prescription of systemic steroids over an extended period of time is rarely warranted due to major side effects (89,119). It seems possible, however, to repeatedly administer short courses of systemic steroids every 6 to 12 months.

Not all patients respond to systemic treatment with corticosteroids—although many of them exhibit typical signs of SND-related olfactory loss. A simple reason for the failure of this treatment might be that their olfactory epithelium has been severely lesioned by the chronic inflammation and/or repetitive URTI (64), which ultimately may lead to degeneration of the olfactory epithelium and its replacement with respiratory mucosa (122).

A number of studies indicate the usefulness of topical steroids (96,114,116,123), also in combination with systemic treatment (124). However, the role of topical steroids in the treatment of SND-related olfactory loss has been seriously questioned (118,120,121,125–128). So far, no factors predicting a favorable response to topical steroids have been identified. A reason why systemic steroids have a higher therapeutic effect than topical steroids (93,121) may relate to the deposition of the

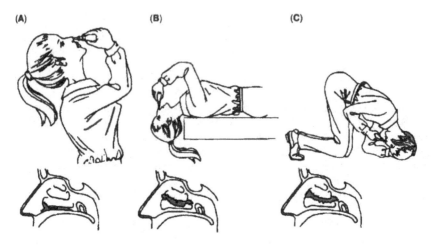

FIGURE 1 Distribution of blue dye in the nasal cavity following administration of nasal sprays. **(A)** Head-tipped-back-position, **(B)** Mygind's position, and **(C)** praying-to-Mecca position. Note the distribution of the spray in the inferior position of the nose in the head-tipped-back-position **(A)**. *Source*: From Refs. 128 and 132.

spray in the nasal cavity. It has been shown that only a small amount of nasally applied sprays reaches the olfactory cleft (129–131). Considering that the dominant function of the nose is the filtering of inspired air, it is easily understood that little or nothing of applied spray reaches the olfactory epithelium. This may be improved slightly by application of sprays in "head-down forward position" (Fig. 1) (118).

Other reasons for the greater efficacy of systemic steroids may relate to the site of action of steroids in SND patients. It has been speculated that the site of inflammation relevant to olfactory loss may not always be in the mucosa but in the central nervous system (133,134). This hypothesis appears particularly attractive in patients who respond to systemic steroids, but have no apparent signs of nasal inflammation and do not respond to locally administered steroids.

In addition to the use of steroids, there are still other therapeutic approaches to the restoration of olfactory loss. They include the use of antileukotrienes (135), sodium citrate (136), saline lavages (137), or approaches that have received less vigorous scientific investigation, e.g., dietary changes (138), acupuncture (139), antiallergy immunotherapy (140), or herbal treatments (141).

CONCLUSIONS

Olfactory dysfunction is frequently associated with chronic or acute SND of allergic, nonallergic, or indeterminate origin. Apart from nasal obstruction, rhinorrhea, and facial pain, this might have further negative impact on the patients' quality of life. In contrast to other causes of olfactory dysfunction (trauma and URTI), SND-related olfactory impairment can be treated successfully in many cases. Thus, it appears worthwhile to focus on olfactory dysfunction in SND patients, especially because treatment of the underlying SND might also improve the olfactory dysfunction. Importantly, olfactory function can also be used as a reliable, validated gauge for either severity of chronic SND or the therapeutic success in the treatment of chronic SND, which, in turn, is typically difficult to assess.

REFERENCES

1. Panel on Communicative Disorders to the National Advisory Neurological and Communicative Disorders and Stroke Council. NIH pub. no. 79-1914, 1979:319.
2. Wysocki CJ, Gilbert AN. National Geographic Smell Survey. Effects of age are heterogeneous. Ann NY Acad Sci 1989; 561:12–28.
3. Hoffman HJ, Ishii EK, MacTurk RH. Age-related changes in the prevalence of smell/taste problems among the United States adult population. Results of the 1994 disability supplement to the National Health Interview Survey (NHIS). Ann NY Acad Sci 1998; 855:716–722.
4. Damm M, Temmel A, Welge-Lüssen A, et al. Epidemiologie und Therapie von Riechstörungen in Deutschland, Österreich und der Schweiz. HNO 2004; 52:112–120.
5. Murphy C, Schubert CR, Cruickshanks KJ, et al. Prevalence of olfactory impairment in older adults. JAMA 2002; 288:2307–2312.
6. Brämerson A, Johansson L, Ek L, et al. Prevalence of olfactory dysfunction: the skövde population-based study. Laryngoscope 2004; 114:733–737.
7. Landis BN, Konnerth CG, Hummel T. A study on the frequency of olfactory dysfunction. Laryngoscope 2004; 114:1764–1769.
8. Hummel T, Nordin S. Olfactory disorders and their consequences for quality of life—a review. Acta Otolaryngol 2005; 125:116–121.
9. Leopold D. Distortion of olfactory perception: diagnosis and treatment. Chem Senses 2002; 27:611–615.
10. Doty RL, Shaman P, Dann M. Development of the University of Pennsylvania Smell Identification Test: a standardized microencapsulated test of olfactory function. Physiol Behav 1984; 32:489–502.
11. Hummel T, Heilmann S, Murphy C. Age-related changes of chemosensory functions. In: Rouby C, Schaal B, Dubois D, et al., eds. Olfaction, Taste and Cognition. New York: Cambridge University Press, 2002:441–456.
12. Deems DA, Doty RL, Settle RG, et al. Smell and taste disorders: a study of 750 patients from the University of Pennsylvania Smell and Taste Center. Arch Otorhinolaryngol Head Neck Surg 1991; 117:519–528.
13. Temmel AF, Quint C, Schickinger-Fischer B, et al. Characteristics of olfactory disorders in relation to major causes of olfactory loss. Arch Otolaryngol Head Neck Surg 2002; 128:635–641.
14. Mott AE, Leopold DA. Update in otolaryngology I: disorders on taste and smell. Med Clin North Am 1991; 75:1321–1353.
15. Cain WS, Gent JF, Goodspeed RB, Leonard G. Evaluation of olfactory dysfunction in the Connecticut Chemosensory Clinical Research Center (CCCRC). Laryngoscope 1988; 98:83–88.
16. Klimek L, Hummel T, Moll B, et al. Lateralized and bilateral olfactory function in patients with chronic sinusitis compared to healthy controls. Laryngoscope 1998; 108:111–114.
17. Lanza DC, Kennedy DW. Adult rhinosinusitis defined. Otolaryngol Head Neck Surg 1997; 117:S1–S7.
18. Fokkens W, Lund V, Bachert C, et al. EAACI position paper on rhinosinusitis and nasal polyps executive summary. Allergy 2005; 60(5):583–601.
19. Engen T. Odor Sensation and Memory. New York: Praeger, 1991.
20. von Skramlik E. Handbuch der Physiologie der niederen Sinne. Leipzig: Georg Thieme, 1926:274–279.
21. Santos DV, Reiter ER, DiNardo LJ, Costanzo RM. Hazardous events associated with impaired olfactory function. Arch Otolaryngol Head Neck Surg 2004; 130:317–319.
22. Lämmle H. Über Geruchsstörungen und ihre klinische Bedeutung. Arch Ohr Nas Kehlk Heilk 1931; 130:22–42.
23. Chalke HD, Dewhurst JR. Coal gas poisoning: loss of sense of smell as a possible contributory factor with old people. Br Med J 1957; 2:1915–1917.

24. Eggert F, Luszyk D, Haberkorn K, et al. The major histocompatibility complex and the chemosensory signalling of individuality in humans. Genetica 1998; 104:265–273.
25. Eklund AC, Belchak MM, Lapidos K, et al. Polymorphisms in the HLA-linked olfactory receptor genes in the Hutterites. Hum Immunol 2000; 61:711–717.
26. Jacob S, McClintock MK, Zelano B, Ober C. Paternally inherited HLA alleles are associated with women's choice of male odor. Nat Genet 2002; 30:175–179.
27. Stern K, McClintock MK. Regulation of ovulation by human pheromones. Nature 1998; 392:177–179.
28. Miwa T, Furukawa M, Tsukatani T, et al. Impact of olfactory impairment on quality of life and disability. Arch Otolaryngol Head Neck Surg 2001; 127:497–503.
29. Kobal G, Hummel C. Cerebral chemosensory evoked potentials elicited by chemical stimulation of the human olfactory and respiratory nasal mucosa. Electroencephalogr Clin Neurophysiol 1988; 71:241–250.
30. Walker JC, Jennings RA. Comparison of odor perception in humans and animals. In: Laing DG, Doty RL, Breipohl W, eds. The Human Sense of Smell. Berlin: Springer, 1991:261–280.
31. Hummel T, Barz S, Lötsch J, et al. Loss of olfactory function leads to a decrease of trigeminal sensitivity. Chem Senses 1996; 21:75–79.
32. Gudziol H, Schubert M, Hummel T. Decreased trigeminal sensitivity in anosmia. ORL J Otorhinolaryngol Relat Spec 2001; 63:72–75.
33. Shusterman D, Murphy MA, Balmes J. Differences in nasal irritant sensitivity by age, gender, and allergic rhinitis status. Int Arch Occup Environ Health 2003; 76:577–583.
34. Doerfler H, Hummel T, Klimek L, Kobal G. Intranasal trigeminal sensitivity in subjects with allergic rhinitis. Eur Arch Otorhinolaryngol 2006; 263:86–90.
35. Landis BN, Hummel T, Hugentobler M, et al. Ratings of overall olfactory function. Chem Senses 2003; 28:691–694.
36. Doty RL, Marcus A, Lee WW. Development of the 12-item cross-cultural smell identification test (CC-SIT). Laryngoscope 1996; 106:353–356.
37. Briner HR, Simmen D. Smell diskettes as screening test of olfaction. Rhinology 1999; 37:145–148.
38. Davidson TM, Freed C, Healy MP, Murphy C. Rapid clinical evaluation of anosmia in children: the Alcohol Sniff Test. Ann NY Acad Sci 1998; 855:787–792.
39. Hummel T, Konnerth CG, Rosenheim K, Kobal G. Screening of olfactory function with a four-minute odor identification test: reliability, normative data, and investigations in patients with olfactory loss. Ann Otol Rhinol Laryngol 2001; 110:976–981.
40. Kobal G, Hummel T, Sekinger B, et al. "Sniffin' Sticks": screening of olfactory performance. Rhinology 1996; 34:222–226.
41. Hummel T, Sekinger B, Wolf S, et al. "Sniffin' Sticks": olfactory performance assessed by the combined testing of odor identification, odor discrimination and olfactory threshold. Chem Senses 1997; 22:39–52.
42. Kobal G, Klimek L, Wolfensberger M, et al. Multicenter investigation of 1,036 subjects using a standardized method for the assessment of olfactory function combining tests of odor identification, odor discrimination, and olfactory thresholds. Eur Arch Otorhinolaryngol 2000; 257:205–211.
43. Kondo H, Matsuda T, Hashiba M, Baba S. A study of the relationship between the T&T olfactometer and the University of Pennsylvania Smell Identification Test in a Japanese population. Am J Rhinol 1998; 12:353–358.
44. Hawkes CH, Shephard BC. Selective anosmia in Parkinson's disease? Lancet 1993; 341:435–436.
45. Koss E, Weiffenbach JM, Haxby JV, Friedland RP. Olfactory detection and recognition in Alzheimer's disease. Lancet 1987; 1:622.
46. Koss E, Weiffenbach JM, Haxby JV, Friedland RP. Olfactory detection and identification performance are dissociated in early Alzheimer's disease. Neurology 1988; 38: 1228–1232.
47. Frasnelli JA, Temmel AF, Quint C, et al. Olfactory function in chronic renal failure. Am J Rhinol 2002; 16:275–279.

48. Hornung DE, Kurtz DB, Bradshaw CB, et al. The olfactory loss that accompanies an HIV infection. Physiol Behav 1998; 15:549–556.
49. Jones-Gotman M, Zatorre RJ. Olfactory identification deficits in patients with focal cerebral excision. Neuropsychologia 1988; 26:387–400.
50. Mesholam RI, Moberg PJ, Mahr RN, Doty RL. Olfaction in neurodegenerative disease: a meta-analysis of olfactory functioning in Alzheimer's and Parkinson's diseases. Arch Neurol 1998; 55:84–90.
51. Daum RF, Sekinger B, Kobal G, Lang CJ. Riechprüfung mit "Sniffin' Sticks" zur klinischen Diagnostik des Morbus Parkinson. Nervenarzt 2000; 71:643–650.
52. Hummel T, Kobal G. Olfactory event-related potentials. In: Simon SA, Nicolelis MAL, eds. Methods and Frontiers in Chemosensory Research. Boca Raton: CRC press, 2001: 429–464.
53. Kobal G, Plattig KH. Methodische Anmerkungen zur Gewinnung olfaktorischer EEG-Antworten des wachen Menschen (Objektive Olfaktometrie). Z EEG-EMG 1978; 9:135–145.
54. Kobal G. Elektrophysiologische Untersuchungen des menschlichen Geruchssinns. Stuttgart: Thieme Verlag, 1981.
55. Picton TW, Hillyard SA. Endogenous event-related potentials. In: Picton TW, ed. EEG-Handbook, Revised Series. Vol. 3. Amsterdam: Elsevier, 1988:361–426.
56. Pause BM, Sojka B, Krauel K, Ferstl R. The nature of the late positive complex within the olfactory event-related potential. Psychophysiology 1996; 33:168–172.
57. Krauel K, Pause BM, Sojka B, et al. Attentional modulation of central odor processing. Chem Senses 1998; 23:423–432.
58. Donchin E, Karis D, Bashore TR, et al. Cognitive psychophysiology and human information processing. In: Coles MGH, Donchin E, Porges SW, eds. Psychophysiology: Systems, Processes and Applications. New York: Guilford Press, 1986.
59. Savic I. Imaging of brain activation by odorants in humans. Curr Opin Neurobiol 2002; 12:455–461.
60. Zald DH, Pardo JV. Functional neuroimaging of the olfactory system in humans. Int J Psychophysiol 2000; 36:165–181.
61. Kettenmann B, Hummel T, Kobal G. Functional imaging of olfactory activation in the human brain. In: Simon SA, Nicolelis MAL, eds. Methods and Frontiers in Chemosensory Research. Boca Raton: CRC press, 2001:477–506.
62. Henkin RI, Levy LM, Lin CS. Taste and smell phantoms revealed by brain functional MRI (fMRI). J Comput Assist Tomogr 2000; 24:106–123.
63. Hummel T, Rothbauer C, Barz S, et al. Olfactory function in acute rhinitis. Ann NY Acad Sci 1998; 855:616–624.
64. Jafek BW, Hartman D, Eller PM, et al. Postviral olfactory dysfunction. Am J Rhinol 1990; 4:91–100.
65. Sugiura M, Aiba T, Mori J, Nakai Y. An epidemiological study of postviral olfactory disorder. Acta Otolaryngol Suppl (Stockh) 1998; 538:191–196.
66. Faulcon P, Portier F, Biacabe B, Bonfils P. Anosmie secondaire à une rhinite aiguë: sémiologie et évolution à propos d'une série de 118 patients. Ann Otolaryngol Chir Cervicofac 1999; 116:351–357.
67. Duncan H. Postviral olfactory loss. In: Seiden AM, ed. Taste and Smell Disorders. New York: Thieme, 1997:72–78.
68. Konstantinidis I, Mueller A, Frasnelli J, et al. Post-infectious olfactory dysfunction exhibits seasonal pattern. Rhinology 2006; 44:135–139.
69. Hummel T, Rothbauer C, Pauli E, Kobal G. Effects of the nasal decongestant oxymetazoline on human olfactory and intranasal trigeminal function in acute rhinitis. Eur J Clin Pharmacol 1998; 54:521–528.
70. Quint C, Temmel AFP, Hummel T, Ehrenberger K. The quinoxaline derivative caroverine in the treatment of sensorineural smell disorders: a proof of concept study. Acta Otolaryngol 2002; 122:877–881.
71. Hummel T, Heilmann S, Hüttenbrink KB. Lipoic acid in the treatment of smell dysfunction following viral infection of the upper respiratory tract. Laryngoscope 2002; 112:2076–2080.

72. Portier F, Faulcon P, Lamblin B, Bonfils P. Sémiologie, étiologie et évolution des paros-mies: à propos de 84 cas. Ann Otolaryngol Chir Cervicofac 2000; 117:12–18.
73. Frasnelli J, Hummel T. Olfactory dysfunction and daily life. Eur Arch Otolaryngol 2004; 262:231–235.
74. Bonfils P, Corre FL, Biacabe B. Semiologie et etiologie des anosmies: a propos de 306 patients. Ann Otolaryngol Chir Cervicofac 1999; 116:198–206.
75. Murphy C, Doty RL, Duncan HJ. Clinical disorders of olfaction. In: Doty RL, ed. Hand-book of Olfaction and Gustation. New York: Marcel Dekker, 2003:461–478.
76. Beidler LM, Smallman RL. Renewal of cells within taste buds. J Cell Biol 1965; 27:263–272.
77. Gradziadei PPC, Monti-Graziadei GA. Continuous nerve cell renewal in the olfactory system. In: Jacobson M, ed. Handbook of Sensory Physiology. Vol. 9. New York: Springer, 1978:55.
78. Reden J, Mueller A, Mueller C, et al. Recovery of olfactory function following closed head injury or infections of upper respiratory tract. Arch Orl 2006; 132:265–269.
79. Henkin RI, Schecter PJ, Friedewald WT, et al. A double-blind study of the effects of zinc sulfate on taste and smell dysfunction. Am J Med Sci 1976; 272:285–299.
80. Yee KK, Rawson NE. Retinoic acid enhances the rate of olfactory recovery after olfac-tory nerve transection. Brain Res Dev Brain Res 2000; 124:129–132.
81. Hendriks APJ. Olfactory dysfunction. Rhinology 1988; 26:229–251.
82. Jafek BW, Murrow B, Linschoten M. Evaluation and treatment of anosmia. Curr Opin Otol Head Neck Surg 2000; 8:63–67.
83. Seiden AM. The initial assessment of patients with taste and smell disorders. In: Seiden AM, ed. Taste and Smell Disorders. New York: Thieme, 1997:4–19.
84. Hughes LF, McAsey ME, Donathan CL, et al. Effects of hormone replacement therapy on olfactory sensitivity: cross-sectional and longitudinal studies. Climacteric 2002; 5:140–150.
85. Dhong HJ, Chung SK, Doty RL. Estrogen protects against 3-methylindole-induced olfactory loss. Brain Res 1999; 824:312–315.
86. Garrett-Laster M, Russell RM, Jacques PF. Impairment of taste and olfaction in patients with cirrhosis: the role of vitamin A. Hum Nutr Clin Nutr 1984; 38:203–214.
87. Kern RC, Conley DB, Haines GK, Robinson AM. Treatment of olfactory dysfunction, II: studies with minocycline. Laryngoscope 2004; 114:2200–2204.
88. Hummel T, Rissom K. Müller A, Reden J, Weidenbecher M, Hüttenbrink KB. "Olfac-tory training" in patients with olfactory loss. Chem Senses 2005; 30:A206–A207.
89. Hotchkiss WT. Influence of prednisone on nasal polyposis with anosmia. Arch Otolar-yngol 1956:478–479.
90. Fein BT, Kamin PB, Fein NN. The loss of sense of smell in nasal allergy. Ann Allergy 1966; 24:278–283.
91. Klimek L, Moll B, Amedee RG, Mann WJ. Olfactory function after microscopic endo-nasal surgery in patients with nasal polyps. Am J Rhinol 1997; 11:251–255.
92. Seiden AM. Olfactory loss secondary to nasal and sinus pathology. In: Seiden AM, ed. Taste and Smell Disorders. New York: Thieme, 1997:52–71.
93. Seiden AM, Duncan HJ. The diagnosis of a conductive olfactory loss. Laryngoscope 2001; 111:9–14.
94. Klimek L, Eggers G. Olfactory dysfunction in allergic rhinitis is related to nasal eosin-ophilc inflammation. J Allergy Clin Immunol 1997; 100:159–164.
95. Seiden AM, Litwin A, Smith DV. Olfactory deficits in allergic rhinitis. Chem. Senses 1989; 14:746–747.
96. Stuck BA, Blum A, Hagner AE, et al. Mometasone furoate nasal spray improves olfac-tory performance in seasonal allergic rhinitis. Allergy 2003; 58:1195.
97. Apter AJ, Mott AE, Frank ME, Clive JM. Allergic rhinitis and olfactory loss. Ann Allergy Asthma Immunol 1995; 75:311–316.
98. Simola M, Malmberg H. Sense of smell in allergic and nonallergic rhinitis. Allergy 1998; 53:190–194.
99. Karlsson G, Holmberg K. Does allergic rhinitis predispose to sinusitis? Acta Otolarn-gyol Suppl 1994; 515:26–29.

100. Wong D, Dolovich J. Blood eosinophilia and nasal polyps. Am J Rhinol 1992; 6:195–198.
101. Cowart BJ, Flynn-Rodden K, McGeady SJ, Lowry LD. Hyposmia in allergic rhinitis. J Allergy Clin Immunol 1993; 91:747–751.
102. Kimmelman CP. The risk to olfaction from nasal surgery. Laryngoscope 1994; 104: 981–988.
103. Stevens CN, Stevens MH. Quantitative effects of nasal surgery on olfaction. Am J Otolaryngol 1985; 6:264–267.
104. Briner HR, Simmen D, Jones N. Impaired sense of smell in patients with nasal surgery. Clin Otolaryngol 2003; 28:417–419.
105. Damm M, Eckel HE, Jungehulsing M, Hummel T. Olfactory changes at threshold and suprathreshold levels following septoplasty with partial inferior turbinectomy. Ann Otol Rhinol Laryngol 2003; 112:91–97.
106. Pfaar O, Hüttenbrink KB, Hummel T. Assessment of olfactory function after septoplasty: a longitudinal study. Rhinology 2004; 42:195–199.
107. Jankowski R, Bodino C. Olfaction in patients with nasal polyposis: effects of systemic steroids and radical ethmoidectomy with middle turbinate resection (nasalization). Rhinology 2003; 41:220–230.
108. Hosemann W, Görtzen W, Wohlleben R, et al. Olfaction after endoscopic endonasal ethmoidectomy. Am J Rhinology 1993; 7:11–15.
109. Rowe-Jones JM, Mackay IS. A prospective study of olfaction following endoscopic sinus surgery with adjuvant medical treatment. Clin Otolaryngol 1997; 22:377–381.
110. Downey LL, Jacobs JB, Lebowitz RA. Anosmia and chronic sinus disease. Otolaryngol Head Neck Surg 1996; 115:24–28.
111. Min YG, Yun YS, Song BH, et al. Recovery of nasal physiology after functional endoscopic sinus surgery: olfaction and mucociliary transport. ORL J Otorhinolaryngol Relat Spec 1995; 57:264–268.
112. Jafek BW, Murrow B, Johnson EW. Olfaction and endoscopic sinus surgery. Ear Nose Throat J 1994; 73:548–552.
113. Fong KJ, Kern RC, Foster JD, et al. Olfactory secretion and sodium, potassium-adenosine triphosphatase: regulation by corticosteroids. Laryngoscope 1999; 109:383–388.
114. Golding-Wood DG, Holmstrom M, Darby Y, et al. The treatment of hyposmia with intranasal steroids. J Laryngol Otol 1996; 110:132–135.
115. Tos M, Svendstrup F, Arndal H, et al. Efficacy of an aqueous and a powder formulation of nasal budesonide compared in patients with nasal polyps. Am J Rhinol 1998; 12:183–189.
116. Mott AE, Cain WS, Lafreniere D, et al. Topical corticosteroid treatment of anosmia associated with nasal and sinus disease. Arch Otolaryngol Head Neck Surg 1997; 123: 367–372.
117. Stevens MH. Steroid-dependent anosmia. Laryngoscope 2001; 111:200–203.
118. Mott AE, Leopold DA. Disorders in taste and smell. Med Clin North Am 1991; 75: 1321–1353.
119. Jafek BW, Moran DT, Eller PM, et al. Steroid-dependent anosmia. Arch Otolaryngol Head Neck Surg 1987; 113:547–549.
120. Heilmann S, Hüttenbrink KB, Hummel T. Local and systemic administration of corticosteroids in the treatment of olfactory loss. Am J Rhinol 2004; 18:29–33.
121. Ikeda K, Sakurada T, Suzaki Y, Takasaka T. Efficacy of systemic corticosteroid treatment for anosmia with nasal and paranasal sinus disease. Rhinology 1995; 33:162–165.
122. Lee SH, Lim HH, Lee HM, et al. Olfactory mucosal findings in patients with persistent anosmia after endoscopic sinus surgery. Ann Otol Rhinol Laryngol 2000; 109:720–725.
123. Meltzer EO, Jalowayski AA, Orgel A, Harris AG. Subjective and objective assessments in patients with seasonal allergic rhinitis: effects of therapy with mometasone furoate nasal spray. J Allergy Clin Immunol 1998; 102:39–49.
124. Aukema AA, Mulder PG, Fokkens WJ. Treatment of nasal polyposis and chronic rhinosinusitis with fluticasone propionate nasal drops reduces need for sinus surgery. J Allergy Clin Immunol 2005; 115:1017–1023.

125. El Naggar M, Kale S, Aldren C, Martin FJ. Effect of Beconase nasal spray on olfactory function in post-nasal polypectomy patients: a prospective controlled trial. J Otolaryngol 1995; 109:941–944.
126. Blomqvist EH, Lundblad L, Bergstedt H, Stjarne P. Placebo-controlled, randomized, double-blind study evaluating the efficacy of fluticasone propionate nasal spray for the treatment of patients with hyposmia/anosmia. Acta Otolaryngol 2003; 123: 862–868.
127. Heilmann S, Just T, Göktas Ö, et al. Untersuchung der Wirksamkeit von systemischen bzw. topischen Corticoiden und Vitamin B bei Riechstörungen. Laryngo-Rhino-Otologie 2004; 86:1–6.
128. Benninger MS, Hadley JA, Osguthorpe JD, et al. Techniques of intranasal steroid use. Otolaryngol Head Neck Surg 2004; 130:5–24.
129. Hardy JG, Lee SW, Wilson CG. Intranasal drug delivery by spray and drops. J Pharmacy Pharmacol 1985; 37:294–297.
130. Newman SP, Moren F, Clarke SW. Deposition pattern from a nasal pump spray. Rhinology 1987; 25:77–82.
131. McGarry GW, Swan IR. Endoscopic photographic comparison of drug delivery by ear-drops and by aerosol spray. Clin Otolaryngol 1992; 17:359–360.
132. Kubba H, Spinou E, Robertson A. The effect of head position on the distribution of drops within the nose. Am J Rhinol 2000; 14:83–86.
133. Roob G, Fazekas F, Hartung HP. Peripheral facial palsy: etiology, diagnosis and treatment. Eur Neurol 1999; 41:3–9.
134. Wolf SR. Idiopathische Fazialisparese. HNO 1998; 46:786–798.
135. Parnes SM, Chuma AV. Acute effects of antileukotrienes on sinonasal polyposis and sinusitis. Ear Nose Throat J 2000; 79:18–20, 24–25.
136. Panagiotopoulos G, Naxakis S, Papavasiliou A, et al. Decreasing nasal mucus Ca++ improves hyposmia. Rhinology 2005; 43:130–134.
137. Bachmann G, Hommel G, Michel O. Effect of irrigation of the nose with isotonic salt solution on adult patients with chronic paranasal sinus disease. Eur Arch Otorhinolaryngol 2000; 257:537–541.
138. Rundles W. Prognosis in the neurologic manifestations of pernicious anemia. Am Soc Hematol 1946; 1:209–219.
139. Tanaka O, Mukaino Y. The effect of auricular acupuncture on olfactory acuity. Am J Chin Med 1999; 27:19–24.
140. Stevenson DD, Hankammer MA, Mathison DA, et al. Aspirin desensitization treatment of aspirin-sensitive patients with rhinosinusitis-asthma: long-term outcomes. J Allergy Clin Immunol 1996; 98:751–758.
141. Marz RW, Ismail C, Popp MA. Wirkprofil und Wirksamkeit eines pflanzlichen Kombinationspräparates zur Behandlung der Sinusitis. Wien Med Wochenschr 1999; 149:202–208.

27

Rhinitis as a Part of Sensory Hyperreactivity Characterized by Increased Capsaicin Cough Sensitivity

Eva Millqvist

Department of Respiratory, Asthma and Allergy Research Group, Medicine and Allergy, The Sahlgrenska Academy at Göteborg University, Göteborg, Sweden

INTRODUCTION

Rhinitis is a common problem among patients in health care. After excluding acute respiratory infections, allergy, nasal polyposis, and other defined disorders, a large number of patients are found to suffer from nonspecific nasal hyperreactivity, vasomotor rhinitis, or idiopathic rhinitis, without known pathophysiology. Among these patients, some complain of hyperreactivity to scents and chemicals such as perfumes, some flowers, tobacco smoke, pesticides, etc. In recent years, it has been possible to identify a new diagnosis for this group, sensory hyperreactivity (SHR) (1–3). This chapter will deal with etiology, prevalence, symptomatology, physiological tests, and treatment of this disorder.

Sensitivity to chemicals in the environment mediated through sensations of odor and sensory irritation (pungency) that evoke certain symptoms, is a common condition today, with various possible etiologies. Sensitivity, especially of the upper airways, to chemicals normally regarded as nontoxic is a common problem frequently reported in population studies (4–8). Airway symptoms induced by inhaled chemicals have been described in different conditions such as multiple chemical sensitivity (9) and sick building syndrome (10), but there has been a lack of objective findings, documented homogenous symptomatology, and known pathophysiology (11). Patients with allergy and asthma also frequently complain of airway symptoms induced by irritants such as car exhausts and perfume, as recorded in standard questionnaires used in conjunction with interviewing patients during their first visit to an allergy center (1,12). However, the pathogenesis behind airway symptoms induced by chemicals and scents in patients with or without allergy is not known.

BACKGROUND

The Sense of Smell and the CCS

Our olfactory system can distinguish between thousands of scents. A large family of olfactory receptors has been identified in rodents and humans, research that was awarded the Nobel Prize (13,14). When a scent is strong enough, not only the olfactory receptors are activated but also the trigeminal afferent C fibers in the nose and eyes. This activation produces what is called the nasal or ocular common chemical sense (CCS), and quite apart from the sense of smell, it also plays a major role in sensitivity to the chemical environment (15,16). This chemical sense, believed to be an important warning system for potentially hazardous chemicals, evokes sensations such as irritation, tickling, burning, warming, cooling, and stinging in the nasal and oral cavities and cornea via nociceptors and the trigeminal nerve and probably also via the vagus nerve (15,17). As many chemicals actually have a smell they may stimulate the olfactory system as well as the CCS, but normally the threshold for the CCS is higher than that for olfaction (18). The CCS handles reactions to chemicals, even those without a smell, including noxious, odorless substances such as some tear gases (e.g., chloroacetophenone and oleoresin capsicum). To differentiate the CCS from olfaction, nasal pungency has been tested in anosmic patients. Nasal pungency thresholds have been shown to be close to eye irritation thresholds and well above odor thresholds for most, but not all, compounds (8,15,16,18). Eye irritation may thus be a good assay for trigeminal chemical sensitivity, because smell does not interfere with it (19). Despite methodological progress, the impact of the trigeminal nerve on chemosensory function has received very limited attention, partially due to the lack of established means for investigating this sensory system.

C-Fiber Receptors

C-fiber receptors are found throughout the upper and lower airways and in the alveoli (20,21). In the upper airways, these receptors originate mainly from the trigeminal nerve and in the lower airway from the vagus nerve. The ophthalmic and the maxillary branches of the trigeminal nerve are responsible for the sensory innervation of the nasal cavity and the eyes. The slow-conducting, sensory, afferent C fibers are small in diameter, unmyelinated, and widely branched. Most C fibers contain neuropeptides such as substance P, neurokinin A, neuropeptide K (all of which are tachykinins), as well as calcitonin gene-related peptide and nerve growth factor (NGF). In both the upper and lower airways, neuropeptides from afferent fibers can cause neurogenic inflammation accompanied by vasodilatation, plasma extravasation, and mucus secretion. The afferent C fibers are involved in centrally mediated reflexes such as sneezing, cough, exocrine secretion, and hypertension. Inhalation of various chemicals and changes in pH, temperature, and osmolarity can activate afferent sensory fibers.

SENSORY HYPERREACTIVITY

SHR is a condition indicated by respiratory symptoms of the upper and lower airways induced by chemicals and scents, in combination with increased cough sensitivity to inhaled capsaicin (1–3,22).

We have previously reported, mainly on a group of women patients, with *symptoms that could be misinterpreted as allergy and/or asthma*, who were referred to our Asthma and Allergy Clinic for investigation of hyperreactive airways (1–3,22). Their commonest symptoms were rhinitis, hoarseness, coughing, dyspnoea, phlegm, and eye irritation, but some also experienced more general symptoms such as fatigue and headache. In most of these patients, the symptoms were induced by chemicals and scents such as perfume, cigarette smoke, paints, exhaust fumes, pesticides, and cleaning agents. These patients suffering from SHR showed no or limited response to antihistamines or nasal/inhaled corticosteroids and β_2-agonists, no bronchial obstruction after provocation with methacholine or histamine, and no signs of immunoglobulin E-mediated allergy. Many of them could not work, and had been on sick leave for long periods, or even granted disability pensions. SHR seems to be a chronic condition, as a recent study showed that a majority of a group of 18 patients demonstrated long-lasting problems (more than five years) with significantly reduced health-related quality of life (HRQL) and increased capsaicin cough sensitivity [Ternesten-Hasséus E, Löwhagen O, Millqvist E. Quality of life and capsaicin sensitivity in patients with airway symptoms induced by chemical agents—five years follow-up, (submitted)]. None of these patients developed allergy, asthma, or any other airway disease. The pathophysiological mechanisms underlying this condition are unclear, and it is sometimes even suggested that the condition is mainly psychosomatic, though no primary psychological mechanisms have been found. However, secondary psychological symptoms are seen, probably because the problems are difficult to deal with. Some patients with chemically induced airway symptoms likely end up visiting otorhinolaryngologists and ophthalmologists, as well as allergists and pulmonologists. Which clinic a patient contacts depends on the medical speciality to which their symptoms are most closely related. Despite the uncertainties in evaluating environmental syndromes, physicians have the duty to take the affected person's problems seriously: these patients are suffering from long-lasting problems that have a major effect on several dimensions of their HRQL [Ternesten-Hasséus E, Löwhagen O, Millqvist E. Quality of life and capsaicin sensitivity in patients with airway symptoms induced by chemical agents—five years follow-up, (submitted)] (23).

The diagnostic criteria for SHR should, as mentioned, first of all include self-reported airway sensitivity to chemicals and scents. To quantify self-reported sensitivity to chemicals and scents in the course of daily activities, a short 11-item chemical sensitivity scale for SHR (CSS-SHR) has been developed. The CSS-SHR shows approximately normal distributions, good reliability, and validity. A cut-off score of greater than or equal to 43 has been suggested for the diagnosis of SHR (24,25).

A suggested marker for SHR is increased cough sensitivity to inhaled capsaicin, compared to healthy subjects and symptom-free asthmatic patients, a sensitivity indicative of C fiber-mediated hypersensitivity of the sensory nerves (Fig. 1) (2,3,22,26). Preinhalation of lidocaine inhibits dose-dependent, capsaicin-induced cough, and other airway and eye symptoms in patients with SHR (2). The patients also experienced a significantly reduced HRQL, according to a general health profile, and there was a good correlation with capsaicin sensitivity (23). The response to inhaled capsaicin is not restricted to lower-airway symptoms, nasal/throat and eye irritation being common as well (Fig. 2), and the patients claim that they recognize the symptoms as "their usual" evoked by chemicals and scents. According to the patients, mucus appears to be produced mainly in the upper airways. These findings are consistent with previous studies, which found that the patients experienced similar difficulties after provocation with perfume (27,28). Interestingly, airway symptoms have been shown to be induced by perfume exposure during bronchial and eye provocation even when olfaction was isolated from exposure, implying that a trigeminal/vagal reflex operates via the respiratory tract or the eye as well (29).

A recent study found that basal levels of NGF in nasal lavage were significantly lower in the SHR patient group than in the control subjects (29). After capsaicin inhalation provocation, the patients showed a significant increase in NGF, which was related to capsaicin cough sensitivity. The symptom scores for rhinitis after the provocations had a strong, though perhaps unsurprising, correlation with an increase in NGF levels, as the nasal mucosa may have produced the factor

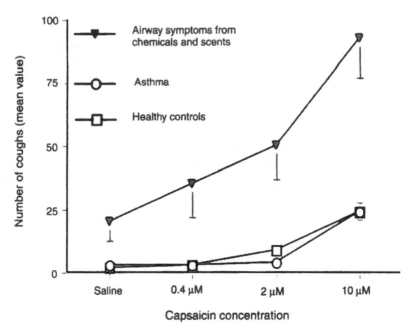

FIGURE 1 Inhalation of capsaicin in increasing concentrations induces an increasing number of coughs in 28 healthy subjects (*squares*), 10 patients with asthma (*circles*), and 10 patients with airway symptoms in response to chemicals and scents (*triangles*). The response of the latter group differs significantly from the others. Results are presented± SEM.

being analyzed. However, the mechanisms underlying the reaction are unclear: it could be reflex-mediated, a small amount of capsaicin could have reached the nose from the back, or some of the nebulized solution could have been dispersed and inhaled through the nose as the patients did not wear nose clips. The results emphasize once more the close connection between the upper and lower airways: an inhalation capsaicin cough test that provoked the lower airways resulted in measurable changes of a neurogenic marker of the upper airways.

CHRONIC COUGH

Coughing is a common clinical problem; when it persists for more than two months, it is generally regarded as chronic (30), though the exact definition of chronic cough varies in the literature. When pulmonary illnesses such as infections, cancer, alveolitis, asthma, and chronic obstructive pulmonary disease are excluded, the reasons for chronic cough may be gastro-esophageal reflux, rhinitis, or postnasal drip (30)—even though the existence of postnasal drip syndrome has been questioned (31). However, differential diagnosis still leaves a group of patients with unexplained cough ("idiopathic cough"), and in specialist cough clinics as many as 40% of patients may be diagnosed with this condition (32,33). Patients with chronic cough are known to have increased capsaicin cough sensitivity (34–36), and this sensitivity seems to be more pronounced when the cough is idiopathic (33). In patients with chronic cough and increased capsaicin cough sensitivity, Cho et al. recently found elevated levels of the neuropeptide substance

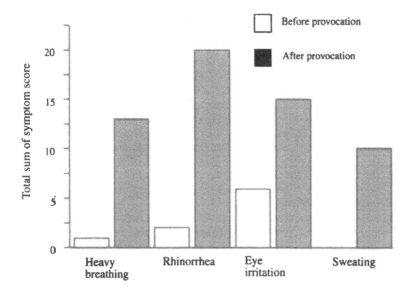

FIGURE 2 Total sum of the four symptom scores (0–3 points for each symptom) in 12 patients with sensory hyperreactivity before inhalation and after provocation with the highest dose of capsaicin (10 μM).

P in nasal lavage fluids (37). Patients with SHR can often also be classified as having chronic cough; longstanding problems with coughing in combination with airway chemical sensitivity and increased capsaicin cough response (38). However, patients with idiopathic chronic cough rarely seem to be questioned about chemical sensitivity as an inducing factor, or about symptoms mimicking asthma. To the best of our knowledge, this approach to chronic cough is seldom or never discussed.

CAPSAICIN

Capsaicin (8-methyl-*N*-vanillyl-6-nonenamide), a noxious and odorless vanilloid, is the pungent ingredient in *Capsicum annum*; it stimulates the nonmyelinated slow C fibers of the sensory nervous system via the genetically identified vanilloid receptor (TRPV1) (39). Capsaicin induces conjunctival irritation, and it is used for self-defense in so-called pepper sprays (40). It is a gastric mucosal irritant, and direct contact with the skin results in a burning sensation followed by a desensitization of the chemosensory afferent C fibers (41). Topically applied capsaicin cream has been used as an analgesic for neuralgias and other painful dermatological conditions (42). In recent years, there has been an increasing interest in capsaicin in pain research (41,43–45).

Capsaicin in Cough Provocations

Capsaicin is well known to induce cough when inhaled, and has often been used in cough provocation models to estimate the sensory neural reactivity of the lower airways (46–48). Stimulation of the afferent C fibers in animals causes bronchoconstriction (49), but in humans this effect of capsaicin provocation is uncertain. A minimal decrease in airway conductance has been found after capsaicin provocation, but with no difference in this response evident among normal, smoking, or asthmatic subjects (46). Several studies have confirmed that this minor, temporary effect probably cannot be detected by spirometry (1,3,22). Increased capsaicin cough sensitivity has been demonstrated in various conditions affecting the upper and lower airways (1,3,34,50–53) and in upper-respiratory infection (54). The cough sensitivity may differ by gender (55,56), and it increases during the pollen season in allergic patients (12). Capsaicin cough sensitivity is decreased in smokers without airway symptoms, supporting the hypothesis that nicotine either inhibits the receptors on the C fibers of the sensory nerves in the respiratory epithelium or induces neuropeptide depletion (57,58). Clinically, this may serve to explain some of the airway symptoms that are often seen after cessation of smoking.

Capsaicin in Nasal Provocations

Capsaicin challenge to the human nose leads to airway sensory nerve activation, and it induces a significant increase in the total protein and lactoferrin contents of nasal lavage fluid after challenge (59). The provocations are also followed by burning, rhinorrhoea, and lacrimation. In allergic rhinitis, enhanced secretory and inflammatory (cellular) responses have been found after local nasal provocation with capsaicin (60,61), and increased nasal sensitivity to capsaicin has been shown during the pollen season (62). Intranasal capsaicin has been used as a treatment of nonallergic rhinitis, indicating a desensitization due to depletion of neuropeptides (63,64).

CAPSAICIN INHALATION TEST IN SHR

An increased cough sensitivity to inhaled capsaicin has been shown in several studies of patients with SHR (1–3,22,23,26). These findings have led to the development of a capsaicin inhalation cough test, now in clinical use at various allergy centers in Sweden (1). Although the test is not specific for the condition, because other airway conditions are also known to be accompanied by an increased capsaicin cough sensitivity (3,34,50–53), recent research has found the test to be valuable in diagnosing SHR. Fifty-two consecutive patients referred for testing with methacholine, mainly due to suspected asthma, were also provoked with inhaled capsaicin in increasing concentrations. A majority of the patients showed no increased sensitivity to methacholine, but did demonstrate SHR and a positive response to capsaicin inhalation testing (22). Ninety-five consecutive patients with upper- and lower-airway problems, who had been admitted for allergy testing, underwent inhalation testing with three different concentrations of capsaicin; of these 95 patients, 15 (16%) were scored high enough on the capsaicin inhalation test to be classified has having SHR (1).

The test uses a stock solution of capsaicin: 1000 µM in ethanol (99.5%). Three aqueous test solutions of 0.4, 2.0, and 10 µM are prepared from the stock solution of capsaicin by dilution with 0.9% saline containing 1% by volume of ethanol. In one challenge, saline and capsaicin of three different concentrations are inhaled by means of a nebulizer. Each 1 mL dose is inhaled through a mouthpiece using tidal volume breathing to completion for six minutes to induce cough, followed by rest for four minutes. The number of coughs is counted for 10 minutes from the start of each provocation dose. The test is regarded as positive when certain levels of coughing are reached. The cut-off values for SHR obtained on a positive capsaicin inhalation test were set to 10, 35, and 55 for 0.4, 2, and 10 µM capsaicin, respectively (1). However, knowledge of the type of inhalation device used, particle size, airflow rate, and inspiratory flow rate are essential when comparing different outcomes of capsaicin-induced cough (38).

Capsaicin (C18H27NO3) has a molecular weight of 305 g, which means that a completed inhalation test represents exposure to 0.00377 g of pure capsaicin. This can be compared with the amount of capsaicin in chili fruits, which range between 0.02% and 1% pure capsaicin. A meal containing 100 g of chilies may contain up to 1 g of pure capsaicin. In some tropical countries, it is estimated that adults consume an average of 3 g of capsaicin per day. However, there are no indications that persons with *respiratory* sensitivity to chemicals should also be intolerant to *ingesting* food with high capsaicin content, though this has yet to be methodically studied.

CONCLUDING REMARKS

Throughout history, many conditions were controversial in the medical establishment until proper diagnostic methods became available, including multiple sclerosis, allergy, and asthma. During the 1940s and 1950s, it was still common to regard these conditions as purely psychosomatic. The more we learn about the underlying mechanisms and understand ways of diagnosing and treating them, the more the diseases have been recognized and studied. However, diagnoses without objective test methods remain a problem, and sometimes these conditions overlap each other. Some patients with multiple chemical sensitivity (MCS) reporting mainly airway symptoms could also be diagnosed with SHR (26), though the MCS criterion of a reported chemical injury as a cause of the problems (9) is not in accordance with SHR. The lack of effective medical treatment of SHR is frustrating for both patient and physician. Despite this shortcoming, "any" correct information about the condition is valuable: any knowledge that helps lessen the uncertainty makes this condition easier for both the patient and the doctor to deal with.

Olfaction and the sense of smell is a highly commercialized field. The fragrance market in the western world is increasing, but not only cosmetics and toiletries are perfumed. Plastics, cars, furniture, and clothes are scented, sometimes to hide or cover an unpleasant smell, or just to attract potential customers. Today, there are no scientific findings that prove whether the exposure to chemicals and artificial scents that our western lifestyle involves could actually be the cause of conditions such as SHR. But for certain, if you have established symptoms with such sensitivity, daily life presents many practical problems and a decreased quality of life.

The expression "united airways" is often used with reference to allergy and asthma, taken together; however, it is probably more or less applicable to most conditions of the airways, including nonallergic reactions to chemicals and scents. Hypothesizing that the airway symptoms found in SHR are due to a neurochemical imbalance, the upper and lower airways could mirror each other in terms of the reflexes of the trigeminal and the vagal nerves—the two main sensory nerves of the airways. Stimulation of nasal sensory nerves is known to be followed by release of substance P that stimulates glandular secretions and leads to pain and congestion (65). In SHR, neuropeptides released in the upper airways may induce symptoms in the lower airways, and vice versa. In patients with chronic cough, there was a fivefold increase of TRPV-1 staining nerve profiles and furthermore, a significant correlation between capsaicin tussive response and the number of TRPV-1 positive nerves (66). Whether there is also an increased expression of TRPV-1 positive nerves in the nasal mucosa in nonallergic rhinitis is not known. In SHR, we hypothesize that such changes have occurred in the upper as well as in the lower airways. Several clues indicate close neural interplay, and future research will probably yield answers to many of the questions that still remain in this field.

REFERENCES

1. Johansson A, Millqvist E, Nordin S, et al. Relationship between self-reported odor intolerance and sensitivity to inhaled capsaicin: proposed definition of airway sensory hyperreactivity and estimation of its prevalence. Chest 2006; 219:1623–1628.
2. Millqvist E. Cough provocation with capsaicin is an objective way to test sensory hyperreactivity in patients with asthma-like symptoms. Allergy 2000; 55(6):546–550.
3. Millqvist E, Bende M, Löwhagen O. Sensory hyperreactivity—a possible mechanism underlying cough and asthma-like symptoms. Allergy 1998; 53(12):1208–1212.
4. Bell IR, Schwartz GE, Peterson JM, et al. Self-reported illness from chemical odors in young adults without clinical syndromes or occupational exposures. Arch Environ Health 1993; 48(1):6–13.
5. Caress SM, Steinemann AC. A review of a two-phase population study of multiple chemical sensitivities. Environ Health Perspect 2003; 111(12):1490–1497.
6. Kreutzer R, Neutra RR, Lashuay N. Prevalence of people reporting sensitivities to chemicals in a population-based survey. Am J Epidemiol 1999; 150(1):1–12.
7. Meggs WJ, Dunn KA, Bloch RM, et al. Prevalence and nature of allergy and chemical sensitivity in a general population. Arch Environ Health 1996; 51(4):275–282.
8. Shusterman D. Odor-associated health complaints: competing explanatory models. Chem Senses 2001; 26(3):339–343.
9. Cullen MR. The worker with multiple chemical sensitivities: an overview. Occup Med 1987; 2(4):655–661.
10. Redlich CA, Sparer J, Cullen MR. Sick-building syndrome. Lancet 1997; 349(9057):1013–1016.
11. Terr AI. Environmental illness. A clinical review of 50 cases. Arch Intern Med 1986; 146(1):145–149.
12. Millqvist E, Johansson A, Bende M. Relationship of airway symptoms from chemicals to capsaicin cough sensitivity in atopic subjects. Clin Exp Allergy 2004; 34(4):619–623.
13. Buck LB. Olfactory receptors and odor coding in mammals. Nutr Rev 2004; 62(11):184–188.
14. Buck LB. The search for odorant receptors. Cell 2004; 116:117–119.
15. Cometto-Muniz JE, Cain WS. Trigeminal and olfactorial sensitivity: comparison of modalities and methods of measurement. Int Arch Environ Health 1998; 71(2):105–110.
16. Cometto-Muniz JE, Cain WS. Relative sensitivity of the ocular trigeminal, nasal trigeminal, and olfactory systems to airborne chemicals. Chemical Senses 1995; 20:191–198.
17. Doty RL. Intranasal trigeminal chemoreception: anatomy, physiology and psychophysics. In: Doty RL, ed. Handbook of Olfaction and Gustation. New York: Marcel Dekker, 1991:821–833.
18. Cometto-Muniz JE, Cain WS, Abraham MH, et al. Sensory properties of selected terpenes. Thresholds for odors, nasal pungency, and eye irritation. Ann NY Acad Sci 1998; 30(855):648–651.
19. Kleno J, Wolkoff P. Changes in eye blink frequency as a measure of trigeminal stimulation by exposure to limonene oxidation products, isoprene oxidation products and nitrate radicals. Int Arch Occup Environ Health 2004; 77(4):235–243.
20. Widdicombe JG. Neurophysiology of the cough reflex. Eur Respir J 1995; 8(7):1193–1202.
21. Widdicombe J. Airway receptors. Respir Physiol 2001; 125(1–2):3–15.

22. Ternesten-Hasseus E, Farbrot A, Löwhagen O, et al. Sensitivity to methacholine and capsaicin in patients with unclear respiratory symptoms. Allergy 2002; 57(6):501–507.
23. Millqvist E, Löwhagen O, Bende M. Quality of life and capsaicin sensitivity in patients with sensory airway hyperreactivity. Allergy 2000; 55(6):540–545.
24. Nordin S, Brämersson A, Liden E, et al. The Scandinavian odor-identification test: development, reliability, validity and normative data. Acta Otolaryngol (Stockh) 1998; 118:226–234.
25. Nordin S, Millqvist E, Lowhagen O, et al. A short chemical sensitivity scale for assessment of airway sensory hyperreactivity. Int Arch Occup Environ Health 2004; 77(4): 249–254.
26. Ternesten-Hasseus E, Bende M, Millqvist E. Increased capsaicin cough sensitivity in patients with multiple chemical sensitivity. J Occup Environ Med 2002; 44(11): 1012–1017.
27. Millqvist E, Bengtsson U, Löwhagen O. Provocations with perfume in the eyes induce airway symptoms in patients with sensory hyperreactivity. Allergy 1999; 54(5):495–499.
28. Millqvist E, Löwhagen O. Placebo-controlled challenges with perfume in patients with asthma-like symptoms. Allergy 1996; 51(6):434–439.
29. Millqvist E, Ternesten-Hasseus E, Ståhl A, et al. Changes in levels of nerve growth factor in nasal secretions after capsaicin inhalation in patients with airway symptoms from scents and chemicals. Environ Health Perspect 2005; 113:849–852.
30. Morice AH, Fontana GA, Sovijarvi AR, et al. The diagnosis and management of chronic cough. Eur Respir J 2004; 24(3):481–492.
31. Morice AH. Post-nasal drip syndrome-a symptom to be sniffed at? Pulm Pharmacol Ther 2004; 17(6):343–345.
32. Chung KF, Widdicombe JG. Cough as a symptom. Pulm Pharmacol Ther 2004; 17(6):329–332.
33. Haque RA, Usmani OS, Barnes PJ. Chronic idiopathic cough: a discrete clinical entity? Chest 2005; 127(5):1710–1713.
34. Choudry NB, Fuller RW. Sensitivity of the cough reflex in patients with chronic cough. Eur Respir J 1992; 5(3):296–300.
35. Nieto L, de Diego A, Perpina M, et al. Cough reflex testing with inhaled capsaicin in the study of chronic cough. Respir Med 2003; 97(4):393–400.
36. O'Connell F, Thomas VE, Pride NB, et al. Capsaicin cough sensitivity decreases with successful treatment of chronic cough. Am J Respir Crit Care Med 1994; 150(2):374–380.
37. Cho YS, Park SY, Lee CK, et al. Elevated substance P levels in nasal lavage fluids from patients with chronic nonproductive cough and increased cough sensitivity to inhaled capsaicin. J Allergy Clin Immunol 2003; 112(4):695–701.
38. Ternesten-Hasséus E, Löwhagen O, Johansson Å, et al. Inhalation method determines outcome of capsaicin inhalation in patients with chronic cough due to sensory hyperreactivity. Pulm Pharmacol Ther 2006; 19:172–178.
39. Caterina MJ, Schumacher MA, Tominaga M, et al. The capsaicin receptor: a heat-activated ion channel in the pain pathway. Nature 1997; 389(6653):816–824.
40. Claman FL, Patterson DL. Personal aerosol protection devices: caring for victims of exposure. Nurse Pract 1995; 20(11 Pt 1):54–56.
41. Szolcsanyi J. Forty years in capsaicin research for sensory pharmacology and physiology. Neuropeptides 2004; 38(6):377–384.
42. Keitel W, Frerick H, Kuhn U, et al. Capsicum pain plaster in chronic non-specific low back pain. Arzneimittelforschung 2001; 51(11):896–903.
43. Chuang HH, Prescott ED, Kong H, et al. Bradykinin and nerve growth factor release the capsaicin receptor from PtdIns(4,5)P2-mediated inhibition. Nature 2001; 411(6840): 957–962.
44. Caterina MJ, Julius D. The vanilloid receptor: a molecular gateway to the pain pathway. Annu Rev Neurosci 2001; 24:487–517.
45. Tominaga M, Julius D. Capsaicin receptor in the pain pathway. Jpn J Pharmacol 2000; 83(1):20–24.
46. Fuller RW, Dixon CM, Barnes PJ. Bronchoconstrictor response to inhaled capsaicin in humans. J Appl Physiol 1985; 58(4):1080–1084.

47. Karlsson JA, Sant'Ambrogio G, Widdicombe J. Afferent neural pathways in cough and reflex bronchoconstriction. J Appl Physiol 1988; 65:1007–1023.
48. Midgren B, Hansson L, Karlsson JA, et al. Capsaicin-induced cough in humans. Am Rev Respir Dis 1992; 146:347–351.
49. Bertrand C, Geppetti P, Graf PD, et al. Involvement of neurogenic inflammation in antigen-induced bronchoconstriction in guinea pigs. Am J Physiol 1993; 265(5 Pt 1): L507–L511.
50. Gordon SB, Curran AD, Turley A, et al. Glass bottle workers exposed to low-dose irritant fumes cough but do not wheeze. Am J Respir Crit Care Med 1997; 156(1):206–210.
51. Fujimura M, Kamio Y, Hashimoto T, et al. Airway cough sensitivity to inhaled capsaicin and bronchial responsiveness to methacholine in asthmatic and bronchitic subjects. Respirology 1998; 3(4):267–272.
52. Doherty MJ, Mister R, Pearson MG, et al. Capsaicin induced cough in cryptogenic fibrosing alveolitis. Thorax 2000; 55(12):1028–1032.
53. Doherty MJ, Mister R, Pearson MG, et al. Capsaicin responsiveness and cough in asthma and chronic obstructive pulmonary disease. Thorax 2000; 55(8):643–649.
54. O'Connell F, Thomas VE, Studham JM, et al. Capsaicin cough sensitivity increases during upper respiratory infection. Respir Med 1996; 90:279–286.
55. Fujimura M, Kasahara K, Kamio Y, et al. Female gender as a determinant of cough threshold to inhaled capsaicin. Eur Respir J 1996; 9(8):1624–1626.
56. Dicpinigaitis PV, Rauf K. The influence of gender on cough reflex sensitivity. Chest 1998; 113(5):1319–1321.
57. Dicpinigaitis PV. Cough reflex sensitivity in cigarette smokers. Chest 2003; 123(3): 685–688.
58. Millqvist E, Bende M. Capsaicin cough sensitivity is decreased in smokers. Respir Med 2001; 95(1):19–21.
59. Philip G, Baroody FM, Proud D, et al. The human nasal response to capsaicin. J Allergy Clin Immunol 1994; 94(6 Pt 1):1035–1045.
60. Sanico AM, Philip G, Proud D, et al. Comparison of nasal mucosal responsiveness to neuronal stimulation in non-allergic and allergic rhinitis: effects of capsaicin nasal challenge. Clin Exp Allergy 1998; 28(1):92–100.
61. Sanico AM, Koliatsos VE, Stanisz AM, et al. Neural hyperresponsiveness and nerve growth factor in allergic rhinitis. Int Arch Allergy Immunol 1999; 118(2–4):154–158.
62. Kowalski ML, Dietrich-Milobedzki A, Majkowska-Wojciechowska B, et al. Nasal reactivity to capsaicin in patients with seasonal allergic rhinitis during and after the pollen season. Allergy 1999; 54(8):804–810.
63. Van Rijswijk JB, Boeke EL, Keizer JM, et al. Intranasal capsaicin reduces nasal hyperreactivity in idiopathic rhinitis: a double-blind randomized application regimen study. Allergy 2003; 58(8):754–761.
64. Blom HM, Severijnen LA, Van Rijswijk JB, et al. The long-term effects of capsaicin aqueous spray on the nasal mucosa. Clin Exp Allergy 1998; 28(11):1351–1358.
65. Tai CF, Baraniuk JN. Upper airway neurogenic mechanisms. Curr Opin Allergy Clin Immunol 2002; 2(1):11–19.
66. Groneberg DA, Niimi A, Dinh QT, et al. Increased expression of transient receptor potential vanilloid-1 in airway nerves of chronic cough. Am J Respir Crit Care Med 2004; 170:1276–1280.

28

Vocal Cord Dysfunction, Gastroesophageal Reflux Disease, and Nonallergic Rhinitis

Ron Balkissoon

Department of Medicine, National Jewish Medical and Research Center, University of Colorado School of Medicine, Denver, Colorado, U.S.A.

INTRODUCTION

What is the association between vocal cord dysfunction (VCD), gastroesophageal reflux disease (GERD), and nonallergic rhinitis?

There are many patients who present with severe asthma that is not responsive to optimum asthma therapy. Such patients are typically evaluated for noncompliance, steroid resistance, complications of asthma such as Churg Strauss or allergic bronchopulmonary mycosis, or evidence of suboptimal control of rhinosinusitis and GERD. More recently, it has been recognized that many patients with difficult-to-control asthma have paradoxical movement of their vocal folds that may mimic symptoms of asthma. The common conditions of GERD and chronic rhinosinusitis, which are known to complicate asthma control, are also major causes for VCD. VCD may mimic or complicate asthma. Identifying this condition early and instituting appropriate therapy can significantly reduce iatrogenic-induced morbidity associated with overuse of systemic corticosteroids.

DEFINITION OF VCD

VCD refers to the paradoxical adduction of the vocal folds during inspiration and/or expiration. Using correct anatomical terms this disorder should be called vocal fold dysfunction. This disorder has been referred to by a variety of names, many reflecting early opinions that this was primarily a functional or conversion disorder—"factitious asthma," Munchausen's stridor, or "hysterical asthma" are just a few examples. More recently, there has been an appreciation of the fact that there can be respiratory symptoms caused by paradoxical adduction of the vocal folds during inspiration and early expiration with or without evidence of the classically described posterior chink (1). Morrison et al. (2) have recently introduced the term "irritable larynx syndrome" to encompass individuals with episodic laryngeal dysfunction triggered by irritant exposures with variable clinical manifestations including VCD, cough, muscle tension dysphonia, and globus sensation. Hence, irritable larynx syndrome and laryngeal dysfunction are terms that are somewhat more inclusive or descriptive of the phenomenon of upper airway compromise masquerading as asthma. Further, there is now a greater appreciation that besides psychological factors, GERD, posterior nasal drainage, and intense irritant exposures can lead to laryngeal hyperresponsiveness.

EPIDEMIOLOGY OF VCD

The exact incidence and prevalence of VCD are unknown. Brugman conducted the most exhaustive and comprehensive literature review with regard to the epidemiology of VCD to date (3). Kenn et al. in Europe reported a 3.1% prevalence of asthma in patients referred to a European pulmonary clinic (4) and 2.5% and 22% incidence in large urban emergency room departments in Philadelphia and Houston, respectively (5,6). Newman et al. conducted a seminal prospective evaluation of 167 patients with a diagnosis of intractable asthma and found that 10% of the patients had VCD alone and 30% of patients had VCD with asthma (7). This is the oft-cited study that reported a high prevalence in females who were health care workers and/or had been previously abused and/or had underlying psychological problems. Brugman describes several other studies that found VCD in 15% of military recruits presenting with exercise-induced dyspnea and in 5% of elite athletes with exercise-induced stridor with a higher percentage (8%) in cold weather athletes, in infants with GERD, and in 10% of approximately 370 pediatric patients referred for severe asthma, and one study that showed 14% had VCD and asthma in a group of adolescents. In fact, VCD occurred more frequently in association with asthma rather than alone (8).

With an ever-increasing number of health care providers having the awareness to look for VCD and perhaps a broader definition of what constitutes VCD, it is now evident that there are a number of groups that appear to be at increased risk for developing VCD beyond abused female health care workers. As outlined above, groups identified that may be at increased risk include elite athletes, military recruits, and individuals who have had high-level irritant exposures (8). Perhaps the most common groups to have VCD are individuals with postnasal drip, GERD, and/or underlying asthma. An examination of the current theories with regard to the pathogenesis of VCD allows one to understand the association between GERD, nonallergic rhinitis/postnasal drip, and asthma in patients with VCD.

PATHOPHYSIOLOGY OF VCD

Structure and Function of the Larynx

The larynx is the gateway to the trachea and consists of nine cartilages bound together by an elastic membrane and moved by a series of muscles (Fig. 1). Two sets of folds (also referred to as cords), the false vocal folds and the true vocal folds form the slit-like opening to the trachea called the glottis. The three major functions of the larynx are to maintain patency of the airway, protect the airway, and produce sound (phonation). The laryngeal muscles coordinate several critical functions, including breathing, swallowing, coughing, phonating, and vomiting, all of which are centrally mediated. The thyroid and cricoid cartilages provide the skeletal support. During inspiration, the cross-sectional area between the vocal cords widens and is augmented during deep inspiration (9). In contrast, the glottis narrows slightly (< 30%) during expiration and may retard expiratory airflow. Closure of the glottis involves actions of the thyroarytenoid, cricoarytenoid lateralis, interarytenoid, and aryepiglottic muscles. The posterior cricoarytenoid muscle is the sole abductor of the arytenoid process, leading to opening of the glottis.

Sensory receptors extending from the nose to the bronchi will detect irritant stimuli, triggering the cough and glottic closure reflexes that are central to protecting the lungs from exogenous noxious agents. The internal branch of the superior

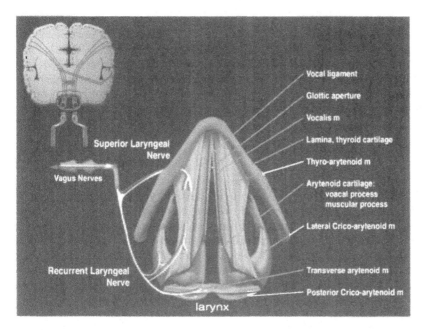

FIGURE 1 Laryngeal anatomy.

laryngeal nerve supplies sensory afferents to the supraglottic larynx (epiglottis, aryepiglottic folds, false cords, and superior surface of the laryngeal ventricle), whereas the recurrent laryngeal nerve supplies sensory afferents for the glottic and subglottic structures (vocal cords, inferior surface of the laryngeal ventricle, and trachea). These nerve impulses are then relayed centrally via the vagus nerve on through the nodose (inferior) ganglion and then the fasciculus solitarus and nucleus solitarus in the medulla. Major projections then enter the reticular formation, an area in the midbrain important for control of respiration. Several other secondary connections to cranial nerve motor nuclei play a role in the laryngeal reflexes. Direct connections to the higher cortical centers remain poorly delineated.

The efferent (motor) fibers start in the somatosensory gyrus and partially decussate before joining the somatic motor nucleus in the medulla. The nucleus ambiguus receives bilateral cortical input as well as sensory input from the nucleus solitarus. This allows the vocal folds to function simultaneously, and it is not possible to dissociate one from the other voluntarily. The cerebellum contributes to fine motor control through fibers to the nucleus solitarus. The nucleus ambiguus relays the motor innervation for the 9th, 10th, and 11th cranial nerves. The superior laryngeal nerve supplies motor innervation to the cricothyroid muscle, an important tensor and adductor of the vocal folds and stabilizer of the larynx during inspiratory abduction. The rest of the motor innervation to the larynx comes from the recurrent laryngeal nerve.

The cough and glottic closure reflexes are not only important for protecting the airway during deglutition, but also in response to potentially noxious inhaled stimuli. Closing the glottic and supraglottic sphincter involves the vocal folds, false folds, and arytenoid cartilages being brought medially to occlude the airway. The aryepiglottic folds shorten, bringing the vertical processes of the arytenoids close to one another and in contact with the epiglottis. The rise in subglottic pressure against a closed glottis is important not only for the cough reflex, but also provides a form of auto positive and expiratory pressure (PEEP) by increasing intra-alveolar pressure. This has been used to advantage by severe asthmatics and those with emphysema to prevent or reduce airway collapse during expiration and thus to promote better emptying. Hence, this mid to late expiratory closure as a means of creating auto PEEP should not be regarded as dysfunctional or maladaptive (10).

Rhinosinusitis, Postnasal Drip, and VCD

Given the role of the larynx to protect the trachea and lungs from noxious inhalants, it is understandable that postnasal drip (from allergic and nonallergic rhinosinusitis) can lead to increased laryngeal sensitivity and consequent laryngeal hyperresponsiveness (2). Bucca et al. (10) followed a group of patients with chronic rhinosinusitis and measured their upper airway hyperresponsiveness by measuring the PC25MIF-50 (i.e., the concentration of methacholine that caused a 25% drop in the mid inspiratory flow midway through the inspiratory effort). This was compared to the PC20 forced expiratory volume in one second (FEV_1), the standard measure of bronchial hyperresponsiveness (BHR). They found that of 88 patients, 76 (86%) had extrathoracic hyperresponsiveness (EA-HR) of whom 46 (52% of the total sample) had both BHR and EA-HR. After treatment with antibiotics and inhaled nasal steroids for two weeks there was a reduction in the EA-HR and BHR. The constant bombardment of the larynx by postnasal drip secretions likely leads to an increased glottic closure response not only to postnasal drip, but also to other noxious stimuli. Bucca et al. proposed that the EA-HR was a product of mediator release from inflammatory cells in the nasal secretions, resulting in mucosal damage that could trigger local reflexes (11,12). Further research, however, is required to elucidate the mechanism of the observed increase in extrathoracic airway hyperresponsiveness and VCD associated with postnasal drip.

Another mechanism by which nonallergic rhinitis may trigger VCD is by alterations in olfaction and/or trigeminal chemoreception, particularly increased chemosensory sensitivity as is sometimes seen after irritant-induced rhinitis. Olfactory triggers may cause augmentation of the glottic closure reflex and trigger VCD attacks at lower odor thresholds than might otherwise occur (13–16).

There are also several reports finding an association between GERD and chronic rhinitis, leading some researchers to speculate that GERD may play a role in the pathogenesis of nonallergic rhinitis (17–23). However, Shaker et al. (24) studied fluctuations in oropharyngeal and esophageal pH and found no difference between vasomotor rhinitis versus controls in a number of acid reflux events in the oropharynx. Similarly, Ulualp et al. (23) found an increased prevalence of acid reflux events in patients with posterior laryngitis, but not chronic rhinosinusitis versus healthy controls. Loehrl et al. (25) compared vasomotor rhinitis with and without GERD to normals with respect to their response to a variety of autonomic reflex tests. According to their interpretation, vasomotor rhinitis subjects with or without GERD showed adrenergic hypoactivity relative to normal controls. Thus, despite possible symptomatic associations, further studies are required to characterize the association (or lack thereof) between GERD and vasomotor rhinitis.

Previous studies have demonstrated that the larynx can be primed by certain agents to become more sensitive to noxious stimuli. Mutoh and Tsubone (26) showed that pre-exposure of a guinea pig model prepared to monitor laryngeal afferent C-fibers had an increased sensitivity to capsaicin and mechanical stretch (laryngeal hyperinflation) after pre-exposure to halothane. These studies were based on the observation that children often develop problems, such as cough, upper airway obstruction, and laryngospasm, following halothane anesthesia. The guinea pig model demonstrated that lower doses of capsaicin were capable of inducing the triggering of the afferent C-fibers after pretreatment of animals with halothane compared to nonhalothane-exposed animals.

GERD, LPR, and VCD

GERD refers to the retrograde flow of gastric contents into the esophagus. GERD is extremely common and the estimated prevalence is 10% to 60% in the general population based on a meta-analysis of studies using pH probes (27), and is reported to be as high as 60% in the asthma population (28–33). The lower esophageal sphincter (LES) is a 3 to 4 cm long segment of tonically contracted smooth muscle at the distal end of the esophagus. The causes for GERD are not completely understood but are likely multifactorial [dietary and other habits (e.g., smoking), body habitus, and anatomical alterations such as hiatal hernias] that ultimately lead to excursions through the physiologically complex anti-reflux barrier at the gastroesophageal junction. Transient lower esophageal sphincter relaxations (tLESRs) are a normal response to gastric distension by food or gas and allow for gas venting (belching). They are increased in frequency and duration in GERD patients (34). LES pressures are generally between 10 and 30 mmHg and various factors such as gastric distension, cholecystokinin, various foods rich in fats, spicy foods, peppermint, alcohol, caffeine, carbonated drinks (increased gas production), smoking, and various drugs will cause transient hypotensive LES pressures that promote reflux (35). During inspiration the diaphragmatic crus tightens around the esophagus and leads to increases in LES pressure (36). If patients have a hiatal hernia with a portion of the stomach above and below the crus, they may suffer from the stretch of the crus. With displacement of the LES above the crus in patients with a hiatal hernia, the contribution from the diaphragm to increase LES during inspiration is lost. Hence, it is not surprising that hiatal hernias also appear to decrease the threshold for eliciting tLESRs in response to gastric distension (37), during normal swallowing and during deep inspiration or with straining [bending, coughing, or the valsalva maneuver (38)].

Even though there is evidence that the presence of acid in the esophagus can cause broncho-constriction and cough, the primary connection between GERD and VCD is laryngopharyngeal reflux (LPR). LPR refers to the retrograde flow of gastric contents, including acid and digestive enzymes such as pepsin, into LP, leading to symptoms of hoarseness, cough, halitosis, dysphagia, throat clearing, and VCD. The epidemiology of LPR is poorly understood, partially because of relatively few studies examining the question but more importantly there are no clear gold standard diagnostic criteria. One study showed that 86% of 105 healthy adults had some signs of reflux on laryngoscopic examination (39).

The refluxate may cause direct damage to the laryngeal mucosa, leading to symptoms. It is important to appreciate that the laryngeal mucosa is different from that of the esophagus and the stomach such that much less acid (and/or pepsin) regurgitation is required to cause significant damage and symptoms. Although it is reported that pH drops below 4 are associated with esophageal damage, it is recognized that the deleterious actions of pepsin can occur with pH levels up to 6 (27). Previous studies have suggested that 50 episodes of reflux are at the upper limits of normal; however, three episodes of laryngeal reflux over a week are capable of leading to significant damage (40–42). The LP does not have the same peristaltic or stripping motion of the esophagus, and hence refluxate materials have greater resident time in the LP to cause damage. It is interesting to note that a number of subjects show signs of laryngeal injury without any evidence of esophagitis compared to GERD patients, suggesting that it requires less exposure to acid and other gastric contents to induce injury of the larynx compared to esophagus. This may indeed help explain the observation that in numerous studies only 30% to 40% of patients with LPR report heartburn (43).

There are now numerous reports linking gastroesophageal reflux and postnasal drip (PND) with VCD (2,38,44–48). As the precise mechanism has not been definitively established, it is presumed that the damage to the laryngeal mucosa leads to an accentuation of the glottic closure reflex. This mechanism is also felt to be important in patients who develop VCD after irritant exposures (1,49–52). Establishing the association between the disorders is instructive in terms of optimal management.

CLINICAL EVALUATION OF VCD

History
Obtaining the history for possible VCD is usually in the context of assessing a patient for refractory asthma or chronic cough. Patients with VCD typically have had a diagnosis of asthma for several years and have required frequent prednisone bursts with only marginal response. They will report often greater difficulty getting air in rather than out and will often point to the throat when asked where it feels like the air cuts off. Many will report audible wheezing during inspiration and/or expiration. Patients with VCD also frequently claim that inhalers cause an increase in their symptoms, whereas nebulized medications provide relief. Because postnasal drip and GERD are common conditions associated with VCD, enquiries regarding allergies, nasal congestion, throat clearing, hoarseness, chronic cough, headaches, heartburn, indigestion, water brash, throat burning, halitosis, increased cough lying flat, and cough worse at night are all clues to PND and/or GERD as likely contributing factors. These patients may report a history of psychological stress or abuse. A more substantial number of patients will have some psychological issues such as anxiety and/or depression as a result of being told they have a condition (asthma) that is potentially life threatening for which they seem to be getting worse and not responding to medicines and their doctors really do not know what to do.

Physical Exam
Further clinical evaluation of these patients involves physical examination and various ancillary tests to confirm paradoxical closure of vocal cords and to rule out other disorders or contributing factors. Physical examination may be relatively unremarkable except for direct detection of laryngeal wheezing and/or stridor, or stigmata of posterior nasal drainage or gastroesophageal reflux (epigastric tenderness). Skin, neurological, and musculoskeletal examinations are helpful to identify lesions that may explain symptoms, as well as signs of rheumatologic or collagen vascular diseases, as a cause of laryngeal dysfunction (relapsing polychondritis and rheumatoid arthritis involvement of the arytenoids).

Ancillary Tests

Spirometry often provides compelling evidence that an upper airway obstructive process may be operative. These patients demonstrate a pattern of variable extra-thoracic airway obstruction on flow–volume loops (truncated inspiratory loop) typically obtained during a period when the patient is symptomatic (Fig. 2).

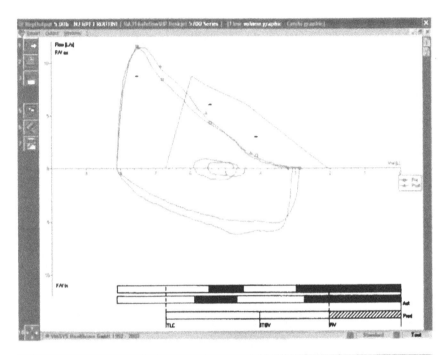

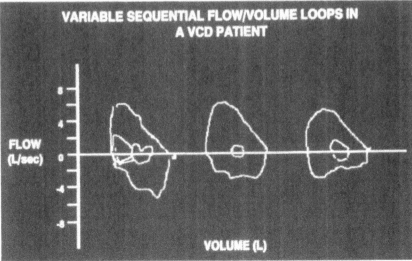

FIGURE 2 Truncated flow–volume loop.

It should be emphasized that true VCD patients may demonstrate flattening in the early segment of the expiratory loop, as well. Recently, Vlahakis et al. (47,53) reported evidence of an inspiratory flow plateau on the open shutter loop during body plethysmography of a patient with laryngoscopy-confirmed VCD. The utility of this noninvasive measurement requires validation. Radiographic studies are generally unhelpful in establishing the diagnosis of VCD, but do help to rule out space-occupying lesions in the upper airway that may be because of neoplasm, infection, or chronic inflammation from various sources.

Although spirometry can be an extraordinarily useful screening tool for VCD, particularly when the patient is symptomatic, direct visualization of the upper airway is the gold standard for making a definitive diagnosis and assessing the nature and severity of the cause of obstruction (Fig. 3). Flexible fibreoptic rhinolaryngoscopy is the typical modality used to evaluate the upper airway. The nasal passages can be visualized for evidence of chronic rhinitis and postnasal drip and chronic inflammation with cobble stoning. The aryepiglottic folds will often demonstrate chronic inflammation and thickening suggestive of LPR (Fig. 4). The vocal folds can have nodules on them. Asking patients to do a variety of maneuvers helps to define their abnormalities. Typically after general visualization of the pharynx, patients are asked to say "EEE": this will normally lead to

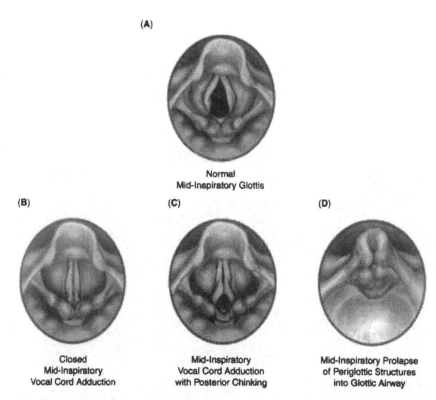

(A)

Normal
Mid-Inspiratory Glottis

(B)   **(C)**   **(D)**

Closed   Mid-Inspiratory   Mid-Inspiratory Prolapse
Mid-Inspiratory   Vocal Cord Adduction   of Periglottic Structures
Vocal Cord Adduction   with Posterior Chinking   into Glottic Airway

FIGURE 3   The appearance of the vocal folds during **(A)** inspiration in a healthy patient and **(B)** during inspiration in a patient with VCD with complete closure of the folds, **(C)** with classic posterior chink and **(D)** with prolapse of the periglottic structures.

(A)   (B)

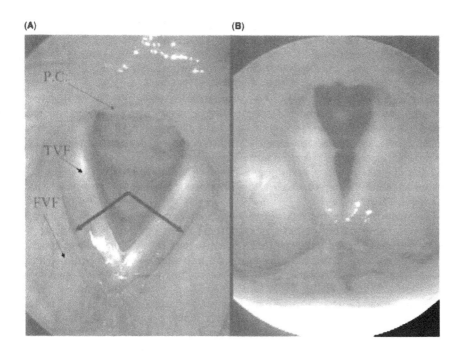

FIGURE 4 **(A)** Demonstration of normal laryngeal ventricles (space between TVF and FVF). **(B)** Obliteration of the ventricles, PC hypertrophy, and moderate vocal fold edema. *Abbreviations:* PC, posterior commissure; TVF, true vocal fold; FVF, false vocal fold. *Source:* From Ref. 54.

adduction of the vocal folds and help to identify patients who may have paralysis of one of the cords by evidence of asymmetric movements. Asking patients then to quietly breath in and out will sometimes bring out the classic paradoxical adduction of the vocal folds. In order to identify vocal fold dysfunction patients may often be asked to do a forced vital capacity maneuver. One often needs to elicit the response by doing provocation studies either with methacholine, with exercise (±cold air) or with irritants such as perfume or cleaning agents containing chlorine or ammonia. Such nonspecific irritant challenges are often based on the history obtained from patients when asked what the typical triggers for their symptoms are. Vocal fold dysfunction should not be considered ruled out until the patients' symptoms have been recreated and patients have direct visualization of their vocal cords during a time they are having their typical symptoms.

Several newer diagnostic tools to document VCD are being studied. Kenn and Hess have examined endospirometry, a technique that combines endoscopy timed with spirometric readings (55). Rigau et al. have examined the use of oscillometry to evaluate VCD (56). Acoustic pharyngometry and air pulse stimulation through a fiberoptic laryngoscope are methods under study but there are no published data as to their utility to date.

Criteria for establishing the diagnosis of GERD remain an area of controversy (57). Symptoms are highly variable and may include heartburn, regurgitation, dysphagia, chest pain, water brash, globus sensation, odynophagia, and nausea. These are relatively nonspecific, and previous studies have shown that only heartburn and acid regurgitation are significantly increased in patients with positive pH probes (58). Even though a symptomatic response to an empiric therapeutic trial with proton pump inhibitors (PPIs) and/or H-2 antagonists may support the presumptive diagnosis of GERD, a meta-analysis found that response to PPIs did not correlate well with ambulatory pH monitoring with a pooled sensitivity of 78% and a specificity of 54% (59). Endoscopy has been suggested as the first diagnostic test, if symptoms suggest a complicated disease process or if patient is at a high risk Barrett's, whereas pH monitoring is useful for confirming reflux in patients not responsive to therapy or who have a compelling history but normal endoscopy (57). Barium and manometry studies are useful for assessing related or distinct motility problems but are relatively insensitive and nonspecific for detecting GERD. The role of other techniques such as wireless endoscopy (pillcam) (60), and esophageal multichannel intraluminal impedance testing (61) for evaluation of GERD require further study.

Diagnostic criteria for LPR have not been firmly established, and most patients are diagnosed on the basis of symptoms and a compatible laryngoscopic exam. Unfortunately, cardinal laryngoscopic features of reflux laryngitis—posterior laryngeal edema, true vocal cord edema, and pseudosulcus—are highly nonspecific (39). Dual level and now tri level pH probes may improve sensitivity and specificity for diagnosing LPR; however, there are no standard criteria, and many authors argue that 24-hour monitoring may be too short and a mark of pH 4 may be too low for the optimum detection of LPR (27,62). Response to an empiric trial of antireflux therapy may be useful to confirm cases but does not rule out LPR.

Differential Diagnosis of VCD

Disorders of laryngeal function may arise as a result of anatomical or neurological dysfunction because of a number of causes. The size and shape of the glottic aperture is influenced by many factors including vocal fold position and motion and the status and function of surrounding supporting structures such as the false folds, epiglottis, and the base of the tongue. Chronic or slowly progressive airflow obstruction at the level of the larynx may be because of vocal cord polyps or granulomas and tumors of the aerodigestive tract, particularly invasive malignancies such as squamous cell carcinomas, lymphomas, or thyroid carcinomas (Table 1). Other etiologies include papilloma formation, leading to internal narrowing in the larynx and trachea or benign thyroid tumors causing extrinsic compression. A significant number of chronic diseases can have laryngeal manifestations including rheumatoid arthritis, lupus, progressive systemic sclerosis, Wegener's granulomatosis, and relapsing polychondritis.

When both recurrent laryngeal nerves are injured, the vocal cords move toward the midline because of persistent action of the cricothyroid muscles. The initial signs of this may be very subtle and only after 10 to 20 years of slowly progressive glottic closure may such patients come to attention. Past history of a thyroidectomy is frequently elicited in these cases. Unilateral vocal cord paralysis (63) is diagnosed more frequently because, for unknown reasons, a patient with such a disorder is prone to aspiration and severe laryngospasm during sleep. In a significant percentage of patients, a search for the cause of this condition fails to uncover a specific etiology. The possibility of cervical or mediastinal malignancy or of aortic aneurysm encroaching on one recurrent laryngeal nerve (usually the left) must be considered (64).

In contrast to the paroxysmal and variable degree of closure noted with VCD, laryngospasm refers to sustained intense, virtually complete closure of the vocal folds following direct laryngeal stimulation by irritants (65). The triggers for

TABLE 1 Differential Diagnosis of Upper Airway Obstructions

Slowly developing upper airway obstruction
Arthritis cricoarytenoid joint
Enlarged tonsils and adenoids or laryngeal obstruction
Esophageal foreign body
Histiocytoma
Laryngeal carcinoma, papilloma, cartilaginous tumors, angioma, cystic hygroma, congenital
   malformations, polyp, granuloma
Malignant metastases to cervical glands
Neurologic disease
Relapsing polychondritis
Thyroid tumors, malignant and benign
Tracheal cyst, stenosis from cylindroma, tracheomalacia
Vocal cord paralysis

Acute onset upper airway obstruction
Foreign bodies
Anesthesia and other states of unconsciousness
Intubation injury
Angioneurotic edema (idiopathic, anaphylactic, and C1-esterase deficiency)
Burn injury
Laryngeal or tracheal trauma
Croup
Epiglottitis
Infections involving surrounding structures
Deep neck infections
Ludwig's angina
Peritonsillar abscess
Retropharyngeal abscess
Malfunction of muscles stabilizing the airways
Syphilitic gumma, tabes dorsalis

---

laryngospasm are not dissimilar from those for VCD, and it may very well be that laryngospasm represents the most severe pathophysiologic consequences of the glottic closure reflex. Intubation, certain anesthetics, GERD, and various other etiologies have been implicated in inducing laryngospasm (66–68).

There are studies emerging that suggest that the larynx can become hypersensitive (2) and may demonstrate evidence of a sensory neuropathy (66) or increases in nerve growth factor (69). Shusterman has demonstrated the increased odor intolerance of individuals with upper airway dysfunction (1,14,16).

Finally, there are functional disorders that must be distinguished from VCD, including spasmodic and muscle tension dysphonia, panic attacks, Munchausen' syndrome (70), and multiple chemical sensitivity (idiopathic environmental intolerance) (71–73) and somatoform disorders (74) that are reported in some individuals.

MANAGEMENT OF VCD

Upper airway obstruction due to laryngeal dysfunction requires the identification of contributing factors (medications, underlying medical problems, psychological factors) and treating these optimally. In addition, teaching patients various laryngeal exercises, a task typically conducted by speech therapists, is of value. For vocal fold paralysis, patients may benefit from surgical fixation of the vocal folds. Understanding the complex nature of the pathophysiology of VCD and laryngeal dysfunction underscores the need for a multidisciplinary approach (75). Physicians (which may include pulmonologists, general internists, otolaryngologists, allergists, occupational medicine specialists, and/or psychiatrists), speech therapists, psychosocial staff, rehabilitation staff, and vocational counselors may all play useful roles in treating these patients.

Speech and language pathologists/therapists provide instruction in techniques of throat relaxation, cough suppression, and throat clearing suppression, and play a central role in the management and follow up of VCD. Too often, however, well meaning but untrained speech therapists meet minimal success when they attempt to apply general therapeutic exercises and techniques that are not specifically targeted for VCD. This circumstance often frustrates the patient and the therapist. Speech therapists may also be helpful in performing controlled irritant challenges where individuals are serially exposed to increasing concentrations of a provocative agent and are coached by the therapist during these exposures on how to control their laryngeal response or how to abort an acute attack.

Psychosocial assessment and treatment is the key in managing these patients because there is generally some degree (though highly variable) of psychological overlay, either pre-existing or as a consequence of developing VCD. Input from psychologists and/or psychiatrists regarding evidence of conversion, panic, anxiety, affective, personality, or post-traumatic stress disorders is helpful (2,75). In addition, patient education and reassurance are extremely important in managing these patients. Follow-up with supportive counseling and the teaching of relaxation and/or biofeedback techniques may also be beneficial. Clinicians should discontinue unnecessary medications such as bronchodilators and steroids, if coexistent asthma has been ruled out. Treatment for associated GERD and/or rhinosinusitis may reduce symptoms.

Treatment for nonallergic rhinitis has been outlined in previous chapters. Treatment for GERD and LPR includes PPIs, ranitidine, and prokinetic agents, in addition to lifestyle measures such as raising the head of the bed, smaller more frequent meals and avoidance of various foods rich in fats, spicy foods, peppermint, alcohol, caffeine, carbonated drinks (increased gas production), and smoking. Treatment for LPR may differ from that for GERD as the goal should be to elevate pH levels above 6 rather than 4, and hence this may require more aggressive therapy with double PPI therapy and use of nighttime H-2 antagonists in addition to pro-kinetic agents (76). Some previous studies have pointed to equal efficacy between lifestyle measures and use of PPIs (77). This points to the importance of eliminating the total refluxate from entering the larynx rather than just the acid component. Hence, for some patients with refractory chronic cough and/or VCD related to LPR, a Nissen Fundiplication may be the optimum treatment. Although the benefits of Nissen Fundiplication for treatment of refractory reflux that is aggravating or mimicking asthma have been previously demonstrated (78,79), the efficacy of this mode of treatment for LPR has not been assessed in clinical trials.

Acute severe episodes of laryngeal dysfunction may generally be controlled and managed with sedation, and/or Heliox (80% helium/20% oxygen) (80,81). Recent studies have suggested that a simple continuous positive airway pressure (CPAP) type device providing intermittent positive pressure can resolve an attack (82). Topical lidocaine applied to the larynx may be useful during acute episodes in selected patients. In severe cases, superior laryngeal blocks with *Clostridium botulinum* toxin have been attempted with variable success (83). This treatment has been more successful for muscle tension dysphonia than for VCD (84).

Tracheotomy has been used for some patients with severe VCD refractory to conventional therapy, but it is rarely (if ever) indicated.

SUMMARY

VCD is often mistaken for asthma and can lead to treatment with corticosteroids and the development of significant side effects. Early and correct diagnosis will avert significant iatrogenic complications. For many individuals, the role of postnasal drip and GERD in the pathogenesis of VCD is central, as they are often associated with VCD and likely lead to increased laryngopharyngeal sensitivity and hyperreactivity. Much needs to be further elucidated in terms of the underlying pathogenesis of VCD. Management of VCD requires identification and treatment of underlying disorders and referral to speech therapists that can teach techniques of throat relaxation, cough suppression, and throat clearing suppression.

REFERENCES

1. Balkissoon R, Shusterman D. Occupational upper airway disorders. Semin Respir Crit Care Med 1999; 20(6):569–580.
2. Morrison M, Rammage L, Emami A. The irritable larynx syndrome. J Voice 1999; 13(3):447–455.
3. Brugman SM. The many faces of vocal cord dysfunction: what 36 years of literature tells us. Am J Respir Crit Care Med 2003; 167(7):A588.
4. Kenn K, Willer G, Bizer C, et al. Prevalence of vocal cord dysfunction in patients with dyspnea. First prospective clinical study. Am J Respir Crit Care Med 1997; 155:A965.
5. Ciccolella DE, Brennan KJ, Borbely B, et al. Identification of vocal cord dysfunction (VCD) and other diagnoses in patients admitted to an inner city university hospital asthma center. Am J Respir Crit Care Med 1997; 155:A82.
6. Jain S, Bandi V, Zimmerman J, et al. Incidence of vocal cord dysfunction in patients presenting to emergency room with acute asthma exacerbation. Chest 1997; 11(4):243S.
7. Newman KB, Mason UG III, Schmaling KB. Clinical features of vocal cord dysfunction. Am J Respir Crit Care Med 1995; 152(4 Pt 1):1382–1386.
8. Brugman S. What's this thing called vocal cord dysfunction. Pulmon Crit Care Update. In press.
9. Baier H, Wanner S, Zarzecki, et al. Relationships among glottis opening, respiratory flow, and upper airway resistance in humans. J Appl Physiol 1977; 43(4):603–611.
10. Bucca C, Rolla G, Scappaticci E, et al. Extrathoracic and intrathoracic airway responsiveness in sinusitis.
J Allergy Clin Immunol 1995; 95(1 Pt 1):52–59.
11. Bucca C, Rolla G, Scappaticci E, et al. Histamine hyperresponsiveness of the extrathoracic airway in patients with asthmatic symptoms. Allergy 1991; 46(2):147–153.
12. Bucca C, Rolla G, Brussino L, et al. Are asthma-like symptoms due to bronchial or extrathoracic airway dysfunction? [see comments]. Lancet 1995; 346(8978):791–795.
13. Shusterman D, Balmes J, Cone J. Behavioral sensitization to irritants/odorants after acute overexposures. J Occup Med 1988; 30(7):565–567.
14. Shusterman D, Balmes J. Measurement of nasal irritant sensitivity to pulsed carbon dioxide: a pilot study. Arch Environ Health 1997; 52(5):334–340.
15. Shusterman D. Critical review: the health significance of environmental odor pollution [see comments]. Arch Environ Health 1992; 47(1):76–87.
16. Shusterman D. Review of the upper airway, including olfaction, as mediator of symptoms. Environ Health Perspect 2002; 110(suppl 4):649–653.
17. Monteiro VR, Sdepanian VL, Weckx L, et al. Twenty-four-hour esophageal pH monitoring in children and adolescents with chronic and/or recurrent rhinosinusitis. Braz J Med Biol Res 2005; 38(2):215–220 [Epub 2005 Feb 15].

18. Loehrl TA, Smith TL, Merati A, et al. Pharyngeal pH probe findings in patients with postnasal drainage. Am J Rhinol 2005; 19(4):340–343.
19. Altman KW, Simpson CB, Amin MR, et al. Cough and paradoxical vocal fold motion. Otolaryngol Head Neck Surg 2002; 127(6):501–511.
20. Peters EJ, Hatley TK, Crater SE, et al. Sinus computed tomography scan and markers of inflammation in vocal cord dysfunction and asthma. Ann Allergy Asthma Immunol 2003; 90(3):316–322.
21. Gilger MA. Pediatric otolaryngologic manifestations of gastroesophageal reflux disease. Curr Gastroenterol Rep 2003; 5(3):247–252.
22. Theodoropoulos DS, Ledford DK, Lockey RF, et al. Prevalence of upper respiratory symptoms in patients with symptomatic gastroesophageal reflux disease. Am J Respir Crit Care Med 2001; 164(1):72–76.
23. Ulualp SO, Toohill RJ, Shaker R. Pharyngeal acid reflux in patients with single and multiple otolaryngologic disorders. Otolaryngol Head Neck Surg 1999; 121(6):725–730.
24. Shaker R, Ren J, Barden E, et al. Pharyngoglottal closure reflex: characterization in healthy young, elderly and dysphagic patients with predeglutitive aspiration. Gerontology 2003; 49(1):12–20.
25. Loehrl TA, Smith TL, Darling RJ, et al. Autonomic dysfunction, vasomotor rhinitis and extraesophageal manifestations of gastroesophageal reflux. Head Neck Surg 2002; 126(126):382–387.
26. Mutoh T, Tsubone H. Hypersensitivity of laryngeal C-fibers induced by volatile anesthetics in young guinea pigs. Am J Respir Crit Care Med 2003; 167(4):557–562.
27. Merati AL, Lim HJ, Ulualp SO, et al. Meta-analysis of upper probe measurements in normal subjects and patients with laryngopharyngeal reflux. Ann Otol Rhinol Laryngol 2005; 114(3): 177–182.
28. Vincent D, Cohen-Jonathan AM, Leport J, et al. Gastro-oesophageal reflux prevalence and relationship with bronchial reactivity in asthma. Eur Respir J 1997; 10(10):2255–2259.
29. Sontag SJ, O'Connell S, Khandelwal S, et al. Most asthmatics have gastroesophageal reflux with or without bronchodilator therapy. Gastroenterology 1990; 99(3):613–620.
30. Harding SM, Guzzo MR, Richter JE. The prevalence of gastroesophageal reflux in asthma patients without reflux symptoms. Am J Respir Crit Care Med 2000; 162(1):34–39.
31. Harding SM. Gastroesophageal reflux: a potential asthma trigger. Immunol Allergy Clin North Am 2005; 25(1):131–148.
32. Harding SM. Recent clinical investigations examining the association of asthma and gastroesophageal reflux. Am J Med 2003; 115(suppl 3A):39S–44S.
33. Field SK, Underwood M, Brant R, et al. Prevalence of gastroesophageal reflux symptoms in asthma. Chest 1996; 109(2):316–322.
34. Mittal RK, Holloway RH, Penagini R, et al. Transient lower esophageal sphincter relaxation. Gastroenterology 1995; 109(2):601–610.
35. Dent J, Dodds WJ, Hogan WJ, et al. Factors that influence induction of gastroesophageal reflux in normal human subjects. Dig Dis Sci 1988; 33(3):270–275.
36. Mittal RK, Rochester DF, McCallum RW. Sphincteric action of the diaphragm during a relaxed lower esophageal sphincter in humans. Am J Physiol 1989; 256(1 Pt 1): G139–G144.
37. Kahrilas PJ, Shi G, Manka M, et al. Increased frequency of transient lower esophageal sphincter relaxation induced by gastric distention in reflux patients with hiatal hernia. Gastroenterology 2000; 118(4):688–695.
38. van Herwaarden MA, Katzka DA, Smout AJ, et al. Effect of different recumbent positions on postprandial gastroesophageal reflux in normal subjects. Am J Gastroenterol 2000; 95(10):2731–2736.
39. Hicks DM, Ours TM, Abelson TI, et al. The prevalence of hypopharynx findings associated with gastroesophageal reflux in normal volunteers. J Voice 2002; 16(4):564–579.
40. Johnston N, Bulmer D, Gill GA, et al. Cell biology of laryngeal epithelial defenses in health and disease: further studies. Ann Otol Rhinol Laryngol 2003; 112(6):481–491.

41. Axford SE, Sharp N, Ross PE, et al. Cell biology of laryngeal epithelial defenses in health and disease: preliminary studies. Ann Otol Rhinol Laryngol 2001; 110(12):1099–1108.
42. Koufman JA, Aviv JE, Casiano RR, et al. Laryngopharyngeal reflux: position statement of the committee on speech, voice, and swallowing disorders of the American Academy of Otolaryngology-Head and Neck Surgery. Otolaryngol Head Neck Surg 2002; 127(1):32–35.
43. Koufman JA. Laryngopharyngeal reflux is different from classic gastroesophageal reflux disease. Ear Nose Throat J 2002; 81(9 suppl 2):7–9.
44. Heatley DG, Swift E. Paradoxical vocal cord dysfunction in an infant with stridor and gastroesophageal reflux. Int J Pediatr Otorhinolaryngol 1996; 34(1–2):149–151.
45. Tilles SA. Vocal cord dysfunction in children and adolescents. Curr Allergy Asthma Rep 2003; 3(6):467–472.
46. Thomas PS, Geddes DM, Barnes PJ. Pseudo-steroid resistant asthma. Thorax 1999; 54(4):352–356.
47. Powell DM, Karanfilov BI, Beechler KB, et al. Paradoxical vocal cord dysfunction in juveniles. Arch Otolaryngol Head Neck Surg 2000; 126(1):29–34.
48. Goldberg BJ, Kaplan MS. Non-asthmatic respiratory symptomatology. Curr Opin Pulm Med 2000; 6(1):26–30.
49. Balkissoon R. Disorders of the upper airway. In: Mason R, et al., eds. Murray and Nadel's: Text Book of Respiratory Medicine. New York: Elsevier, 2005.
50. Perkner JJ, Fennally K, Balkissoon R, et al. Irritant-associated vocal cord dysfunction. J Occup Environ Med 1998; 40(2):136–143.
51. Balkissoon R. Occupational upper airway disease. Clin Chest Med 2002; 23(4):717–725.
52. Ayres JG, Gabbott PL. Vocal cord dysfunction and laryngeal hyperresponsiveness: a function of altered autonomic balance? Thorax 2002; 57(4):284–285.
53. Vlahakis NE, et al. Diagnosis of vocal cord dysfunction: the utility of spirometry and plethysmography. Chest 2002; 122(6):2246–2249.
54. Belafsky PC. Abnormal endoscopic pharyngeal and laryngeal findings attributable to reflux. Am J Med 2003; 115(3A):90S–96S.
55. Kenn K, Hess MM. Vocal cord dysfunction—a "solely pneumatologic" illness? Hno 2004; 52(2):103–109.
56. Rigau J, Farre R, Trepat X, et al. Oscillometric assessment of airway obstruction in a mechanical model of vocal cord dysfunction. J Biomech 2004; 37(1):37–43.
57. DeVault KR, Castell DO. Updated guidelines for the diagnosis and treatment of gastro-esophageal reflux disease. Am J Gastroenterol 2005; 100(1):190–200.
58. Klauser AG, Schindlbeck NE, Muller-Lissner SA. Symptoms in gastro-oesophageal reflux disease. Lancet 1990; 335(8683):205–208.
59. Numans ME, Lau J, de Wit NJ, et al. Short-term treatment with proton-pump inhibitors as a test for gastroesophageal reflux disease: a meta-analysis of diagnostic test characteristics. Ann Intern Med 2004; 140(7):518–527.
60. Iddan G, Meron G, Glukhovsky A, et al. Wireless capsule endoscopy. Nature 2000; 405(6785):417.
61. Tutuian R, Vela MF, Balaji NS, et al. Esophageal function testing with combined multichannel intraluminal impedance and manometry: multicenter study in healthy volunteers. Clin Gastroenterol Hepatol 2003; 1(3):174–182.
62. Vaezi MF, Schroeder PL, Richter JE. Reproducibility of proximal probe pH parameters in 24-hour ambulatory esophageal pH monitoring. Am J Gastroenterol 1997; 92(5):825–829.
63. Clerf LH. Unilateral vocal cord paralysis. J Am Med Assoc 1953; 151(11):900–903.
64. Parnell FW, Brandenburg JH. Vocal cord paralysis. A review of 100 cases. Laryngoscope 1970; 80(7):1036–1045.
65. Nishino T. Physiological and pathophysiological implications of upper airway reflexes in humans. Jpn J Physiol 2000; 50(1):3–14.
66. Lee B, Woo P. Chronic cough as a sign of laryngeal sensory neuropathy: diagnosis and treatment. Ann Otol Rhinol Laryngol 2005; 114(4):253–257.
67. Poelmans J, Tack J. Extraoesophageal manifestations of gastro-oesophageal reflux. Gut 2005; 54(10):1492–1499.

68. Riley RH, Musk MT. Laryngospasm induced by topical application of lignocaine. Anaesth Intensive Care 2005; 33(2):278.
69. Millqvist E, Ternesten-Hasseus E, Stahl A, et al. Changes in levels of nerve growth factor in nasal secretions after capsaicin inhalation in patients with airway symptoms from scents and chemicals. Environ Health Perspect 2005; 113(7):849–885.
70. Leo RJ, Konakanchi R. Psychogenic respiratory distress: a case of paradoxical vocal cord dysfunction and literature review. Prim Care Compan J Clin Psychiatr 1999; 1(2):39–46.
71. Tarlo SM, Poonai N, Binkley K, et al. Responses to panic induction procedures in subjects with multiple chemical sensitivity/idiopathic environmental intolerance: understanding the relationship with panic disorder. Environ Health Perspect 2002; 110(suppl 4):669–671.
72. Poonai NP, Antony MM ,Binkley KE, et al. Psychological features of subjects with idiopathic environmental intolerance. J Psychosom Res 2001; 51(3):537–541.
73. Poonai N, Antony MM ,Binkley KE, et al. Carbon dioxide inhalation challenges in idiopathic environmental intolerance. J Allergy Clin Immunol 2000; 105(2 Pt 1):358–363.
74. Bailer J, Witthoft M, Paul C, et al. Evidence for overlap between idiopathic environmental intolerance and somatoform disorders. Psychosom Med 2005; 67(6):921–929.
75. Andrianopoulos MV, Gallivan GJ, Gallivan KH. PVCM, PVCD, EPL, and irritable larynx syndrome: what are we talking about and how do we treat it? J Voice 2000; 14(4):607–618.
76. El-Serag HB, Lee P, Buchner A, et al. Lansoprazole treatment of patients with chronic idiopathic laryngitis: a placebo-controlled trial. Am J Gastroenterol 2001; 96(4):979–983.
77. Steward DL, Wilson KM, Kelly DH, et al. Proton pump inhibitor therapy for chronic laryngo-pharyngitis: a randomized placebo-control trial. Otolaryngol Head Neck Surg 2004; 131(4):342–350.
78. Sontag SJ, O'Connell S, Khandelwal S, et al. Asthmatics with gastroesophageal reflux: long term results of a randomized trial of medical and surgical antireflux therapies. Am J Gastroenterol 2003; 98(5):987–999.
79. Field SK, Gelfand GA, McFadden SD. The effects of antireflux surgery on asthmatics with gastroesophageal reflux. Chest 1999; 116(3):766–774.
80. Reisner C, Borish L. Heliox therapy for acute vocal cord dysfunction. Chest 1995; 108:1477.
81. Reybet-Degat O. Pathology of craniocervical junction and sleep disorders. Rev Neurol (Paris) 2001; 157(11 Pt 2):S156–S160.
82. Archer GJ, Hoyle JL, McCluskey A, et al. Inspiratory vocal cord dysfunction, a new approach in treatment. Eur Respir J 2000; 15(3):617–618.
83. Altman JS, Benninger MS. The evaluation of unilateral vocal fold immobility: is chest X-ray enough?. J Voice 1997; 11(3):364–367.
84. Bielamowicz S, Gupta A, Sekhar LN. Early arytenoid adduction for vagal paralysis after skull base surgery. Laryngoscope 2000; 110(3 Pt 1):346–351.

29 The Nonallergic Rhinitis of Chronic Fatigue Syndrome

James N. Baraniuk

Department of Medicine, Division of Rheumatology, Immunology and Allergy, and Georgetown University Proteomics Laboratory, Georgetown University Medical Center, Washington, D.C., U.S.A.

Uyenphuong Ho Le

Department of Medicine, Drexel University, Philadelphia, Pennsylvannia, U.S.A.

INTRODUCTION

Rhinitis is present in 74% ± 3% (range 66–80%) of chronic fatigue syndrome (CFS) subjects (1–3). These subjects will be an increasing component of the patient mix seen by the allergist and rhinologist. This is unavoidable, as switching of drugs to over-the-counter status and the introduction of generic medications will lead to more widespread access to satisfactory treatment of allergic rhinitis (AR). Rhinitis subjects who fail self-medication and primary health care treatment plans will have severe AR and the nonallergic rhinitis (NAR) syndromes that we have discussed in this book. A significant number of these "treatment failures" will have additional complaints that are commonly, but mistakenly, interpreted as being of "allergic" or "atopic" origin. Many of these subjects will have CFS, fibromyalgia (FM), or one of their spectra of overlapping, associated illnesses. These subjects and their nonallergic disorders are the future for our clinical practices.

CFS is characterized by a severe, sudden onset fatigue lasting at least six months that leads to significant disability with a decrement in work productivity and strain on the ability to perform activities of daily living (4). No other medical or psychiatric condition may be present to explain the fatigue. This excludes most chronic illnesses such as thyroid, diabetes, and other endocrinopathies, and cerebrovascular, cancer, autoimmune, and other inflammatory conditions. In addition to severe fatigue, there must be new onset of ancillary symptoms lasting for at least six months. At least four of the following eight symptoms must be present: sore throat, sore lymph nodes, sore muscles (myalgia), sore joints without swelling or redness (arthralgia), new onset headaches, neurocognitive disability with difficulty in concentrating and perceived short-term memory loss (brain fog), sleep disturbances, and exertional exhaustion. The latter is one of the stronger ancillary criterion predictors. It is readily identified in subjects who perform exercise of any type that is more than their usual daily exertion and who then develop a relapse in their condition with extreme exhaustion that may send them to their bed for several days with severe fatigue, pain (the first five minor criteria), and disordered neurocognitive function. These criteria were first selected by consensus after statistical review of a large number of cases, and have subsequently been validated in epidemiological studies (5–8).

Associated disorders include FM (9), post-traumatic fatigue syndrome, irritable larynx, irritable bowel, irritable bladder, irritable vagina (vulvodynia) (10), and other nonspecific "functional" disorders of neural regulation and hyperalgesia

(11). The American College of Rheumatology case designation criteria for FM rely on pain and tenderness (12). The symptom of pain must be present continuously for at least three months and affect all four quadrants of the body. This means left and right sides above and below the waist plus the axial skeleton. The axial skeletal pain can involve the neck, thoracic and lower spine, ribs (costochondritis), and sternum. The sign of hyperalgesia, or tenderness, is pain elicited by pressure. The standard research criterion is to induce pain by pressing with one's thumbs over "tender points" (formerly trigger points) until the thumbnail blanches (about 4 kg of pressure) (13). The subject must complain of pain at ≥ 11 of 18 traditional, standardized tender points. These are located bilaterally at the occiput, cervical spine, supraspinatus, trapezius, anterior ribs, lateral epicondyle, gluteus maximus, greater trochanter, and medial knee. This type of analysis of hyperalgesia is essentially passé, as administration of deep pressure using the thumb causes pain that the subject cannot control (14). As a result, anxious subjects have a higher number of positive tender points compared to healthy control (HC) subjects. Once one painful point has been pushed, the patient has a higher probability of anxiously preparing for more pain and is more likely to complain of a painful response (15). Pressure at the patient's thumb nails and at two other random spots, rather than the "classical trigger points," may be sufficient to identify those with lower deep pressure–induced hyperalgesia (16).

Randomized delivery of different deep tissue pressures in double-blind pain testing paradigms is far superior for detecting hyperalgesia, as the elements of anxiety and predictability are reduced (15). These types of studies have demonstrated that FM is related to intrinsic spinal cord mechanisms of hyperalgesia. FM subjects have larger flare responses to intradermal injections of capsaicin, indicating hyperactivity of transient receptor potential vanilloid 1 ion channel–bearing nociceptive neurons with an increase in their release of calcitonin gene-related peptide (CGRP) that is responsible for the flare (17–19). At the spinal cord level, there is dysregulation of nociceptive afferent signaling to dorsal horn substantia gelatinosa interneurons and secondary, ascending pain neurons. These signals are not "gated" or blocked because of opioid or other spinal cord inhibitory dysfunction, or reduced brainstem to spinal cord descending inhibitory, antinociceptive aminergic (norepinephrine, dopamine, serotonin) pathways. Because FM and CFS overlap significantly with many subjects having both syndromes, it is highly likely that an analogous type of neural dysfunction plays a role in their concomitant nasal pathophysiology. The same type of neural dysfunction in visceral, mucosal organs may also explain irritable syndromes of the airways, gastrointestinal, and genitourinary systems.

The CFS and FM case designation criteria are also met by many subjects who developed similar symptoms following the Persian Gulf War of 1990 to 1991 (20–22). This suggests a pathophysiological overlap between these syndromes.

CLINICAL INVESTIGATION

As clinicians in a joint Allergy and Rheumatology clinic specializing in FM, we had many FM subjects referred for allergy evaluations. CFS was more common than FM, as about two-thirds of CFS subjects met criteria for FM (Table 1). Hyperalgesia (tenderness) was present as tested by manual thumb pressure (~4 kg) or graded increases in pressure (dolorimetry) (2). The majority complained of "sinus" problems. CFS subjects had higher Rhinitis Scores, and about half had positive skin tests (2). However, they did not have typical symptoms of histamine-induced itch,

TABLE 1 Chronic Fatigue Syndrome (CFS) and Other Symptom Complexes in Mucosal and Somatic Organs in 138 Healthy Control and 125 CFS Subjects

Questionnaires and subsets of questionnaire items	Items (n)	Control mean± SEM (n)	CFS mean± SEM (n)
Fibromyalgia (American College of Rheumatology criteria)		0% (57)	28.7% (66)[a]
Widespread pain		0% (57)	52% (66)[a]
Manual tender point count	18	7.1±0.9 (46)	12.3±0.9 (36)[a]
Dolorimetry tender point count	18	3.7±0.5 (105)	9.0±0.7 (65)[b]
Dolorimetry pain threshold (kg)	—	7.41±2.51 (105)	5.12±0.31 (65)[b]
Rhinitis Score	40	7.43±0.76	15.97±0.82[a]
Irritant Rhinitis Score	72	8.95±0.83	15.75±0.99[a]
Tobacco Score	88	10.33±1.13	24.12±1.71[a]
Self-report of "Sinusitis"	1	29.2% (106)	69.2% (65)[b]
Systemic complaints	52	7.9±0.8 (106)	25.6±1.3 (65)[b]
Neurocognitive system	4	0.59±0.10	3.10±0.16[a]
Ear, nose, and throat system	6	0.62±0.09	2.50±0.16[a]
"Dyspnea"/pulmonary system	9	0.36±0.07	2.33±0.19[a]
Gastrointestinal system	8	0.52±0.12	3.05±0.24[a]
Bladder system	5	0.99±0.08	2.15±0.14[a]
Musculoskeletal system	10	0.94±0.13	4.79±0.21[a]
Irritable bowel syndrome	8	5.8%	44.0%[a]

Significant ANCOVA followed by two-tailed unpaired Student's *t*-test: [a]$p < 0.0001$; [b]$p < 10^{-6}$.
Abbreviations: ANCOVA, Analysis of covariance.

TABLE 2 Psychometric Comparison of Control and Chronic Fatigue Syndrome Populations [Mean± SEM, (Number Analyzed)]

Questionnaire	Control (n)	CFS (n)
Minnesota Heart Score	11.5±1.7 (102)	8.1±2.3 (63)
Beck Depression Index	6.3±0.7 (104)	13.6±1.0 (62)[a]
State-Trait Anger Expression Inventory	32.2±1.3 (68)	40.8±1.8 (48)[b]
McGill Pain Score	1.2±0.3 (62)	4.8±1.5 (20)[b]
McGill Present Pain Index	0.94±0.24 (31)	2.64±0.28 (11)[a]
McGill Visual Analog Scale	1.05±0.34 (31)	5.05±0.68 (10)[a]
McGill Total Pain Score	2.63±0.71 (62)	16.15±2.33 (20)[a]
McGill Affective Score	0.47±0.18 (62)	3.75±0.68 (20)[a]
McGill Sensory Score	2.6±1.0 (31)	14.9±2.2 (11)[a]
Multidimensional Fatigue Inventory	(n = 66)	(n = 23)
General fatigue	9.49±0.54	15.48±0.85[a]
Physical fatigue	8.1±0.5	12.7±0.9[a]
Reduced activity	8.3±0.5	11.7±0.9[b]
Reduced motivation	8.0±0.4	11.4±0.9[b]
Mental fatigue	9.0±0.6	13.3±1.0[b]
SF-36	(n = 102)	(n = 65)
Physical function	61.3±3.4	41.9±3.5[b]
Social function	52.0±3.9	38.8±3.9[c]
Role functioning physical	44.2±4.6	16.5±3.6[b]
Role functioning emotional	50.5±4.6	39.1±5.1
Mental health	56.7±2.7	50.5±3.1
Energy/vitality	38.3±2.9	24.0±2.6[b]
Bodily pain	50.1±3.8	30.9±3.2[b]
General health perception	49.4±3.2	29.7±2.8[b]

[a]Unpaired Student's *t*-tests: [a]$p < 0.01$; [b]$p < 0.0001$; [c]$p < 10^{-6}$.

sneeze, watery rhinorrhea, or eosinophilia. Therefore, AR and atopy were unlikely to explain their diverse sets of symptoms. Instead, a pattern of nasal sensitivity to irritant substances leading to sensations of congestion ± rhinorrhea has emerged. CFS subjects had more facial tenderness than HC or acute sinusitis subjects (23). This was associated with "functional" syndromes of irritable bowel, irritable bladder, and other mucosal disorders.

CFS and control subjects were compared for a wide range of psychometric parameters (Table 2). The groups were equally sedentary to ensure that aerobic exercise did not skew the normal responses (Minnesota Heart Score) (24). CFS has significantly more complaints of depression (25,26), pain (27), all categories of fatigue (28), physical functioning, and quality of life (SF-36) (29,30). Anxiety and anger (31) were greater in CFS subjects. By using a nominal (yes vs. no) scoring system, it was found that CFS subjects had significantly more qualitative complaints than controls (2). The ability of irritants to stimulate sensations of congestion and nasal discharge (32) and sensitivity to tobacco smoke (33) were generally increased in CFS, but were not present in all of the CFS population. Anxiety has already been shown to be significantly greater in women with either allergic or idiopathic NAR compared to control subjects (34). CFS/FM subjects had greater hyperalgesia, higher prevalence of interstitial cystitis and irritable bladder symptoms (35), and dyspnea (36). Potential theories to explain the symptom complex included atopy, inflammation, viral infection, and autonomic and nociceptive nerve dysfunction. Investigations of these mechanisms are described in the rest of this chapter.

ATOPY IN CFS

The notion that atopy was increased in prevalence and was causative of CFS (2) began with allergy skin test data from 24 (37) and 28 (38) subjects, and these tests were positive in 50% and 53%, respectively. These rates were higher than the rates of 20% to 30% that had been published for the previous decade (39–43). CFS subjects complained of skin rashes, urticaria, rhinitis, asthma, and drug and food reactions. These conditions were designated as "atopic," even though there were no other confirmatory or provocation testing to evaluate IgE-mediated mechanisms. CFS subject complaints were lumped together, and the authors concluded that 83% to 90% of CFS subjects were "atopic." This was probably not justified because nonallergic syndromes such as maculopapular skin rashes, "hives" described by the patients or physicians, NAR, nonallergic asthma, non-IgE drug idiosyncratic or expected pharmacological reactions, and food intolerances would have all been included in these "atopic disorders" (44). IgE was not compared between the CFS and local control populations. The long differential diagnosis of inflammatory eosinophilic, chronic nonallergic rhinosinusitis, and neutrophilic chronic infectious rhinosinusitis was not investigated. Noninflammatory rhinitides related to hormonal, neural, sympathetic, parasympathetic [cholinergic rhinitis (45)], and nociceptive ("vasomotor rhinitis," idiopathic rhinitis) neural dysfunctions (46) were not investigated. As early as 1992, Metzger's group had proposed that NAR was the most likely diagnosis (1). This finding was largely ignored as investigators stampeded to the TH2 dysfunction hypothesis of CFS pathology.

If TH2-IgE mechanisms are responsible for CFS rhinitis, then it is reasonable to expect that typical antiallergy therapies would improve the conditions. This expectation was false in CFS. Both antihistamines (terfenadine) (38) and topical nasal glucocorticoids (47) had no effect on the presumed "allergic rhinitis" of CFS. This implies that TH2–IgE–mast cells–eosinophil pathways do not contribute to either CFS or its associated rhinitic syndrome.

We investigated this problem further by assessing the constellation of symptoms in CFS, AR, and control groups, and the rates of positive allergy skin tests and elevated IgE levels. CFS and HC subjects retrospectively scored the severities of 30 skin, eye, and airway symptoms over the past six months using an Airway Symptoms Severity Questionnaire (2,48,49). The severity of each symptom was scored as none (score = 0), mild (1), moderate (2), or severe (3). This questionnaire was validated by prospectively assessing changes in symptoms prior to, during, and after periods of seasonal AR, and following the emergency room treatment of acute asthma. The score was modified by adding the level of trivial complaints, which prevented a "floor" effect when subjects had minimal symptoms that were not persistent or disabling enough to be considered "mild." There was no ceiling effect, as the category of "extremely severe" was not statistically valid by Cronbach's α testing. A score of 13 for the nose, sinus, and throat questions was defined as an "abnormal" or "positive" Rhinitis Score. This score exceeded the 95th percentile for a negative control group ($n = 79$), who had no AR, sinusitis, FM, or CFS and who were recruited for a separate protocol where rhinitis and skin testing status were not used as inclusion or exclusion criteria.

Allergy Skin Test Results

Skin testing was positive for at least two allergens plus histamine in 39% of 92 CFS, 50% of 139 HC, and 100% of AR subjects ($n = 27$). Rates for CFS and normal groups were not significantly different (χ^2).

Rhinitis Classification

Rhinitis Scores less than and greater than or equal to 13, and positive or negative allergy skin tests were used to classify CFS and control subjects into different subsets of rhinitis (2). (i) NAR was defined by negative allergy skin tests with positive histamine response plus a positive Rhinitis Scores ≥ 13. (ii) AR had positive allergy

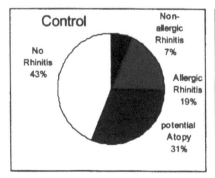 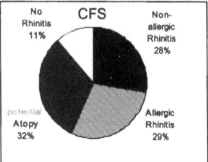

FIGURE 1   Comparison of rhinitis types in control and chronic fatigue syndrome (CFS) groups. There were significantly more subjects with negative Rhinitis Scores (no rhinitis and potential atopy) in the control group. In contrast, the high Rhinitis Scores found in the CFS group lead to higher prevalences of nonallergic and allergic rhinitis. *Abbreviation:* CFS, chronic fatigue syndrome.

TABLE 3 Rhinitis Scores and IgE for Each Rhinitis Type in the Control and Chronic Fatigue Syndrome Populations

Rhinitis type	Group	Rhinitis Score mean± SEM (n^a)	Serum (IgE) IU/mL mean± SEM (n^a)
All	Control	6.8± 0.6 (149)[b]	121.5± 17.3 (126)
All	CFS	17.3± 0.9 (119)[b]	136.1± 43.1 (107)
NAR	Control	20.4± 2.8 (8)	45.1± 11.0 (7)
NAR	CFS	20.1± 1.3 (27)	73.0± 14.4 (27)
AR	Control	19.6± 1.4 (23)	177.0± 29.2 (17)
AR	CFS	21.8± 1.0 (28)	182.4± 49.8 (23)
PotAt	Control	3.7± 0.7 (38)[c]	188.6± 43.8 (36)
PotAt	CFS	6.1± 0.7 (31)[c]	106.3± 42.0 (26)
NoRh	Control	2.5± 0.4 (54)[d]	61.6± 17.0 (49)
NoRh	CFS	6.3± 1.2 (11)[d]	110.8± 24.6 (7)

[a]Different numbers of subjects completed Rhinitis Scores and phlebotomy.
[b]$p < 0.0000001$ by two-tailed unpaired Student's t-test.
[c]$p = 0.017$ by unpaired Student's t-test.
[d]$p = 0.003$ by unpaired Student's t-test. Some seemingly significant differences were due to small sample sizes.
Abbreviations: AR, allergic rhinitis; NAR, nonallergic rhinitis; NoRh, no Rhinitis group; PotAt, potential atopy.

skin tests with positive Rhinitis Scores. (iii) Potential atopy subjects had positive allergy skin tests with negative Rhinitis Scores. This implied allergen sensitization without significant nasal symptoms. (iv) The no Rhinitis group had negative allergy skin tests and Rhinitis Scores. The distributions of these groups were compared between CFS and HC groups (Fig. 1). Subjects were not aware that the purpose of the investigation was to assess rhinitis. The significantly higher RhSc in the CFS population led to higher percentages of NAR and AR subjects. However, there were no differences in the frequencies of allergy skin tests. Stratification by serum IgE concentrations also showed no significant differences between normal and CFS subsets (Table 3) (50).

In multivariate analysis, a positive Rhinitis Score was more predictive of CFS ($p < 0.000001$) than a positive allergy skin test result (not significant). The absence of a relationship between CFS and allergy skin test results (2) combined with the similar distributions of IgE concentrations (Table 3) (50) in CFS and control populations confirmed that atopy was not more frequent in CFS. Stratification by Rhinitis Score and allergy skin test status did not generate any differences between CFS and control subgroups. The hypothesis that atopy was responsible for CFS (37,51) was not supported by these data.

MUCOSAL INFLAMMATION

An alternative hypothesis was that CFS rhinitis was the result of airway inflammation. The hypothesis was derived from the original cardinal features of CFS that resembled those of an infectious illness (e.g., myalgias, sore throat, fatigue, and sensation of fever). Initial studies described the illness in terms of an epidemic. This led to the conclusion that CFS was initiated and perpetuated by an infectious agent (52–56). If so, then vascular, glandular, and cellular inflammatory changes characteristic of viral or immune etiologies were predicted.

The initial impression of potential viral epidemics as a cause of CFS was disproven by epidemiologic studies. Fukuda et al. at the Centers for Disease Control and Prevention investigated a series of cases reported by a single physician in a rural Michigan town (57). The residents of two towns within the epidemic region were selected as the cases, and the residents of two distant towns were selected as controls. There were two noteworthy results. First, there was no difference between the prevalence of prolonged fatigue (8% related to chronic disease, affective disorder, or idiopathic fatigue) or CFS (2%) between the two sets of residents. This first formal case–control study of CFS revealed that there was no epidemic at all. Instead, a "pseudo-epidemic" was identified. The rate of CFS was equal and relatively high in both populations. Active surveillance for CFS by the informed physician identified a "disease cluster," whereas the same prevalence was present in the other towns where there was no active surveillance. This study also found that the minimum prevalence of CFS in the four rural Michigan towns was greater than 1%, much higher than previous estimates. One reason for this increased prevalence was that the new, less restrictive 1994 definition of CFS was used (4). These prevalence figures have been supported by other community-based studies in Chicago, Seattle, and Witchita, Kansas (7,58). A population-based study on a cohort of HMO patients estimated a lower point prevalence for CFS (0.1–0.2%) (59), but patients with chronic complaints were excluded from enrollment.

Chronic viral infections by Epstein–Barr virus (EBV) (60) were suggested because of the similarity of CFS to cases of prolonged infectious mononucleosis. Early studies found high titers of antibodies to EBV in CFS subjects (6). Further studies showed that antibody titers for EBV, human herpes virus 6 (HHV-6), cytomegalovirus (CMV), varicella, enteroviruses, and retroviruses lacked sensitivity and specificity for CFS (61). Elevated titers to numerous ubiquitous infectious agents weakened the hypothesis that any single virus provoked CFS. In addition, high viral titers have also been reported in subjects living under high-stress conditions, such as the caregivers to Alzheimer patients (62–68). This suggested that chronic physiological stressors may modulate immune responses in a wide variety of situations. Finally, CFS overlaps with other syndromes. Chronic viral and immune aberrations have been postulated to cause only CFS, and not the overlapping illnesses of FM, somatoform disorders, irritable bowel syndrome (IBS), migraine headaches, interstitial cystitis, and neurally mediated hypotension that are so common in the CFS population.

If active inflammation is responsible for CFS rhinitis, then changes in vascular, glandular, and cellular biomarkers should be present. Nasal lavage fluid was assessed in CFS, active AR, cystic fibrosis, rhinovirus infections, and HC subjects (Table 4) (3). AR had significantly higher total protein, IgG (vascular permeability), 7F10-mucin (submucosal gland serous cell mucin), eosinophil cationic protein, and neutrophil elastase than the HC and CFS groups (3,69). Cystic fibrosis patients with chronic infectious rhinosinusitis had significantly higher 7F10-mucin, Alcian Blue positive acidic mucin (submucosal gland mucous cells), and elastase. In a separate study, control subjects were inoculated with *Rhinovirus Hanks* (70). Vascular exudation of albumin and IgG was increased four to sevenfold on days 3 and 4, followed by fourfold increase in sIgA. Gel phase acid mucins and interleukin-8 (IL-8) levels were increased twofold. Again, these values were significantly different from the noninfected HC and CFS groups.

These data reduce the likelihood that AR, eosinophilic NAR or sinusitis, chronic infectious sinusitis, or humoral or other immunodeficiencies contribute to CFS rhinitis. However, there may be slight mucous hypersecretion and mucosal friability (increased free hemoglobin in nasal lavage fluid) compared to HC

TABLE 4 Concentrations of Baseline Nasal Mucus Constituents in Lavage Fluid from CFS, Allergic Rhinitis, Cystic Fibrosis, and Normal Control Subjects [10 min Collections; Mean± SEM (n)]

Mucus constituents	Normal	CFS	Allergic rhinitis	Cystic fibrosis
Total protein (µg/mL)	340± 75 (21)	331± 47 (52)	645± 103 (23); $p=0.023^a$	509± 74 (7)
IgG (µg/mL)	28.8± 4.7 (25)	22.8± 3.0 (38)	58.3± 11.8 (34); $p=0.045^a$	15.0± 3.2 (7)
Lysozyme (µg/mL)	30.4± 3.31 (15)	27.7± 1.8 (43)	40.8± 5.9 (10)	30.8± 2.9 (7)
7F10-mucin (mU/mL)	42.0± 7.6 (22)	72.4± 17.0 (47)	112.0± 30.1 (21); $p=0.027^a$	119± 20 (7); $p=0.0012^a$
Alcian blue staining acid mucin (µg/mL)	364± 60 (44)	385± 62 (44)	373± 125 (8)	684± 119 (7); $p=0.04^a$
ECP (ng/mL)	3.30± 1.26 (11)	11.26± 5.54 (24)	79.55± 22.72 (9); $p=0.0016$	Not done
Elastase (ng/mL)	233± 28 (9)	213± 16 (9)	304± 45 (7); $p=0.03^b$	301± 12 (7); $p=0.0025^b$

[a]Mann-Whitney U tests.
[b]Fisher's exact test compared to normal values.
Abbreviations: CFS, chronic fatigue syndrome; ECP, eosinophil cationic protein.

subjects (71,72). Patterns of mast cells, eosinophils, IgE-immunoreactive cells, and mucin mRNA expression were not different between normal and idiopathic rhinitis subjects (73,74). Factors that have been proposed, but not confirmed, to distinguish AR from idiopathic NAR include mucosal goblet cell number, a 23 kDa protein in nasal lavage fluid, plasma histamine, IgD, and soluble *fas* (75–78). These changes are of interest because there is a high probability that the NAR of CFS is analogous to "vasomotor" or idiopathic rhinitis.

Differences in cytokine levels would implicate inflammatory mechanisms in CFS. However, there were no differences from control values in baseline nasal lavage fluid for nerve growth factor, tumor necrosis factor–α (TNF-α), or IL-8 (79)

TABLE 5 Cytokines in Control and CFS Subjects [mean± SEM (n)]

	Control[a]	CFS[a]	Acute sinusitis	Active allergic rhinitis
Total protein (µg/mL)	414± 68 (65)	388± 54 (79)	942± 400 (12)[b]	342± 51 (15)
Hemoglobin (µg/mL)	2.5± 0.6 (65)	2.3± 0.9 (76)	3.8± 1.5 (10)	1.9± 1.0 (13)
NGF (pg/mL)	69.1± 26.8 (41)	81.5± 24.3 (47)	45.1± 20.8 (10)	52.6± 31.6 (13)
TNF-α (pg/mL)	15,119± 5,441 (64)	9,509± 3,591 (78)	61,606± 26,984 (11)[c]	2,864± 1,212 (13)
IL-8 (pg/mL)	4.170± 1.718 (63)	7.029± 2.540 (78)	103.856± 49.801 (10)[d]	14.859± 7.908 (14)

[a]There were no significant differences between control and CFS results in these or log transformed data (geometric means).
[b]$p=0.01$.
[c]$p=0.00003$.
[d]$p=0.00000002$ for Acute Sinusitis compared to Control.
Abbreviations: CFS, chronic fatigue syndrome; NGF, nerve growth factor; TNF-α, tumor necrosis factor–α; IL, interleukin; SEM, Standard error of the mean.

(Table 5). In contrast, the positive control of acute sinusitis had significantly higher total protein, TNF-α, and IL-8. These were not higher in active AR, perhaps because of the ongoing allergically triggered secretion of copious volumes of plasma and glandular mucus components that diluted these mediators in active disease.

DYSAUTONOMIA IN CFS

CFS and FM subjects have significant autonomic dysfunction. This has been demonstrated by heart rate variability (80,81), neurally mediated hypotension on tilt table testing (82), and impaired sympathetic response to stressors such as exercise, muscle contraction, noise, and other stimuli (83,84). These data generated the hypothesis that dysautonomia with a blunted sympathetic response to stressors and generalized elevation in parasympathetic influences contribute to FM and CFS pathophysiology.

Dysautonomia has been identified in IBS and migraine headaches (85–88). These syndromes have increased prevalences in CFS and FM. Migraine headaches have baseline sympathetic hypofunction and instability of sympathetic responses (87–92). Nociceptive nerve axon responses with the release of the potent vasodilator CGRP are also implicated in the migraine family of headaches.

In IBS, specific abnormalities in the central sympathetic and parasympathetic autonomic nervous systems can predict diarrhea-predominant versus constipation-predominant subtypes (93–96). Gastrointestinal epithelial enterochromaffin cells act as sensory transducers, which activate intrinsic and extrinsic primary afferent neurons of the submucosal and myenteric plexuses. Serotonin (5-hydroxytryptamine; 5-HT) is the predominant neurotransmitter. 5-HT activates 5-HT(1P) receptors on primary submucosal plexus afferent neurons. 5-HT acting at 5-HT4 receptors enhances the release of neurotransmitters to generate prokinetic reflex pathways. Signaling to the central nervous system and myenteric neurotransmission are mediated via 5-HT3 receptor pathways. Dysfunction of these systems may lead to the subtypes of IBS (97). Potentiation of 5-HT release or receptor activation may account for diarrhea-predominant IBS. Reduced release of 5-HT or desensitization of 5-HT receptors may lead to constipation-predominant IBS. This latter syndrome is of importance as the 5-HT may also play an important role in responses. Constipation-predominant IBS may be related to the development of Parkinson disease in later life (98). Because Parkinson's is not associated with the CFS spectrum of illnesses, it is unlikely that 5-HT and 5-HT4 receptor dysfunctions are responsible for CFS.

Intestinal smooth muscle dysmotility in IBS is also generalized to smooth muscle dysmotility throughout the entire body. This includes the bladder, lung, and esophagus (99–102). Numerous studies have shown that IBS is characterized by increased visceral nociception (103). However, the crampy pain may be due to a distinct central activation of pain pathways, whereas the diarrhea/constipation component appears to be the result of dysmotility mediated by the intrinsic intestinal submucosal and myenteric plexuses. A similar relationship exists between esophageal motor tone and visceral nociception. Esophageal spasm (nutcracker esophagus) can cause noncardiac chest pain that must be carefully distinguished from coronary artery disease and atypical angina.

These studies suggest that there may be a significant neurological dissociation between the mechanisms of the pain and hyperalgesia in FM, fatigue in CFS, and generalized autonomic dysfunction. Each of these symptom complexes may represent different expressions of the same underlying pathological responses to physiological stressors in subjects with differing environmental backgrounds. Multigenic, haplotypic single nucleotide polymorphisms and early life trauma–related gene silencing mechanisms may play modulatory or permissive roles.

Adrenal Function

CFS and FM subjects have deficient morning cortisol surges that are compatible with tertiary adrenal insufficiency and are reminiscent of the findings in atypical seasonal depression in the winter, dysthymia, and less common chronic fatigue states (104). These changes are opposite to those seen in melancholic depression, which is characterized by increased stress system activity (105). Adrenal insufficiency occurs in response to exercise in FM, as cortisol levels fall paradoxically rather than rise in response to physical exertion (106). This postexercise adrenal insufficiency, as well as the decreased sympathetic response to exercise, could be responsible for the severe postexertional fatigue of these syndromes. Because of the complexity and plasticity of the Hypothalamic-pitiutary-adernal (HPA) axis, it may be more appropriate to emphasize the similarities between the HPA axis in these conditions rather than the minor differences: all are characterized by both an underactive and blunted "stress response." It is possible that these disturbances are surrogate markers of central nervous system dysfunction in the dopaminergic mesocorticolimbic system or the reticular activating system (104).

Sympathetic Nervous System Responses to Isometric Handgrip

Isometric handgrip contraction is a simple, well-understood way to stimulate systemic sympathetic reflexes. The strong sympathetic discharge causes vasoconstriction of all tissue vascular beds including the nasal sinusoids (107–110). In an initial pilot study, six control and five CFS subjects contracted a hand dynamometer to maximum strength (111). After a 30-minute rest period, they sat relaxed for a five minute "sham" contraction with the dynamometer in their hands. Vital signs and acoustic rhinometry variables were averaged for the sham period. Acoustic rhinometry measured the minimum cross-sectional area of the anterior nasal valve (narrowest point, Amin) and airspace volume of the anterior 8 cm of the nasal cavity (112). Subjects then contracted the dynamometer at 30% of maximum strength for as long as possible (1.5–2.5 minutes; no difference between CFS and control subjects).

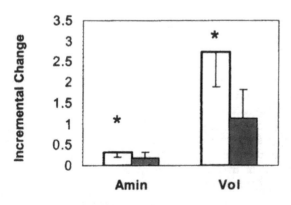

FIGURE 2 Acoustic rhinometry. The incremental changes in Amin and airspace volume (vol) are shown between an isometric handgrip at 30% of maximum and a relaxed "sham contraction." Changes were significant (*$p < 0.05$) for control subjects (white bars) but not chronic fatigue syndrome subjects (black bars).

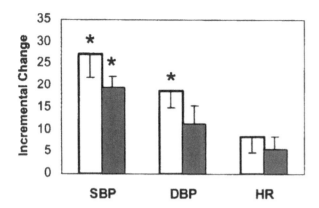

FIGURE 3   Vital signs. The incremental change between isometric and sham handgrip contractions are shown for SBP and DBP and heart rate. The asterisks indicate $p < 0.01$ for the incremental changes. *Abbreviations*: SBP, systolic blood pressure; DBP, diastolic blood pressure; HR, heart rate.

The final "peak" measurements taken before each subject reached exhaustion and the incremental differences from the average for the "sham" period were calculated. Both the minimum cross-sectional area and nasal cavity volumes were significantly increased in the control subjects, but incremental changes were not significant for CFS (Fig. 2). The control subjects had significantly increased diastolic and systolic blood pressures, but not heart rates (Fig. 3). There were no significant changes in vital signs in these CFS subjects, or in a larger group that has been tested subsequently. These data are consistent with decreased sympathetic function in CFS. Alternative sites for reflex dysfunction following isometric forearm muscle contraction include defective sensing of contracted muscle length, ischemia, or acidosis (113,114); spinal cord or brain stem coordination of sympathetic outflow, efferent post-ganglionic norepinephrine or neuropeptide Y (NPY) vasoconstrictor release; and insensitivity of α-adrenergic receptors or absent signal transduction in arterial smooth muscle leading to reduced sympathetic vasoconstriction. Multiple other molecular targets are conceivable.

Systemic parasympathetic dysfunction may contribute to CFS pathophysiology based on heart rate variability studies (80,81), increased cholinergic reactivity in the subset of "runners" with excessive reflex rhinorrhea (45), and increased vasoactive intestinal peptide–immunoreactive, noncholinergic neurons described in "vasomotor" rhinitis (115).

NOCICEPTIVE DYSFUNCTION IN CFS RHINITIS

The studies of baseline nasal lavage fluid cited above demonstrated that there were limited differences between HC and CFS subjects, but very significant differences from the inflammatory syndromes of AR, cystic fibrosis, and viral infections. Nociceptive nerve function was assessed by hypertonic saline (HTS) provocation. HTS mimics the effects of capsaicin, and is desensitized by capsaicin pretreatment (116). In allergic, nonallergic, and postviral asthma and rhinitis, HTS causes exaggerated effects or mucosal hyperresponsiveness (117). HTS may lead to nociceptive nerve depolarization by acting on chloride ion channels to directly depolarize

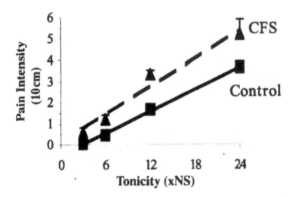

FIGURE 4 Pain intensity after unilateral hypertonic saline. Chronic fatigue syndrome (▲, ---, $n=10$) had significantly greater pain intensity (first pain) than control subjects (■, —, $n=29$) ($p=0.01$). *Abbreviation:* CFS, chronic fatigue syndrome. *Source:* Permission from Baraniuk MD.

nociceptive nerves, or by osmotically drawing water out of epithelial cells causing them to shrink and so activate transient receptor potential ion channels or adjacent chemosensitive/mechanicothermal C-fibers (118). Dry powders such as mannose, the high osmolarity induced by the sudden release of pollen components upon hydration on the nasal mucosa, and inhaled irritants on particulate material may activate additional mechanisms (119–123). Irritant hyperresponsiveness occurs in both allergic and nonallergic subjects (117), with glandular exocytosis being stimulated by a potential nociceptive nerve axon responses mechanism (124). Other mucosal irritants may activate additional mechanisms that remain to be determined.

Unilateral HTS Nasal Provocations
Unilateral HTS provocations were performed in CFS subjects (112,124). Sensations and secretions were assessed from the ipsilateral, challenged nostril, and the contralateral nostril (125).

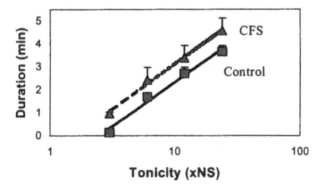

FIGURE 5 Pain duration after unilateral hypertonic saline. The duration of the paresthetic second pain was significantly longer ($p=0.008$) in chronic fatigue syndrome than control subjects. The log-linear relationships were high significant ($r^2 > 0.98$ for each line). *Abbreviation:* CFS, chronic fatigue syndrome. *Source:* Permission from Baraniuk MD.

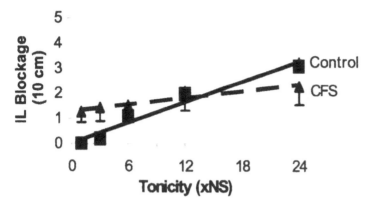

FIGURE 6 Nasal blockage. The chronic fatigue syndrome (CFS) group had a significantly greater sensation of nasal blockage after challenge with 0.9% (normal) saline. The control group had a dose-dependent increase in blockage, while there was no significant change in the CFS group. *Abbreviation:* CFS, chronic fatigue syndrome. *Source:* Courtesy of James N. Baraniuk MD.

Pain

HTS caused an immediate, intense, but short-lived (up to 20 seconds), burning (Fig. 4) that was followed by a more prolonged dose-dependent paresthetic, dull ache (Fig. 5). Curiously, the former showed a linear dose response ($r^2 > 0.94$ for each line), whereas the latter was log-linear ($r^2 > 0.98$), suggesting two distinct mechanisms. These two sensations may be analogous to the First and Second Pain mediated by Type Aδ and C nociceptive fibers (126). Pain intensity ($p = 0.01$ by Analysis of covariance (ANCOVA) and duration ($p = 0.008$) were significantly higher for CFS than control subjects, ANCOVA indicating nociceptive dysfunction in CFS.

Nasal Obstruction

Self-reported sensations of blockage were higher in CFS ($p < 0.000001$) than controls after the first normal saline provocation (Fig. 6). The control subjects had a

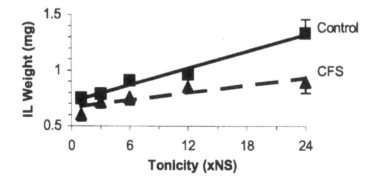

FIGURE 7 Weight of returned nasal lavage fluid. Significant nasal secretion occurred in the control group since the weight of fluid increased to above the amount sprayed into each nostril (1 mL). Chronic fatigue syndrome subjects did not provide a significant amount of fluid suggesting net mucosal absorption. *Abbreviation:* CFS, chronic fatigue syndrome. *Source:* Courtesy of James N. Baraniuk MD.

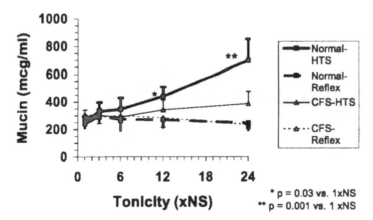

FIGURE 8 Nasal lavage mucin. The normal control subjects had an hypertonic saline dose-dependent increase in mucin secretion (—). They had no significant contralateral reflex (---). The chronic fatigue syndrome subjects had no ipsilateral (—) or contralateral (...) secretion. *Abbreviation:* CFS, chronic fatigue syndrome; HTS, hypertonic saline. *Source:* Courtesy of James N. Baraniuk MD.

significant HTS dose response with increasing obstruction. In contrast, the CFS response was significantly blunted. This suggested that CFS subjects could not effectively detect or report changes in blockage compared to the controls. The sensation of nasal obstruction did not change on the contralateral side for either group.

Rhinorrhea
The weight of nasal lavage fluid increased in HTS dose-dependent fashion in control subjects. However, there was almost a net loss of fluid in the CFS subjects. This suggested absorption of lavage fluid by the mucosa (Fig. 7).

7F10-mucin (Fig. 8) and the submucosal gland serous cells markers urea (Fig. 9) and lysozyme (not shown) were secreted in HTS dose-dependent fashion

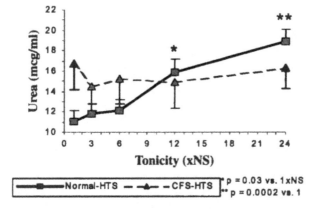

FIGURE 9 Nasal lavage urea. Hypertonic saline induced a dose-dependent secretion of urea from submucosal gland serous cells in normal subjects (—, ■). In contrast, the chronic fatigue syndrome group had higher initial urea levels but not dose response (---, ▲). *Abbreviations:* CFS, chronic fatigue syndrome; HTS, hypertonic saline. *Source:* Courtesy of James N. Baraniuk MD.

in normal subjects, but only on the ipsilateral side. There was no contralateral reflex secretion. In the CFS group at the baseline, urea was significantly elevated in the CFS group compared to controls, whereas 7F10-mucin was the same as in controls. HTS did not cause ipsilateral or contralateral secretion of urea or 7F10-mucin. These findings indicated that the mechanisms responsible for normal submucosal gland exocytosis were highly disrupted in CFS.

There were no changes in albumin or IgG during HTS provocations at these levels of induced pain. This indicates that the direct effect of HTS or nociceptive axon responses do not increase plasma exudation in either normal or CFS subjects.

CONCLUSION

Functional differences between nonallergic, idiopathic, and CFS rhinitis; inflammatory rhinitis; and normal control subjects have been discussed. Idiopathic "vasomotor" and CFS rhinitis are associated with decreased sympathetic responses. HTS induced dose responses for sensations of pain, nasal obstruction, and rhinorrhea in CFS subjects, having significantly higher responses. This was in striking contrast to the function of the nasal mucosa. Normal subjects appeared to develop noncholinergic, nociceptive nerve axon responses that led to glandular exocytosis without vascular permeability or plasma exudation. In contrast, the CFS subjects had increased mucin and urea at baseline, but no significant secretory responses to HTS. These studies cannot be generalized to all groups of nonallergic noninflammatory rhinitis. However, they provide a strong indication that functional defects in nociceptive nerve function, axon responses, and potentially other mechanisms will be identified as additional, carefully phenotyped, clinical subsets of patients are studied in a rigorous, systematic fashion.

Unfortunately, the attitudes of physicians toward CFS, NAR, and functional disorders such as IBS are highly stigmatized (127). Physicians tend to stereotype this group of their patients as having certain undesirable traits. The stereotyping was because of the lack of a precise bodily location; the reclassification of the syndrome over time; transgression of social roles, with patients seen as failing to conform to the work ethic, and "sick role"; and conflict between doctor and patient over causes and management. These factors lead to severe difficulties and even outright rejection for many general practitioners in managing patients with CFS. The same can be said of idiopathic rhinitis. The physicians would not consider referral for mental health interventions because they were not familiar with the interventions or thought them unavailable or unnecessary. This was despite the recognition of the critical roles of social and psychological factors in these patients' well being. Sadly, doctors' beliefs served as barriers to patient treatment. Negative stereotyping of patients and the absence of awareness about the best currently available medical evidence regarding CFS and NAR translated into ignorance and lack of confidence in current management strategies. These barriers are a formidable challenge in dealing with these syndromes that are "all in the patient's head." This is a start, however, as the supracervical structure is the anatomical location of the upper airways and most of the body's neurons. Widespread dispersal of newer evidence of proteomic, functional magnetic resonance, and other brain imaging studies, and hopefully the introduction of novel, effective drugs will be required to overcome these medical biases and improve the lot of this misunderstood group of patients and their enigmatic disorders.

ACKNOWLEDGMENTS

This work was supported by U.S. Public Health Service Awards RO1 AI42403, M01-RR13297, and P50 DC000214.

REFERENCES

1. Cleveland CH Jr., Fisher RH, Brestel EP, Esinhart JD, Metzger WJ. Chronic rhinitis: an underrecognized association with fibromyalgia. Allergy Proc 1993; 13:263–267.
2. Baraniuk JN, Clauw DJ, Gaumond E. Rhinitis symptoms in chronic fatigue syndrome. Ann Allergy Asthma Immunol 1998; 81:359–365.
3. Baraniuk JN, Clauw D, Yuta A, et al. Nasal secretion analysis in allergic rhinitis, cystic fibrosis, and nonallergic fibromyalgia/chronic fatigue syndrome subjects. Am J Rhinol 1998; 12:435–440.
4. Fukuda K, Straus SE, Hickie I, et al. The chronic fatigue syndrome: a comprehensive approach to its definition and study. Ann Intern Med 1994; 121:953–959.
5. Reeves WC, Lloyd A, Vernon SD, et al. Identification of ambiguities in the 1994 chronic fatigue syndrome research case definition and recommendations for resolution. BMC Health Serv Res 2003; 3:25.
6. Wagner D, Nisenbaum R, Heim C, Jones JF, Unger ER, Reeves WC. Psychometric properties of the CDC Symptom Inventory for assessment of Chronic Fatigue Syndrome. Popul Health Metr 2005; 3:8.
7. Reeves WC, Wagner D, Nisenbaum R, et al. Chronic fatigue syndrome—a clinically empirical approach to its definition and study. BMC Med 2005; 3:19.
8. Taylor RR, Jason LA. Chronic fatigue, abuse-related traumatization, and psychiatric disorders in a community-based sample. Soc Sci Med 2002; 55:247–256.
9. White KP, Speechley M, Harth M, Ostbye T. Co-existence of chronic fatigue syndrome with fibromyalgia syndrome in the general population. A controlled study. Scand J Rheumatol 2000; 29:44–51.
10. Baraniuk JN. Neurogenic inflammation. In: Leppert PC, Turned ML, eds. Vulvodynia: Toward Understanding a Pain Syndrome. Proceedings from the Workshop, April 14–15, 2003, supported by the National Institute of Child Health and Human Development (NICHD), the Office of Research on Women's Health, and the Office of Rare Diseases, 2004:16–18; http://www.nichd.nih.gov/publications/pubs/final_vulvodynia_report.pdf
11. Baraniuk JN. CFS and overlapping conditions. CFS Res Rev 2004; 6–9.
12. Wolfe F, Smythe HA, Yunus MB, et al. The American College of Rheumatology 1990 Criteria for the Classification of Fibromyalgia. Report of the Multicenter Criteria Committee. Arthritis Rheum 1990; 33:160–172.
13. Wolfe F, Ross K, Anderson J, Russell IJ, Hebert L. The prevalence and characteristics of fibromyalgia in the general population. Arthritis Rheum 1995; 38:19–28.
14. Petzke FR, Khine A, Clauw DJ. Pain sensitivity in patients with fibromyalgia (FM): expectancy effects on pain measurements [abstr]. Arthritis Rheum 1999; 42:S342.
15. Gracely RH, Geisser ME, Giesecke T, et al. Pain catastrophizing and neural responses to pain among persons with fibromyalgia. Brain 2004; 127:835–843.
16. Petzke F, Ambrose K, Gracely RH, Clauw DJ. What do tender points measure? [abstr]. Arthritis Rheum 1999; 42:S342.
17. Littlejohn GO. Balanced treatments for fibromyalgia. Arthritis Rheum 2004; 50: 2725–2729.
18. Caterina MJ. Vanilloid receptors take a TRP beyond the sensory afferent. Pain 2003; 105:5–9.
19. Weidner C, Klede M, Rukwied R, et al. Acute effects of substance P and calcitonin gene-related peptide in human skin: a microdialysis study. J Invest Dermatol 2000; 115:1015–1020.
20. Fukuda K, Nisenbaum R, Stewart G, et al. Chronic multisymptom illness affecting air force veterans of the gulf war. JAMA 1999; 280:981–988.

21. Baraniuk JN, Casado B, Maibach H, Clauw DJ, Pannell LK, Hess S. A chronic fatigue syndrome related proteome in cerebrospinal fluid. BMC Neurol 2005; 5:22.
22. Clauw DJ, Engel CC Jr., Aronowitz R, et al. Unexplained symptoms after terrorism and war: an expert consensus statement. J Occup Environ Med 2003; 45:1040–1048.
23. Naranch K, Park Y-J, Repka-Ramirez SM, Velarde A, Clauw D, Baraniuk JN. A tender sinus does not always mean sinusitis. Otolaryngol Head Neck Surg 2002; 127:387–397.
24. Folsom AR, Caspersen CJ, Taylor HL, et al. Leisure time physical activity and its relationship to coronary risk factors in a population-based sample. The Minnesota Heart Survey. Am J Epidemiol 1985; 121:570–579.
25. Beck AT, Ward CH, Mendelson M, Mock J, Erbaugh J. An inventory for measuring depression. Arch Gen Psychiatr 1961; 4:561–571.
26. Beck AT, Epstein N, Brown G, Steer RA. An inventory for measuring clinical anxiety: psychometric properties. J Consult Clin Psych 1988; 56:893–897.
27. Melzack R. The short-form McGill pain questionnaire. Pain 1987; 30:191–197.
28. Smets EM, Garssen B, Bonke B, De Haes JC. The Multidimensional Fatigue Inventory (MFI) psychometric qualities of an instrument to assess fatigue. J Psychosom Res 1995; 39:315–325.
29. Ware JE, Sherbourne CD. The MOS 36-item short-form health survey (SF-36): I. Conceptual framework and item selection. Medical Care 1995; 30:473–483.
30. Ware JE, Kosinski M, Keller SD. Anonymous-Physical and Mental Health Summary Scales: A User's Manual. Boston: The Health Institute, 1994.
31. Spielberger CD, Gorsuch RC, Lushene RE, et al. Manual for the State Trait Anxiety Inventory (Form Y). Palo Alto, CA: Consulting Psychologists, 1983:1996.
32. Baraniuk JN, Naranch K, Maibach H, Clauw D. Irritant rhinitis in allergic, nonallergic, control and Chronic Fatigue Syndrome populations. J CFS 2000; 7:3–31.
33. Baraniuk JN, Naranch K, Maibach H, Clauw D. Tobacco sensitivity in chronic fatigue syndrome. J CFS 2000; 7:33–52.
34. Addolorato G, Ancona C, Capristo E, et al. State and trait anxiety in women affected by allergic and vasomotor rhinitis. J Psychosom Res 1999; 46:283–289.
35. Clauw DJ, Schmidt M, Radulovic D, Singer A, Katz P, Bresette J. The relationship between fibromyalgia and interstitial cystitis. J Psychiatr Res 1997; 31:125–131.
36. Naranch K, Singer A, Gaumond E, et al. Dyspnea in fibromyalgia (FM) and chronic fatigue syndrome (CFS). Am J Respir Crit Care Med 1999; 103:A763.
37. Straus SE, Dale JK, Wright R, Metcalfe DD. Allergy and chronic fatigue syndrome. J Allergy Clin Immunol 1988; 81:791–794.
38. Steinberg P, McNutt BE, Marshall P, et al. Double-blind placebo-controlled study of efficacy of oral terfenadine in the treatment of chronic fatigue syndrome. J Allergy Clin Immunol 1996; 97:119–126.
39. Chan-Yeung M, Vedal S, Lam S, Enarson D. Immediate skin reactivity and its relationship to age, sex, smoking, and occupational exposure. Arch Environ Health 1985; 40:53.
40. Gergen PJ, Turkeltaub PC, Kovar Mg. The prevalence of allergic skin test reactivity to eight common aeroallergens in the U.S. population: results from the second National Health and Nutrition Examination Survey. J Allergy Clin Immunol 1987; 80:669.
41. Aberg N, Hesselmar B, Aberg B, Eriksson B. Increase of asthma, allergic rhinitis and eczema in Swedish schoolchildren between 1979 and 1991. Clin Exp Allergy 1995; 25:815–819.
42. Barbee RA, Halonen M, Lebowitz M, Burrows B. Distribution of IgE in a community population sample: correlations with age, sex, and allergen skin test reactivity. J Allergy Clin Immunol 1981; 68:106–111.
43. Droste JHJ, Kerkhof M, de Monchy JGR, Schouten JP, Rijcken B, Dutch ECRHS Group. Association of skin test reactivity, specific IgE, and eosinophils with nasal symptoms in a community-based population study. J Allergy Clin Immunol 1996; 97:922–932.
44. Middleton E, Reed CE, Ellis EF, Adkinson NF, Yunginger JW, Busse WW. Allergy Principles and Practice. 4th ed. St. Louis, MO: Mosby, 1993.
45. Stjarne P, Lundblad L, Lundberg JM, Anggard A. Capsaicin and nicotine sensitive afferent neurones and nasal secretion in healthy human volunteers and in patients with vasomotor rhinitis. Br J Pharmacol 1989; 96:693–701.

46. Mygind N, Naclerio RM, eds. Allergic and Nonallergic Rhinitis. Philadephia, W.B. Saunders PA, 1993.
47. Kakumanu SS, Mende CN, Lehman EB, Hughes K, Craig TJ. Effect of topical nasal corticosteroids on patients with chronic fatigue syndrome and rhinitis. J Am Osteopath Assoc 2003; 103:423–427.
48. Wasserfallen JB, Gold K, Schulman KA, Baraniuk JN. Development and validation of a rhinoconjunctivitis and asthma symptom score for use as an outcome measure in clinical trials. J Allergy Clin Immunol 1997; 100:16–22.
49. Wasserfallen JB, Gold K, Schulman KA, Baraniuk JN. Item responsiveness of a rhinitis and asthma symptom score during a pollen season. J Asthma 1999; 36:459–465.
50. Repka-Ramirez MS, Naranch K, Park Y-J, Velarde A, Clauw D, Baraniuk JN. IgE levels are the same in chronic fatigue syndrome (CFS) and control subjects when stratified by allergy skin test results and rhinitis types. Ann Allergy Asthma Immunol 2001; 87: 218–221.
51. Manu P, Lane TJ, Matthews DA. The pathophysiology of chronic fatigue syndrome; confirmations, contradictions, and conjectures. Int J Psychiatr Med 1992; 22:397–408.
52. Khan AS, Heneine WM, Chapman LE, et al. Assessment of a retroviral sequence and other possible risk factors for the chronic fatigue syndrome in adults. Ann Int Med 1993; 118:241–245.
53. Wray BB, Gaughf C, Chandler FW, et al. Detection of Epstein–Barr virus and cytomegalovirus in patients with chronic fatigue. Ann Allergy 1993; 71:223–226.
54. Levy JA. Part III: viral studies of chronic fatigue syndrome. Clin Inf Dis 1994; 18(suppl 1):S117–S120.
55. Barker E, Fujimura SF, Fadem MB, Landay AL, Levy JA. Immunologic abnormalities associated with chronic fatigue syndrome. Clin Inf Dis 1994; 18(suppl 1):S136–S141.
56. Anon. Inability of retroviral tests to identify persons with chronic fatigue syndrome, 1992. MMWR 1993; 42:189–190.
57. Fukuda K, Wilson L, Dobbins J. A community-based study of unexplained prolonged and chronic fatiguing illness in a rural area of Michigan [abstr]. AACFS Proc 1994.
58. Jason L, Taylor R, Wagner L, et al. A pilot study estimating rates of chronic fatigue syndrome from a community based sample [abstr]. AACFS Proc 1994.
59. Buchwald D, Umali P, Umali J, et al. Chronic fatigue and the chronic fatigue syndrome: prevalence in a Pacific Northwest health care system. Ann Intern Med 1995; 123:81–88.
60. Ablashi DV. Viral studies of chronic fatigue syndrome. Clin Infect Dis 1994; 18(suppl 1):S130–S133.
61. Straus SE. Studies of herpesvirus infection in chronic fatigue syndrome. Ciba Found Symp 1993; 173:132–197.
62. Schulz R, Visintainer P, Williamson GM. Psychiatric and physical morbidity effects of care giving. J Gerontol 1990; 45:181–191.
63. Irwin M, Brown M, Patterson T, Hauger R, Mascovich A, Grant I. Neuropeptide Y and natural killer cell activity: findings in depression and Alzheimer caregiver stress. FASEB J 1991; 5:3100–3107.
64. Mills PJ, Adler KA, Dimsdale JE, et al. Vulnerable caregivers of Alzheimer disease patients have a deficit in beta 2-adrenergic receptor sensitivity and density. Am J Geriatr Psychiatr 2004; 12:281–286.
65. Glaser R, Sheridan J, Malarkey WB, MacCallum RC, Kiecolt-Glaser JK. Chronic stress modulates the immune response to a pneumococcal pneumonia vaccine. Psychosom Med 2000; 62:804–807.
66. Bauer ME, Vedhara K, Perks P, Wilcock GK, Lightman SL, Shanks N. Chronic stress in caregivers of dementia patients is associated with reduced lymphocyte sensitivity to glucocorticoids. J Neuroimmunol 2000; 103:84–92.
67. Glaser R, MacCallum RC, Laskowski BF, Malarkey WB, Sheridan JF, Kiecolt-Glaser JK. Evidence for a shift in the Th-1 to Th-2 cytokine response associated with chronic stress and aging. J Gerontol A Biol Sci Med Sci 2001; 56:M477–M482.
68. Stowell JR, Kiecolt-Glaser JK, Glaser R. Perceived stress and cellular immunity: when coping counts. J Behav Med 2001; 24:323–339.

69. Yuta A, Ali M, Sabol M, Gaumond E, Baraniuk JN. Mucoglycoprotein hypersecretion in allergic rhinitis and cystic fibrosis. Am J Physiol 1997; 273:L1203–L1207 (Lung Cell Mol Physiol 17).

70. Yuta A, van Deusen M, Gaumond E, et al. Rhinovirus infection induces mucus hypersecretion. Am J Physiol 1998; 274:L1017–L1023 (Lung Cell Mol Physiol 18).

71. Naranch K, Repka-Ramirez SM, Park Y-J, et al. Differences in baseline nasal secretions between chronic fatigue syndrome (CFS) and control subjects. J CFS 2002; 10:3–15.

72. Park Y-J, Repka-Ramirez SM, Naranch K, Velarde A, Clauw D, Baraniuk JN. Nasal lavage concentrations of free hemoglobin as a marker of microepistaxis during nasal provocation testing. Allergy 2002; 57:329–335.

73. Aust MR, Madsen CS, Jennings A, Kasperbauer JL, Gendler SJ. Mucin mRNA expression in normal and vasomotor inferior turbinates. Am J Rhinol 1997; 11(4):293–302.

74. Blom HM, Godthelp T, Fokkens WJ, et al. Mast cells, eosinophils and IgE-positive cells in the nasal mucosa of patients with vasomotor rhinitis. An immunohistochemical study. Eur Arch Otorhinolaryngol 1995; 252(suppl 1):S33–S39.

75. Zielinski A. A comparative immunological study of vasomotor rhinitis and pollinosis. J Investig Allergol Clin Immunol 1996; 6:261–265.

76. Kato M, Hattori T, Ito H, et al. Serum-soluble Fas levels as a marker to distinguish allergic and nonallergic rhinitis. J Allergy Clin Immunol 1999; 103:1213–1214.

77. Iguchi Y. Differentiation between allergic rhinitis and vasomotor rhinitis by electrophoretic evaluation of the protein in pituita. Nippon Jibiinkoka Gakkai Kaiho 1995; 98:410–420.

78. Berger G, Moroz A, Marom Z, Ophir D. Inferior turbinate goblet cell secretion in patients with perennial allergic and nonallergic rhinitis. Am J Rhinol 1999; 13:473–477.

79. Repka-Ramirez MS, Naranch K, Park Y-J, Clauw D, Baraniuk JN. Cytokines in nasal lavage fluids from acute sinusitis, allergic rhinitis, and chronic fatigue syndrome subjects. Allergy Asthma Proc 2002; 23:185–190.

80. Glass JM, Lyden AK, Petzke F, et al. The effect of brief exercise cessation on pain, fatigue, and mood symptom development in healthy, fit individuals. J Psychosom Res 2004; 57:391–398.

81. Stein PK, Domitrovich PP, Ambrose K, et al. Sex effects on heart rate variability in fibromyalgia and Gulf War illness. Arthritis Rheum 2004; 51:700–708.

82. Rowe PC, Bou-Holaigah I, Kan JS, Calkins H. Is neurally mediated hypotension an unrecognised cause of chronic fatigue? Lancet 1995; 345:623–624.

83. Qiao ZG, Vaery H, Merkrid L. Electrodermal and microcirculatory activity in patients with fibromyalgia during baseline, acoustic stimulation and cold pressor tests. J Rheumatol 1993; 18:1383–1389.

84. Elam M, Johansson G, Wallin BG. Do patients with primary fibromyalgia have an altered muscle sympathetic nerve activity? Pain 1993; 48:371–375.

85. Mayer EA, Raybould HE. Role of visceral afferent mechanisms in functional bowel disorders. Gastroenterology 1990; 99:1688–1704.

86. Lynn R, Friedman L. Irritable bowel syndrome. N Engl J Med 1993; 329:1940–1945.

87. Buzzi M, Bonamini M, Cerbo R. The anatomy and biochemistry of headache. Funct Neurol 1993; 8:395–402.

88. Pogacnik T, Sega S, Pecnik B, Kiauta T. Autonomic function testing in patients with migraine. Headache 1993; 33:545–550.

89. Pareja JA. Chronic paroxysmal hemicrania: dissociation of the pain and autonomic features. Headache 1995; 35:111–113.

90. Zigelman M, Appel S, Davidovitch S, Kuritzky A, Zahavi I, Akselrod S. The effect of verapamil calcium antagonist on autonomic imbalance in migraine: evaluation by spectral analysis of beat-to-beat heart rate fluctuations. Headache 1994; 34:569–577.

91. Prusinski A, Trzos S, Rozentryt P, et al. Studies of heart rhythm variability in migraine. Preliminary communication. Neurol Neurochir Pol 1994; 28:23–27.

92. Appel S, Kuritzky A, Zahavi I, Zigelman M, Akselrod S. Evidence for instability of the autonomic nervous system in patients with migraine headache. Headache 1992; 32:10–17.

93. Aggarwal A, Cutts TF, Abell TL, et al. Predominant symptoms in irritable bowel syndrome correlate with specific autonomic nervous system abnormalities. Gastroenterology 1994; 106:945–950.

94. McAllister C, Fielding JF. Patients with pulse rate changes in irritable bowel syndrome. Further evidence of altered autonomic function. J Clin Gastroenterol 1988; 10:273–274.

95. Fukudo S, Suzuki J. Colonic motility, autonomic function, and gastrointestinal hormones under psychological stress on irritable bowel syndrome. Tohoku J Exp Med 1987; 151:373–385.

96. Whitehead WE, Holtkotter B, Enck P. Tolerance for rectosigmoid distension in irritable bowel syndrome. Gastroenterology 1990; 98:1187–1192.

97. Gershon MD. Review article: serotonin receptors and transporters–roles in normal and abnormal gastrointestinal motility. Aliment Pharmacol Ther 2004; 20(suppl 7):3–14.

98. Chaudhuri KR, Yates L, Martinez-Martin P. The non-motor symptom complex of Parkinson's disease: a comprehensive assessment is essential. Curr Neurol Neurosci Rep 2005; 5:275–283.

99. White AM, Stevens WH, Upton AR, et al. Airway responsiveness to inhaled methacholine in patients with irritable bowel syndrome. Gastroenterology 1991; 100:68–74.

100. Kellow JE, Eckersley GM, Jones M. Enteric and central contributions to intestinal dysmotility in irritable bowel syndrome. Dig Dis Sci 1992; 37:168–174.

101. Whorwell PJ, Clouter C, Smith CL. Oesophageal motility in the irritable bowel syndrome. Br Med J 1981; 282:1101–1102.

102. Whorwell PJ, Lupton EW, Erduran D, et al. Bladder smooth muscle dysfunction in patients with irritable bowel syndrome. Gut 1986; 27:1014–1017.

103. Adam V. Visceral Perception. In: Understanding Internal Cognition. New York: Plenum Press, 1998:1–232.

104. Chrousos GP, Gold PW. The concepts of stress and stress system disorders. Overview of physical and behavioral homeostasis. JAMA 1992; 267:1244–1252.

105. Griep EN, Boersma JW, de Kloet ER. Altered reactivity of the hypothalamic-pituitary-adrenal axis in the primary fibromyalgia syndrome. J Rheumatol 1993; 20:469–474.

106. van Denderen JC, Boersma JW, Zeinstra P, et al. Physiological effects of exhaustive physical exercise in primary fibromyalgia syndrome (PFS): is PFS a disorder of neuroendocrine reactivity? Scand J Rheumatol 1993; 21:35–37.

107. Wilde AD, Cook JA, Jones AS. The nasal response to isometric exercise. Clin Otolaryngol 1995; 20:345–347.

108. Wilde AD, Cook JA, Jones AS. The nasal response to isometric exercise in non-eosinophilic intrinsic rhinitis. Clin Otolaryngol 1996; 21:84–86.

109. Baraniuk J. Cardiovascular effects of an isometric training program. Faculty of Medicine, University of Manitoba, 1979.

110. Khurana RK, Setty A. The value of the isometric hand-grip test–studies in various autonomic disorders. Clin Autonom Res 1996; 6:211–218.

111. Park Y-J, Naranch K, Repka-Ramirez SM, Clauw D, Baraniuk JN. Sympathetic dysfunction demonstrated by isometric handgrip responses in CFS. American Association for Chronic Fatigue Syndrome. Seattle, WA (oral presentation), January, 2001.

112. Baraniuk JN, Ali M, Naranch K. Hypertonic saline nasal provocation and acoustic rhinometry. Clin Exp Allergy 2002; 32:543–550.

113. Tominaga M, Caterina MJ, Malmberg AB, et al. The cloned capsaicin receptor integrates multiple pain-producing stimuli. Neuron 1998; 21:531–543.

114. Caterina MJ, Leffler A, Malmberg AB, et al. Impaired nociception and pain sensation in mice lacing the capsaicin receptor. Science 2000; 288:306–313.

115. Kurian SS, Blank MA, Sheppard MN. Vasoactive intestinal polypeptide (VIP) in vasomotor rhinitis. Clin Biochem 1983; 11:425–427.

116. Togias A, Lykens K, Kagey-Sobotka A, et al. Studies on the relationships between sensitivity to cold, dry air, hyperosmolar solutions, and histamine in the adult nose. Am Rev Respir Dis 1990; 141:1428–1433.

117. Sanico AM, Philip G, Proud D, Naclerio RM, Togias A. Comparison of nasal mucosal responsiveness to neuronal stimulation in non-allergic and allergic rhinitis: effects of capsaicin nasal challenge. Clin Exp Allergy 1998; 28:92–100.

118. Liedtke W, Tobin DM, Bargmann CL, Friedman JM. Mammalian TRPV4 (VR-OAC) directs behavioral responses to osmotic and mechanical stimuli in Caenorhabditis elegans. PNAS 2003; 100:14531–14536.

119. Baraniuk JN, Esch RE, Buckley CE III. Pollen grain column chromatography. J Allergy Clin Immunol 1988; 81:1126–1134.
120. Baraniuk JN, Bolick M, Buckley CE III. Pollen grain column chromatography: a novel method for separation of pollen wall solutes. Ann Botany 1990; 66:321–329.
121. Baraniuk JN, Bolick M, Esch R, Buckley CE. Quantification of pollen solute release using pollen grain column chromatography. Allergy 1992; 47:411–417.
122. Peterson B, Saxon A. Global increases in allergic respiratory disease: the possible role of diesel exhaust particles. Ann Allergy Asthma Immunol 1996; 77:263–268.
123. Bell IR, Baldwin CM, Schwartz GE. Illness from low levels of environmental chemicals: relevance to chronic fatigue syndrome and fibromyalgia. Am J Med 1998; 105:74S–82S.
124. Baraniuk JN, Petrie KN, Le U, et al. Neuropathology in rhinosinusitis. Am J Respir Crit Care Med 2005; 171:5–11.
125. Baraniuk JN, Ali M, Yuta A, Fang SY, Naranch K. Hypertonic saline nasal provocation stimulates nociceptive nerves, substance P release, and glandular mucous exocytosis in normal humans. Am J Respir Crit Care Med 1999; 160:655–662.
126. Dray A, Urban L, Dickenson A. Pharmacology of chronic pain. TIPS 1994; 15:190–197.
127. Raine R, Carter S, Sensky T, Black N. General practitioners' perceptions of chronic fatigue syndrome and beliefs about its management, compared with irritable bowel syndrome: qualitative study. BMJ 2004; 328:1354–1357.

Rhinitis and Sleep Apnea

Maria T. Staevska

*Allergology and Clinical Immunology, Clinic of Asthma, Medical University of Sofia,
University Hospital "Alexandrovska," Sofia, Bulgaria*

James N. Baraniuk

*Department of Medicine, Division of Rheumatology, Immunology and Allergy,
and Georgetown University Proteomics Laboratory, Georgetown University
Medical Center, Washington, D.C., U.S.A.*

INTRODUCTION

Up to one-third of the population may have some degree of abnormal breathing
during sleep (1). Sleep fragmentation and microarousals unfavorably influence
daytime energy levels, mood, and daytime function (2,3). Causes include the common cold, allergic and inflammatory nonallergic rhinitis, and hyperactive nasal
posture reflexes with exaggerated nasal airflow obstruction when recumbent (4).
Atopic dermatitis and asthma are also associated with disordered sleep breathing
(DSB). Pharyngeal risk factors, such as obesity, chronic adenoid and tonsil
hypertrophy, and excessive relaxation of the supraglottic musculature also promote closure of the nasal, pharyngeal, and laryngeal airways. These more severe
airway obstruction syndromes may affect 2% to 4% of the populace. The links
between different phenotypes of rhinitis and sleep disturbances will be discussed
by beginning with the effects of inflammation on normal sleep patterns, classifications of sleep pathology, pathophysiological mechanisms, and diagnostic and
treatment regimens.

PHASES OF SLEEP

Sleep is divided into two phases (5), one of which is nonrapid eye movement sleep
(NREMS; "quiet sleep") that has four stages in humans. Of these, two stages of deep
refreshing sleep are characterized by high amplitude, low frequency (0.5–4 Hz)
delta wave electroencephalographic (EEG) activity. Brain metabolic rate is
decreased during NREMS. This may provide a restorative period of brain activity
and the restful sensations of a good night's sleep.

The other phase is rapid eye movement sleep (REMS; paradoxical or dream
sleep). REMS accounts for about 25% of sleep time in humans (5). Endogenous type
1 interferons α and β and other cytokines act in the central nervous system to
shorten the duration of REM sleep and to increase δ-wave amplitude. The prolonged NREM and shortened REM provide a longer duration of low brain
metabolism rate and restorative sleep. The period of inactivity may be beneficial
by decreasing muscle activity and diverting energy and metabolic reserves to ther-
moregulation (e.g., fever) and tissue healing processes. Circadian changes in mRNA
and protein expression in the suprachiasmatic nucleus of the hypothalamus, liver,
and other tissues support these inflammation- and infection-related alterations (6).

Transport of these peripheral blood cytokines and other factors across the blood–brain barrier into the central nervous system activates systems in the hypothalamus, median eminence, organum vasculosum of the lamina terminalis, and other sleep regulatory centers. Positive feedback loops between nerve growth factor, interleukin (IL)-1, and tumor necrosis factor (TNF)-α promote slow wave sleep (NREMS) (5). Nuclear Factor-κB (NF-κB) is the critical transcription factor central to the induction of these pro-somnogenic cytokines. These activate the actual mediators of NREM sleep: growth hormone–releasing hormone (GHRH), nitric oxide, adenosine, and prostagladin D2 (PGD2) (7).

The production of sleep-regulating cytokines is linked to infection, the innate immune system, and inflammation (5). Factor sleep (factor S) was discovered in the 1970s and was chemically identified as fragments of bacterial peptidoglycan that were very similar to muramyl dipeptide, the active agent of Freund's adjuvant (8). These bacterial cell wall fragments activate the nucleotid-binding oligomerization domain (NOD) family of proteins in macrophages to stimulate IL-1β. IL-1β is somnogenic and pyrogenic in femtomolar concentrations. IL-6, TNF-α, and other cytokines share these endogenous pyrogenic properties and may mediate the sleep disruption and daytime somnolence common to many low-grade inflammatory conditions. For example, infusion of antibodies to TNF-α in arthritis improves daytime somnolence in arthritis (9). These cytokines are synthesized by a wide array of cell types, including airway epithelium, fibroblasts, and leukocytes that are activated in allergic rhinitis, sinusitis, nasal polyps, and the eosinophilic, neutrophilic, and mixed inflammatory subsets of nonallergic rhinitis. Therefore, periods of short term (e.g., acute sinusitis), intermittent (e.g., a short season of pollenosis), and persistent (e.g., house dust mite allergy, NARES, and chronic rhinosinusitis) somnolence and daytime malaise are to be anticipated in these cytokine-laden disorders.

Disruption of NREM sleep and its restorative physiological processes may play a major role in the symptomatology of sleep-disordered breathing (SDB) and obstructive sleep apnea (OSA). IL-4, IL-10, soluble TNF-α receptors, and the stress hormones, CRH and cortisol (and by implication, systemic glucocorticoids), decrease NREM sleep (5–8). In allergic rhinitis, this produces a paradoxical conflict of cytokine effects. The TH2-type cytokines will reduce restorative NREM sleep, whereas IL-1β, IL-6, TNF-α, and others will attempt to prolong NREM sleep. The result may be the "allergic fatigue syndrome" (Melvin Danzig, personal communication, 1997) (10,11). Chronic fatigue syndrome (CFS) has been proposed to have a TH2-cytokine bias based on in vitro studies (12), although there is little evidence to support a pro-atopic bias in the clinical manifestations of this disorder. In fact, the nonallergic rhinitis of CFS is characterized by normal distributions of IgE and the absence of eosinophilia rather than the anticipated TH2-driven clinical manifestation of atopy (11,13–17).

SDB AND OSAS

SDB is the general term applied to all forms of dysfunctional airflow obstruction syndromes during sleep. SDB is a large entity encompassing a variety of conditions of sleep-related regular respiratory disturbances. One algorithm proposes a continuum of intermittent snoring → persistent or habitual snoring → upper airway resistance syndrome → mild obstructive sleep apnea syndrome (OSAS) → severe OSAS → obesity → Pickwickian hypoventilation syndrome (18). However, this linear progression has not been clearly identified in prospective longitudinal studies.

TABLE 1 Tentative Criteria for Sleep Apnea in Adults

At least one of the following three observations:
  Patient complaints of unintentional sleep episodes during wakefulness,
    daytime sleepiness, unrefreshing sleep, fatigue, or insomnia.
  Patient wakes up at night with breath holding, gasping, or choking.
  Bed partner observes symptoms of loud snoring and/or breathing interruptions.
Polysomnographic recording shows the following:
  Five or more scoreable respiratory events per hour of sleep (hypopnea, respiratory effort-related
    arousals, apnea, or other events).
  Evidence of respiratory effort (diaphragmatic contraction and decreased intrathoracic pressure
    by esophageal manometry) during all or part of each respiratory event.
Symptoms cannot be explained by another sleep disorder, medical condition, mental disorder,
  medication, substance abuse, or dependence.

Snoring

The mildest form of SDB is snoring. It may be intermittent to persistent (nightly). It generally has no detrimental effect on an individual's health. Snoring affects 35% of the middle-aged population including 44% of men and 28% of women. Prevalence increases with age (19). Snoring is produced by turbulent airflow through partially collapsed pharyngeal walls that cause vibration of the soft palate. Nasal polyps, hypertrophied turbinates, and nasal septal deviation are often found. A population-based cohort study indicated that nocturnal nasal congestion had a significant odds ratio of 4.9 for habitual snoring (19).

Obstructive Sleep Apnea Syndrome

OSAS is defined as (i) complete or partial collapse of the upper airways during sleep with consequent cessation of breathing despite ongoing respiratory effort (OSA), plus (ii) coexistent daytime somnolence (disabling symptomatology) (Table 1) (20). Less well-established criteria have been proposed for children (Table 2), as there are few standardized normative studies, and the differential diagnosis may be different from adults. These guidelines will be subject to periodic revision.

Apnea

It is defined as cessation of airflow for at least 10 seconds. It may be central, obstructive, or mixed. Central sleep apnea is rare and is due to absence of brainstem-derived respiratory efforts. OSA is much more common and results from complete obstruction of the upper airways despite persistent ventilatory effort. Hypopnea results from incomplete upper airway obstruction. It is defined by at least a 30% reduction of airflow. The apnea–hypopnea index (AHI) is the average number of apnea and hypopnea events per hour of sleep. AHI <5 is considered normal. OSA is defined by AHI $\geq$ 5. This is generally associated with a 4% decrease in oxygen saturation (Medicare definition of sleep apnea). OSA is divided into three severity levels: (i) mild with AHI of 5 to 15, (ii) moderate with AHI of 15 to 30, and (iii) severe with AHI >30. Apnea and hypopnea always cause arousal. These repetitive arousals cause sleep fragmentation that leads to daytime sleepiness. OSA together with daytime sleepiness defines OSAS (20).

Risk factors include rhinitis, obesity, increased neck circumference, aging, male sex, acromegaly (21), hypothyroidism, and relatively rare craniofacial

TABLE 2   Tentative Criteria for Sleep Apnea in Children

The caregiver reports snoring and/or labored or obstructed breathing during sleep
The caregiver observes at least one of the following:
Paradoxical inward rib cage motion during inspiration
Movement arousals
Diaphoresis
Neck hyperextension during sleep
Excessive daytime sleepiness, hyperactivity, or aggressive behavior
Slow rate of growth
Morning headaches
Secondary enuresis
Polysomnography shows:
At least one obstructive event (poorly defined because of limited studies) in at least two respiratory cycles per hour of sleep, plus one of (a) or (b):
a) One of the following: frequent arousals from sleep associated with respiratory effort; or arterial oxygen desaturation in association with apnea; or hypercapnia during sleep; or markedly negative esophageal pressure (intrathoracic pressure) variations
b) Periods of hypercapnia and/or desaturation during sleep associated with snoring, paradoxical inward rib cage motion during inspiration, and at least one or more of the following: frequent arousals from sleep; or markedly negative esophageal pressure swings
Symptoms cannot be explained by another sleep disorder, medical condition, mental disorder, medication, substance abuse, or dependence

abnormalities (22). Risks because of rhinitis, obesity, and hypothyroidism may be actively reduced by diet and medical treatments. Increased nasal airflow obstruction was not thought to be a risk factor because early studies did not demonstrate a linear correlation between nasal resistance measured by rhinomanometry and the severity of OSAS (22–24). However, more recent stepwise multiple regression analyses that accounted for other risk factors and more precise clinical phenotyping identified daytime nasal obstruction as an independent risk factor for OSAS. Nasal obstruction had a weaker correlation than cephalometric landmarks, obesity, and male sex, but was stronger than age (25,26). The role of nasal obstruction in the genesis of SDB has been confirmed in other studies (27–29).

OSAS is an important health problem. Its prevalence is at least 4%. Two kinds of clinical sequelae are associated with the disorder. Neuropsychiatric complications include sleepiness, depression, cognitive dysfunction, disruption of professional, family and social life, and inattention that can result in road and industrial accidents. Cardiovascular complications include pulmonary and systemic hypertension because of chronic sleep-related hypoventilation, congestive heart failure, coronary heart disease, myocardial infarction, and stroke (30).

OSAS may be the result of chronic nasal inflammatory conditions with elevated levels of cytokines and inflammatory mediators. Asthma may be more severe and difficult to control if OSAS is present. Nasal continuous positive airway pressure (nCPAP) can improve both the OSAS and the asthma (31,32). The inflammatory mediators generated during OSA may contribute to the cardiovascular and asthmatic complications (33). The cause(s) of the OSA-related inflammation and its role in rhinitis are still open to debate (please see below).

Pickwickian Syndrome

At the far end of the spectrum is Pickwick or obesity-hypoventilation syndrome. This is the most severe form of SDB and is characterized by persistent hypoxia and hypercapnia, high morbidity and mortality. Its potential relationship to the "blue bloater" is intriguing.

OTHER SLEEP-DISORDERED BREATHING SYNDROMES

Respiratory Effort–Related Arousal

A subgroup of patients has excessive daytime sleepiness because of repetitive nocturnal arousals, but without apnea, hypopnea, or oxygen desaturation. In these cases, the airflow channel of the nocturnal polysomnogram shows less severe inspiratory flow limitation. Inspiratory esophageal pressures indicate repetitive, increased upper airway resistance. The respiratory efforts aimed at overcoming this increased upper airway resistance result in transient arousals. The term "respiratory effort–related arousal" (RERA) is applied to this event.

Upper Airways Resistance Syndrome

Guilleminault et al. noted that the repetitive RERAs were pathognomonic for a condition they termed "upper airways resistance syndrome" (UARS) (34). As nasal resistance is responsible for at least 40% of total airway resistance, its increase could result in UARS. UARS is the mildest form of SDB and shows better sleep fragmentation responses with treatment of nasal congestion than other OSA (27,35). Like OSAS, UARS is characterized by excessive daytime sleepiness and fitful sleep. However, snoring is not present in all patients. Although UARS was often placed between snoring and OSAS in a linear paradigm of disease progression, it is more likely to be a distinct disorder (36). Unlike OSAS, UARS patients are predominantly nonobese, younger women with histories of fainting, cold extremities, low blood pressure, and postural hypotension (36). These patients frequently complain of sleep-onset insomnia, fatigue, headaches, depression, irritable bowel syndrome (IBS), bruxism (teeth grinding), gastroesophageal reflux disease, and rhinitis (37). The arousal threshold for increased inspiratory effort is elevated in OSAS, but is lower than normal in UARS. As a result, UARS patients wake up very easily in response to even mild increases in respiratory effort. Guilleminault et al. hypothesize that different functional, arousal pathways are dysfunctional in the two syndromes. Blunted mechanoreceptor responses predominate in OSAS patients, whereas UARS patient have intact or even increased sensitivity of their mechanoreceptor systems (36).

Delta sleep is decreased in OSAS. In contrast, UARS patients have relatively increased delta sleep, percentage of sleep spent in alpha rhythms, and evidence of "alpha–delta sleep." This EEG pattern occurs when alpha rhythms of wakefulness intrude into the slow-wave delta rhythm that characterizes deep sleep. This EEG finding is not a feature of OSAS. Curiously, "alpha–delta sleep" is widespread in disorders characterized by chronic fatigue. These include CFS, fibromyalgia, migraine/tension headache syndrome, IBS, and temporomandibular joint syndrome. Gold et al. demonstrated a correlation between UARS and increasing prevalence of alpha–delta rhythm, IBS, headache, and sleep-onset insomnia.

Subjects with OSAS had low correlations with these conditions. Rhinitis was present in about 30% of UARS patients included in this study (37).

Sensory Sensitization Dysfunctional Disorder

Levander examined the pathophysiology of otherwise unexplained somatic dysfunctional disorders such as CFS, fibromyalgia, migraine/tension headache syndrome, IBS, temporomandibular joint syndrome, dry eyes and mouth syndrome (SICCA syndrome), gastralgia, interstitial cystitis, chronic prostatitis, vestibulitis syndrome, and nonallergic rhinitis (38). There is extensive overlap between these syndromes, including noninflammatory rhinitis in 73% of CFS subjects (11). It is tempting to speculate that UARS is part of the spectrum of "sensory sensitization dysfunction disorders." Coexisting nonallergic rhinitis could be an additional aggravating factor for UARS, resulting in increased inspiratory effort because of nasal obstruction.

PHARYNGEAL PATHOPHYSIOLOGY

The pharynx is a complex structure that regulates airflow, swallowing, and phonation. Its actions open the airway to allow breathing and phonation and close the airway to prevent aspiration and allow swallowing, and synchronize these functions with other components of the nasopharynx, oropharynx, and laryngopharynx (Fig. 1). The nasopharynx is the area between the nasal turbinates and

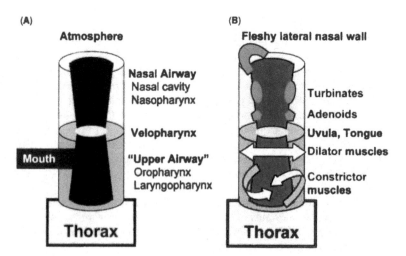

FIGURE 1 Functional anatomy. Soft tissue is shown in shades of gray from the nasal, pharyngeal "upper airway," mouth, and intrathoracic airways (thorax). The lumen is in black. (A) The nasal airway consists of the parallel nasal cavities and posterior nasopharynx. The narrowest cross-section is at the level of uvula and soft palate (velopharynx). The oropharynx and laryngopharynx form the traditional "upper airway" according to thoracic investigators. The mouth forms an outlet when the nasal airway is obstructed. The mouth is not included on subsequent diagrams. (B) The functional components of nasal and pharyngeal airways are shown. The fleshy lateral nasal wall and inferior turbinate form the anterior nasal valve. Adenoids and the rest of the ring of Waldeyer can form space-occupying lesions obstructing airflow. Posterior collapse of the relaxed uvula, soft palate, and tongue can obstruct the laryngeal airway. Dilator and constrictor muscles control the flow of air and fluids through the supraglottic region, esophagus and larynx.

hard palate. The oropharynx is the space between the hard palate and epiglottis. The laryngopharynx is also called hypopharynx. It is situated between the base of the tongue and the larynx. The narrowest portion of the pharynx is the retropalatal region of the oropharynx or velopharynx. The oropharynx has no bony structural support and is the most easily collapsible part of the airway. The normal pharynx has an elliptical cross-sectional area with a major lateral diameter. The pharynx walls are composed of dilator and constrictor muscles, lymphoid tissue, and pharyngeal mucosa. Parapharyngeal fat pads are present in the velopharynx and retroglossal oropharynx (18,39,40). The dilator muscles are activated at the start of inspiration. They buttress the upper airway walls to counter the negative intraluminal pressure generation during inspiration by subsequent diaphragmatic contraction (41). The constrictor muscles participate in expiration to counter the positive intraluminal pressure of exhaled air. During sleep, the dilator muscles have reduced tone that leads to the normal nocturnal narrowing of the pharynx. Their tone is maintained in response to relative hypoventilation and higher $PaCO_2$ setpoint for chemoreceptors during sleep. The carotid body, mucosal and other afferents, brainstem nuclei coordination of input, and activation of efferent reflexes that modify muscle tone make sleep a vulnerable period regarding upper airway stability.

Remmers et al. identified the oropharynx as the exact location of collapse in OSA. They proposed that the collapse resulted from an imbalance of the negative intraluminal pressure of inspiration with decreased buttressing opposing forces from the pharyngeal dilator muscles (42). OSA patients have narrower pharyngeal airways than normal subjects because of genetic or obesity-related structural abnormalities. These factors change the longest diameter of the pharyngeal cross-sectional area to an anterior–posterior orientation, making it more round and susceptible to lateral wall collapse. Other factors that tend to narrow the pharyngeal airway include neck flexion, jaw opening, gravity, and surface adhesive forces. OSA patients may maintain patency of their anatomically narrower airway through higher activity of their dilator muscles (43). However, physiological dilator muscle hypotonia occurs during sleep. Their force may drop below the intraluminal pressure leading to nocturnal pharyngeal obstruction. Environmental factors that can further attenuate dilator muscle activation are alcohol, sleep deprivation, sedatives, and anesthesia.

Mezzanote et al. showed that pharyngeal obstruction is the primary defect in OSA as opposed to reflex or arousal response abnormalities (44). This can be modeled by representing the pharynx as an elastic tube. The tube's cross-sectional area (patency) is determined by the transmural pressure (P_{tm}). P_{tm} represents the balance between the negative intraluminal pressure ($P_{il} <$ atmospheric pressure) during inspiration and the negative constriction pressure (i.e., positive dilation pressure) created by contraction of the surrounding dilator muscles (P_{surr}). Contraction of the constrictor muscles is defined to cause an increase in the positive value of P_{surr}, whereas their relaxation and the contraction of the dilator muscles leads to a negative value. As a result, P_{tm} is determined by the subtraction of two negative values ($P_{tm} = P_{il} - P_{surr}$) (Fig. 2). Healthy subjects maintain sufficient dilator muscle tone to create a net positive transmural pressure of 0 to $+10\,cmH_2O$ during sleep ($P_{il} - P_{surr} = P_{tm} > 0\,cmH_2O$) (44).

The airway will collapse when the transmural pressure (P_{tm}) drops below zero. This occurs when the pressure generated by the dilator muscles of the surrounding tissues (P_{surr}) moves towards zero and is unable to prevent airway collapse. The exact value of P_{surr} at the time of collapse (i.e., no airflow) is called

Patmosphere = 0 cmH₂O
Pintralumemal = P$_{il}$

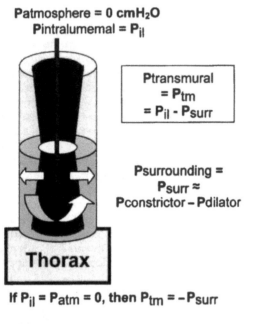

Ptransmural
= P$_{tm}$
= P$_{il}$ - P$_{surr}$

Psurrounding =
P$_{surr}$ ≈
Pconstrictor – Pdilator

Thorax

If P$_{il}$ = P$_{atm}$ = 0, then P$_{tm}$ = – P$_{surr}$

FIGURE 2 Pharyngeal transmural pressure. The pharynx is the source of obstruction in sleep disordered breathing. The net pressure of the surrounding tissue on the airway lumen (P_{surr}) is determined by the active contractions of the constrictor and dilator muscles, and passive factors such as the space-occupying fat pads and gravity's effects on cervical tissues (jowls). The intralumenal pressure (P_{il}) is determined by the flow of air, phase of respiration, and degree of obstruction. In the special case where there is no airflow, P_{il} will equal atmospheric pressure ($0 \, cmH_2O$). The transmural pressure (P_{tm}) can then be measured by balloon manometry as the numerical opposite of the pressure exerted on the balloon by the surrounding tissues (P_{surr}).

the critical closure pressure (P_{crit}). P_{crit} exceeds $-41 \, cmH_2O$ in awake healthy subjects. In contrast, P_{crit} ranges from -17 to $-41 \, cmH_2O$ in awake OSA patients (30).

During sleep in normal subjects, dilator muscle hypotonia causes P_{crit} to rise to $-13 \, cmH_2O$ (30). This is still sufficient to maintain a patent airway. In contrast, sleeping apneic patients have lax dilator muscle tone and higher P_{surr} values than normal sleeping subjects (Fig. 3). Their dilator muscles are unable to maintain airway patency. P_{crit} increases with more severe sleep apnea. Asymptomatic snorers have P_{crit} of approximately $-6.5 \, cmH_2O$ (30). P_{crit} in UARS patients is about $-4.0 \, cmH_2O$ (40). Sleep apnea subjects with hypopnea, but no apnea, have P_{crit} of $-1.6 \, cmH_2O$ (30). Patients with frank apneas have P_{crit} of $+2.5 \, cmH_2O$ (6). As a result, OSASs may be considered a condition resulting from pathologically elevated P_{crit} during sleep. P_{crit} is an important index, because it defines the lowest level of nCPAP that will keep the upper airways patent (30).

The "Starling resistor" model can be applied to the upper airways (24). Under conditions of flow limitation, the maximal inspiratory flow is determined by the change in pressure between the upstream (i.e., nasal passage) pressure and that at the most collapsible site of the upper airway. The downstream (tracheal) pressure generated by diaphragmatic inspiration does not affect this relationship. That means at the beginning of an inspiratory effort, the rate of airflow will increase in proportion to the increasing intraluminal pressure. However, when P_{crit} is reached, the airway cross-sectional diameter is maximized and airflow will remain constant. Airflow will not increase even if the intrathoracic, diaphragmatic driving pressure is raised. This plateau leads to the characteristic flattened shape of the flow versus pressure curve and inspiratory flow–volume loop.

Inspiratory airway flow limitation is a very sensitive marker of elevated pharyngeal intraluminal airflow resistance (Fig. 4). The maximal intraluminal

(A)
Contract Dilator Muscles
Anterior Uvula & Tongue
$P_{tm} = P_{il} - P_{surr} \gg 0$ cmH$_2$O
Patent Airway

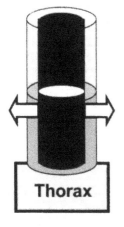

(B)
Contract Constrictor Muscles
Retroversion of Uvula & Tongue
$P_{tm} = P_{il} - P_{surr} \ll 0$ cmH$_2$O
Airway Closure

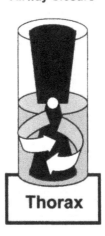

FIGURE 3   Pharyngeal muscle actions. (A) Dilator muscles are attached to bony and mucosal surfaces. Their contraction pulls the pharynx open. When the uvula, soft palate, and tongue are in anterior positions that do not block the velopharynx, the dilator muscles and surrounding tissues will generate a larger magnitude pressure (P_{surr}) than the intralumenal pressure (P_{il}) and so will increase the transmural pressure (P_{tm}) leading to airway patency. (B) The more concentric pharyngeal constrictor muscles combined with the potential posterior movement of the uvula, soft palate, and tongue will generate a small magnitude P_{surr}, so that P_{tm} will be less than 0 cmH$_2$O. Airway closure will result.

pressure depends on two factors. The first is the transmural pressure discussed above. The second is the resistance of the upstream segment, that is, the nasal and nasopharyngeal sections of the upper airways. An increase in airflow velocity in an attempt to maintain the intraluminal pressure actually results in a paradoxical drop in pressure and pharyngeal collapse because of the Bernoulli effect (41). Under these circumstances, the higher air velocity leads to a reduction in the pressure exerted against the airway walls.

Any pathologic event that increases nasal resistance can limit maximal upper airways airflow and contribute to OSA and UARS (Fig. 5). This includes all obstructive conditions of the nasal cavity such as nasal septum deviation, hypertrophy of the inferior turbinates, stenosis of the nasal valve, nasal polyps, the nasal congestion characteristic of rhinitis, and adenoidal hypertrophy (45). One response to nasal airflow obstruction is to switch to unstable oral breathing. However, this may eliminate effective nasal reflexes and facilitate SDB (29).

Complete closure of pharyngeal "upper airway" causes apnea. Apnea leads to hypoxia and hypercapnia. These chemical changes stimulate increased respiratory efforts that can provoke an arousal from sleep. The arousal itself stimulates pharyngeal dilator muscle activity that can restore airway patency. The repetitive nature of these events leads to fragmented sleep, disrupted sleep architecture, intermittent hypoxia and hypercapnia, and adrenergic stimulation (33). The

(A)   (B)

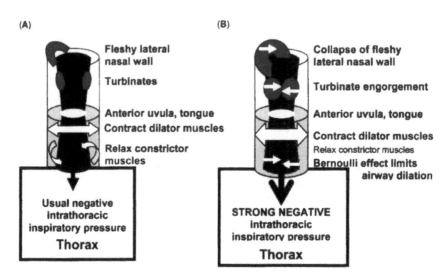

FIGURE 4   Inhalation. **(A)** Negative intrathoracic pressure draws air through the nasal and pharyngeal airway. This is facilitated by coordinated contraction of the dilator and relaxation of the constrictor muscles. **(B)** Forced inspiratory efforts are induced by stronger diaphragmatic, intercostal, and accessory muscle actions that generate a strong negative intrathoracic pressure. The pharyngeal muscle balance swings towards dilator muscle activity. These forces' efforts may occur as a result of pharyngeal obstruction, exercise, or during peak nasal inspiratory flow measurements. Peak flow increases rapidly at the outset, but then reaches a plateau. Further effort causes collapse of the fleshy lateral nasal wall with obstruction of the anterior nasal valve, followed by engorgement of the inferior, then middle turbinate that narrows the nasal cleft. The negative intrathoracic pressure causes an increase in the velocity of airflow, but no net change in resistance. The rapidly moving air produces Bernoulli effects that exert negative pressures on the nasal and pharyngeal walls, and buffer the actions of the dilator muscles. Each of these events can exacerbate nasopharyngeal airflow resistance and lead to sleep disordered breathing.

periods of high airway resistance result in a significant numbers of cortical arousals, sleep fragmentation, and subsequent daytime sleepiness.

NASAL AIRFLOW RESISTANCE IN OSA

The Starling resistor model of the upper airway has been examined by anterior rhinomanometry in 37 normal subjects and 53 patients with OSA (24). Nasal resistance was increased in patients compared to the normal group, even though there was no linear correlation with apnea severity. In contrast, there were no differences in nasal resistance in 71 OSA patients and 70 non-OSA heavy snorers (23). This may have been because chronic nasal airflow obstruction is a strong risk factor for snoring (19). Patients with SDB and impaired nasal patency had significantly more subjective nighttime dyspneic episodes and higher apnea index scores, but no significant differences in the numbers of hypopneas or SaO_2 (46). A population-based sample of 911 subjects was assessed by anterior rhinomanometry (22). There was no relationship between nasal resistance and sleep indices. In post hoc analysis, the subset with allergic rhinitis and nasal congestion was 1.8 times more likely to have an AHI >1 than nonallergic subjects. Anterior rhinomanometry was tested in the seated and supine positions and demonstrated nasal

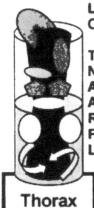

Lax lateral nasal wall
Obstructed anterior
nasal valve
Turbinate hypertrophy
Nasal polyps
Adenoidal hyperplasia
Autonomic instability
Rostral palate & tongue
Fat pads
Loss of dilator tone
  Increased constrictor
  muscle tone

Thorax | **Vocal cord dysfunction**

FIGURE 5 Sources of nasal and pharyngeal obstruction. Anterior nasal obstruction is because of collapse of the fleshy lateral nasal wall, obstruction of the anterior nasal valve, turbinate hypertrophy including autonomic dysfunction with paradoxical vascular engorgement, and nasal polyps. These factors may play roles in upper airway respiratory arousal syndrome. Nasopharyngeal adenoid hyperplasia is a significant cause in children. Posterior collapse of the soft palate and tongue contribute to hypopharyngeal obstruction. Cervical and peripharyngeal fat pads are an important cause in obesity. Muscular imbalance with decreased dilator muscle and increased constrictor muscle activity may be more important in myopathic diseases.

obstruction in 44% of 36 consecutive OSA patients (33). Again, there was no significant correlation between nasal resistance and the degree of OSA.

A prospective study of 541 unselected, consecutive snorers used rigorous clinical phenotyping, posterior rhinomanometry while awake, and sleep polysomnography to assess the relationships between nasal airflow resistance and sleep apnea (25). Rigorous entry criteria for OSA (AHI >15) were met by 259 out of 541 patients (48%). OSA patients had significantly higher nasal resistance than the non-OSA patients. Subjects with nasal resistances $\geq 3\,kPa/L/sec$ were more prevalent in OSA group, with a significant odds ratio of 2.2. Stepwise multiple linear regression analysis ranked the explained variances (R^2) of AHI as hyoid bone position 6.2%, obesity 4.6%, male sex 3.0%, nasal obstruction 2.3%, increasing age 1.3%, and mandibular characteristics 0.9%. Subsequently, an association was discovered between nasal resistance and the cross-sectional area of the pharyngeal airway at the base of the tongue in the supine position (47). Nasal resistance and the change into a relaxed mandibular position during recumbency were independent predictors of AHI among patients with normal body mass index. The authors considered the possibility that there are several subtypes of OSAS with different pathogenic factors. In some, nasal mucosal receptors may regulate pharyngeal dilator muscle activity. These studies support the hypothesis that nasal obstruction and impaired pharyngeal patency are risk factors for OSA.

EXPERIMENTAL NASAL OBSTRUCTION

Early studies of partial or complete nasal obstruction identified the positive relationship between nasal obstruction and SDB. Acute viral rhinitis can lead to poor quality of sleep and obstructive sleep apnea in some infants (48). Nasal obstruction was produced by inflating intranasal balloon canula in 10 healthy men. Full night recordings of sleep stages and breathing rhythms were assessed before and during nasal obstruction. A significantly increased length of time was spent in stage I NREM light sleep with reduced duration of deep sleep. Apneic events were significantly more frequent during nasal obstruction. The apneas caused a twofold increase in cortical arousals and awakenings. Ear lobe oxymetry in four subjects demonstrated 255 episodes of oxygen desaturation with SaO_2 < 90% during sleep with nasal obstruction compared to 27 times during control sleep. These results were confirmed in eight normal subjects who had bilateral nasal packing in a crossover study design (49). Nasal packing after polypectomy or septoplasty was associated with significantly increased number, frequency, and duration of nocturnal cortical arousals (50). Bilateral nasal occlusion caused significantly more apneic events than unilateral obstruction in 10 normal young adults (51). Nonapneic microarousals and the amount of wake time during sleep were also increased. Packing both nostrils with petrolatum-impregnated gauze caused significant increases in sleep latency, REM latency, and a trend towards lighter sleep and less slow-wave and REM sleep (52). The number of apneas, hypopneas, and minutes of obstructive events per hour of sleep were also significantly increased.

A clinically relevant nasonasal and nasobronchial reflex occurs after surgery, and in particular nasal surgery. Intra- or post-operative apnea should be an indication for immediate sleep studies. Complete nasal obstruction caused by nasal packing increases SDB (53). The effects vary from patient to patient and depend on age and individual anatomy. Patients with preexisting OSAS and anatomical alterations such as severe nasal septal deviation can develop severe complications. Nasal obstruction can activate central reflex mechanisms that increase the negative inspiration pressure in the hypopharynx, promote the transition from transnasal to transoral breathing, and increase the likelihood of pharyngeal collapse. Pre- and post-operative polysomnography has been advocated to determine if nasal and pharyngeal surgery was beneficial or induced any worsening of OSA.

Reflex-mediated protection of the hypopharyngeal–glottic airway is compromised in the prone sleeping position during active sleep. This swallowing reflex is impaired in OSAS (54). Defective swallowing reflexes can affect otherwise healthy infants who are exposed to minute pharyngeal fluid volumes of 0.4 mL (55). Swallowing and arousal are crucial to prevent stimulation of the laryngeal chemoreflex with airway closure. This is because the swallowing rate is reduced significantly, and there is no compensatory increase in arousal during prone sleeping. The reduction in airway protective reflexes may be one mechanism for the increased risk of sudden infant death syndrome in the prone position.

SUBJECTIVE "CONGESTION" VS. OBJECTIVE MEASURES OF NASAL AIRWAY DIMENSIONS AND "OBSTRUCTION"

Much confusion has been caused by assuming that subjective complaints of nasal congestion, fullness, and obstruction to airflow are equivalent to objective measures of nasal dimensions and the flow dynamics through narrowed and dilated nasal cavities (56). Schumacher has focused attention on this languid lingo and called for specific definitions combined with precise use of these terms (57). Nowhere is this more apparent than in the objective evaluation of nasal function in OSA. This syndrome has been defined objectively with relatively little credence given to the subjective nasal complaints. This is unlike most of the other nonallergic inflammatory and noninflammatory rhinitis syndromes.

"REVERSIBLE" NASAL OBSTRUCTION VS. "NONREVERSIBLE" NASAL OBSTRUCTION: THE DEFINING ROLE OF α-ADRENERGIC AGONISTS

The objective role of nasal airway dimensions (nasal obstruction to airflow) has been studied in snoring subjects by using oxymetazoline nasal decongestant spray. Initial unblinded studies suggested that improvements in snoring and apnea were helpful in deciding which snoring subjects would benefit from surgery (58). The results of this simple anecdote-based unblinded type of analysis have been shown to be unreliable for identifying OSA and demonstrating the need for surgery.

The effects of oxymetazoline in snoring and nonsnoring subjects demonstrate this point. Posture influences nasal airway resistance when measured by both anterior and posterior rhinomanometry (59). Moving from the seated to recumbent position increased nasal airflow resistance by 50%. Oxymetazoline was given to decongest the nasal mucosa. Recumbent airway resistance was improved in the nonsnoring subjects. However, the large magnitude increase in resistance was no different in the snoring group. This indicated that the nonsnorers may have "reversible obstruction." The mechanism may be vasodilation and engorgement of the nasal venous sinusoids. The α-agonist–mediated vasoconstriction of the arteriovenous anastomoses and venous sinusoids likely caused thinning of the nasal mucosa with an increase in nasal airway dimensions and decreased airflow resistance. However, snorers did not have a response to oxymetazoline. This suggested "irreversible obstruction." The mucosal thickness did not decrease suggesting that inflammatory cells, fibrosis, glandular hypertrophy, anatomical, or other nonvascular causes of α-agonist–resistant wall thickening were present. This may also be considered "restriction" because the cross-sectional area for airflow through the bony and mucosal box of the nasal cavity was limited. These changes in snorers did not predict the presence of OSA.

Analysis of nasal dimensions after topical α-agonist decongestion has not been fully exploited. There remains a need for further evaluations of phenotypically distinct subsets of rhinitis and different severities of OSA subjects (60).

INFLAMMATION

Patterns of cytokeratin (CK) expression are unique to specific cell types in the epithelia from different organs, and are altered during mucosal inflammation (61). CK expression was examined in uvula biopsies in SDB (62). The patient group had a significant reduction of CK13-immunoreactive material compared to nonsnoring control subjects. Basal cell CK14 and suprabasal cell CK4 were present in all subjects of less than 60 years. CK10 was absent from all epithelial samples. Acanthosis of the uvular epithelium was found only in the apnea group (62).

Acanthosis is the limited detachment of squamous epithelial cells from each other. As in the skin, this may represent generalized inflammation of the uvular mucosa (63). This finding was associated with general flattening of basement membrane architecture. Normally, the mucosal surface is ruggose, as the basement membrane undulates between connective tissue papillae that project towards the surface deep crevasses between these papillae. This surface has a large basement membrane surface area. This provides a large area for the exchange between the interstitial fluid and overlying salivary uvular epithelial lining fluid (64). The stratified squamous epithelium will also have a deep and complex composition of basal-to-mature surface cells. However, acanthosis was associated with the loss of this undulating landscape and so the "flattening" of the basement membrane in apneic compared to nonsnoring subjects (63). Flattening means a loss of total basement membrane area. As a result, there is decreased area for anchorage of surface epithelium and, by inference, a substantial loss in the total number of epithelial cells. A decrease in the large basement membrane surface area also suggests a net loss in the epithelial surface area available for the exchange of nutrients and inflammatory cells between the interstitial fluid and overlying salivary epithelial lining fluid. Similar, but less extreme changes are seen during normal aging.

Acanthosis was associated with changes in the types of inflammatory cells in the lamina propria. There were diffuse increases in CD3+ and B-lymphocytes of apneic compared to nonsnoring subjects (62,63). CD4+ and CD8+ T-lymphocytes have been present in surgically removed tissue, with CD4+ and CD25+ cells in the muscular layers of the soft palate and tonsillar pillars of OSAS patients (65). Other hypopharyngeal regions show a predominance of CD8+ T-cells (66). CD4+ and CD8+ cell numbers were correlated with body weight in OSAS suggesting a relationship with obesity, adiponectin, and other adipose cell hormones (65,67). The proportions of neutrophils were increased, and macrophages decreased in induced sputum samples from OSAS, with no changes in total eosinophils or lymphocytes (68).

Most of the studies dealing with pharyngeal airway trauma have examined the musculature of the uvula. However, both hypertrophy (69,70) and atrophy with disruption of muscle bundles (71–73) have been reported. Histological evidence of submucosal gland hypertrophy, ductal dilation, focal squamous metaplasia, extensive vasodilation, and edema of the lamina propria may also be present, although the prevalence has not been assessed or correlated with the severity of the sleep obstruction (69,74).

An increased density of abnormal nerve endings has been found in the soft palate mucosa of patients with sleep apnea and habitual snorers (75). This may be related to an increase in the parasympathetic vasodilating neurotransmitter vasoactive intestinal peptide that has been found in nasal lavage of OSA subjects (76). However, denervation may occur in muscular layers (65). Sleep apnea subjects also had significantly higher total cell counts, percentage of polymorphonuclear cells, and concentrations of bradykinin in the lavage fluid (76). Activated circulating leukocytes with increased expression of intracellular adhesion molecule-1 (ICAM-1) and elevated circulating levels of IL-6, IL-8, monocyte chemoattractant protein 1, erythropoietin, and vascular endothelial growth factor have been found (66,77). Exhaled air condensates also showed increased indicators of inflammation and oxidant stress including reactive oxidant species, nitric oxide, pentane, and 8-isoprostane in OSA patients compared to normal control subjects (33,78,79). These proinflammatory changes improve with nCPAP therapy (80).

Similar mediators act in allergic rhinitis, asthma, and inflammatory nonallergic disorders. Even though eosinophils were not associated with sleep apnea per se, NARES subjects also suffer from increased rates of sleep apnea compared to healthy control subjects (81). There is some evidence that OSA is associated with more severe asthma and that both improve with nCPAP therapy (31,32). Proinflammatory changes in OSA may increase cardiovascular morbidity and mortality (33).

Vibrational trauma induced by severe snoring may be one cause of these histological changes. Extrapolation to encompass the entire circumference of the oropharyngeal wall raises the possibility of generalized mucosal swelling and thickening. The invaginating tissue may impinge on the cross-sectional area for airflow and promote upper airway occlusion (82). These findings are consistent with the Starling resistor model described above, as a narrower airway would generate a higher resistance during inhalation during sleep. This would increase the magnitude of the negative intraluminal pressure and promote upper airway collapse (83).

Rhinitis and Nasal Obstruction

Positional changes in nasal airflow resistance occur in normal subjects. Recumbency increases total nasal resistance. However, both allergic and nonallergic rhinitis subjects have larger magnitude changes in total nasal resistance between the upright (low resistance) and supine (high resistance) positions than healthy control subjects (84). These findings suggest that increased nasal obstruction (85) may be more critical for DSB than the etiology of the rhinitis.

Idiopathic nonallergic rhinitis subjects have sympathetic, but not parasympathetic, dysfunction when assessed by tilt table and other methods (86). Oxymetazoline, exercise, and other sympathetic stimuli may induce paradoxical nasal and potentially pharyngeal vasodilation with airflow obstruction in this syndrome (87,88). Reduced sympathetic vasoconstrictor activity would accentuate postural nasal reflexes and dependent blood redistribution to the cephalic vessels during sleep.

These augmented effects may be implied from the mechanisms regulating nasal hysteresis during inhalation and exhalation through the nose. Nasal inspiratory airflow can be measured by peak nasal inspiratory flow. Once inhalation is started, the airflow rapidly reached a maximum and plateaus at that rate (Fig. 4). Additional respiratory muscle effort to increase nasal airflow has no effect. Instead, the negative intrathoracic pressure of inhalation is transmitted to the nostril where the negative pressure contributes to the collapse of the fleshy lateral wall of the anterior nasal valve. This effect varies between subjects based on the compliance of this wall. Elderly subjects are more subject to these soft tissue effects and obstruction. The net effect is an increase in nasal airflow resistance with no change in flow rate. The effects at the anterior nasal valve account for about half of the total nasal airflow resistance.

The collapse of the anterior nasal valve is followed closely in time by collapse of the airway at the anterior end of the inferior turbinate. Subsequently, the body of the inferior turbinate and middle turbinate occludes the region of the middle meatus.

During exhalation, these collapsed nasal airways are pushed open by the positive pressure of the lung elastic recoil. These changes from negative nasal air pressure of inspiration to positive pressure during exhalation may have direct effects on the degree of engorgement of the erectile vessels of the mucosa. The negative air pressure may increase the volume of blood in the sinusoids, whereas the high exhalation pressures may force blood out of the turbinates.

This novel "bellows" mechanism is based on statistical models of nasal airflow through different segments of the nose (89). Teleologically, this physiological mechanism may be designed to protect the nasal mucosal epithelium from the deleterious shearing forces and Bernoulli effects generated by negative airway pressures. These effects serve as a model for the pharyngeal collapse during inspiration in OSA. They may be particularly applicable to subjects with autonomic dysfunction and UARS (34).

Allergic Rhinitis

It has been associated with difficulty in falling asleep, nocturnal awakenings, excessive daytime sleepiness, periodic breathing, and hypo- and hyperpneic episodes (3). Microarousals were 10-fold more frequent than in normal subjects. Nasal resistance and the number of obstructive apneas were significantly higher during ragweed season compared to after the season in seven seasonal allergic rhinitis subjects (90). Correlations were more significant for males than for females. Oxygen desaturation was milder in allergic rhinitis–related apnea than more severe OSAS patients.

Allergic rhinitis subjects with and without mild sleep apnea were assessed for airway dimensions while awake using acoustic rhinometry. The subset with sleep apnea had significantly smaller nasal cavity dimensions (e.g., lower minimum cross-sectional area and volumes) than those without no sleep disturbances (35). Oxymetazoline increased nasal dimensions in the allergic rhinitis subjects with no sleep apnea, but had no effect when sleep apnea was present. These changes may be exacerbated during sleep and contribute to nocturnal nasal obstruction.

Atopic children may be of particular risk for SDB. A self-response questionnaire was presented to 11,114 parents of randomly selected four- to seven-year-old children in Singapore (91). Snoring and habitual snoring were reported in 28.1% and 6.0% of the children, respectively. On multivariate logistic regression analysis, snoring was significantly associated with male gender, race, atopy (asthma, allergic rhinitis, or atopic dermatitis), maternal atopy (allergic rhinitis or atopic dermatitis), maternal smoking, and breastfeeding. Habitual snoring was significantly associated with obesity (odds ratio; 95% confidence interval: 3.75; 1.67–8.42), allergic rhinitis (2.90; 2.06–4.08), atopic dermatitis (1.80; 1.28–2.54), maternal smoking (2.22; 1.09–4.53), and breastfeeding (1.49; 1.11–1.98). Atopy was the strongest risk factor for habitual snoring, with the odds ratios increasing with concomitant atopic asthma, allergic rhinitis, and dermatitis (7.45; 3.48–15.97). Atopic children require additional screening for snoring, habitual snoring, and other features of OSAS.

TREATMENT OF SDB

Nasal Continuous Positive Airway Pressure

Night ventilation with nCPAP is the gold standard for treatment of moderate and severe OSAS (80). The flow generator provides air under positive pressure through a nasal or facial mask. The pressure (P_{crit}) is determined during polysomnography and ranges from 4 to 20 cmH$_2$O (33,80). This provides a "pneumatic splint" of the upper airways. This splinting is especially important if there is collapse of the lateral, fleshy wall of the anterior nasal valve because of loss of facial muscle tone or facial obesity.

Short-term administration of nCPAP between 0 and 20 cmH_2O in normal supine subjects caused significant pressure-dependent decreases of cardiac output and stroke volume with an increase in total peripheral resistance (92). Analysis of heart rate variability (the frequency of variation in the EKG R-R intervals) indicated significant baroreflex mediated decreases in both parasympathetic and sympathetic neural outputs. nCPAP decreased nasal airflow resistance in both snoring [$45\% \pm 4\%$ (SEM); $n = 70$; $p < 0.05$] and nonsnoring ($30\% \pm 4\%$; $n = 11$; $p < 0.05$) groups of nonapneic subjects (59). Baroreflex sensitivity during sleep was decreased in nonapneic snoring subjects but not in normal healthy controls (93). nCPAP prevented excessive baroreflex fluctuations. Unlike OSA patients, there were no changes in blood pressure in nonapneic snoring subjects.

nCPAP caused direct mechanical compression of the upper esophagus that reduced nocturnal, recumbent gastroesophageal reflux (94). It remains unclear if nasal or hypopharyngeal reflexes were involved. Previously reported reflex-mediated increases in lower esophageal sphincter constriction were not found. Impairments of the upper esophageal swallowing reflex that occur in OSAS may be reversed by nCPAP (54).

Compliance with nCPAP treatment can be relatively low because of undesirable side effects. These include nasal congestion, rhinorrhea, crusted nose, epistaxis, sneezing, and dryness. Nasal congestion and rhinorrhea may be worsened by breathing cold dry air. Heated, humidified air can improve patient comfort and efficacy (95). Nasal steroids, decongestants, anticholinergic agents, allergy shots, house dust mite and other allergen avoidance, and surgical correction of severe anatomical obstructions can serve as useful adjunctive treatment to improve compliance and outcomes with nCPAP therapy (16,80). Many of these modalities have not been tested in sleep apnea.

Some OSAS patients do not benefit from nCPAP, but instead appear to develop nasal inflammation in response to the positive nasal airway pressure (96). It has been hypothesized that this subgroup may develop upregulated inflammatory cytokine (IL-3, IL-4, IL-6, IL-8, and IL-13) and T cell adhesion molecule (ICAM-1) expression. An alternative hypothesis is that these subjects may have more severe OSA with preexistent inflammation and relative steroid resistance. This would be compatible with similar nasal, sinus, and asthmatic inflammatory conditions.

External Nasal Splints

These bandage-like splints have been widely used by professional athletes and others to improve the nasal inspiratory flow of air. External nasal splints decrease nasal resistance at rest and during isometric exercise, but have little proven value when performing isotonic exercise such as running (97). They may improve snoring in nonapneic subjects (98) and provide a small ancillary benefit to nCPAP for sleep-related breathing (99).

Nasal Steroids

Subjective scores of nasal congestion and sleep were significantly improved in 20 perennial allergic rhinitis patients in a double-blind, placebo-controlled trial (4100) using topical corticosteroid spray (fluticasone propionate). Daytime sleepiness also improved, but did not achieve significance ($p = 0.08$). Unfortunately, no objective measurements of sleep and nasal obstruction were included in the study. Subjective outcomes were assessed using the Epworth Sleepiness Scale, Functional Outcomes of Sleep Questionnaire, Rhinoconjunctivitis Quality of Life Questionnaire, and a daily diary for nasal symptoms, sleep problems, and daytime fatigue records (101). Budesonide significantly improved daytime fatigue, somnolence, and quality of sleep. Treatment with triamcinolone nasal spray for three weeks had similar, statistically beneficial effects on sleep quality (102). The subjective effects of fluticasone propionate on nocturnal symptoms were significantly greater than with montelukast (103).

The effects on the AHI were assessed in 23 snorers with rhinitis and OSA using a crossover design (104). Fluticasone propionate significantly decreased AHI [median (quartile range): 11.9 (22.6)] compared to placebo [20 (26.3); $p < 0.05$]. Thirteen snorers had significant apnea (AHI >10/hr) whereas 10 did not. An open label study of budesonide in 14 children with allergic rhinitis demonstrated that hypopneic episodes were most significantly improved (7.5/hr reduced to 0.9/hr; $p = 0.003$) (105). AHI was also decreased significantly from 10.7 to 5.8 in 13 children with OSA related to adenoidal and tonsillar hypertrophy (106). Oxygen desaturation and respiratory movement/sleep arousals were also improved by the topical nasal fluticasone propionate compared to the placebo treatment. There were no changes in adenoid sizes.

Azelastine antihistamine nasal spray significantly improved subjective sleep scores in 24 allergic rhinitis subjects but had no effects on nasal congestion or daytime sleepiness (107).

Furosemide nasal spray may be useful as an adjunctive therapy, as it decreases nasal airflow resistance (108). It has not been tested in OSA.

Surgery is an option with uvulopalatoplasty in adults, with adenoidectomy and tonsillectomy in children being the most common procedures (30). If there are significant nasal anatomical deviations with obstruction to airflow, then partial inferior turbinectomy and potentially septoplasty may be of some limited value.

Adenoidectomy is the most beneficial surgery for children who have sleep apnea (109). The operation reduced the number of episodes of rhinosinusitis per year ($p < 0.001$) and polysomnographically determined obstructive sleep disorders ($p < 0.008$) compared to the year before surgery in 37 children (mean age 6).

Injection of elongated uvulas with a mixture of ethanol and glucocorticoid has been proposed as a limited and potentially outpatient procedure (110). In simple snoring, the uvula length was reduced from 11 to 8.5 mm, and the visual analog scale for snoring (VAS) was reduced from 7/10 to 2/10. In OSAS, the uvula was reduced from 15 to 10 mm, the VAS was reduced from 10/10 to 4/10, and the AHI improved from 35.3 to 26.1 after treatment. It was not clear if uvula length correlated with any of the indices or the severity of the OSA.

Other Potential Treatments

Ipratropium bromide is a reasonable adjunctive treatment in patients with excessive nasal and nasopharyngeal glandular secretion. It has not been tested in OSA. Oral and topical α1- and α2-adrenergic agonists may be useful for assessing the "reversible" component to nasal obstruction. However, they should be avoided because of their hypertensive potential in any group at risk for cardiac disease. Nasal saline sprays and gels, or potentially nebulized water humidification, may reduce drying complaints associated with nCPAP. The absence of other treatments specific to nonallergic rhinitis and lack of understanding of the uvulopalatal and other inflammatory mechanisms associated with DSB syndromes are a major hindrance in advancing therapeutic progress.

CONCLUSIONS

OSA is largely the result of nasal and pharyngeal abnormalities. The full differential diagnosis and pathogenic factors are not yet fully worked out. The influence of the nose on pharyngeal collapse is apparent from the "Starling resistor" model of the extrathoracic airway as a collapsible tube. The nose does not collapse, but instead the wall thickens from vascular engorgement to decrease the cross-sectional area for airflow. Nasal reflexes likely play an important role in maintaining pharyngeal patency. Artificial nasal obstruction clearly induced SDB. However, there was no linear correlation of nasal resistance with apnea severity in either OSAS or non-OSAS patients. OSAS is defined by OSA plus daytime somnolence.

Overall, nasal obstruction is an independent but relatively weak risk factor for OSA. However, increased nasal resistance was a stronger, independent predictor in a nonobese subgroup of OSA patients with less severe sleep disorders. UARS may be subdivided into two main subtypes: obese, heavy snorers at risk for OSAS and nonobese, nonsnoring patients that may have functional somatic syndromes. The latter group appears to have a strong link with nonallergic rhinitis and potentially the CFS spectrum of illnesses.

nCPAP is the "gold-standard" for treatment as it pressurizes the nasopharyngeal airway and prevents its physical collapse because of obesity or muscle relaxation. Nasal steroid sprays are an important adjunctive therapy as inflammation appears to a common component of OSA. The steroids reduce nasal inflammation and improve sleep quality, nocturnal arousals, daytime sleepiness, and fatigue. OSA subjects with coexisting allergic rhinitis improve after nasal steroids, successful allergen avoidance, and allergy shots.

ACKNOWLEDGMENTS

This work is supported by U.S. Public Health Service Awards RO1 AI42403, M01-RR13297, and P50 DC000214.

REFERENCES

1. Frank-Piskorska A. Sleep related breathing disorders in allergology practice. Przegl Lek 2002; 59:457–461.
2. Martin SE, Wraith PK, Deary IJ, et al. The effect of nonvisible sleep fragmentation on daytime function. Am J Resir Crit Care Med 1997; 155:1596–1601.
3. Lavie P, Gertner R, Zomer J. Breathing disorders in sleep associated with "microarousals" in patients with allergic rhinitis. Acta Otolaryngol 1981; 92:529–533.
4. Craig TJ, McCann JL, Gurevich F, Davies MJ. The correlation between allergic rhinitis and sleep disturbance. J Allergy Clin Immunol 2004; 114:S139–S145.
5. Majde JA, Krueger JM. Links between the innate immune system and sleep. J Allergy Clin Immunol 2005; 116:1188–1198.
6. Lowery PL, Takahashi JS. Mammalian genetic advances in sleep research and their relevance to sleep medicine. Sleep 2005; 28:357–367.

7. Obal F Jr., Kreuger JM. Biochemical regulation of non-rapid-eye-movement sleep. Front Biosci 2003; 8:520–550.
8. Opp MR. Cytokines and sleep: the first 100 years. Brain Behav Immun 2004; 18:295–297.
9. Vgontzas AN, Zoumakis E, Lin HM, Bixler EO, Trakada G, Chrousos GP. Marked decrease in sleepiness in patients with sleep apnea by etanercept, a tumour necrosis factor-alpha antagonist. J Clin Endocrinol Metab 2004; 89:4409–4414.
10. Chester AC. Symptoms of rhinosinusitis in patients with unexplained chronic fatigue or bodily pain: a pilot study. Arch Intern Med 2003; 163:1832–1836.
11. Baraniuk JN, Clauw DJ, Gaumond E. Rhinitis symptoms in chronic fatigue syndrome. Ann Allergy Asthma Immunol 1998; 81:359–365.
12. Majde KA, Krueger JM. Neuroimmunology of sleep. In: D'heanen H, ed. Textbook of Biological Psychiatry. London: John Wiley & Sons, 2002:1247–1257.
13. Baraniuk JN, Clauw DJ, MacDowell-Carneiro A-L, et al. Serum IgE concentrations in chronic fatigue syndrome. J CFS 1998; 4:13–21.
14. Baraniuk JN, Clauw DJ, Yuta A, et al. Nasal secretion analysis in allergic rhinitis, cystic fibrosis and fibromyalgia / chronic fatigue syndrome subjects. Am J Rhinol 1998; 12:435–440.
15. Repka-Ramirez MS, Naranch K, Park Y-J, Velarde A, Clauw D, Baraniuk JN. IgE levels are the same in Chronic Fatigue Syndrome (CFS) and control subjects when stratified by allergy skin test results and rhinitis types. Ann Allergy Asthma Immunol 2001; 87:218–221.
16. Naranch K, Repka-Ramirez SM, Park Y-J, et al. Differences in baseline nasal secretions between Chronic Fatigue Syndrome (CFS) and control subjects. J CFS 2002; 10:3–15.
17. Repka-Ramirez MS, Naranch K, Park Y-J, Clauw D, Baraniuk JN. Cytokines in nasal lavage fluids from acute sinusitis, allergic rhinitis, and Chronic Fatigue Syndrome subjects. Allergy Asthma Proc 2002; 23:185–190.
18. Bonekat HW, Hardin KA. Severe upper airway obstruction during sleep. Clin Rev Allergy Immunol 2003; 25:191–210.
19. Young T, Finn L, Palta M. Chronic nasal congestion at night is a risk factor for snoring in a population—based cohort study. Arch Intern Med 2001; 161:1514–1519.
20. Anon. American Academy of Sleep Medicine. Sleep related breathing disorders in adults: recommendations for syndrome definition and measurement techniques in clinical research. Sleep 1999; 22:667–689.
21. Fatti LM, Scacchi M, Pincelli AI, Lavezzi E, Cavagnini F. Prevalence and pathogenesis of sleep apnea and lung disease in acromegaly. Pituitary 2001; 4:259–262.
22. Young T, Finn L, Kim H. Nasal obstruction as a risk factor for sleep-disordered breathing. J Allergy Clin Immunol 1997; 99:S757–S762.
23. Atkins M, Taskar V, Clayton N, et al. Nasal resistance in obstructive sleep apnea. Chest 1994; 105:1133–1135.
24. Blakley BW, Mahowald MW. Nasal resistance and sleep apnea. Laryngoscope 1987; 97:752–754.
25. Lofaso F, Coste A, d'Ortho MP, et al. Nasal obstruction as a risk factor for sleep apnoea syndrome. Eur Respir J 2000; 16:639–643.
26. Liistro G, Rombaux P, Belge C, et al. High Mallampati score and nasal obstruction are associated risk factors for obstructive sleep apnoea. Eur Respir J 2003; 21:248–252.
27. Chen W, Kushida CA. Nasal obstruction in sleep-disordered breathing. Otolaryngol Clin North Am 2003; 36:437–460.
28. Meltzer E. Does rhinitis compromise night-time sleep and daytime productivity? Clin Exp All Rev 2002; 2:67–72.
29. Verse T, Pirsig W. Impact of impaired nasal breathing on sleep—disordered breathing. Sleep Breath 2003; 7:63–76.
30. Sher AE. An overview of sleep disordered breathing for the otolaryngologist. Ear Nose Throat J 1999; 78:694–708.
31. Chan CS, Woolcock AJ, Sullivan CE. Nocturnal asthma: role of snoring and obstructive sleep apnea. Am Rev Respir Dis 1988; 137:1502–1504.
32. Bohadana AB, Hannhart B, Teculescu DB. Nocturnal worsening of asthma and sleep-disordered breathing. J Asthma 2002; 39:85–100.

33. Qureshi A, Ballard RD, Nelson HS. Obstructive sleep apnea. J Allergy Clin Immunol 2003; 112:643–651.
34. Guilleminault C, Stoohs R, Clerk A, et al. A cause of daytime sleepiness: the upper airway resistance syndrome. Chest 1993; 104:781–787.
35. Houser SM, Mamikoglu B, Aquino BF, et al. Acoustic rhinometry findings in patients with mild sleep apnea. Otolaryngol Head Neck Surg 2002; 126:475–480.
36. Guilleminault C, Chowdhuri S. Upper airway resistance syndrome is a distinct syndrome. Am J Respir Crit Care Med 2000; 161:1413–1416.
37. Gold AR, Dipalo F, Gold MS, et al. The symptoms and signs of upper airway resistance syndrome: a link to the functional somatic syndromes. Chest 2003; 123:12–14.
38. Levander H. Sensory sensitization, Part II: pathophysiology in dysfunctional disorders. Understanding the inner life of the nerve pathways may explain hitherto unexplainable symptoms. Lakartidningen 2003; 100:1618–1619.
39. Rama AN, Tekwani SH, kushida CA. Sites of obstruction in obstructive sleep apnea. Chest 2002; 122:1139–1147.
40. Gold AR, Marcus CL, Dipalo F, Gold MS. Upper airway collapsibility during sleep in upper airway resistance syndrome. Chest 2002; 121:1531–1540.
41. Ayappa I, Rapoport DM. The upper airway in sleep: physiology of the pharynx. Sleep Med Rev 2003; 7:9–33.
42. Strohl KP, Hensley MJ, Hallett M, et al. Activation of upper airway muscle before onset of inspiration in normal humans. J Appl Physiol 1980; 49:638–642.
43. Remmers JE, de Groot WJ, Sauerland EK, et al. Pathogenesis of upper airway occlusion during sleep. J Appl Physiol 1979; 46:931–938.
44. Mezzanote WS, Tangel DJ, White DP. Waking genioglossal electromyogram in sleep apnea patients versus normal controls (a neuromuscular compensatory mechanism). J Clin Invest 1992; 89:1571–1579.
45. De Vito A, Berrettini S, Carabelli A, et al. The importance of nasal resistance in obstructive sleep apnea syndrome: a study with positional rhinomanometry. Sleep Breath 2001; 5:3–11.
46. Duchna HW, Rasche K, Orth M, et al. Anamnestic and polygraphic parameters in obstructive sleep apnea syndrome patients with reduced nasal respiration during the day in comparison with obstructive sleep apnea patients with normal nasal respiration. Wien Med Wochenschr 1996; 146:348–349.
47. Virkkula P, Hurmerinta K, Loytonen M, et al. Postural cephalometric analysis and nasal resistance in sleep-disordered breathing. Laryngoscope 2003; 113:1166–1174.
48. Zwillich CW, Pickett C, Hanson FN, et al. Disturbed sleep and prolonged apnea during nasal obstruction in normal men. Am Rev Respir Dis 1981; 124:158–160.
49. Olsen KD, Kern EB, Westbrook PR. Sleep and breathing disturbance secondary to nasal obstruction. Otolaryngol Head Neck Surg 1981; 89:804–810.
50. Taasan V, Wynne JW, Cassisi N, et al. The effect of nasal packing on sleep-disordered breathing and nocturnal oxygen desaturation. Laryngoscope 1981; 91:1163–1172.
51. Lavie P, Fischel N, Zomer J, et al. The effects of partial and complete mechanical occlusion of the nasal passages on sleep structure and breathing in sleep. Acta Otolaryngol 1983; 95:161–166.
52. Suratt PM, Turner BL, Wilhoit SC. Effect of intranasal obstruction on breathing during sleep. Chest 1986; 90:324–329.
53. Dreher A, de la Chaux R, Grevers G, Kastenbauer E. Influence of nasal obstruction on sleep-associated breathing disorders. Laryngorhinootologie 1999; 78:313–317.
54. Okada S, Ouchi Y, Teramoto S. Nasal continuous positive airway pressure and weight loss improve swallowing reflex in patients with obstructive sleep apnea syndrome. Respiration 2000; 67:464–466.
55. Jeffery HE, Megevand A, Page H. Why the prone position is a risk factor for sudden infant death syndrome? Pediatrics 1999; 104:263–269.
56. Corey JP, Houser SM, Ng BA. Nasal congestion: a review of its etiology, evaluation, and treatment. Ear Nose Throat J 2000; 79:690–693.
57. Schumacher MJ. Nasal congestion and airway obstruction: the validity of available objective and subjective measures. Curr Allergy Asthma Rep 2002; 2:245–251.

58. Fairbanks DN. Predicting the effect of nasal surgery on snoring: a simple test. Ear Nose Throat J 1991; 70:50–52.
59. Desfonds P, Planes C, Fuhrman C, Foucher A, Raffestin B. Nasal resistance in snorers with or without sleep apnea: effect of posture and nasal ventilation with continuous positive airway pressure. Sleep 1998; 21:625–632.
60. Mamikoglu B, Houser SM, Corey JP. An interpretation method for objective assessment of nasal congestion with acoustic rhinometry. Laryngoscope 2002; 112:926–929.
61. Moll R, Franke WW, Schiller DL. The catalog of human cytokeratins: patterns of expression in normal epithelia, tumors and cultured cells. Cell 1982; 31:11–24.
62. Paulsen FP, Steven P, Tsokos M, et al. Upper airway epithelial structural changes in obstructive sleep-disordered breathing. Am J Respir Crit Care Med 2002; 166:501–509.
63. Sekosan M, Zakkar M, Wenig BL, Olopade CO. Inflammation in the uvula mucosa of patients with obstructive sleep apnoea. Laryngoscope 1996; 106:1018–1020.
64. Kobayashi K, Miyata K, Iino T. Three-dimensional structure of the connective tissue papillae of the tongue in newborn dogs. Arch Histol Jpn 1987; 50:347–357.
65. Boyd JH, Petrof BJ, Hamid Q, Fraser F, Kimoff RJ. Upper airway muscle inflammation and denervation changes in obstructive sleep apnea. Am J Respir Crit Care Med 2004; 170:541–546.
66. Bergeron C, Kimoff J, Hamid Q. Obstructive sleep apnea syndrome and inflammation. J Allergy Clin Immunol 2005; 116:1393–1396.
67. Series F, Chakir J, Boivin D. Influence of weight and sleep apnea status on immunologic and structural features of the uvula. Am J Respir Crit Care Med 2004; 170:1114–1119.
68. Salerno FG, Carpagnano E, Guido P, et al. Airway inflammation in patients affects by obstructive sleep apnea syndrome. Respir Med 2004; 98:25–28.
69. Stauffer JL, Buick MK, Bixler EO, et al. Morphology of the uvula in obstructive sleep apnoea. Am Rev Respir Dis 1989;140:724–728.
70. Iannaccone S, Ferini-Strambi L, Nemni R, Smirne S. Neurogenic effects on the palatopharyngeal muscle in patients with obstructive sleep apnoea: a muscle biopsy study. J Neurol Neurosurg Psychiatr 1993; 56:426–427.
71. Woodson BT, Garancis JC, Toohill RJ. Histopathologic changes in snoring and obstructive sleep apnoea syndrome. Laryngoscope 1991; 101:1318–1322.
72. Friberg D, Ansved T, Borg K, Carlsson-Nordlander B, Larsson H, Svanborg E. Histological indications of a progressive snorers disease in an upper airway muscle. Am J Respir Crit Care Med 1998; 157:586–593.
73. Hamans EP, Van Marck EA, De Backer WA, Creten W, Van de Heyning PP. Morphometric analysis of the uvula in patients with sleep-related breathing disorders. Eur Arch Otorhinolaryngol 2000; 257:232–236.
74. Friberg D, Gazelius B, Lindblad LE, Nordlander B. Habitual snorers and sleep apnoics have abnormal vascular reactions of the soft palatal mucosa on afferent nerve stimulation. Laryngoscope 1998; 108:431–436.
75. Friberg D, Gazelius B, Hokfelt T, Nordlander B. Abnormal afferent nerve endings in the soft palatal mucosa of sleep apnoics and habitual snorers. Regul Pept 1997; 71:29–36.
76. Rubinstein I. Nasal inflammation in patients with obstructive sleep apnea. Laryngoscope 1995; 105:175–177.
77. Dyugoskaya L, Lavie P, Lavie L. Increased adhesion molecule expression and production of reactive oxygen species in leukocytes of sleep apnea patients. Am Respir Crit Care Med 2002; 165:934–939.
78. Lavie L. Obstructive sleep apnoea syndrome—an oxidative stress disorder. Sleep Med Rev 2003; 7:35–51.
79. Carpagnano GE, Kharitonov SA, Resta O, Foschino-Barbaro MP, Gramiccioni E, Barnes PJ. Increased 8-isoprostane and interleukin-6 in breath condensate of obstructive sleep apnea patients. Chest 2002; 122:1162–1167.
80. Hollandt JH, Mahlerwein M. Nasal breathing and continuous positive airway pressure (CPAP) in patient with obstructive sleep apnea (OSA). Sleep Breath 2003; 7:87.

81. Kramer MF, de la Chaux R, Fintelmann R, Rasp G. NARES: a risk factor for obstructive sleep apnea? Am J Otolaryngol 2004; 25:173–177.

82. Bradley TD, Brown IG, Grossman RE, et al. Pharyngeal size in snorers, nonsnorers, and patients with obstructive sleep apnea. N Engl J Med 1986; 315:1327–1331.

83. Gleadhill IC, Schwartz AR, Schubert N, Wise RA, Permutt S, Smith PL. Upper airway collapsibility in snorers and in patients with obstructive hypopnea and apnea. Am Rev Respir Dis 1991; 143:1300–1303.

84. Stroud RH, Wright ST, Calhoun KH. Nocturnal nasal congestion and nasal resistance. Laryngoscope 1999; 109:1450–1453.

85. Meltzer EO. Introduction: stuffy is also related to sleepy and grumpy—the link between rhinitis and sleep-disordered breathing. J Allergy Clin Immunol 2004; 114(5 suppl):S133–S134.

86. Woodson BT, Brusky LT, Saurajen A, Jaradeh S. Association of autonomic dysfunction and mild obstructive sleep apnea. Otolaryngol Head Neck Surg 2004; 130:643–648.

87. Papon J-F, Brugel-Ribere L, Fodil R, et al. Nasal wall compliance in vasomotor rhinitis. J Appl Physiol 2006; 100:107–111.

88. Jaradeh SS, Smith TL, Torrie L, et al. Autonomic nervous system evaluation in patients with vasomotor rhinitis. Laryngoscope 2000; 110:1828–1831.

89. Brugel-Ribere L, Fodil R, Coste A, et al. Segmental analysis of nasal cavity compliance by acoustic rhinometry. J Appl Physiol 2002; 93:304–310.

90. McNicholas WT, Tarlo S, Cole P, et al. Obstructive apneas during sleep in patients with seasonal allergic rhinitis. Am Rev Respir Dis 1982; 126:625–628.

91. Chng SY, Goh DY, Wang XS, Tan TN, Ong NB. Snoring and atopic disease: a strong association. Pediatr Pulmonol 2004; 38:210–216.

92. Valipour A, Schneider F, Kossler W, Saliba S, Burghuber OC. Heart rate variability and spontaneous baroreflex sequences in supine healthy volunteers subjected to nasal positive airway pressure. J Appl Physiol 2005; 99:2137–2143.

93. Gates GJ, Mateika SE, Basner RC, Mateika JH. Baroreflex sensitivity in nonapneic snorers and control subjects before and after nasal continuous positive airway pressure. Chest 2004; 126:801–807.

94. Fournier MR, Kerr PD, Shoenut JP, Yaffe CS. Effect of nasal continuous positive airway pressure on esophageal function. J Otolaryngol 1999; 28:142–144.

95. Winck JC, Delgado JL, Almeida JM, Marques JA. Heated humidification during nasal continuous positive airway pressure for obstructive sleep apnea syndrome: objective evaluation of efficacy with nasal peak inspiratory flow measurements. Am J Rhinol 2002; 16:175–177.

96. Shadan FF, Jalowayski A, Fahrenholz J, Dawson A, Kline L. Differential gene expression in the T-helper lymphocytes of obstructive sleep apnea patients treated with nasal continuous positive airway pressure (nCPAP). Med Hypotheses 2004; 63:630–632.

97. Wilde AD, Ell SR. The effect on nasal resistance of an external nasal splint during isometric and isotonic exercise. Clin Otolaryngol 1999; 24:414–416.

98. Pevernagie D, Hamans E, Van Cauwenberge P, Pauwels R. External nasal dilation reduces snoring in chronic rhinitis patients: a randomized controlled trial. Eur Respir J 2000; 15:996–1000.

99. Gosepath J, Amedee RG, Romantschuck S, Mann WJ. Breathe right nasal strips and the respiratory disturbance index in sleep related breathing disorders. Am J Rhinol 1999; 13:385–389.

100. Craig TJ, Teets S, Lehman EB, Chinchilli VM, Zwillich C. Nasal congestion secondary to allergic rhinitis as a cause of sleep disturbance and daytime fatigue and the response to topical nasal corticosteroids. J Allergy Clin Immunol 1998; 101:633–637.

101. Hughes K, Glass C, Ripchinski M, et al. Efficacy of the topical nasal steroid budesonide on improving sleep and daytime somnolence in patients with perennial allergic rhinitis. Allergy 2003; 58:380–385.

102. Mintz M, Garcia J, Diener P, Liao Y, Dupclay L, Georges G. Triamcinolone acetonide aqueous nasal spray improves nocturnal rhinitis-related quality of life in patients

treated in a primary care setting: the Quality of Sleep in Allergic Rhinitis study. Ann Allergy Asthma Immunol 2004; 92:255–261.

103. Ratner PH, Howland WC III, Arastu R, et al. Fluticasone propionate aqueous nasal spray provided significantly greater improvement in daytime and nighttime nasal symptoms of seasonal allergic rhinitis compared with montelukast. Ann Allergy Asthma Immunol 2003; 90:536–542.

104. Kiely JL, Nolan P, McNicholas WT. Intranasal corticosteroid therapy for obstructive sleep apnoea in patients with co-existing rhinitis. Thorax 2004; 59:50–55.

105. Mansfield LE, Diaz G, Posey CR, Flores-Neder J. Sleep disordered breathing and day-time quality of life in children with allergic rhinitis during treatment with intranasal budesonide. Ann Allergy Asthma Immunol 2004; 92:240–244.

106. Brouillette RT, Manoukian JJ, Ducharme FM, et al. Efficacy of fluticasone nasal spray for pediatric obstructive sleep apnea. J Pediatr 2001; 138:838–844.

107. Golden S, Teets SJ, Lehman EB, et al. Effect of topical nasal azelastine on the symptoms of rhinitis, sleep, daytime somnolence in perennial allergic rhinitis. Ann Allergy Asthma Immunol 2000; 85:53–57.

108. Cavaliere F, Masieri S. Furosemide protective effect against airway obstruction. Curr Drug Targets 2002; 3:197–201.

109. Ungkanont K, Damrongsak S. Effect of adenoidectomy in children with complex pro-blems of rhinosinusitis and associated diseases. Int J Pediatr Otorhinolaryngol 2004; 68:447–451.

110. Wu MD, Kimura M, Kusumi T, Taguchi A, Nakayama M, Inafuku S. "Restricted ablation" of elongated uvula mucosa by the injection of the ethanol/steroid mixture: a new treatment for snoring and OSAS. Nippon Jibiinkoka Gakkai Kaiho 2005; 108:15–19.

Index

About the Editors

JAMES N. BARANIUK is Asssociate Professor, Department of Medicine, Georgetown University Medical Center, Washington, D.C. Dr. Baraniuk's areas of expertise include neuroimmune regulation of mucosal function in rhinitis, sinusitis, asthma, and chronic fatigue syndrome.

DENNIS SHUSTERMAN is Professor, Department of Medicine, University of Washington, Seattle. Dr. Shusterman received the M.P.H. degree from the University of California, Berkeley, and the M.D. degree from the University of California, Davis.